Imaging Non-traumatic Abdominal Emergencies in Pediatric Patients

Vittorio Miele • Margherita Trinci
Editors

Imaging Non-traumatic Abdominal Emergencies in Pediatric Patients

Springer

Editors
Vittorio Miele
Department of Emergency Radiology
S. Camillo Hospital
Rome
Italy

Margherita Trinci
Department of Emergency Radiology
S. Camillo Hospital
Rome
Italy

ISBN 978-3-319-41865-0 ISBN 978-3-319-41866-7 (eBook)
DOI 10.1007/978-3-319-41866-7

Library of Congress Control Number: 2016958305

Printed on acid-free paper

This Springer imprint is published by Springer Nature
The registered company is Springer International Publishing AG Switzerland
The registered company address is Gewerbestrasse 11, 6330 Cham, Switzerland

Dedicated to our Colleagues, who are true professionals, dear friends, work and life mates

Foreword

Pediatric radiology, despite being recognized as an imaging subspecialization, in many countries does not have a strong presence in either undergraduate or postgraduate radiology education programs.

The aim of this book is to offer a reference text for radiologists and student radiologists working within general imaging departments and highlights unique aspects of pediatric radiology practice. In many cases, general radiologists have inadequate contact with pediatric radiology during their course of training. Pediatricians and surgeons, who wish to understand the indications, limitations, and clinical applications of imaging will also gain value from this book. Usually, pediatricians lack not only the ability to interpret the images, but also awareness about the importance of a finding for the next step toward a diagnosis and thus for treatment.

The editors, Dr. V. Miele and Dr. M. Trinci, have been very efficacious in engaging several national specialists in the field, to contribute to different chapters and I would like to congratulate them for the quick and brilliant harmonization of the editorial preparation of this second book on emergencies. The first one was *Imaging Trauma and Polytrauma in Pediatric Patients* (Springer, 2015).

The goal of this second book is to deliver again a comprehensive text on the clinical application of radiology in a pediatric population. As in the first book, this goal is obtained by providing information on ways to enhance the performance and interpretation of images, and to avoid technical and interpretative errors: far greater emphasis is placed on radiation-dose reduction techniques.

The initial chapter provides exhaustive instruction for studying neonatal acute abdomen, while reducing radiation exposure and presents hands-on protocols for imaging. In the succeeding chapters, abnormal findings are described and illustrated for pediatric acute abdomen, neonatal and pediatric GU emergencies, and critical issues in pediatric emergencies.

Importantly, when writing this text, the authors tried to provide a description of all pediatric imaging techniques or provide answers to all imaging dilemmas, even if many of these will be dependent upon local expertise, radiographic equipment, and availability of alternative imaging modalities.

The diagnostic strategies used for children differ from those used for adults in many points. Children and adolescents are not simply small adults; they suffer from different diseases and require different treatments. The same is true where imaging is concerned. The diagnostic approaches – using identical diagnostic instruments – are different; the care prior to, during, and following the examination differs from that of adults. One of the most important aspects is radiation protection, as children are particularly sensitive to ionizing radiation and, with their longer life expectancy, can also expect to accumulate a higher dose from natural and artificial – above all medical – causes. The latter increase the individual risk of malignant diseases. The best radiation protection is the justification of an examination employing ionizing radiation (X-rays, CT scan). This is realized by establishing strict indications and, on the other hand, if possible, by replacing ultrasonography or magnetic resonance imaging for X-rays or CT. In addition to the aspect of radiation protection, however, there is also a physical reason for the great value of ultrasonography in pediatric radiology. High frequencies allow for high diagnostic quality but results in less penetration depth. Given the lesser body volume of children, higher frequencies can be used in them. This is one of the reasons why ultrasonography is of greater value in pediatric radiology than in adult radiology. Therefore, diagnostic flow charts produced from adult imaging cannot be directly applied to pediatric radiology.

As in the first highly successful book, the main emphasis is put on the actual role of cross-sectional imaging methods in conjunction with standard radiography. This volume covers our current knowledge and new visions into the crucial role that radiological imaging plays in the appropriate management of infants and children with acute abdominal diseases.

In summary, this book strives to update the current knowledge on non-traumatic abdominal emergencies in children. Equipment continues to improve; new technologies continue to develop; and the clinical applications of radiology continue to evolve. It is necessary that radiologists meet the challenge of applying these new technologies and applications to the care of pediatric patients.

I am confident that this book will again inspire great interest among both general and specialized pediatric radiologists, as well as among neonatologists, pediatricians, and pediatric surgeons.

Paolo Tomà
Diagnostic Imaging Department,
Children's Hospital Bambino Gesù,
S. Onofrio Square, Rome, Italy

Contents

Part IV Critical Issues in Pediatric Emergencies

Part I

Neonatal Acute Abdomen

Intestinal Stenosis and Atresia

1

Vittorio Miele, Claudia Lucia Piccolo, Valeria Saracco, Maria Napoletano, Margherita Trinci, and Luca Brunese

1.1 Esophageal Atresia and Tracheoesophageal Fistula

Esophageal atresia (EA), isolated or associated with tracheoesophageal fistula (TEF), was first described by Thomas Gibson in 1697, but it was only in 1941 that Cameron Haight performed the first successful surgical repair of this anomaly (Mortell and Azizkhan 2009; Pinheiro et al. 2012).

The overall incidence is approximately 1:3–5000 live-born infants (de Jong et al. 2010). In the majority of cases, it is sporadic, but the incidence is higher in twins, 2.56 higher than in singletons (Seo et al. 2010; Holland and Fitzgerald 2010).

These pathological entities represent a complex of congenital anomalies characterized by an incomplete formation of the primitive esophagus or by an abnormal communication between the trachea and esophagus.

The pathologic mechanism behind this malformation is still unknown, although it is thought to be a developmental disorder involving the division of the primitive foregut into trachea and esophagus occurring since the fourth week of gestation (Cumming 1975). There are three main theories explaining this phenomenon: the first theory states that the evagination of the tracheal diverticulum begins with the primitive digestive tube, which, growing in the caudal direction very quickly, results into a separation of trachea from esophagus, which is still part of the digestive tube. According to this mechanism, the tracheoesophageal malformation results from a tracheal growth failure.

The second theory postulates the formation of a septum in the coronal plane of the primitive digestive tube, which separates the trachea ventrally and the esophagus dorsally; a failure in this process might result into a tracheoesophageal malformation. The third theory combines the previous two, suggesting that the growth of the tracheal diverticulum occurs together with the separation of the digestive tube, resulting in the final separation of the trachea from the esophagus. The loss of a portion of the previously formed tube due to a regression toward the main part of the embryo may result in the EA (Ioannides and Copp 2009).

Some reports described this entity occurring as a multifactorial complex, involving both genetic and environmental factors; 6–10% of patients

V. Miele (✉) • V. Saracco • M. Trinci
Department of Emergency Radiology, S. Camillo Hospital, Rome, Italy
e-mail: vmiele@sirm.org

C.L. Piccolo • L. Brunese
Department of Medicine and Health Sciences, University of Molise, Campobasso, Italy

M. Napoletano
Division of Radiology, Department of Surgical and Biomedical Sciences, S. Maria della Misericordia Hospital, S. Andrea delle Fratte, Perugia, Italy

V. Miele, M. Trinci (eds.), *Imaging Non-traumatic Abdominal Emergencies in Pediatric Patients*,
DOI 10.1007/978-3-319-41866-7_1

have a defined genetic syndrome (Genevieve et al. 2007). There are also molecular and morphogenic factors related to EA, such as apoptosis, the Sox2, Shh, Gli-2, Gli-3, and FOX genes, and the transcription factors Nkx2.1 and Tbx4. A failure in the expression of one of these genes or in their apoptotic programs could be responsible for EA (El-Gohary et al. 2010; Shaw-Smith 2010). Furthermore, environmental factors increasing the risk to develop EA have been described; for example, maternal alcohol and smoking, maternal exposure to methimazole and diethylstilbestrol (DES), exogenous sex hormones, infectious disease, and maternal diabetes are severe factor risks. A role for vitamin A deficiency has been suggested in the development of EA/TEF, since it caused severe congenital anomalies in the offspring of pregnant rats, including agenesis of the lung and TEF (Di Gianantonio et al. 2001; Nora et al. 1976; Wong-Gibbons et al. 2008; Felix et al. 2007).

As evident, no specific environmental risk factors has been identified.

In 25 % of cases, this anomaly is associated with other gastrointestinal malformations, such as pyloric stenosis, annular pancreas, imperforate anus, and the VACTERL complex (vertebral, anal, cardiac, tracheal, esophageal, renal, and limb anomalies), which is the best known group of anomalies associated with EEA/TEF.

Other recognized associations are trisomy 18 and 21, CHARGE syndrome, and Potter syndrome.

1.2 Classification

The classification of EA anomalies is based on the location of atresia and the presence of any associated tracheoesophageal fistula.

The first classification was described by Vogt in 1929 and then modified by Gross in 1953. According to the last one, five types of congenital EA are possible (Fig. 1.1):

- Type A: pure esophageal atresia without fistula.
- Type B: esophageal atresia with a fistula between the trachea and the proximal esophageal pouch.
- Type C: esophageal atresia with fistula between the trachea or the main bronchus and the distal esophageal segment.
- Type D: esophageal atresia with both proximal and distal fistulas.
- Type E: tracheoesophageal fistula "H or N" shaped without atresia. It is called N-type fistula because it courses obliquely from the esophagus upward to the trachea. Most of them are at thoracic inlet (T2–T3).

Type C is by far the most common, occurring in 82–86 % of cases. Then we have type A atresia (8–9 % of cases), followed by type E (6 % of cases). The less common are type B and C occurring in about 1 % of cases (Spitz 2007).

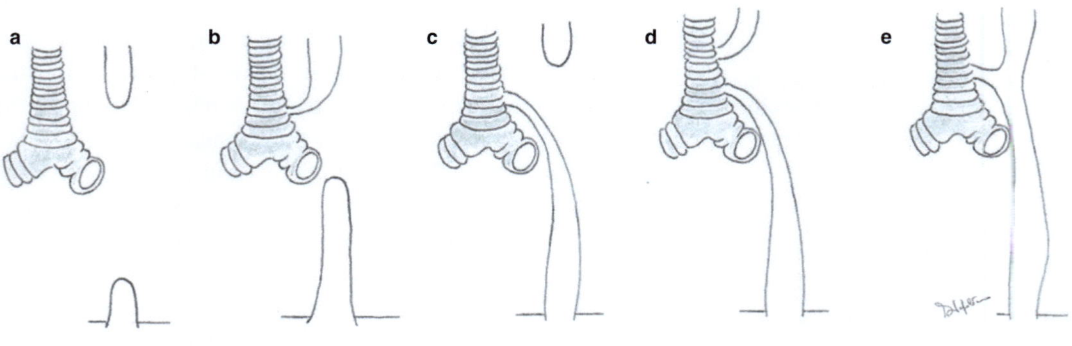

Fig. 1.1 These drawings show the five types of EA/TEF. In (**a**) pure esophageal atresia; in (**b**) and (**c**), respectively, it is associated with a proximal or distal fistula with the trachea or main bronchus. In (**d**) there are both the fistulas and in (**e**) you can find a tracheoesophageal fistula without esophageal atresia

1.3 Diagnosis

1.3.1 Prenatal Diagnosis

US, performed between the 16th and 20th week of gestation, can demonstrate the presence of polyhydramnios, reduced intraluminal liquid, and the absence of gastric bubble, signs suggesting EA, although they are not specific criteria, reporting a PPV of 44 % and 56 %, respectively.

The so-called upper pouch sign, the dilatation of the upper blind fundus of the atresic esophagus, may be observed during fetal deglutition at the 32nd gestational week (Holland and Fitzgerald 2010; Houben and Curry 2008); nevertheless this sign could not be observed also in experienced hands.

In the presence of a high US suspicion of EA/TEF, MR can be performed, having a sensitivity of 100 % to diagnose these anomalies: the diagnostic criterion is represented by the lack of visualization of the intrathoracic region of the esophagus (Pinheiro et al. 2012; Houben and Curry 2008).

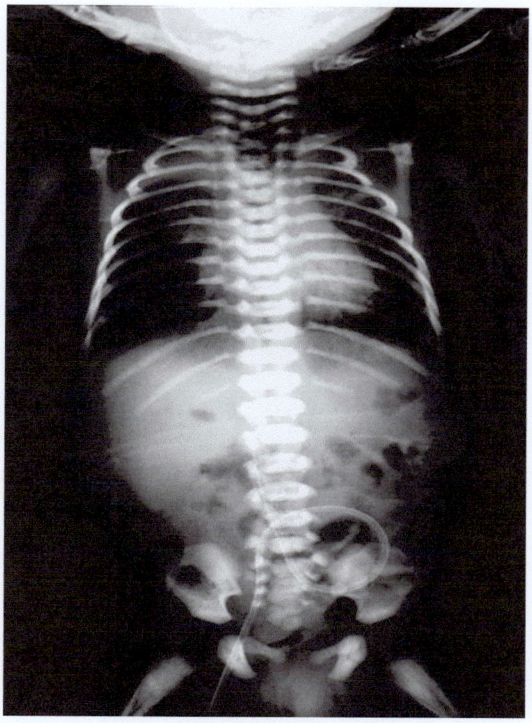

Fig. 1.2 Esophageal atresia: abdomen x-ray shows air-filled dilated proximal esophageal pouch. The presence of air in the bowel suggests a distal tracheoesophageal fistula

1.3.2 Neonatal Diagnosis

1.3.2.1 Clinical Findings

The impossibility to pass a catheter beyond 11 or 12 cm is the primary sign of EA in the delivery room (Lahdes-Vasama et al. 2009).

In the nursery room, the inability to swallow saliva or milk, aspiration during early feeding, or cyanosis can make us to suspect the presence of EA. In type E atresia, the clinical diagnosis may be performed later in years because of delayed symptoms such as cough while swallowing, distended abdomen, and recurrent pneumonia.

1.3.2.2 Diagnostic Imaging

Plain X-ray

The confirmation requires an anteroposterior and lateral chest radiography revealing the proximal blind pouch distended with air (Fig. 1.2). The abdomen must always be included in the radiograph to find out air in the gastrointestinal tract, in cases of distal fistula. In fact, in types A and B, there is no any sign of gas in stomach and intestinal tract (Fig. 1.3), whereas in types C and D, we can observe gas distending the bowel loops (Fig. 1.4) (Berrocal et al. 1999a).

A paramount detail to convey to the surgeon is the position of the aortic arch, because it helps to choose the best surgical approach; when chest x-ray does not recognize the side of the arch, it is indicated to perform an echocardiography to plan the surgical method and to prognosticate the outcome; in fact a right-sided aortic arch (2.5 % of cases) implies a very challenging repair requiring a left thoracotomy.

Radiographically, it can be possible to recognize the type of EA by advancing a radiopaque feeding tube through the nose to the level of atresia (Fig. 1.5); the tube will stop and curl coming in front of a blind end. The proximal pouch may be distended by a gentle injection of air or a little amount (1–2 ml) of water-soluble contrast medium via the tube (Fig. 1.5).

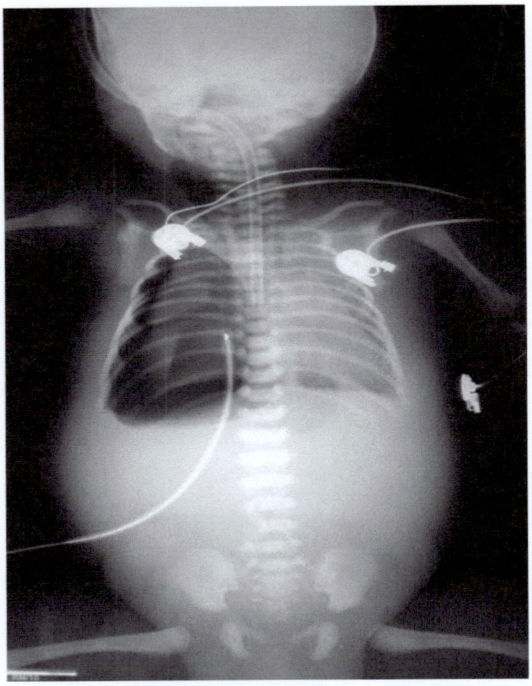

Fig. 1.3 Esophageal atresia with upper fistula. The nasogastric tube stops in the upper esophagus. Associated findings are right pneumothorax and left pneumonia. No gas in the abdomen

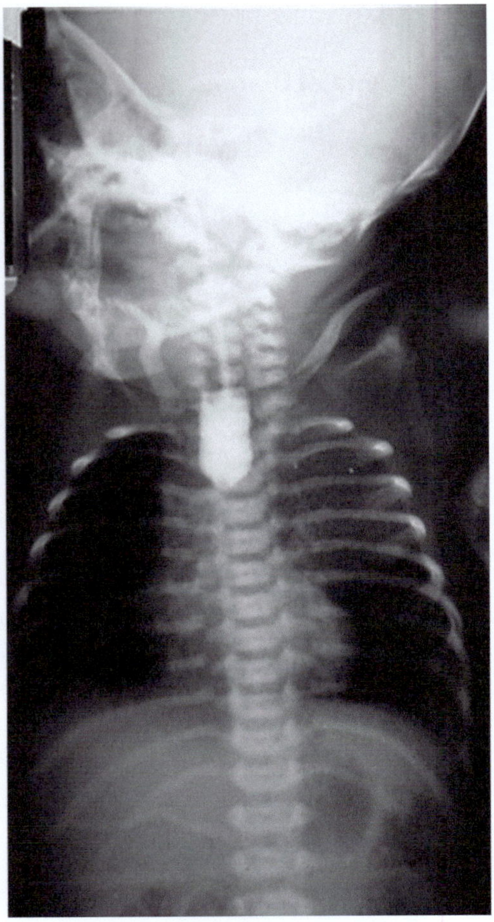

Fig. 1.4 Esophageal atresia with lower fistula along with pneumonia of the upper left lobe. Esophagogram shows a distended proximal pouch

Isolated long-gap EA (>2 vertebral bodies or a gap >3 cm) is associated with 13 pairs of ribs.

When a fistula occurs, atelectasis and pneumonia of the upper right lobe are detected in 50 % of cases (see Figs. 1.3 and 1.4).

When type E is suspected, the best way to demonstrate the fistula is to perform a tube esophagogram under fluoroscopic guidance. It is always preferable to use an iodinate nonionic water-soluble contrast material, diluted with water at 50 %. It is administered both directly and through a nasogastric tube located at the gastroesophageal junction. The patient is in right lateral position, with the lower limb slightly raised with respect to the upper limb, in order to promote the opacification of the tracheoesophageal fistula, running upward and rightward (Fig. 1.6). The contrast media must be aspirated back immediately at the end of the examination.

Iodinated water-soluble contrast media is usually preferred to the diluted barium because the latter one could cause a severe respiratory distress if aspirated, being a quickly solidifying substance.

During the preoperative period, it has been proposed to perform tracheobronchoscopy to vcarina, to recognize other anomalies, and to occlude the TEF with a balloon, in order to improve the mechanical ventilation and to avoid gastric distension and gastroesophageal reflux.

1.4 Treatment

In the absence of severe malformations, the primary correction of EA and TEF is the best treatment option. In some cases the primary anastomosis cannot be performed because of a "long gap" separating the two ends of the esoph-

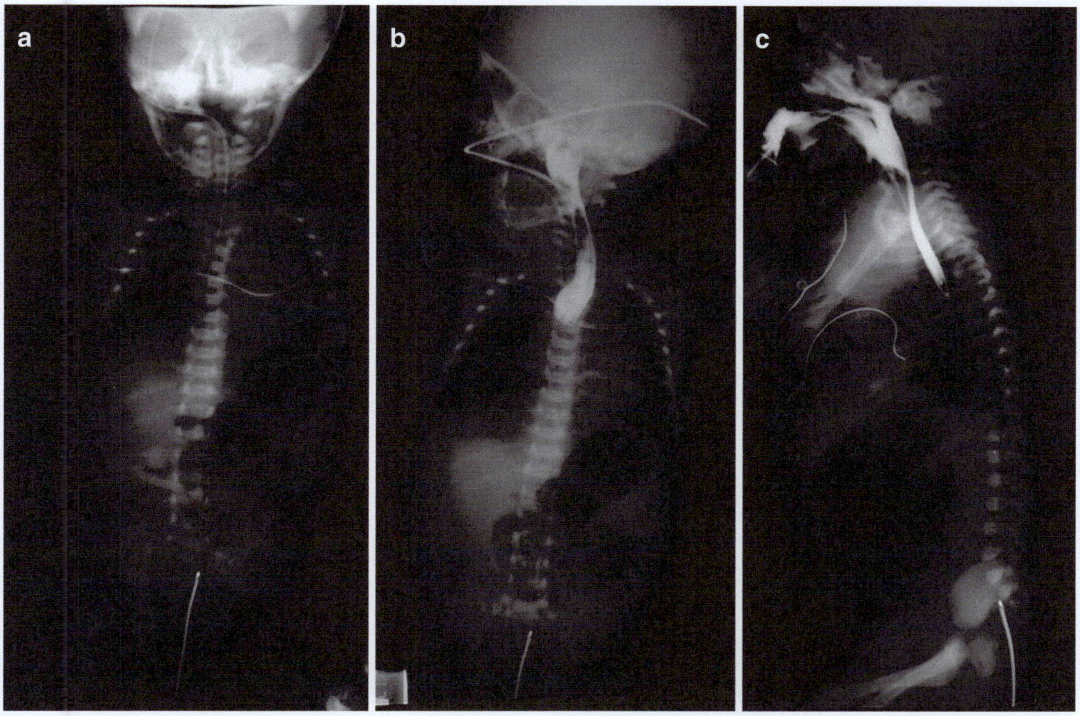

Fig. 1.5 Esophageal atresia with lower fistula. (**a**) Frontal radiograph shows the nasogastric tube arresting within the upper esophageal pouch. It is clearly depicted in air distention of the stomach and jejunum. (**b**, **c**) Esophagogram shows a complete upper esophageal obstruction

agus; to overcome these difficult cases, many options have been suggested, such as the Livaditis myotomy, the Foker technique, and the extensive mobilization of the distal segment through the diaphragmatic hiatus. Nevertheless, some complications may occur if the anastomosis is tailored under tension, such as gastroesophageal reflux, esophageal stricture, and a high leak rate (Seitz et al. 2006; Sharma et al. 2000; Alabbad et al. 2009).

In type A the surgical approach consists of tailoring of a gastrostomy for feeding and a suctioning of the blind pouch to protect the airways. The following options for reconstructions involve or a delayed primary repair using the native esophagus or its replacement using colon or stomach.

In type E the operation requires a neck dissection to expose the anomaly, then the division and the repair of the fistula. This technique is characterized by a quite high risk of recurrent laryngeal nerve injury; in the recent years, an Nd:YAG laser has been used for this purpose, although new data are necessary because experience is limited and it is not widely recommended.

During the postoperative period, if the esophageal anastomosis has been performed under tension, the patient is electively paralyzed and ventilated for 5–7 days. If a transanastomotic feeding tube has been inserted, the feeding usually starts 48 h after the surgery and proceeds very slowly (Alabbad et al. 2009). Only when the child starts to swallow, the oral feeding may start. The primary complications after surgery are represented by the leak and stenosis of anastomosis (Fig. 1.7), esophageal dysmotility, gastroesophageal reflux, fistula recurrence, scoliosis, and respiratory disorders.

Some patients may have an uneventful postoperative period, whereas others may come across some respiratory or esophageal disorders that can affect their ability to develop adaptive behaviors.

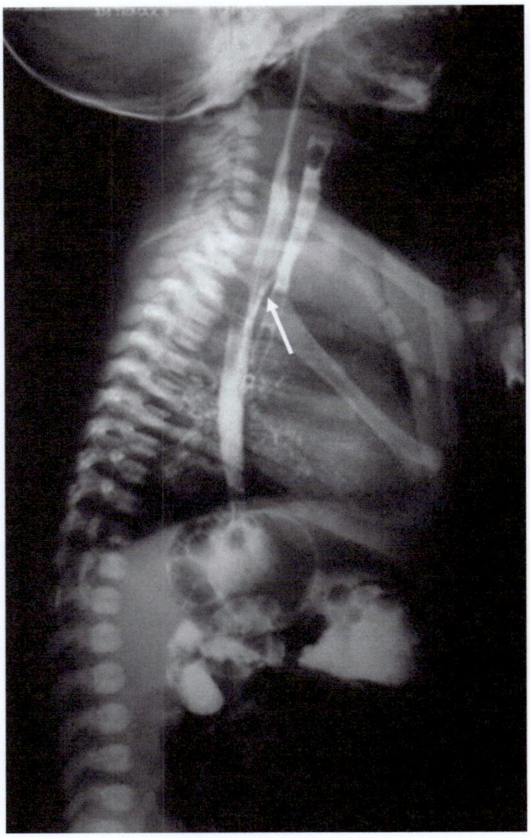

Fig. 1.6 Tracheoesophageal fistula without atresia. Esophagogram shows a communication between the thoracic esophagus and trachea (*white arrow*). Contrast media fill the whole tracheobronchial tree

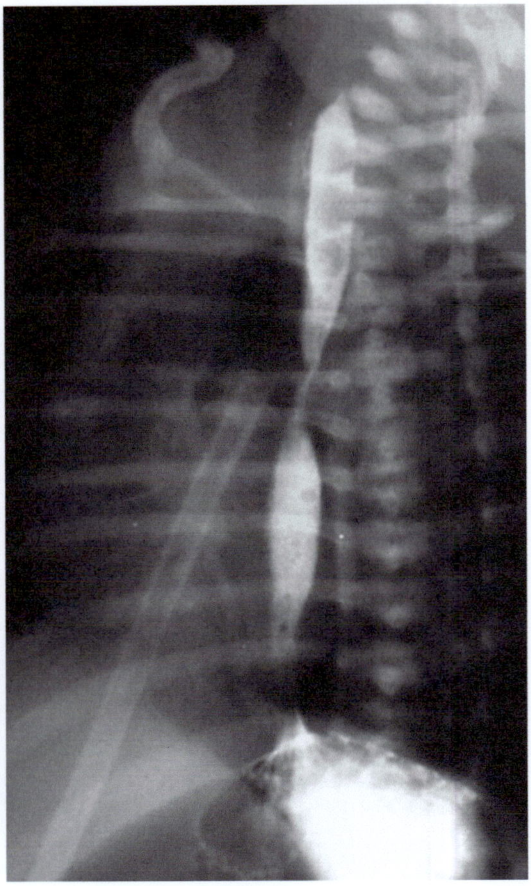

Fig. 1.7 Esophageal atresia: esophagogram shows a postsurgery stenosis

1.5 Esophageal Stenosis and Webs

They are considered as a variant of esophageal atresia and are often associated with TEF.

Congenital stenosis often appears as a 2–3 mm constriction in the middle or distal esophagus. Their differential diagnosis must include gastroesophageal reflux, surgery-related strictures, and corrosive ingestion.

Congenital webs are identified on barium enema studies as smooth and thin defect in the esophagus and can be located at the same level of the fistula.

1.6 Stomach

A complete gastric agenesis never occurs. Microgastria, a congenitally small stomach, is a very rare condition occurring both isolated and in association with other anomalies, especially the heterotaxia syndrome with asplenia. At imaging the typical finding is represented by an enlarged esophagus with a small midline stomach (Applegate et al. 1999).

A complete obstruction involving the gastric outlet is very rare, except when caused by extrinsic conditions, such as congenital peritoneal bands exercising pressure on gastric walls or by pancreatic tissue within gastric wall (Berrocal et al. 1999a).

Gastric atresia is also a rare condition, accounting for <1 % of all congenital intestinal obstructions, and it is typically localized to the antrum or pyloric region. It is thought to be a consequence of localized vascular occlusion in fetal life rather than to failed bowel canalization, mainly because of the absence of epithelial perforation in the stomach as in the esophagus and duodenum.

Pyloric atresia is divided into three types: (1) complete atresia with no connection between the stomach and duodenum, (2) complete atresia with a fibrous band connecting the stomach and duodenum, and (3) gastric membrane or a diaphragm.

Clinical presentation is characterized by nonbilious vomiting within the first few hours after delivery and abdominal distention (Moore 1989).

It can be familial or associated with epidermolysis bullosa.

Its diagnosis requires an abdomen x-ray showing the so-called single bubble sign, caused by the distention of the stomach close to the obstruction with the absence of gas in bowel lumen. Contrast media is not needed.

The partial gastric outlet obstruction is commonly caused by incomplete prepyloric diaphragm, antral stenosis, aberrant pancreatic tissue in gastric antrum, and antral duplication cysts.

At abdomen x-rays, it is possible to detect gastric distention with small amount of gas within the small bowel, depending on the site of the obstruction.

Barium enema and US can help to identify the defect; in fact barium enhances the presence of *membranes* as thin (2–3 mm) and linear filling defects interrupting the barium column, resulting in "pseudo double bulb" appearance, because the inflowing barium outlines at first the space between the antrum and the pylorus and then the duodenal bulb (Clements et al. 1979).

When the stomach is filled with clear fluid, US can detect the membrane as an echogenic band extending centrally from the lesser to greater curvatures in the prepyloric region (Chew et al. 1992 Van Winckel et al. 1994).

The aberrant pancreatic tissue can be found more commonly in the gastric antrum and may cause intermittent obstruction because it prolapses into the pylorus. Contrast media is able to highlight a smooth, dome-shaped filling defect of 1–3 cm with a central umbilication on the larger curvature (Lai and Tompkins 1986).

Gastric duplication accounts for about 7 % of gastrointestinal tract duplications. Most of them are located on the greater curvature and are noncommunicating. The clinical symptoms depend on their size, their location, and the presence of any communication with any tract of digestive tube.

They are usually found out during childhood with vomiting and abdominal pain, although most of them are asymptomatic.

Abdomen x-ray and contrast enema can display a paragastric mass displacing the stomach, but US, CT, or MRI can better detect a well-defined cystic mass close to the greater curvature, appearing at sonogram having an echogenic inner rim with a hypoechoic outer muscle layers.

1.7 Duodenum

1.7.1 Complete Duodenal Obstruction

Complete duodenal obstruction is generally caused by duodenal atresia, resulting from a defect of recanalization during the 9th–11th week of gestation; it does not seem to be related to intrauterine vascular insults, as occurs in lower small bowel atresia.

It is characterized by a reported incidence of about 1:5000–10,000 live births, with most recent data indicating 0.9 per 10,000 (Best et al. 2012).

Unlike other intestinal atresia, it is often associated with other congenital anomalies, such as congenital heart disease, additional intestinal atresia, VACTERL syndrome, malrotation, annular pancreas, biliary tract and mandibulofacial anomalies, and trisomy 21, which is present in almost 30 % of cases (Hertzberg and Bowie 1990).

Four main types of duodenal atresia have been described (Fig. 1.8): type I is characterized by a complete mucosal membrane or a diaphragm

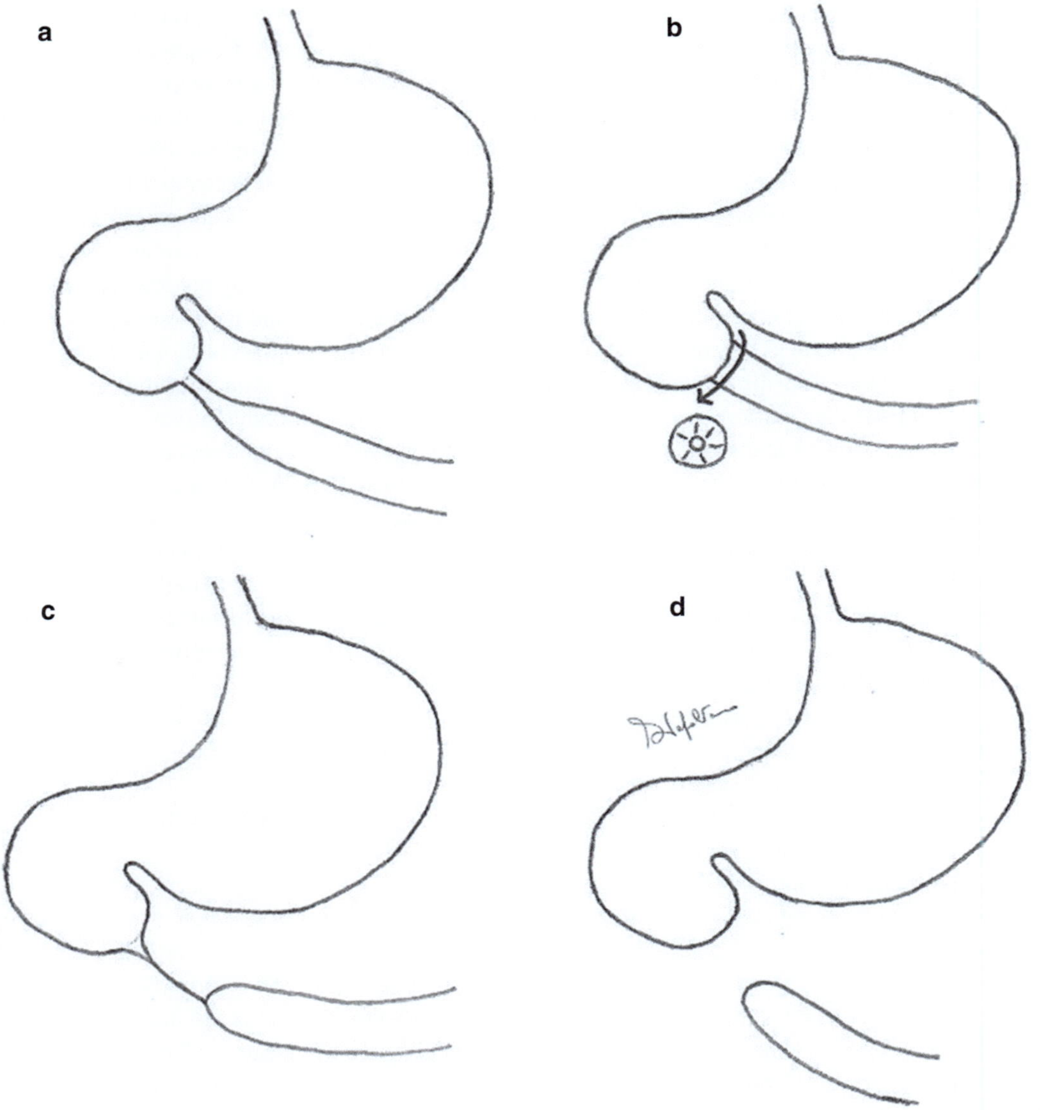

Fig. 1.8 These drawings show the main types of duodenal atresia. In (**a**–**b**) there is a complete mucosal membrane or a diaphragm within the muscularis with an intact serosa, thus maintaining the continuity of the bowel. In (**c**) there is a fibrous cord linking the two duodenal segments. In (**d**) does not consider any connection between the proximal and distal segments of the duodenum

within the muscularis with an intact serosa, thus maintaining the continuity of the bowel. In type 2 there is a fibrous cord linking the two duodenum segments that are discontinuous. Type 3 does not consider any connection between the proximal and distal segments of the duodenum. In type IV we have multiple atretic segments such as a "string of sausages" (Grosfeld et al. 1979).

Other causes of duodenal obstruction are annular pancreas, midgut volvulus, duodenal web, Ladd bands, and pre-duodenal portal vein.

Annular pancreas is an abnormal portion of pancreatic tissue arising from the head and encircling the second part of duodenum forming a ring; when a complete ring is formed, a total and severe duodenal obstruction occurs, while if the ring is incomplete, obstructive symptoms may occur later in life (Norton et al. 1992).

Midgut volvulus is the most dramatic result of intestinal malrotation, and, when present, its radiographic findings are indistinguishable from duodenal atresia in such cases. As a consequence, any duodenal obstruction presenting at birth must be considered as a midgut volvulus until proved otherwise (Berrocal et al. 1999a).

1.8 Diagnosis

1.8.1 Clinical Manifestations

The initial manifestation is often specific, usually polyhydramnios due to the infant's inability to swallow and to absorb the amniotic fluid. After birth, the typical manifestation is vomiting, which is delayed until after the first feeding, and bilious, because the obstruction is located beyond the ampulla of Vater.

The vomiting is going to increase dramatically thereafter. Abdominal distention and feeding difficulties are often associated (Brantberg et al. 2002).

1.8.2 Diagnostic Imaging

Perinatal US can detect the presence of polyhydramnios, which is an early clue to the possibility of duodenal atresia since about 15% of neonates showing this finding will have a gastrointestinal anomaly and about 80% of cases with duodenal atresia have polyhydramnios. An important US finding, detected both ante- and postnatally, is the "double bubble" sign indicating the distention of proximal duodenum and stomach associated with lack of gas in the lower bowel (Correia-Pinto and Ribeiro 2014).

In cases of complete duodenal atresia, no gas will be detected distal to the proximal duodenum. This is the classic finding discovered on abdomen x-ray also (Fig. 1.9), and when it is present, no other radiographic studies are required.

Contrast media diluted with water at 50% and administered via a nasogastric tube shows gastric and duodenal distention without any sign of contrast media in the distal duodenum (Fig. 1.10). Nevertheless, the upper gastrointestinal study is not indicated when the abdomen x-ray does not show any certain sign of duodenal obstruction, because the administration of contrast media may lead to aspiration.

It is important to notice that this sign is also present in other conditions, such as intestinal malrotation; for this reason, some authors suggested performing contrast enema to make sure of the right diagnosis, since in intestinal atresia a microcolon of disuse would be found, while a malpositioned colon and cecum would suggest a malrotation (Laya et al. 2015; Strouse 2008).

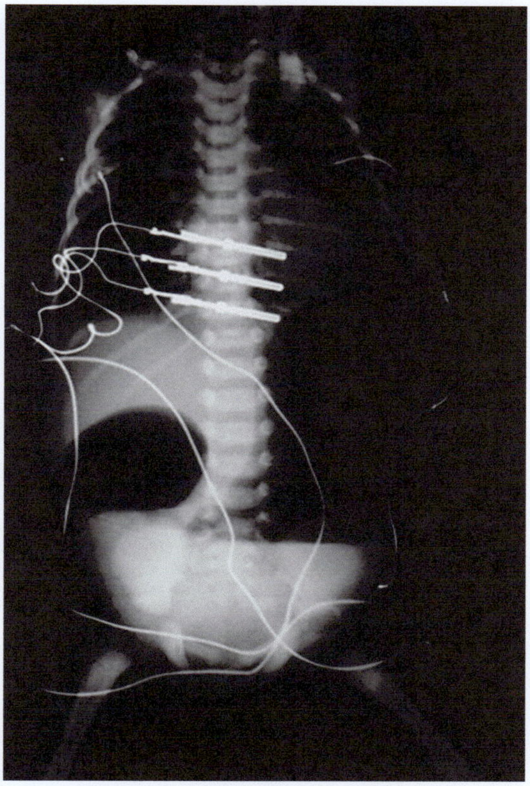

Fig. 1.9 Frontal x-ray depicts a markedly distended stomach and duodenum (double bubble sign), without evidence of gas in the rest of bowel tract, typical of duodenal atresia

1.9 Treatment

A naso- or orogastric tube is placed in order to decompress the stomach and to reduce the risk of aspiration; intravenous fluids are given to support vital functions.

Once obtained the hemodynamical stability, the little patient can undergo the surgical repair, via laparotomy or laparoscopy, performing a duodenoduodenostomy or a duodenojejunostomy. While operating, it is always fundamental to rule out other gastrointestinal anomalies, such as malrotation, bowel atresia, or annular pancreas (Son et al. 2015; van der Zee 2011).

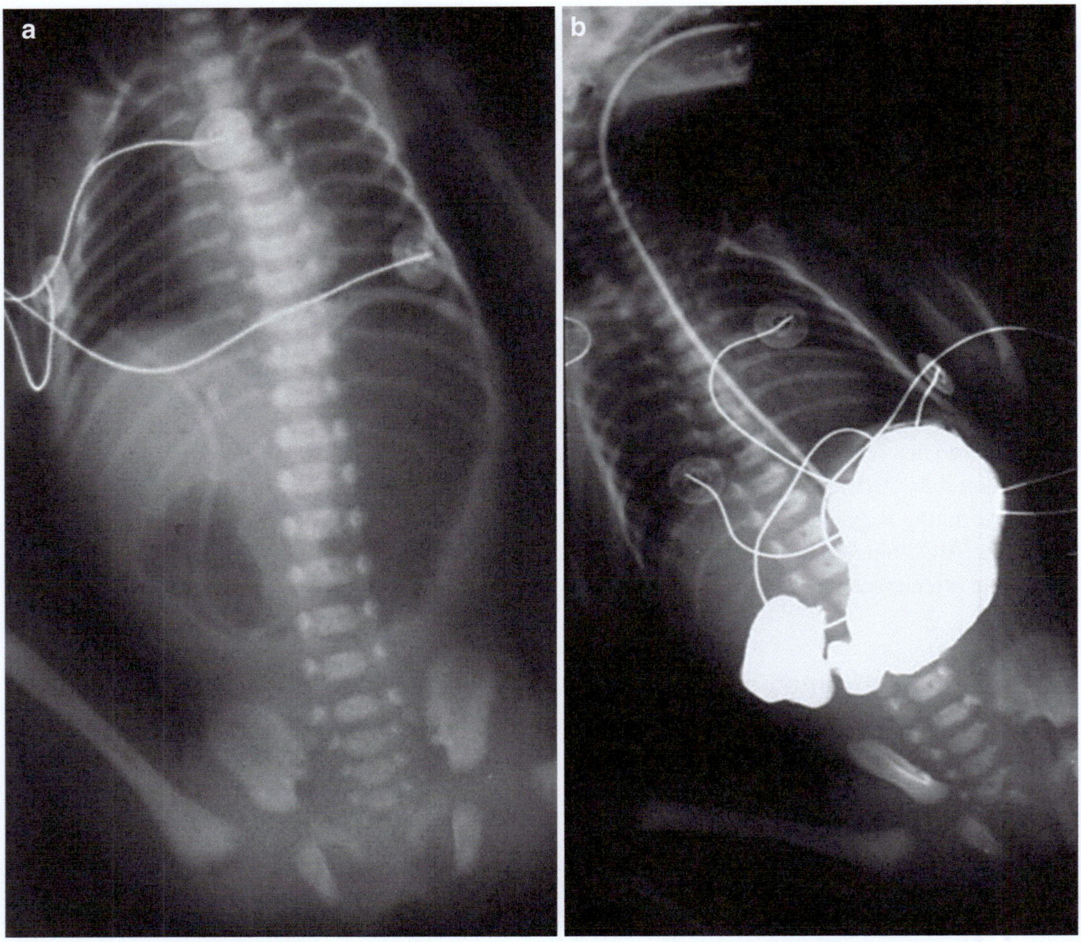

Fig. 1.10 (**a**) Plain film shows gas distention of the stomach and proximal duodenum; no gas is seenthe rest of the abdomen. (**b**) Barium study confirms the duodenal atresia with the double bubble sign

Long-term outcome is very favorable with survival rates of about 90 %. Among the causes of morbidity and mortality, associated anomalies and ultrashort bowel syndrome have to be mentioned, requiring long-term parenteral nutrition.

1.10 Partial Duodenal Obstruction

1.10.1 Duodenal Stenosis and Duodenal Web

Partial duodenal obstruction can be caused by duodenal stenosis and web, Ladd bands, annular pancreas, midgut volvulus, pre-duodenal portal vein, and duplication cyst.

As seen in patients with duodenal atresia, also in *duodenal stenosis*, the radiologic sign of "double bubble" is present, but in this case, a small amount of gas in the lower gastrointestinal tract is visible (Fig. 1.11).

Performing UGI studies is useful and is performed with an iodinated water-soluble contrast media diluted with water at 50 %, administered via a nasogastric tube. It allows to visualize a slow progression of contrast media through the stenotic segment of the duodenum to the distal bowel; in addition, it is helpful to differentiate it from a midgut volvulus in which the small intestine twists like a corkscrew around the superior mesenteric artery. This finding can be visualized by performing color Doppler US also, recognizing the so-called whirlpool sign of a midgut vol-

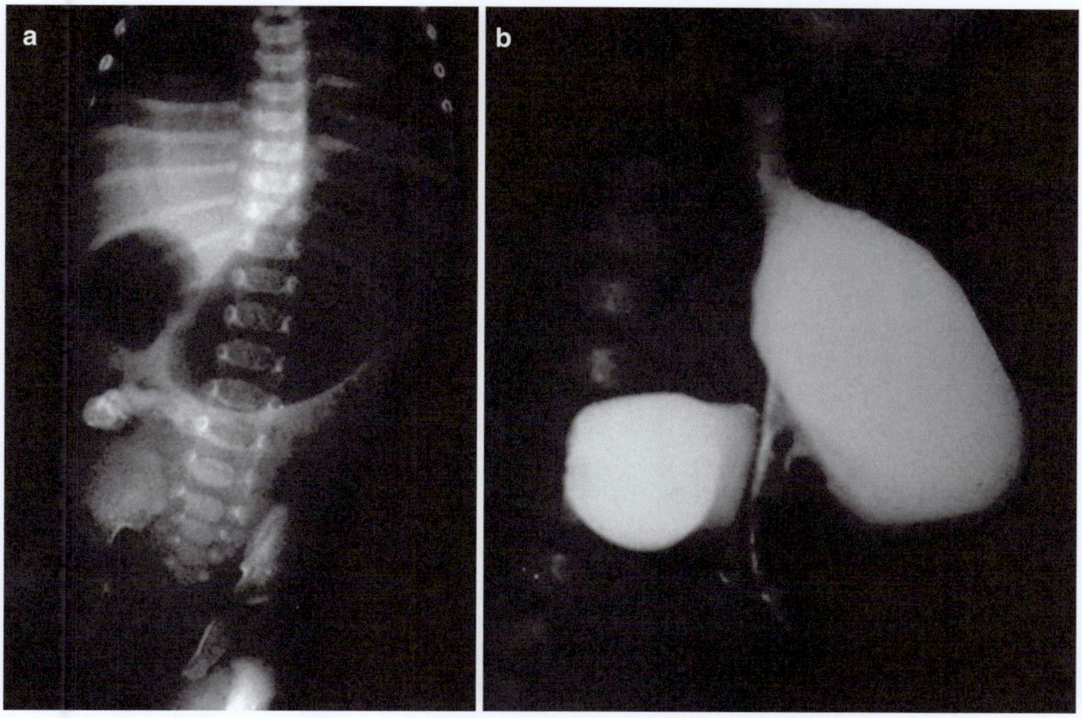

Fig. 1.11 (**a**) Radiograph performed before shows gas distension of the stomach and of the proximal aspect of the duodenum; note the presence of little amount of air in the intestinal loops (**b**) Barium study depicts a severe duodenal stenosis with the double bubble sign

volulus, characterized by the clockwise wrapping of the superior mesenteric vein and the mesentery around the superior mesenteric artery (Materne 2001).

Duodenal webs are small congenital obstructive membranes of the mucosa and submucosa layers, with a central pinhole opening representing the functional web.

They occur because of an incomplete bowel lumen recanalization during the eighth to tenth week of gestation. They are typically located in the second portion of the duodenum (85–90 % of cases), less frequently in the third and fourth portion.

Their incidence is approximately 1:10,000–40,000 live births. In the majority of cases, they are congenital, although some reports suggest they can be a complication of a long-term therapy with nonsteroidal anti-inflammatories. They are often associated with other congenital conditions, such as malrotation, trisomy 21, annular pancreas, and congenital heart disease.

Prenatal US can show polyhydramnios and growth failure, associated with a dilated stomach.

After birth, clinical presentations usually consist of vomiting, food refusal, and failure to thrive; in some reports gastrointestinal bleeding has been described (Nagpal et al. 1993; Al Shahwani et al. 2013).

Abdominal x-rays may demonstrate a double bubble sign or be normal, while upper GI series may reveal the "wind-sock sign," which is the result of the long-term pressure of peristalsis against the stenotic portion of the duodenum, leading to distal stretching of the web, creating an intraluminal pseudodiverticulum. The finding is characterized by a thin radiolucent membrane representing barium filling the lumen and around the diaphragm.

Because of the partial obstruction, these congenital anomalies may be diagnosed later in life with respect to those with duodenal atresia, or they are diagnosed incidentally because the patient undergoes examinations for other reasons.

1.10.2 Treatment

Surgical options are duodenoduodenostomy or duodenotomy with web lysis, via laparotomy or laparoscopy. When proximal duodenal lumen is equal or exceeds 5 cm, it can be possible to choose for imbrications or tapering duodenoplasty (Sarin et al. 2012). Possible complications after surgery are bleeding and pancreatitis, whereas the endoscopic approach may lead to incomplete repair of the web. In the presence of malrotation, Ladd procedures are to be performed.

The general outcome is good and, as for other gastrointestinal malformations, depends mainly on associated congenital anomalies (Escobar et al. 2004).

1.11 Jejunum and Ileum

Jejunoileal atresias are commonly caused by an intrauterine ischemic insult, related to a vascular cause or secondary to a volvulus, intussusception, malrotation, or intestinal strangulation via a hernia. Also maternal smoking and cocaine abuse have been indicated as possible causes of intestinal atresia.

Their incidence is about 1:50,000–10,000 live births, affecting both sexes equally.

They can affect the small bowel everywhere, although the distal portion of the ileum is the most involved (Baglaj et al. 2008).

The association with other congenital malformations is less common, and, when present, cystic fibrosis and malrotation are the most commonly associated conditions.

A form of hereditary intestinal atresia is the multiple intestinal atresia (HMIA), a severe variant firstly described in 1970 by Mishalany and Der Kaloustian and Guttman et al. This is an autosomal recessive disorder affecting multiple bowel segments from the pylorus to the rectum, with long intestinal segments frequently occluded. It occurs commonly in French Canadians and can be associated with combined immunodeficiency. Studies reported a linkage with the mutation of tetratricopeptide repeat domain-7A (TTC7A) gene, fundamental for the development of the thymus and intestinal epithelium. This condition is characterized by a poor outcome since after surgical repair, the patients keep on having low gastrointestinal functions although preserving the intestinal length to avoid the short gut syndrome (Ali et al. 2011).

Intestinal stenoses mainly result from three causes: external compression, intramural narrowing from the rest of heterotypic tissue, and incompletely perforated intraluminal web. Extrinsic compressions are most commonly confined to the duodenum, resulting from peritoneal bands or annular pancreas (Free and Gerald 1968).

1.11.1 Classification

The classification of jejunoileal atresia was firstly provided by Louw and then refined by Martin and Zerella and by Grosfield et al. The classification considers four types of intestinal atresia based on anatomic features. Type I is characterized by a mucosa and submucosa web with continuity of the proximal and distal muscular layers with an intact mesentery. Type II consists of a fibrous cord connecting the atretic bowel ends. Type III has two subtypes: in the IIIa form, there is an atretic segment with a mesenteric defect "V shaped" also and IIIb is the so-called apple-peel deformity, in which you have a proximal jejunal atresia with an extensive mesenteric defect with the bowel wrapped around a single artery. Type IV describes multiple atresias appearing like a "string of sausage" (Grosfeld et al. 1968) (Fig. 1.12).

1.11.1.1 Clinical Presentation

The typical presentation is a newborn in the first 1–2 days of life with bilious vomiting and abdominal distention which depends on the location of atresia, with more distal lesions having more distentions. Infants may experience hyperbilirubinemia and feeding difficulties also. A history of maternal polyhydramnios is often associated. In more distal lesions, meconium may not pass; in more proximal lesions meconium may pass because of generation of success entericus (Frischer and Azizkhan 2012).

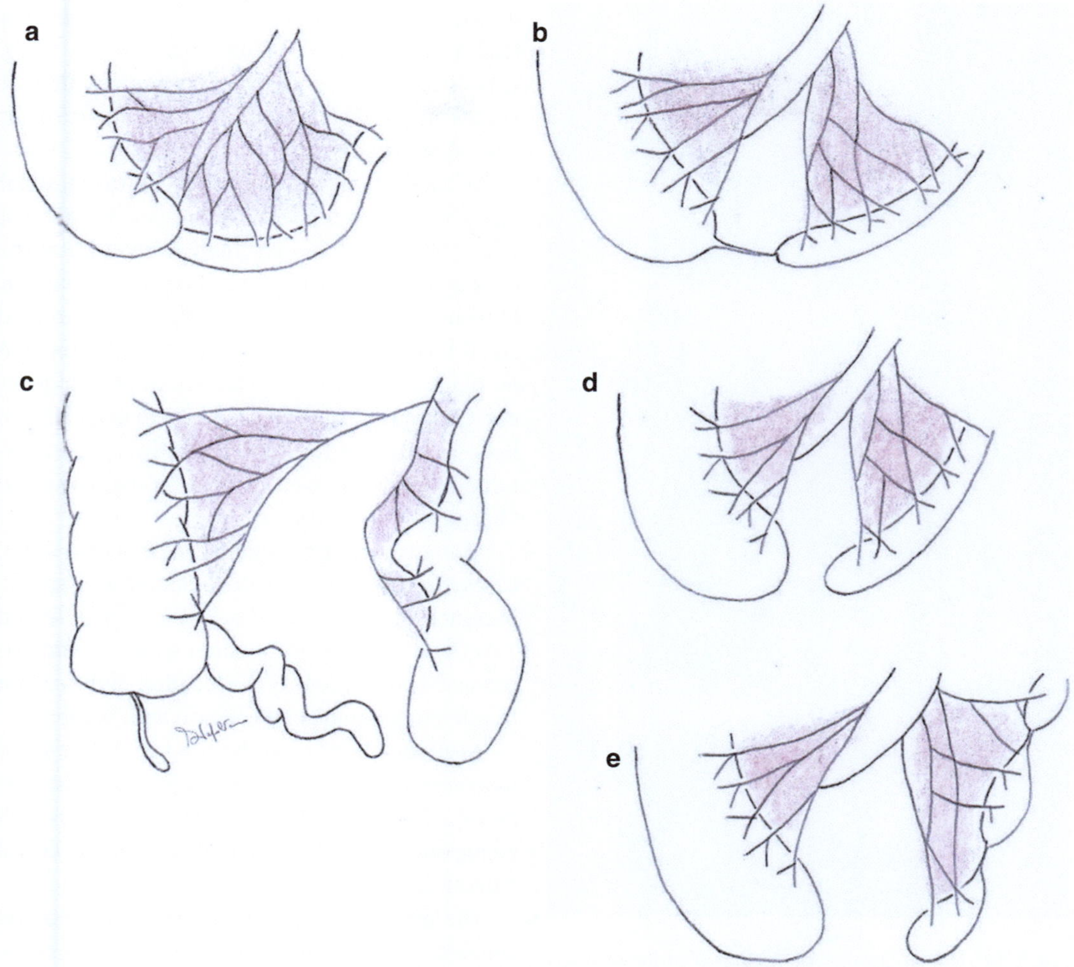

Fig. 1.12 These drawings show the four types of jejunoileal atresia, note the lost of mesenteric integrity and the presence of multiple stenoses

1.11.1.2 Diagnosis

Prenatal ultrasound may show dilated, echogenic bowel and maternal polyhydramnios in about one-third of cases. In ultrasound uncertain cases, MRI can be performed.

Postnatally, the first step to perform is an abdomen x-ray which reveals several dilated bowel loops, more than the double bubble of duodenal atresia but less than in the lower obstructions (Fig. 1.13). Typical is the so-called triple bubble sign, indicating the dilatation of stomach, duodenum, and proximal jejunum; the disproportionate dilatation of the bowel proximal to the atresia results in a bulbous contour suggestive of congenital small bowel obstruction (Fig. 1.14).

In cases of partial obstruction, a small amount of air can be observed distally; in some cases, a little amount of air can be injected through a nasogastric tube to discriminate between a partial and a total obstruction. In isolated duodenum of jejunal atresia, the colon is normal in size because of intestinal secretions by the distal bowel loops making a normal caliber colon; instead, in ileal atresia the colon is diffusely reduced in caliber (functional microcolon), well demonstrable by performing a contrast enema (Morris et al. 2016; Berrocal et al. 1999b).

The fluoroscopic gastrointestinal study is performed as already described earlier; the enema can show a distal unused colon (microcolon)

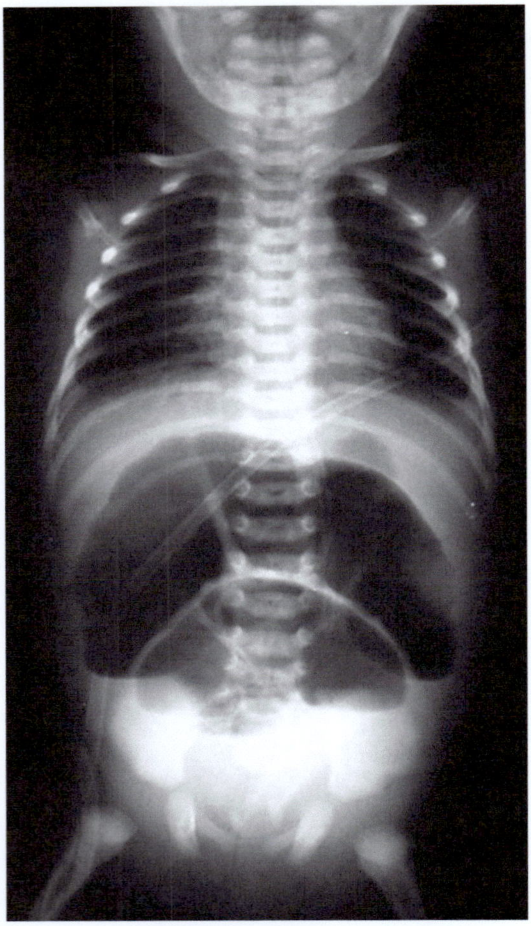

Fig. 1.13 Jejunal atresia. Air distention of the stomach and first jejunal loops, with signs of obstruction

which is not in its right position in the abdomen, leading to some grades of malrotation (Fig. 1.15). It is often easy to observe the retrograde flow of enema in the distal ileum until the site of ill or jejunal atresia.

In most instances an upper gastrointestinal study is not required before surgical repair; but when performed it may help to exclude other obstructive disorders (i.e., meconium ileus or Hirschsprung's disease), especially when dilated small bowel or the colon cannot be differentiated on plain radiography. If meconium ileus is present, Gastrografin can be used as enema which can help to evacuate the meconium, being a hypertonic solution, as well as make a diagnosis (Di Giacomo et al. 2015).

Moreover, contrast media can be performed in cases of partial obstruction, demonstrating the presence and the grade of stenosis (Figs. 1.16 and 1.17) or a mucosal web with a small opening. It can also help to identify the location of the cecum to rule out anomalies of rotation and fixation.

Also sonography can be used to differentiate meconium ileus and ill atresia, because the former is characterized by dilated loops filled with echogenic material, while in ill atresia, the bowel content is echo-poor.

The presence of intraperitoneal calcifications suggests a meconium peritonitis as a consequence of intrauterine intestinal perforation and

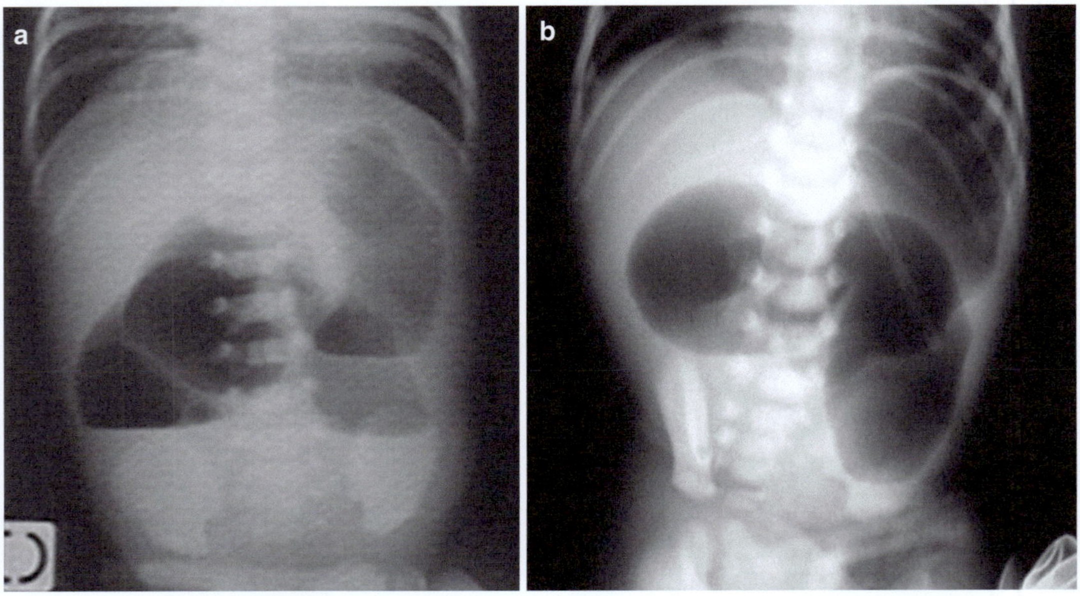

Fig. 1.14 (a–b) Frontal plain films show jejunal atresia along with intestinal occlusion. "Triple bubble" sign (b)

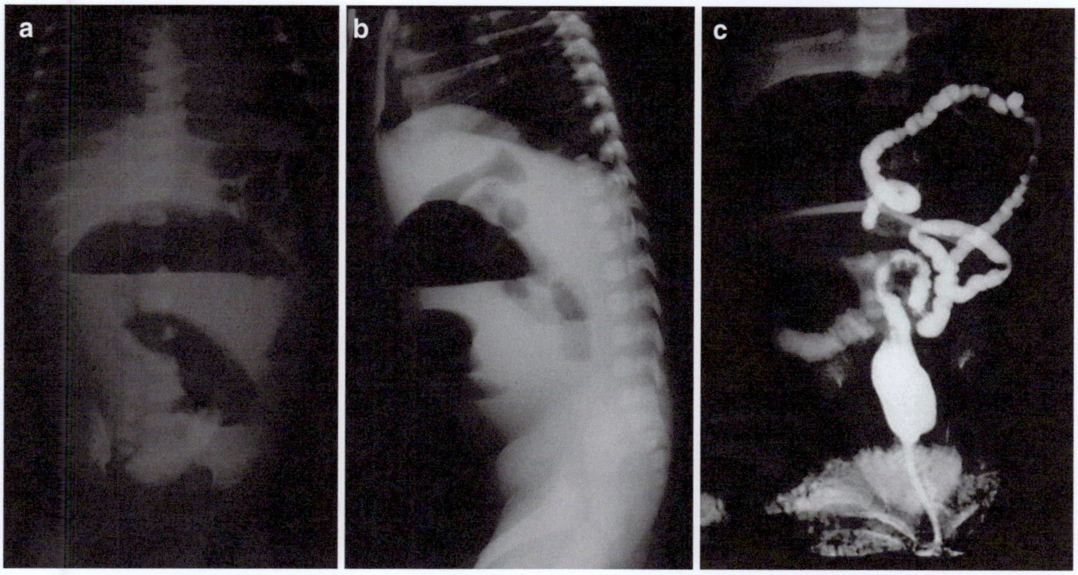

Fig. 1.15 Multiple intestinal atresias. (**a**, **b**) Frontal and lateral radiographs show intestinal obstruction with air-fluid levels. (**c**) Barium enema study demonstrates an unused microcolon occupying the left abdomen

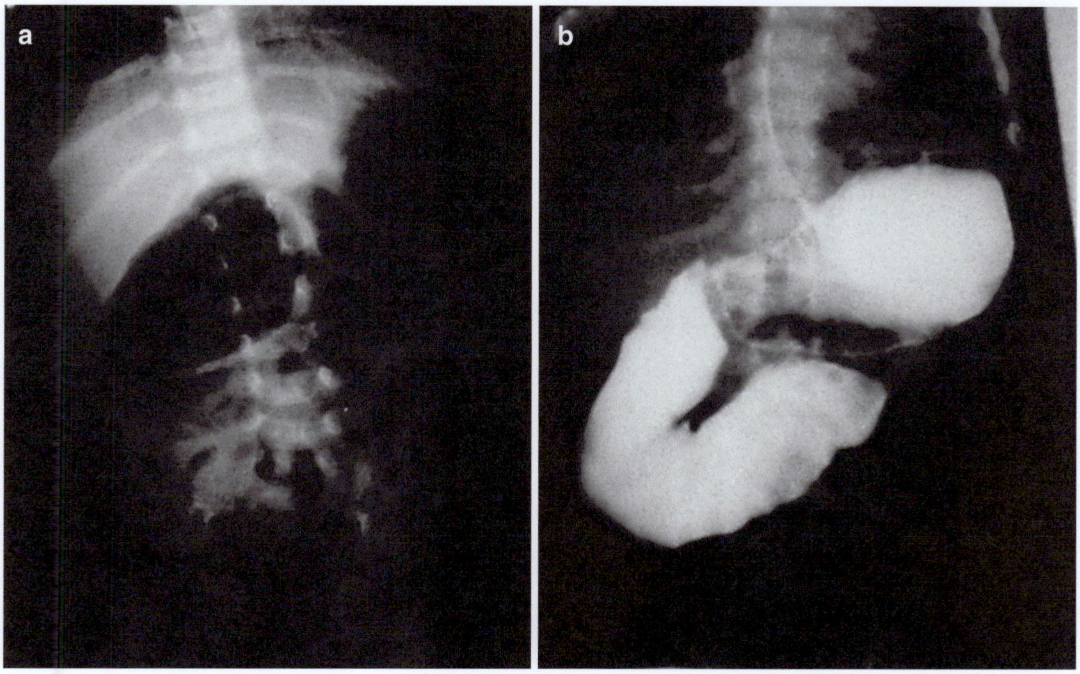

Fig. 1.16 (**a**) Radiograph shows dilatation of the stomach and duodenal loop. Gas is seen in jejunal loops. (**b**) Barium study demonstrated a jejunal stenosis at the level of Treitz ligament

can be seen in 12% of cases (Frischer and Azizkhan 2012); intestinal perforation can occur also after birth (Fig. 1.18).

The "apple-peel" syndrome is characterized by proximal jejunal atresia with the absence of mid-small intestine and the dorsal mesentery as a

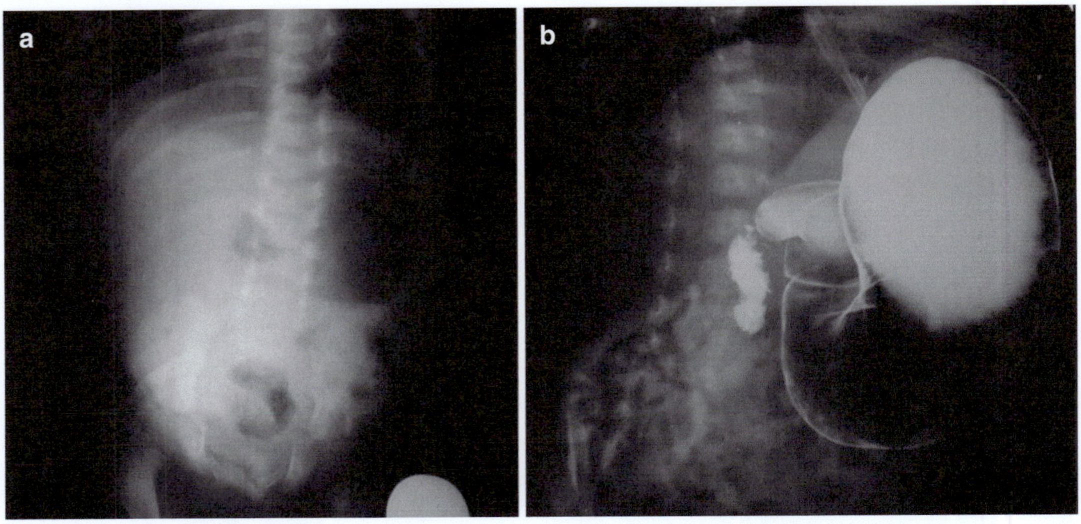

Fig. 1.17 (**a**) Abdominal plain radiogram shows a dilated stomach and irregular distribution of the air in the abdomen; (**b**) after a barium enema study one can observe a dilated stomach and proximal duodenum, with air in the distal bowel loops, suggesting a duodenal stenosis

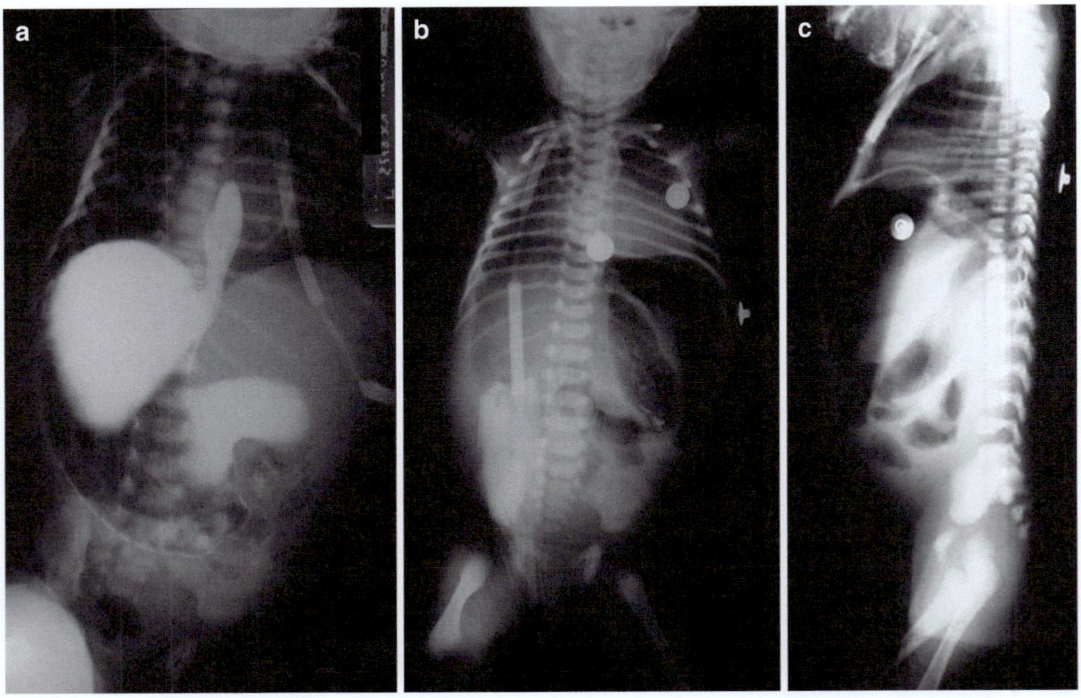

Fig. 1.18 (**a**) The fluoroscopic gastrointestinal study shows a duodenal stenosis because of dilatation of the stomach and proximal duodenum. (**b**, **c**) The same patient in AP and LL projections: intestinal perforation is evident also

consequence of intrauterine occlusion of the distal superior mesenteric artery. Therefore, the distal bowel derives its bloody supply from the proximal superior mesenteric artery and the distal small bowel spirals around its single vascular supply resembling an apple peel.

1.11.1.3 Treatment

At first, infant needs to be stabilized and needs of a nasogastric tube to decompress the stomach and to minimize the aspiration. Broad-spectrum antibiotics must be administered. Surgical repair can be performed both laparoscopically and via laparotomy. The choices of operation depend on the pathological findings, associated alterations (malrotation, volvulus, gastroschisis, meconium peritonitis), and the length of the remaining bowel. In patients with a normal length remaining bowel, a resection of the atretic loop can be performed; in case with a short bowel left, a proximal tapering enteroplasty or intestinal plication has been proposed to preserve bowel length (Juang and Snyder 2012).

For these patients, it is also of utmost importance to document a complete distal patency; therefore, an intraluminal catheter and a saline solution flush can often identify additional distal atresias. In fact, while a primary resection or a tapering enteroplasty is needed for the initial atresia, in cases of multiple atresias, the distal ones are not distended; a direct end-to-end anastomosis without resection for type II or IIIA distal atresia separated by a cord or a gap or an enterotomy and web excision with traverse closure of the enterotomy for distal type I web are acceptable.

Postoperative complications are anastomotic leak, infection, and short gut syndrome. These patients may suffer from feeding intolerance also, especially in the presence of meconium peritonitis, short bowel syndrome, and luminal discrepancy (Wang et al. 2014).

The prognosis is good with >90 % of survival; the prognosis for those suffering of short gut syndrome depends on the length of the remaining bowel, the dependence on parenteral nutrition, and the presence of the ileocecal valve (Calisti et al. 2012).

1.12 Colon

Colonic atresia is relatively less common compared to ileal atresia and is one of the rarest causes of neonatal intestinal obstructions, having an incidence of 5–15 % of all intestinal atresias.

It is usually caused by a fetal extrinsic mesenteric vascular obstruction associated with internal hernia, volvulus, and intussusception or strangulation.

An intraluminal vascular obstruction has also been advocated as a possible cause of CA. Some authors proposed the theory of emboli that, originating from the placenta and reaching the fetal mesenteric circulation, may cause intrinsic vascular obstruction bypassing the lung circulation (Etensel et al. 2005; Erskine 1970).

Puri and Fujimoto stated that multiple intestinal atresias may derive from a malformative process of the gastrointestinal tract (Puri and Fujimoto 1988).

Varicella has been claimed to play a role in the pathogenesis of CA; in fact it seems that it might cause an injury to the enteric plexus leading to poor blood vessel development and ischemic condition, resulting in intestinal atresia (Sauve and Leung 2003).

In about two thirds of cases, it has been reported as an isolated anomaly, although it can be associated with other congenital anomalies, in particular fixation and malrotation. In fact it seems that, causing problems related with location and formation of proximal and distal segments, they both cause CA or are caused by colonic atresia (Landes et al. 1994; Sarin 2000; Benawra et al. 1981).

It commonly affects the colon proximal to the splenic flexure. Atresias affecting the ascending colon are often indistinguishable from obstructions of the distal ileum.

Affected neonates complain with abnormal abdominal distention, vomiting, and failure to pass meconium. The differential diagnosis includes ileal atresia, meconium ileus or peritonitis, functional immaturity of the colon, and Hirschsprung's disease (Berrocal et al. 1999b).

1.12.1 Classification

The classification of CA was firstly provided by Louw and then refined by Marin and Zerella and Grosfeld (Grosfeld et al. 1979; Louw 1967; Martin and Zerella 1976). It consists of four types of CA: type I represents a mucosal defect with an intact mesentery. Type II is characterized by a fibrous cord connecting the atretic bowel ends. Type IIIa consists of an atretic segment with a "V-shaped" mesenteric defect; type IIIb is the so-called apple-peel deformity in which we have a proximal colonic atresia, and the distal bowel is supplied by a single retrograde blood vessel. In type IV there are multiple atretic segments.

1.12.2 Diagnosis

Prenatal US shows a characteristic finding of a colon with apparent haustra and showing an intestinal coursing at the periphery of the abdomen (Anderson et al. 1993).

Plain radiography shows features of low intestinal obstruction with air-fluid levels due to retained meconium, multiple dilated bowel loops, and the absence of air in the rectum. The colon proximal to the point of atresia is disproportionately dilated, and a mottled pattern of gas and feces can be identified.

Colonic enema study has been already described: enema typically shows a distal unused colon (microcolon) (Fig. 1.15c) with obstruction to the retrograde flow of contrast medium at the site of atresia with the more proximal dilated colon ending in a blind pouch. Nevertheless, it cannot define the length of bowel involved nor whether a proximal lesion exists (Winters et al. 1992).

Performing enema, different radiological signs have been described; that is, in type I defect, it can be observed the "wind-sock sign" because the contrast media pushes against the membrane. In type III there is the "hook" sign described on the microcolon sign (Azzie et al. 2002; Blair and Jamieson 2001).

US findings of atretic colon include dilation of the distal small bowel and proximal colon whose content appears markedly echogenic due to the retained meconium. The differential diagnosis between small bowel and colonic obstruction can be performed only if the distal portions of the colon are visualized and appear collapsed (Pasto et al. 1984).

1.12.3 Treatment

Previous studies recommended resection with primary anastomosis for lesions located close to the splenic flexure and colostomy with delayed anastomosis for atresia distal to this point (Coran and Eraklis 1969; Schiller et al. 1979).

In the recent years, it has been proposed to perform resection and primary anastomosis, regardless of the location of the atresia, when the newborn's condition permits: in fact the distal and proximal ends close to the atresia are different for innervation, vascularity, and size (Pohlson et al. 1988).

Cox et al. proposed that this approach could be safely performed with a diameter variance of 3:1 (proximal:distal) and without other distal mechanical obstructions (Cox et al. 2005).

In the absence of small bowel atresias, the normal length of small intestine can guarantee a normal bowel function.

When the ileocecal valve is intact, colonic atresia may appear as a closed loop obstruction with a high risk of perforation (Watts et al. 2003).

Regarding survival and postoperative complications, CA is the most favorable type of intestinal atresias. In these cases the overall mortality is 10 % or less; nevertheless, delayed diagnosis (>4 days) may result in a very high rate of mortality, about 100 % (Karnak et al. 2001; Tao et al. 1987).

1.13 Anorectal Malformations

Anorectal malformations (ARMs) comprise a wide group of congenital anomalies involving the distal anus, the rectum, and the genitourinary tract. The estimated incidence is about 1:5000 live births, affecting males and females with a similar frequency. Most of them are represented by imperforate anus with the distal enteric component ending blindly (atresia) or through a fistula into the genital or urinary tract or into the perineum. They are usually associated with other congenital anomalies in up to 70 % of cases, such as cardiac, vertebral (i.e., genesis and atresia of the sacrum, vertebral dysplasia, and tethered cord syndrome), renal, and limb anomalies.

In particular, urogenital anomalies are the most common encountered in up to 60% of patients complaining with hydronephrosis and vesicoureteral reflux (Berrocal et al. 1999b; Levitt and Peña 2007).

1.13.1 Embryology

In the early embryonic like the development of the anorectum, the urogenital sinus and the caudal neural tube are strictly related. In fact, between the fourth and sixth week of gestation, the primitive hindgut and the allantois (primitive urogenital sinus) enter into the cloaca, and the urorectal septum develops some infoldings of the lateral cloacal walls. At the same time, the developing neural tube and the mesodermal compartment, growing longitudinally, are responsible for the initial curvature of the embryo; therefore, the distance between the cloacal membrane and the tip of the urorectal septum is reduced. At the end of week 7, the urorectal septum and the cloacal membrane are located at the same level. The cloaca is then divided into a ventral part (the urogenital sinus) and a dorsal part (the rectum and proximal anal canal). Between them, the tip of the urorectal septum becomes the perineal area. At this time, the cloacal membrane ruptures and opens two orifices in the perineum: one ventral or urogenital and one dorsal or anal. Simultaneously, a secondary occlusion of the anorectal canal takes place which then will rupture and recanalize by apoptosis at the end of week 8 (Nievelstein et al. 1993, 1998, 2002).

Anomalies in the development of the anorectal septum are the most involved in the ARMs.

They are divided into two main groups depending on the period in which the anomalies occur; the anomalies characterized by an early abnormal development of the dorsal part of the cloaca and the cloacal membrane typically manifest as an ectopic anal orifice or fistula. Those anomalies due to a later abnormal recanalization of the secondary occluded anal orifice manifest as abnormal anus in a normal position.

1.13.2 Classification

The best known classification of ARMs is that provided by Wingspread in 1984, which divides these anomalies into three groups, low, intermediate, or high, depending on the location of the rectal pouch with respect to the puborectal sling (Stephens et al. 1988).

A low-type ARM is defined as a rectal pouch located below the level of the puborectal muscle.

An intermediate- or high-type ARM is characterized by a rectal pouch located at or above the level of the puborectal sling.

In 2005 the Krickenbeck Conference established a new classification depending on the presence or absence of fistulas and their location, as well as the position of the rectal pouch. This classification provides five types of fistulas: rectoperineal, rectovestibular, rectourethral bulbar, rectourethral prostatic, and rectovesical. The rectovaginal fistula is a variant of cloacal anomaly (Holschneider et al. 2005).

While the Wingspread classification indicates the location of the rectal pouch, the Krickenbeck's one gives anatomic evaluation about the rectal pouch but also indications about any fistulas. This is an important finding for the surgeon who can anticipate the extent of mobilization of the atretic rectal segment and define the most appropriate surgical approach.

Finally there is the one provided by Gans, which is the simplest and most used. This classification comprised three types of ARMs: *rectal atresia*, in which the anus is open but the rectum above the anus is atretic and no fistula is present. Then we have the *ectopic anus*, occurring when the terminal bowel fails to descend causing lack of communication with the anus. As a consequence, the rectum opens via a fistula at an abnormal location, such as the vestibule, vagina, urethra, bladder, and cloaca. In i*mperforate anus* the distal bowel ends blindly without any fistula (Gans 1970) (Figs. 1.19 and 1.20).

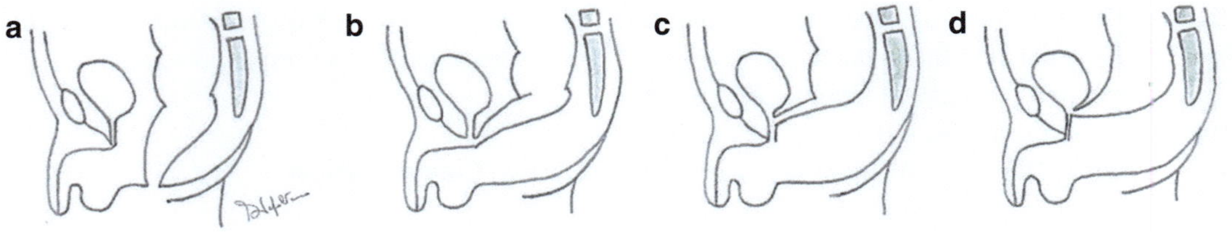

Fig. 1.19 These drawings show the different types of male ARMs with or without *rectal atresia* and with or whithout the presence of a rectal fistula with the urinary tract. The anus can be ectopic or imperforate

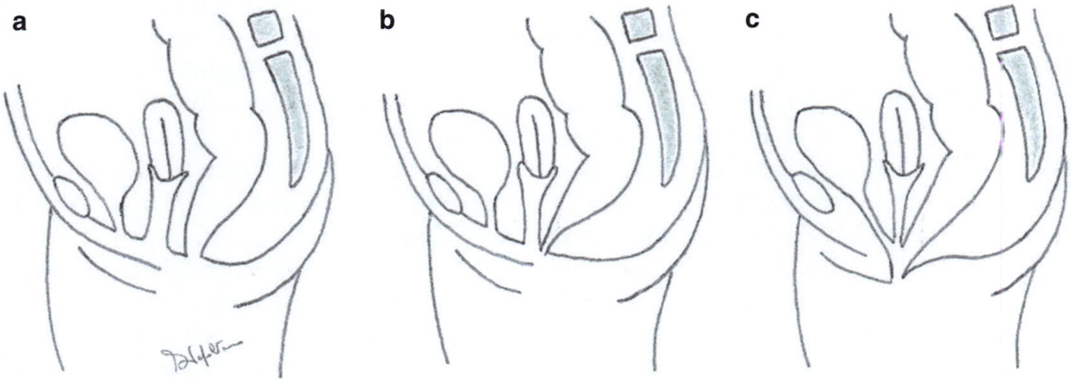

Fig. 1.20 These drawings show the different types of female ARMs with anorectal agenesia or rectal atresia with or without fistula. In the most complex malformation there is a common outlet: the cloaca

1.13.3 Diagnosis

A prenatal diagnosis is very difficult to reach, occurring in about 16% of cases. Associated findings are oligohydramnios, abdominal or pelvic cystic masses, fetal ascites, hydronephrosis, and intestinal distention. In the presence of a distended bladder with oligohydramnios, a possible ARM should be considered.

When multiple pelvic cystic structures are observed in a female fetus, one may take in mind it could correspond to a distended bladder or a unique or septate fluid-filled vagina; therefore a cloacal anomaly should be suspected. The differential diagnosis includes hydrometrocolpos related to imperforate hymen (Bischoff et al. 2010; Calvo-Garcia et al. 2011).

Fetal MR imaging in the third trimester of gestation can help confirm ARMs. In a normal fetus, urine has signal intensity similar to that of fluid, whereas normal meconium appears hyperintense on T1-weighted images and hypointense on T2-weighted images. In some fetuses with ARMs, mainly long common-channel cloacal anomalies in females and some rectourinary fistulas in males, increased signal intensity in the rectum, and decreased signal intensity in the bladder can be observed on T2-weighted images as a result of the mixing of urine and meconium.

Nevertheless, in the majority of cases, ARMs are diagnosed at birth. All diagnostic techniques can be used (Miele et al. 2006; Miele and Di Giampietro 2014). In infants with a rectoperineal or a rectovestibular fistula (external fistulas), the diagnosis of a low type of ARM is evident, and a perineal surgical procedure can be performed early. If no external fistula is evident, the passage of meconium through the vagina or with the urine may become evident after 24–48 h of life, delaying the diagnosis of an intermediate or high type of ARM (Alamo et al. 2010).

There are different opinions about the most useful imaging studies to perform in neonates with ARMs. Imaging studies in the first 2 days of life include radiography of the thorax, spine, and pelvis with cardiac, perineal, abdominal, pelvic, and spine US to detect possible associated anomalies.

In the past the invertography was performed to determine the level of atresia (Fig. 1.21); nowadays its use is to be discouraged as it causes unuseful stress. In fact, during invertogram, the baby keeps on crying causing obliteration of the lower rectum because of the contraction of puborectalis sling, and the rectum, being pushed into a cephalic direction, causes an error in ARM classification (Niedzielski 2005).

In the presence of fistula, in invertogram this one becomes the highest point of the rectum, and some gas may escape causing less distention of the rectum.

In a prone cross-table lateral view with babies heat in genupectoral position, the fistula becomes the lowest point and the rectum is better distended with a better delineation of rectal gas (Fig. 1.22).

The "M line" runs horizontally through the junction of the lower third and upper two thirds of the ischium; it describes the level of the puborectal sling, and it is used to classify lesions as high, intermediate, or low on lateral radiographs.

Plain radiography of the thorax, spine, and pelvis in the anteroposterior and lateral views allow identification of associated cardiac, costal, and vertebral anomalies (Narasimha Rao et al. 1983).

Perineal US is an excellent technique for evaluating the distance between the rectum distal pouch and the perineum and even the location of any rectourogenital fistulas (Figs. 1.23 and 1.24) (Niedzielski 2005; Oppenheimer et al. 1983). It is usually performed with a 10–12-MHz high-resolution linear array transducer by using the transperineal approach, with the child in a supine position and the pelvis and legs elevated. The distance between the rectal pouch and the anus is measured in the midline sagittal plane through the perineum. A distance of greater than 15 mm indicates a high type of ARM, whereas a distance of less than 15 mm suggests a low type of malformation (Haber et al. 2007; Haber 2009).

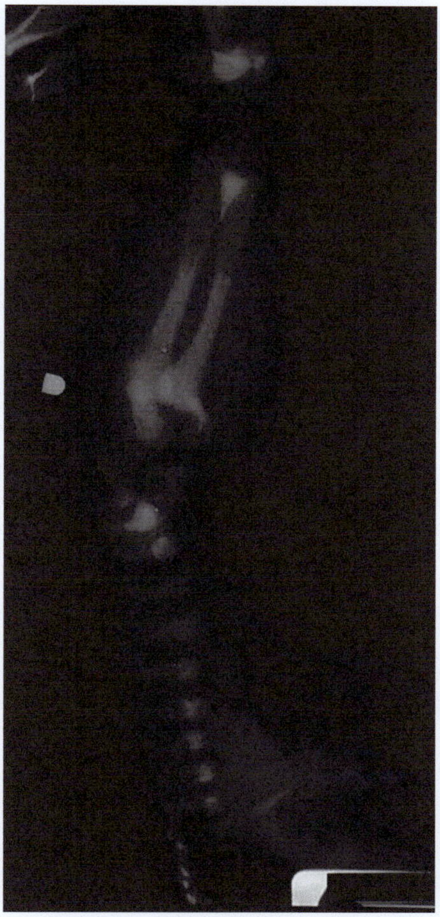

Fig. 1.21 Anorectal atresia. Invertogram. A small metal object is fixed to the anal dimple

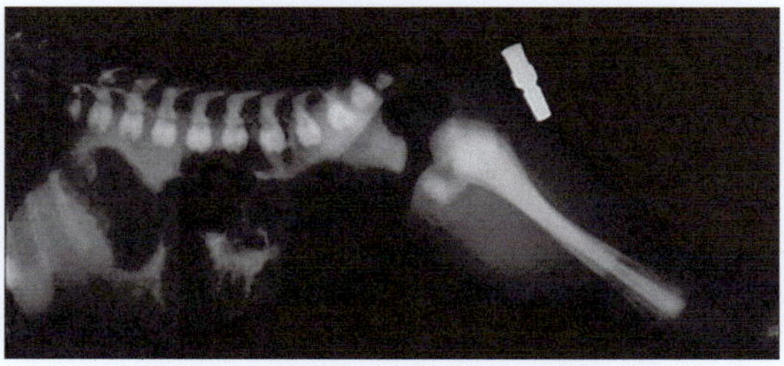

Fig. 1.22 Anorectal atresia. Lateral radiograph shows a distended rectal pouch. A small metal object is fixed to the anal dimple

Nevertheless, differentiation between a low and a high lesion in a relatively low position may be difficult, and any crying by the patient can increase the intra-abdominal pressure, displacing

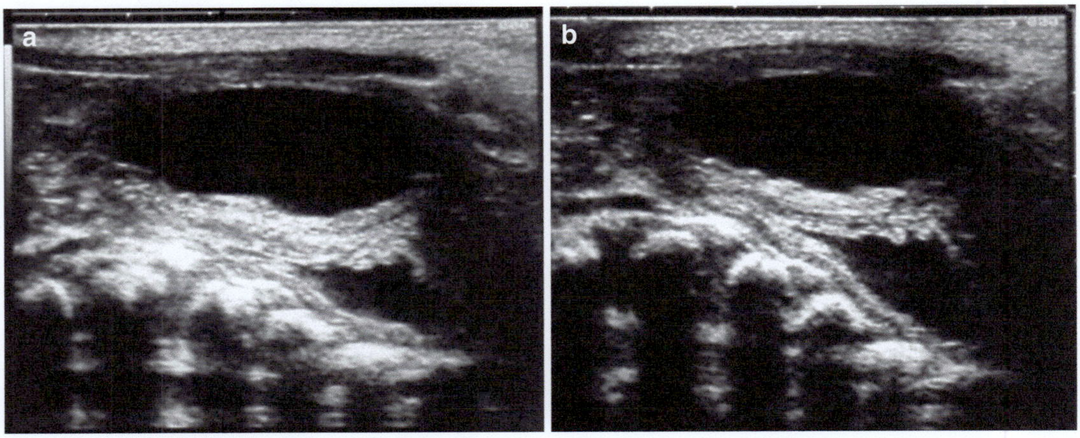

Fig. 1.23 Anorectal atresia with bladder fistula. (**a**) US shows a fluid-filled urinary bladder and a not-distended rectal pouch behind. (**b**) During the urinary bladder voiding phase, you can observe the filling of rectal pouch, indicating a communication between the rectum and bladder

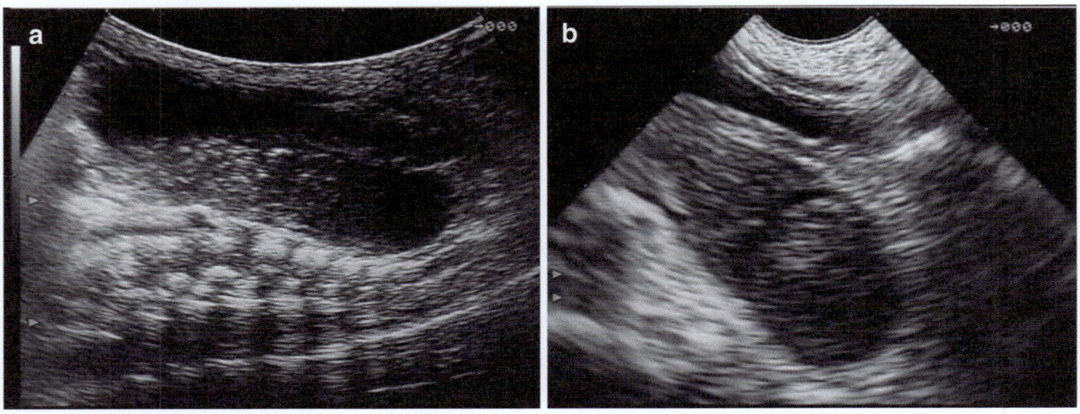

Fig. 1.24 Anorectal atresia with bladder fistula. (**a**) US shows a fluid-filled urinary bladder and a rectal pouch distended by corpuscolated material backward (**b**) During the urinary bladder voiding phase, you can observe the additional filling of rectal pouch, indicating a communication between the rectum and bladder

the distal rectal pouch to the perineum and shortening this distance. Fistulas may be identified as linear tracts connecting the rectal pouch to the bladder, urethra, or posterior wall of the vagina.

Abdominal US evaluation of the urinary tract is limited in the first 24 h after birth, because the physiologic dehydration and the reduced urinary output cause the lack of upper tract dilatation. However, detection of any genitourinary anomalies requires a voiding cystourethrography (Boemers et al. 1999).

Spinal US provides accurate information about the morphology and integrity of the sacrum and distal vertebral column, allowing identification of the level of the medullary cone and demonstration of any presacral mass. In these cases complementary spinal MR imaging is mandatory.

Cystography and/or colostography are routinely performed to delineate associated fistulas between rectum and urinary tract as well as vesicoureteral reflux (Figs. 1.23 and 1.24).

CT and MR are the techniques of choice to delineate pelvic anatomy, in particular the puborectalis sling and the external sphincter. In neonates with ARMs, a combined protocol of pelvic and spinal MR would be acceptable (Figs. 1.25 and 1.26).

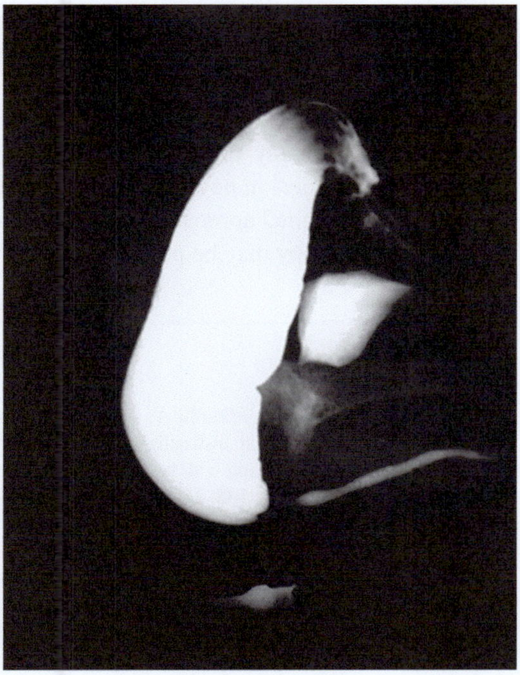

Fig. 1.25 Anorectal malformation. Image from colostography depicts a rectourethral fistula and anal atresia

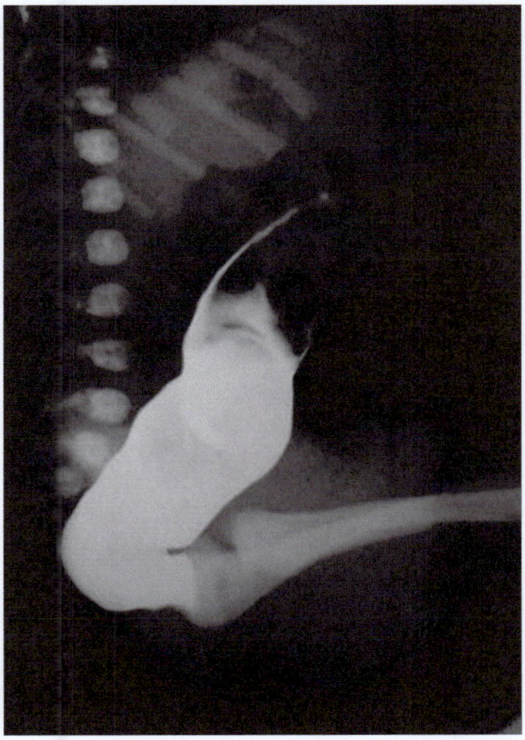

Fig. 1.26 Colostography shows an anorectal atresia with perineal fistula

Boys presenting with ARM usually show other genital anomalies like hypospadias, micropenis, and ambiguous genitalia. MR imaging typically displays normal sphincteric development with the anterior part of the rectum anteriorly dislocated and a rectoperineal fistula.

Male patients commonly suffer from the high or intermediate form of ARM, with a rectourethral fistula and almost normal perineal and gluteal anatomy with a well-developed levator ani and sphincteric muscle at MR imaging (Ratan et al. 2004; Peña and Hong 2000).

In girls, any perineal or vestibular fistula can be well diagnosed at clinical examination. This is a low type of ARM, in which rectum and vagina are well separated in most of cases.

The most common anomaly depicted at MR imaging is the rectovestibular fistula, in which both levator ani and external sphincter are well developed.

Cloacal anomaly is well diagnosed at clinical inspection, where a unique opening is seen for rectum, vagina, and urethra, but it is more difficult to delineate at MR because of the association of other genital anomalies, such as hydrocolpos, and a septum in uterus and vagina. However, MR can show an underdeveloped levator ani muscle which appears even atrophic along with a nonvisible external anal sphincter (Nievelstein et al. 1993; Peña and Hong 2000).

The most frequent clinical syndromes associated with ARMs are the VACTERL syndrome, the caudal regression syndrome, and the Currarino syndrome.

The prevalence of VACTERL is about 1.10,000–40,000 live births, and in most of cases, it is sporadic.

Its diagnosis can be suspected in the presence of US findings of a single umbilical artery and polyhydramnios along with vertebral, renal, limb, and cardiac malformations. These patients have a high prevalence of spinal dysraphism, tethered cord syndrome, and genitourinary conditions. In these cases MR imaging is mandatory.

Caudal regression syndrome is a neural tube defect presenting with developmental anomalies of the distal spine along with complete or partial agenesis of the os sacrum and pelvic deformity and anomalies affecting the neural tube, gastrointestinal and genitourinary tract, limbs, and heart. Clinically patients suffer from a complete neurological deficit as well as no control of the bladder and bowel.

Prenatal US findings show interruption of the distal spine because of the absence of thoracic and lumbar vertebrae or the sacrum with fusion of pelvic bones and typical frog-like position of lower limbs (Solomon 2011; Solomon et al. 2011; Kuo et al. 2007). Also in this case, MR imaging is required after birth to find out the level of spinal agenesis.

Currarino syndrome was first described in 1981 to describe the association of ARM, sacrococcygeal defect, and a presacral mass (teratoma, dermoid cyst, meningocele, neuroenteric cyst) responsible for a tethered cord syndrome.

This is an autosomal dominant disorder with incomplete penetrance. Patients usually present with intractable constipation (Currarino et al. 1981; Alamo et al. 2013).

Lateral x-ray depicts the sacral anomaly with preservation of the first sacral vertebra and dysplasia of the last sacral vertebrae, with a sickle or scimitar appearance. MR imaging well depicts the presacral mass, the tethered cord, and the high atrophy of the sphincteric muscle.

1.13.4 Treatment

The mainstay of therapy is to obtain a good quality of life with acceptable levels of bowel control and normal sexual and reproductive abilities.

The low-type ARM can be managed early with opening of the rectal pouch and ligature of the fistula, when present.

The intermediate and high-type ARMs are treated with colostomy at first and then with a definitive repair at a later age, by performing a posterior sagittal anorectoplasty alone or along with laparoscopic rectoplasty in a second intervention (deVries and Peña 1982; Georgeson et al. 2000). Prior the definitive repair, a high-pressure distal colostogram is required to confirm the level of rectal atresia and to identify any fistulous tract. Through a Foley catheter, a water-soluble contrast medium is injected under mild pressure to inflate its balloon and occlude the stoma. The injection should be continued until the patient starts voiding to increase the possibility to visualize the fistula (Gross et al. 1991; Gupta and Guglani 2005).

High fistulas, mainly the rectourethral prostatic or the rectovesical in boys, are very difficult to visualize on a sagittal approach, so that a laparotomy or laparoscopy may be performed.

References

Al Shahwani N, Mandhan P, Elkadhi A, Ali MJ, Latif A (2013) Congenital duodenal obstruction associated with Down's syndrome presenting with hematemesis. J Surg Case Rep 2013(12). pii: rjt108. doi:10.1093/jscr/rjt108

Alabbad SI, Ryckman J, Puligandla PS, Shaw K, Nguyen LT, Laberge JM (2009) Use of transanastomotic feeding tubes during esophageal atresia repair. J Pediatr Surg 44:902–905

Alamo L, Laswad T, Schnyder P et al (2010) Fetal MRI as complement to US in the diagnosis and characterization of anomalies of the genito-urinary tract. Eur J Radiol 76(2):258–264

Alamo L, Meyrat BF, Meuwly JY, Meuli RA, Gudinchet F (2013) Anorectal malformations: finding the pathway out of the labyrinth. Radiographic 33:491–512

Ali YA, Rahman S, Bhat V, Al Thani S, Ismail A, Bassiouny I (2011) Hereditary multiple intestinal atresia (HMIA) with severe combined immunodeficiency (SCID): a case report of two siblings and review of the literature on MIA, HMIA, and HMIA with immunodeficiency over the last 50 years. BMJ Case Rep. doi:10.1136/bcr.05.2010.3031. pii: bcr0520103031

Anderson N, Malpas T, Robertson R (1993) Prenatal diagnosis of colon atresia. Pediatr Radiol 23:63–64

Applegate KE, Goske MJ, Pierce G, Murphy D (1999) Situs revisited: imaging of the heterotaxy syndrome. RadioGraphics 19:837–852; discussion, 853–854

Azzie G, Craw S, Beasley SW (2002) Colonic atresia: from suspicion to confirmation on pre-operative radiology. J Paediatr Child Health 38:518–520

Baglaj M, Carachi R, Lawther S (2008) Multiple atresia of the small intestine: a 20-year review. Eur J Pediatr Surg 18:13–18

Benawra R, Puppala BL, Mangurten HH, Booth C, Bassuk A (1981) Familial occurrence of congenital colonic atresia. J Pediatr 99:435–436

Berrocal T, Torres I, Gutierrez J, Prieto C, del Hoyo ML, Lamas M (1999a) Congenital anomalies of the upper gastro-intestinal tract. Radiographics 19:855–872

Berrocal T, Lamas M, Gutieerrez J, Torres I, Prieto C, del Hoyo ML (1999b) Congenital anomalies of the small intestine, colon, and rectum. Radiographics 19(5): 1219–1236

Best KE, Tennant PW, Addor MC, Bianchi F, Boyd P, Calzolari E et al (2012) Epidemiology of small intesti-

nal atresia in Europe: a register based study. Arch Dis Child Fetal Neonatal Ed 97(5):F353–F358
Bischoff A, Levitt MA, Lim FY, Guimarães C, Peña A (2010) Prenatal diagnosis of cloacal malformations. Pediatr Surg Int 26(11):1071–1075
Blair GK, Jamieson DH (2001) Colon atresia-type III. J Pediatr Surg 36:530–531
Boemers TM, Beek FJ, Bax NM (1999) Guidelines for the urological screening and initial management of lower urinary tract dysfunction in children with anorectal malformations: the ARGUS protocol. BJU Int 83(6):662–671
Brantberg A, Blaas HG, Salvesen KA, Haugen SE, Møllerlokken G, Eik-Nes SH (2002) Fetal duodenal obstructions: increased risk of prenatal sudden death. Ultrasound Obstet Gynecol 20(5):439–446
Calisti A, Olivieri C, Coletta R, Briganti V, Oriolo L, Giannino G (2012) Jejunoileal atresia: factors affecting the outcome and long-term sequelae. J Clin Neonatol 1(1):38–41
Calvo-Garcia MA, Kline-Fath BM, Levitt MA et al (2011) Fetal MRI clues to diagnose cloacal malformations. Pediatr Radiol 41(9):1117–1128
Chew AL, Friedwald JP, Donovan C (1992) Diagnosis of congenital astral web by ultrasound. Pediatr Radiol 22:342–343
Clements JL, Jinkins JR, Torres WE et al (1979) Antral mucosal diaphragm in adults. AJR Am J Roentgenol 133:1105–1109
Coran AG, Eraklis AJ (1969) Atresia of the colon. Surgery 65:828–831
Correa-Pinto J, Ribeiro A (2014) Congenital duodenal obstruction and double-bubble sign. N Engl J Med 371(11):e16
Cox SG, Numaouglu A, Millar AJW, Rode H (2005) Colonic atresia: spectrum of presentations and pitfalls in management. A review of 14 cases. Pediatr Surg Int 21:813–818
Cumming WA (1975) Esophageal atresia and tracheoesophageal fistula. Radiol Clin N Am 13:277–285
Currarino G, Coln D, Votteler T (1981) Triad of anorectal, sacral, and presacral anomalies. AJR Am J Roentgenol 137(2):395–398
de Jong EM, Felix JF, de Klein A, Tibboel D (2010) Etiology of esophageal atresia and tracheoesophageal fistula: "mind the gap". Curr Gastroenterol Rep 12:215–222
deVries PA, Peña A (1982) Posterior sagittal anorectoplasty. J Pediatr Surg 17(5):638–643
Di Giacomo V, Trinci M, Van der Byl G, Catania VD, Calisti A, Miele V (2015) Ultrasound in newborns and children suffering from nontraumatic acute abdominal pain: imaging with clinical and surgical correlation. J Ultrasound 18:385–393. doi:10.1007/s40477-014-0087-4. Epub 2014 Apr 9
Di Gianantonio E, Schaefer C, Matroiacovo PP et al (2001) Adverse effects of prenatal methimazole exposure. Teratology 64:262–266
El-Gohary Y, Gittes GK, Tovar JA (2010) Congenital anomalies of the esophagus. Semin Pediatr Surg 19:186–193
Erskine JM (1970) Colonic stenosis in the newborn: the possible thromboembolic etiology of intestinal stenosis and atresia. J Pediatr Surg 5:321–333
Escobar MA, Ladd AP, Grosfeld JL, West KW, Rescorla FJ, Scherer LR 3rd et al (2004) Duodenal atresia and stenosis: long-term follow-up over 30 years. J Pediatr Surg 39(6):867–871
Etensel B, Temir G, Karkiner A et al (2005) Atresia of the colon. J Pediatr Surg 40:1258–1268
Felix JF, Steegers-Theunissen RP, de Walle HE, de Klein A, Torfs CP, Tibboel D (2007) Esophageal atresia and tracheo-esophageal fistula in children of women exposed to diethylstilbestrol in utero. Am J Obstet Gynecol 197:e31–e35
Free EA, Gerald B (1968) Duodenal obstruction in the newborn due to annular pancreas. Am J Roentgenol 103(2):321–325
Frischer JS, Azizkhan RG (2012) Jejunoileal atresia and stenosis. In: Coran AG (ed) Pediatric surgery, 7th edn. Elsevier Saunders, Philadelphia
Gans SL (1970) Classification of anorectal anomalies: a critical analysis. J Pediatr Surg 5:511–513
Genevieve D, de Pontual L, Amiel J, Sarnacki S, Lyonnet S (2007) An overview of isolated and syndromic esophageal atresia. Clin Genet 71:392–399
Georgeson KE, Inge TH, Albanese CT (2000) Laparoscopically assisted anorectal pull-through for high imperforate anus: a new technique. J Pediatr Surg 35(6):927–930, discussion 930–931
Grosfeld JL, Ballantine TVN, Shoemaker R (1968) Operative management of intestinal atresia and stenosis based on pathologic findings. J Pediatr Surg 14:368–375
Grosfeld JL, Ballantine TV, Shoemaker R (1979) Operative management of intestinal atresia and stenosis based on pathologic findings. J Pediatr Surg 14(3):368–375
Gross GW, Wolfson PJ, Pena (1991) An augmented-pressure colostogram in imperforate anus with fistula. Pediatr Radiol 21(8):560–562
Gupta AK, Guglani B (2005) Imaging of congenital anomalies of the gastrointestinal tract. Indian J Pediatr 72:403–414
Haber HP (2009) Ultrasonography of imperforate anus in neonate: an approach correlated with current surgical concepts. Ultraschall Med 30(2):189–195
Haber HP, Seitz G, Warmann SW, Fuchs J (2007) Transperineal sonography for determination of the type of imperforate anus. AJR Am J Roentgenol 189(6):1525–1529
Hertzberg BS, Bowie JD (1990) Fetal gastrointestinal abnormalities. Radiol Clin N Am 28:101–114
Holland AJ, Fitzgerald DA (2010) Oesophageal atresia and trachea-esophageal fistula: current management strategies and complications. Pediatr Respir Rev 11:100–106, quiz 106–107
Holschneider A, Hutson J, Peña A et al (2005) Preliminary report on the international conference for the development of standards for the treatment of anorectal malformations. J Pediatr Surg 40(10):1521–1526

Houben CH, Curry JI (2008) Current status of prenatal diagnosis, operative management and outcome of esophageal atresia/tracheo-esophageal fistula. Prenat Diagn 28:667–675
Ioannides AS, Copp AJ (2009) Embryology of esophageal atresia. Semin Pediatr Surg 18:2–11
Juang D, Snyder CL (2012) Neonatal bowel obstruction. Surg Clin North Am 92(3):685–711
Karnak I, Ciftci AO, Senocak ME, Tanyel FC, Buyukpamukcu N (2001) Colonic atresia: surgical management and outcome. Pediatr Surg Int 17:631–635
Kuo MF, Tsai Y, Hsu WM, Chen RS, Tu YK, Wang HS (2007) Tethered spinal cord and VACTERL association. J Neurosurg 106(3 Suppl):201–204
Lahdes-Vasama TT, Sihvonen R, Iber T (2009) Perforation of the upper and lower segments of atretic esophagus (type C) secondary to nasogastric tube insertion. Pediatr Surg Int 25:537–538
Lai ECS, Tompkins RK (1986) Heterotopic pancreas: review of 26-year experience. Am J Surg 151:697–700
Landes A, Shuckett B, Skarsgard E (1994) Non-fixation of the colon in colonic atresia: a new finding. Pediatr Radiol 24:167–169
Laya BF, Andres MM, Conception NDP, Dizon RH (2015) Patterns of microcolon: imaging strategies for diagnosis of lower intestinal obstruction in neonates. J Am Osteopat Coll Radiol 4(1):1–11
Levitt MA, Peña A (2007) Anorectal malformations. Orphanet J Rare Dis 2:33
Louw JH (1967) Resection and end-to-end anastomosis in the management of atresia and stenosis of the small bowel. Surgery 62:940–950
Martin LW, Zerella JT (1976) Jejunoileal atresia: a proposed classification. J Pediatr Surg 11:399–403
Materne R (2001) The duodenal wind sock sign. Radiology 218(3):749–750
Miele V, Di Giampietro I (2014) Diagnostic imaging in emergency. Salute Soc (2EN): 127–138. doi:10.3280/SES2014-002010EN
Miele V, Andreoli C, Grassi R (2006) The management of emergency radiology: key facts. Eur J Radiol 59:311–314. Epub 2006 Jun 27
Moore CCM (1989) Congenital gastric outlet obstruction. J Pediatr Surg 24:1241–1246
Morris G, Kennedy A Jr, Cochran W (2016) Small bowel congenital anomalies: a review and update. Curr Gastroenterol Rep 18:16. doi:10.1007/s11894-016-0490-4
Mortell AE, Azizkhan RG (2009) Esophageal atresia repair with thoracotomy: the Cincinnati contemporary experience. Semin Pediatr Surg 18:12–19
Nagpal R, Schnaufer L, Altschuler SM (1993) Duodenal web presenting with gastrointestinal bleeding in a seven-month-old infant. J Pediatr Gastroenterol Nutr 16(1):90–92
Narasimha Rao KL, Prasad GR, Katariya S, Yadav K, Mitra SK, Patak IC (1983) Prone cross table lateral view: an alternative to the invertogram in imperforate anus. AJR Am J Roentgenol 140:227–229
Niedzielski JK (2005) Invertography versus ultrasonography and distal colostography for the determination of bowel skin distance in children with anorectal malformations. Eur J Pediatr Surg 15(4):262–267
Nievelstein RA, Hartwig NG, Vermeij-Keers C, Valk J (1993) Embryonic development of the mammalian caudal neural tube. Teratology 48(1):21–31
Nievelstein RA, van der Werff JF, Verbeek FJ, Valk J, Vermeij-Keers C (1998) Normal and abnormal embryonic development of the anorectum in human embryos. Teratology 57(2):70–78
Nievelstein RA, Vos A, Valk J, Vermeij-Keers C (2002) Magnetic resonance imaging in children with anorectal malformations: embryologic implications. J Pediatr Surg 37(8):1138–1145
Nora JJ, Nora AH, Pervinche AG, Ingram JV, Fountain AK, Peterson MJ (1976) Congenital abnormalities and first trimester exposure to progestagen/oestrogen (letter). Lancet 1:313–314
Norton KI, Tenreiro R, Rabinowitz JG (1992) Sonographic demonstration of annular pancreas and a distal duodenal diaphragm in a newborn. Pediatr Radiol 22:66–67
Oppenheimer DA, Carroll BA, Shochat SJ (1983) Sonography of imperforate anus. Radiology 148:127–128
Pasto ME, Deiling JM, O'Hara AE, Rifkin MD, Goldberg BB (1984) Neonatal colonic atresia: ultrasound findings. Pediatr Radiol 14:346–348
Peña A, Hong A (2000) Advances in the management of anorectal malformations. Am J Surg 180(5):370–376
Pinheiro PFM, Simoes AC, Pereira RM (2012) Current knowledge on esophageal atresia. World J Gastroenterol 18(28):3662–3672
Pohlson EC, Hatch EI Jr, Glick PL, Tapper D (1988) Individualized management of colonic atresia. Am J Surg 155:690–692
Puri P, Fujimoto T (1988) New observations on the pathogenesis of multiple intestinal atresias. J Pediatr Surg 23:221–225
Ratan SK, Rattan KN, Pandey RM, Mittal A, Magu S, Sodhi PK (2004) Associated congenital anomalies in patients with anorectal malformations: a need for developing a uniform practical approach. J Pediatr Surg 39(11):1706–1711
Sarin YK (2000) Pyloric atresia associated with intestinal atresias. Indian Pediatr 37:205–207
Sarin YK, Sharma A, Sinha S, Deshpande VP (2012) Duodenal webs: an experience with 18 patients. J Neonatal Surg 1(2):20
Sauve RS, Leung AK (2003) Congenital varicella syndrome with colonic atresias. Clin Pediatr (Phila) 42:451
Schiller M, Aviad I, Freund H (1979) Congenital colonic atresia and stenosis. Am J Surg 138:721–724
Seitz G, Warmann SW, Schaefer J, Poets CF, Fuchs J (2006) Primary repair of esophageal atresia in extremely low birth weight infants: a single-center experience and review of the literature. Biol Neonate 90:247–251
Seo J, do Kim Y, Kim AR, Kim DY, Kim SC, Kim IK et al (2010) An 18-year experience of tracheoesophageal fistula and esophageal atresia. Korean J Pediatr 53:705–710

Sharma AK, Shekhawat NS, Agrawal LD, Chaturvedi V, Kothari SK, Goel D (2000) Esophageal atresia and tracheoesophageal fistula: a review of 25 years' experience. Pediatr Surg Int 16:478–482

Shaw-Smith C (2010) Genetic factors in esophageal atresia, trachea-esophageal fistula and the VACTERL association: roles for FOXF1 and the 16q24.1 FOX transcription factor gene cluster, and review of the literature. Eur J Med Genet 53:6–13

Solomon BD (2011) VACTERL/VATER association. Orphanet J Rare Dis 6:56–67

Solomon BD, Raam MS, Pineda-Alvarez DE (2011) Analysis of genitourinary anomalies in patients with VACTERL (vertebral anomalies, anal atresia, cardiac malformations, tracheo-esophageal fistula, renal anomalies, limb abnormalities) association. Congenit Anom (Kyoto) 51(2):87–91

Son TN, Liem NT, Kien HH (2015) Laparoscopic simple oblique duodenoduodenostomy in management of congenital duodenal obstruction in children. J Laparoendosc Adv Surg Tech A 25(2):163–166

Spitz L (2007) Oesophageal atresia. Orphanet J Rare Dis 2:24

Stephens FD, Smith ED, Paoul NW (1988) Anorectal malformations in children: update 1988. Liss, New York

Strouse PJ (2008) Malrotation. Semin Roentgenol 43(1):7–14

Tao HA, Lin CC, Huang FY, Yeh ML, Shih SL (1987) Congenital atresia of the colon: a case report. Acta Pediatr Sin 28:120–122

van der Zee DC (2011) Laparoscopic repair of duodenal atresia: revisited. World J Surg 35(8):1781–1784

Van Winckel MAJM, Afschrift MB, Vande Walle JGJ (1994) Ultrasound diagnosis of a prepyloric diaphragm. J Clin Ultrasound 22:141–143

Wang J, Du L, Cai W, Pan W, Yan W (2014) Prolonged feeding difficulties after surgical correction on intestinal atresia: a 13-year experience. J Pediatr Surg 49(11):1593–1597

Watts AC, Sabharwal AJ, MacKinlay GA, Munro FD (2003) Congenital colonic atresia: should primary anastomosis always be the goal? Pediatr Surg Int 19:14–17

Winters WD, Weinberger E, Hatch EI (1992) Atresia of the colon in neonates: radiographic findings. AJR 159:1273–1276

Wong-Gibbons DL, Romitti PA, Sun L, Moore CA, Reefhuis J, Bell EM, Olshan AF (2008) Maternal periconceptional exposure to cigarette smoking and alcohol and esophageal atresia +/– trachea-esophageal fistula. Birth Defects Res A Clin Mol Teratol 82:776–784

2 Intestinal Malrotation and Volvulus

Viola Valentini, Claudia Lucia Piccolo, Maria Napoletano, Rosanna Mamone, Massimo Zeccolini, and Vittorio Miele

2.1 Definition

Intestinal malrotation is a congenital abnormal position of the bowel within the peritoneal cavity secondary to an arrest of normal rotation of any part of the intestinal tract. Malrotation is accompanied by abnormal bowel fixation by mesenteric bands or the absence of fixation of portions of the bowel (malfixation), leading to increased risks of bowel obstruction and midgut volvulus. Because the mesentery contains the vessels supplying and draining the small bowel, in the case of twisting on its axis, intestinal necrosis may occur in a very short time, making malrotation with volvulus an acute surgical emergency.

V. Valentini (✉) • V. Miele
Department of Emergency Radiology, S. Camillo Hospital, Rome, Italy
e-mail: violavalentini@libero.it

C.L. Piccolo
Department of Medicine and Health Sciences, University of Molise, Campobasso, Italy

M. Napoletano
Division of Radiology, Department of Surgical and Biomedical Sciences, S. Maria della Misericordia Hospital, S. Andrea delle Fratte, Perugia, Italy

R. Mamone
Department of Radiology, Santobono Pediatric Hospital, Naples, Italy

M. Zeccolini
Department of Radiology, Pausilipon Pediatric Oncologic Hospital, Naples, Italy

2.2 Embryologic Origins

The embryo's gut develops from the yolk sac, which early divides into three sections: the foregut, supplied by the celiac artery; the midgut, extending from the duodenum at the insertion of bile duct to the distal transverse colon, supplied by the superior mesenteric artery (SMA); and the hindgut, supplied by the inferior mesenteric artery (Fig. 2.1).

The midgut is divided into a cephalad, prearterial portion, and a caudad, post-arterial portion by the SMA and the vitelline duct (Snider and Chaffin 1954). The cephalad midgut gives rise to the distal duodenum, jejunum, and proximal ileum. The caudad midgut contributes to the distal ileum, cecum, appendix, and ascending and first two-thirds of transverse colon.

Between the 4th and the 12th week of gestation, the gut lengths rapidly, and, after a series of complex rotations, it undergoes fixation in the normal position in the abdomen (Fig. 2.2).

First the duodenum rotates 90° counterclockwise to a position at the right of the SMA, while the colon rotates 90° to a location to the left of SMA. At 6 weeks the midgut herniates in a U-shaped loop into the umbilical cord, where the duodenum rotates counterclockwise another 90°. At 10 weeks the gut returns to the abdominal cavity where the duodenum completes its final 90° rotation, until the duodenojejunal junction is located to the left of the spine, while the colon

V. Miele, M. Trinci (eds.), *Imaging Non-traumatic Abdominal Emergencies in Pediatric Patients*,
DOI 10.1007/978-3-319-41866-7_2

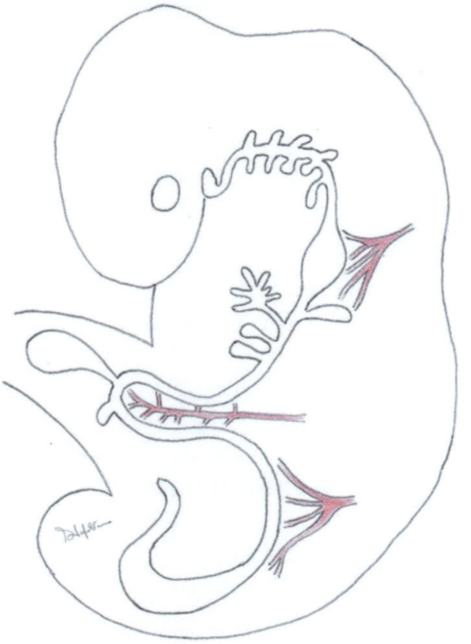

Fig. 2.1 The embryo's three gut sections, foregut, midgut, and hindgut, and their vascular supplying

rotates 180° until the cecum is located in the right lower quadrant.

Throughout the remainder of gestation and postnatally for the first few months of life, further elongation of the cecum and fixation of the gut occur. The ascending and descending colons are anchorated to the right and left abdominal gutters. The small bowel's broad mesenteric attachment, extending from the ligament of Treitz – that anchorates the duodenojejunal junction (DDJ) in the upper left abdomen – to the ileocecal valve in the lower right abdomen, stabilizes its position and prevents volvulus (Fig. 2.3).

2.3 Classification and Physiopathology

The term "malrotation" applies not to a single distinct entity, but rather to a continuum of intestinal anomalies reflecting a failure occurring at any time in the embryologic development of the midgut. This can result in an appearance ranging from complete midgut malrotation to normal anatomy except for a high-riding cecum in the right upper right quadrant. In the majority of cases, malrotation involves both the small and large bowel.

Different patterns of malrotation can be categorized on the bases of the timing of the developmental failure (Long and Markowitz 1996).

Non-rotation: this is the most common positional anomaly, reflecting an early failure of rotation. The initial 90° rotation has occurred with the duodenum lying right of the SMA and the distal colon left to the SMA. The first and second parts of the duodenum are normally positioned, but the third and fourth parts descend vertically along the right side of the SMA. The small bowel is located at the right and the colon lies to the left of the midline (Figs. 2.3b and 2.4).

Incomplete rotation: failure during the final 180° counterclockwise rotation of the small bowel and/or of the colon. The resultant abnormality varies from complete non-rotation to normal. Abnormally rotated bowel does not develop a normal mesenteric attachment, leading to the risk of volvulus that varies with the degree of mesenteric attachment (Fig. 2.4b).

Reversed rotation: the caudal midgut (cecocolic loop) returns to the abdominal cavity first, and the duodenum rotates clockwise rather than counterclockwise. As a result, the duodenum courses anterior to SMA rather than posterior, and the colon (ascending and transversus) courses posterior rather than anterior.

The abnormally positioned right colon can have aberrant attachments to the right upper quadrant retroperitoneum, known as Ladd's bands (Fig. 2.5). These peritoneal bands, crossing anterior to the bowel rather than posterior to it, may cause intestinal obstruction, most frequently by impinging the third portion of the duodenum.

In malrotation, the proximity between the DDJ and the cecum, the two fixation points of the small bowel, results in a short mesenteric root, predisposing the malfixated midgut to rotate around the axis of the superior mesenteric artery. This twisting causes an obstruction of the bowel lumen, of lymphatic and venous drainage, and, eventually, of arterial supply, leading to extensive intestinal necrosis, which can be fatal.

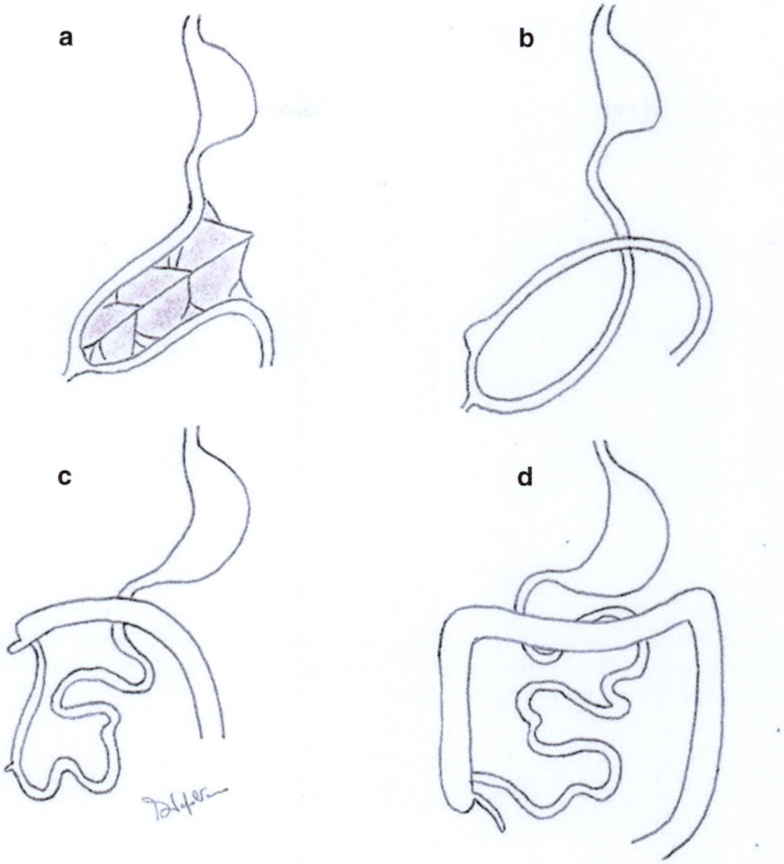

Fig. 2.2 The stages of normal intestinal rotation during embryologic development. (**a**) Lateral view of the midgut loop before rotation. (**b**) Lateral view after the first 180° counterclockwise rotation around the mesenteric vessel axis. (**c**) Frontal view after complete midgut 270° rotation. (**d**) Frontal view of the final intestinal location, after elongation of the cecum and fixation of the gut

Malrotation, in itself, is not a surgical emergency; however, it does indicate a potential propensity to volvulus, a true life-threatening emergency.

2.4 Epidemiology and Clinical Presentation

Malrotation occurs in approximately 1 in 500 live births

Malrotation of the bowel is always present in patients with congenital defects of the abdominal wall, such as omphalocele, gastroschisis, or diaphragmatic hernia (Fig. 2.6). It is often associated with a number of syndromes and anatomic anomalies, mostly gastrointestinal, such as jejunal and duodenal stenosis, annular pancreas, Hirschsprung disease, and intussusception. It is very common in patients with heterotaxy syndrome.

Malrotation is usually diagnosed in newborns and young infants; up to 75 % of symptomatic cases occur soon after birth and up to 90 % within the first year of life (Torres and Ziegler 1993). The classical clinical manifestation is bilious vomiting, with or without abdominal distension, associated with either duodenal obstructive bands or midgut volvulus (Strouse 2008). In 62 % of newborns presenting with bilious vomiting, the cause is not an anatomic obstruction, but imaging can be useful to exclude malrotation (Strouse 2004).

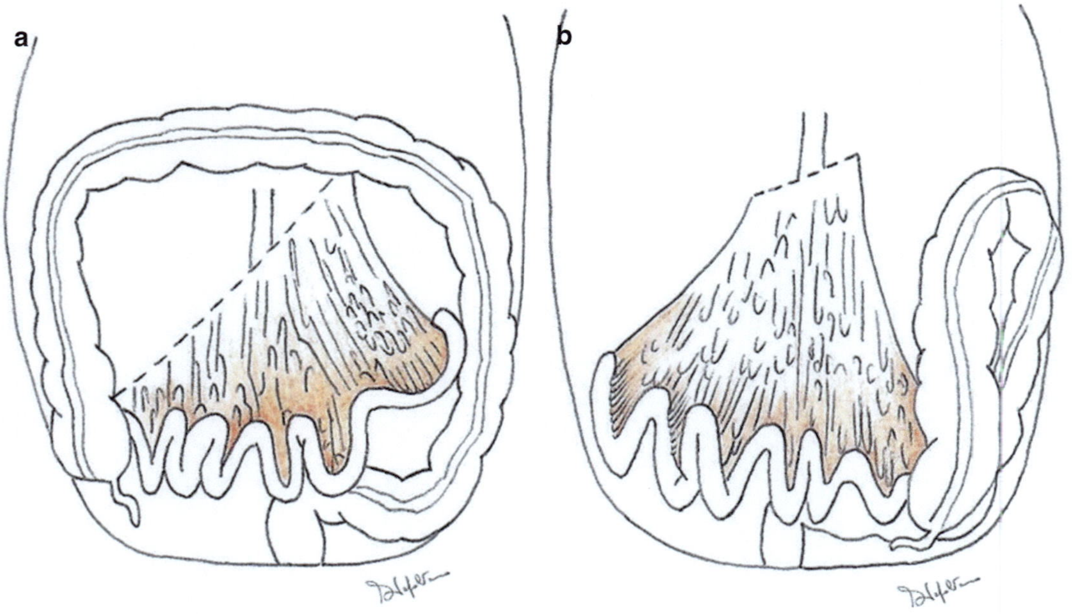

Fig. 2.3 (**a**) The small bowel has a broad mesenteric attachment, extending from the DDJ in the upper left abdomen to the ileocecal valve in the lower right abdomen. (**b**) In malrotation, the root of the small bowel mesentery is narrow, predisposing to intestinal volvulus

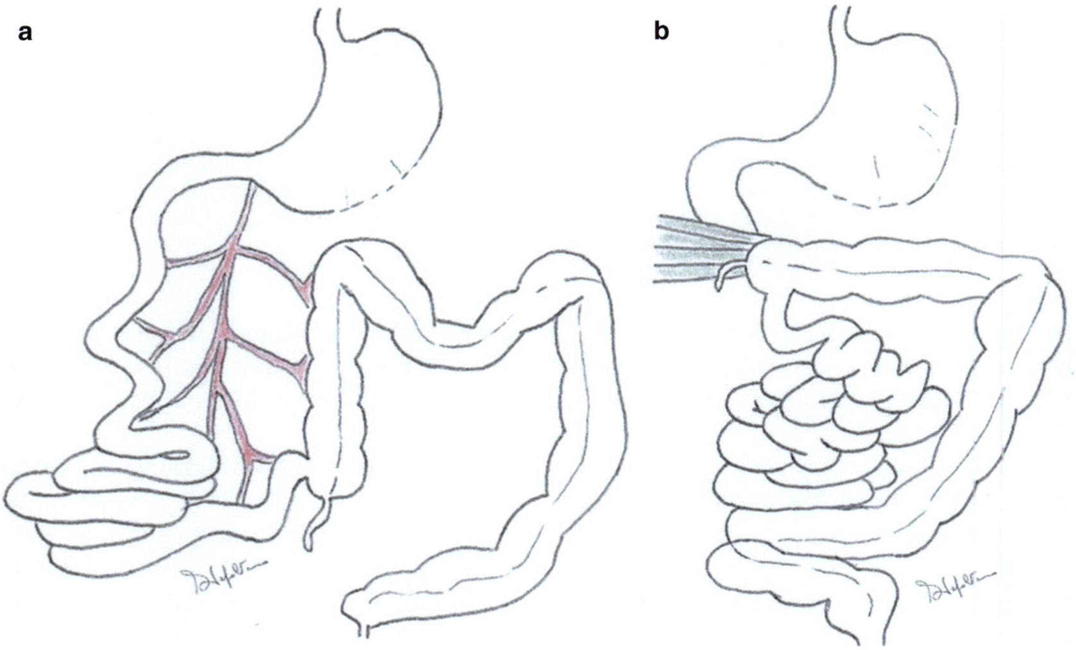

Fig. 2.4 (**a**) Non-rotation. (**b**) Incomplete rotation

In intestinal volvulus diagnosis must be made promptly and children must undergo surgery without delay. Mortality in affected newborns is 3–5 % (Applegate et al. 2006).

Patients with malrotation who do not develop volvulus at birth may remain asymptomatic for the rest of their lives. Most of patients who present with intestinal obstruction later in life do so

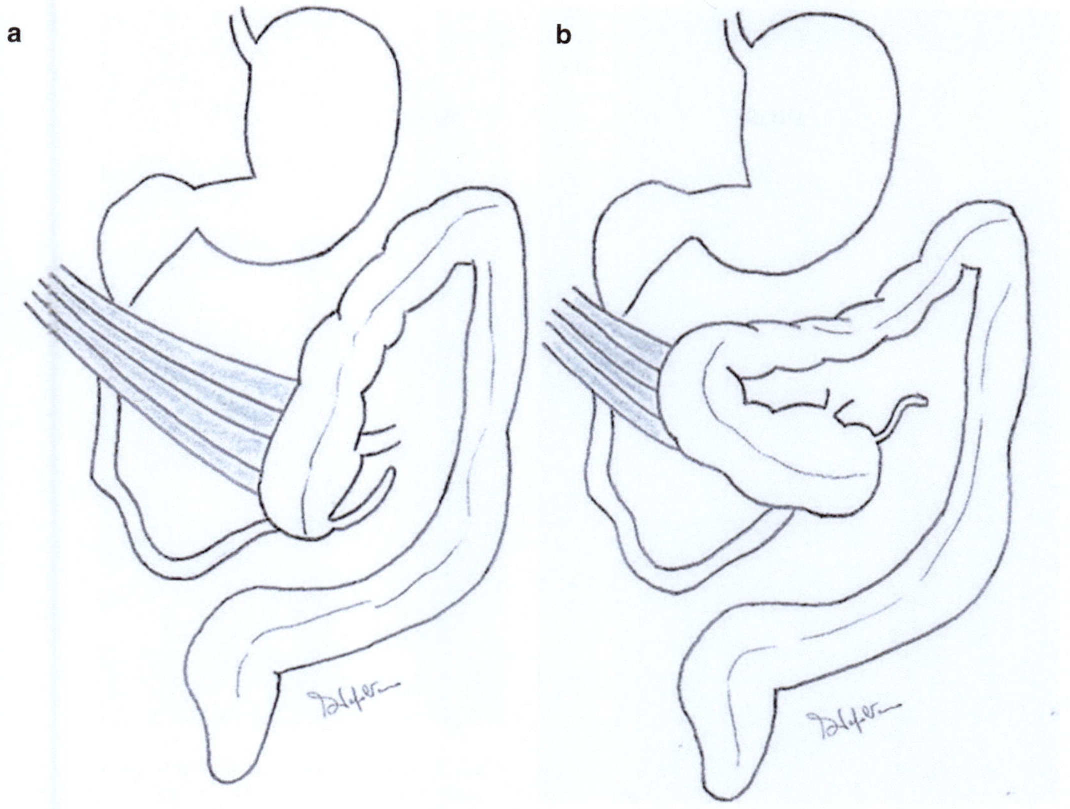

Fig. 2.5 Ladd's bands

because of crossing peritoneal bands. Malrotation beyond infancy may have unusual clinical manifestations that vary from acute abdominal pain and vomiting to mild intermittent pain and malabsorption. The incidental diagnosis of malrotation is not uncommon, especially in adults (Zissin et al. 1999).

2.5 Imaging

2.5.1 Abdominal Radiograph

Abdominal plain radiographs are usually the initial diagnostic procedure obtained. They are usually nonspecific, but they help to exclude other etiologies and to guide further investigations. In the setting of a neonate with bilious vomiting, the bowel gas pattern will help to differentiate distal from proximal obstruction. The most common intestinal gas pattern in malrotation is normal. If the loops are distended, radiographs may occasionally show the small bowel on the left and the colon on the right, suggesting a positional anomaly (Fig. 2.7). In the case of severe duodenal obstruction due to volvulus or Ladd's bands, the classical appearance of "double bubble sign" may be seen, gas-filled, dilated stomach and duodenal bulb, with little gas in the distal bowel. If the obstruction is complete, this pattern is indistinguishable from duodenal atresia and other causes of congenital duodenal obstruction (Fig. 2.8).

Radiographic findings in midgut volvulus can be ambiguous: the abdomen might be gasless, there might be dilatation of numerous small bowel loops simulating a distal small bowel obstruction, and the volvulized bowel can determine some mass effect in the mid-abdomen. The presence of intestinal pneumatosis or free intraperitoneal air is extremely rare, but represents a poor prognostic sign.

If the radiographs are normal or nonspecific, a contrast-enhanced examination should be performed.

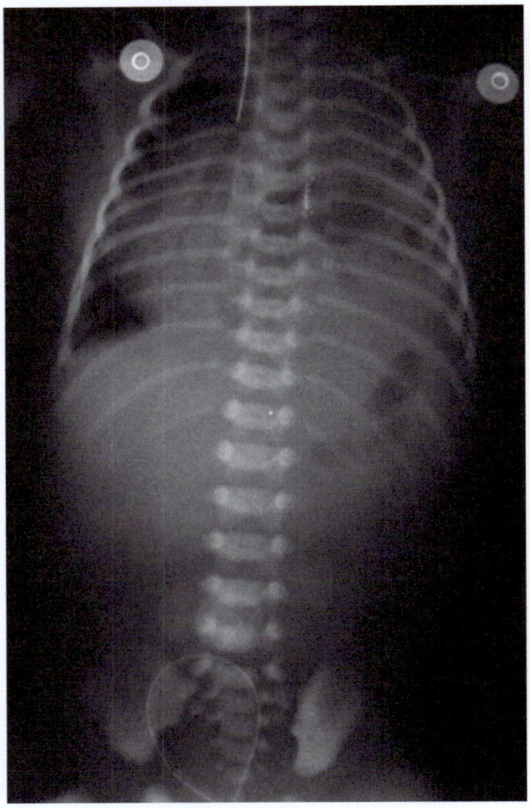

Fig. 2.6 Plain radiograph shows herniation of the bowel in the left chest cavity, with displacement of the heart, in diaphragmatic hernia

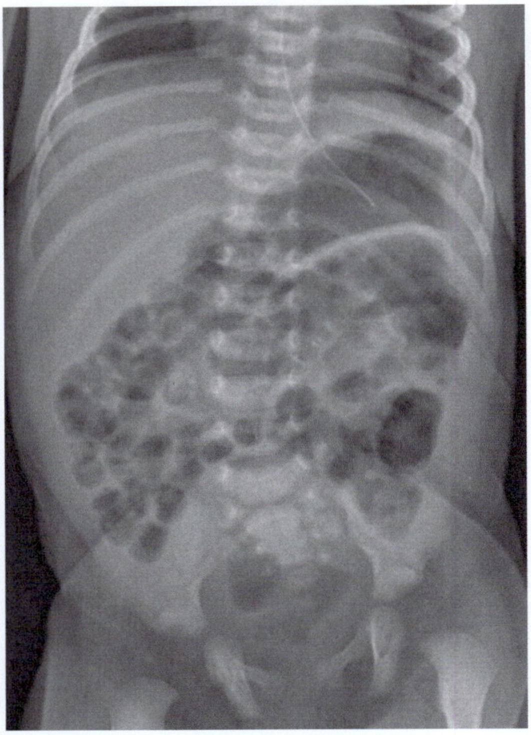

Fig. 2.7 Abnormal position of air-distended bowel loops on plain radiograph, suggesting malrotation at 12 days of age. The small bowel is located in the right side of the abdomen and the large bowel in the left side on frontal view

2.5.2 Fluoroscopic-Guided Contrast Studies

Contrast studies are the gold standard for the evaluation of intestinal malrotation, with or without volvulus or Ladd's band obstruction. The procedures can be performed with barium, but, in pediatric imaging, it is preferable to use diluted water-soluble nonionic iodinated contrast agents, when the risk of a potential perforation is suspected. Using a nasogastric tube aids in delivering and controlling the administration of contrast from above.

2.5.2.1 Upper GI Tract Examination

The contrast small intestinal series remains the mainstay for radiologic diagnosis of malrotation and volvulus. Upper GI is fast and accurate in locating duodenojejunal junction, which is the key landmark in the upper GI tract examination and easily demonstrates a duodenal obstruction (Sizemore et al. 2008). The DDJ is normally positioned to the left of the left pedicle at the level of duodenal bulb on frontal views and posterior on the lateral views. The duodenal sweep is usually smooth and "C" shaped, and the jejunum is usually in the upper left quadrant (but a different position of the jejunum by itself is not an indication of malrotation). In the case of malrotation, the upper GI series shows a malposition of the DDJ, low-positioned and to the right of the spine or midline from an anteroposterior view and anteriorly positioned on a lateral view (Fig. 2.9). Both frontal and lateral views are crucial to define the position of the DDJ. Orienting the patient left side down allows contrast material to pool in the gastric cavity, and subsequent rotation into right prone oblique position allows contrast material to move into the duodenum. The lateral view pro-

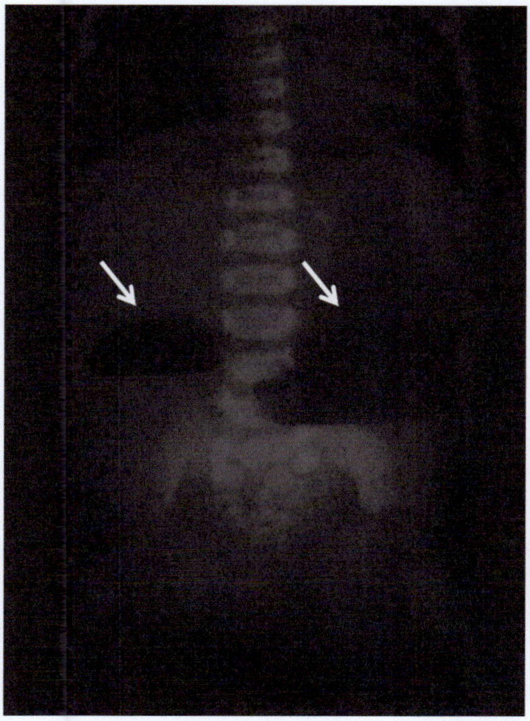

Fig. 2.8 "Double bubble" sign, with air-fluid levels in distended stomach and duodenum (*arrows*), is a nonspecific sign of proximal bowel obstruction. Constricting Ladd's band is indistinguishable from atresia and other causes of congenital duodenal obstruction on plain radiographs

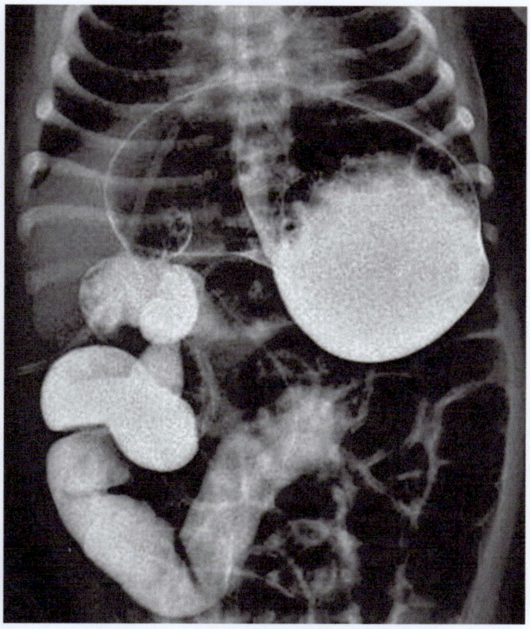

Fig. 2.9 Upper GI series shows malrotated stomach and small bowel in a 17-day-old newborn. Note the abnormal position of the duodenojejunal junction (*arrow*) to the right of the spine on frontal view

vides confirmatory information on the duodenal course.

It is important to localize precisely the DDJ during fluoroscopic observation of the first pass of contrast along the duodenal sweep, because it can be easily obscured by contrast in the antrum or jejunum. In children with acute duodenal obstruction, the upper GI series may depict a Z-shaped duodenum in the presence of obstructing peritoneal bands or a duodenojejunal corkscrew twist in the presence of volvulus. The corkscrew sign (spiral sign), visualized both in frontal and lateral views, illustrates a spiral configuration of the fourth portion of the duodenum and the proximal jejunum (Ortiz-Neira 2007) (Fig. 2.10). Dilatation of the proximal duodenum is often associated. Midgut volvulus involves the entire length of the small bowel, with the exception of the first and second duodenal portions.

Due to the relative laxity of peritoneal ligaments in infants, the DDJ position is variable (Koch et al. 2016), and it can easily be inferiorly displaced by a dilated stomach or intestinal segment or by an enteric feeding tube, carrying the risk of malrotation overdiagnosis (Katz et al. 1987). Radiological false-positive rate for UGI series showing malrotation may be as high as 15 % (Applegate et al. 2006), so in equivocal cases, when the diagnosis of malrotation does not match with the clinical history and physical examination, a contrast enema and eventually a repeat of the UGI series might be prudent.

2.5.2.2 Contrast Enema

Abnormal position of the cecum can be found in 80–87 % of surgically proven cases of malrotation (Applegate et al. 2006). Malrotation of the colon alone is much rarer than that limited to the small bowel or that of the small and large bowel together. Enema, performed using iodinated hydrosoluble contrast material diluted at 10 % in 1,000 ml of warm water, can be useful to localize the cecum (Figs. 2.11 and 2.12) and thereby define distal end

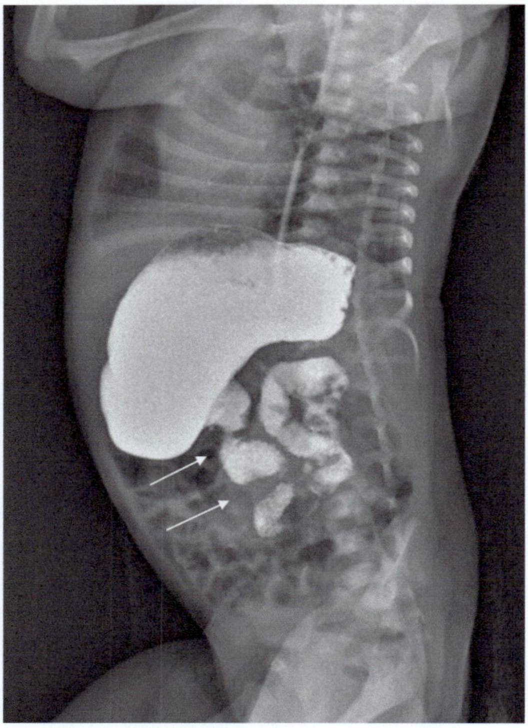

Fig. 2.10 Corkscrew sign. Upper GI series performed with iodinated water-soluble contrast agent shows a dilated stomach and a spiral appearance of the distal duodenum and the proximal jejunum (*arrows*) on the lateral view in malrotation pattern

of the mesenteric attachment of the midgut. The shorter the distance between the DDJ and the cecal apex, the shorter the length of the small bowel mesentery and the greater the risk of volvulus. Approximately 20 % of individuals with malrotation have a normally positioned cecum (Katz et al. 1987); thus normal cecal position does not rule out the diagnosis of malrotation (Slovis and Strouse 2009). Contrast enema is rarely used alone; nevertheless, documentation of frankly abnormal cecal position in the setting of an equivocal upper GI might be of benefit (Fig. 2.13).

In infants and older children who present with vomiting, enema may reveal a distal bowel obstruction due to an acute bowel volvulus (Fig. 2.14).

2.5.2.3 Ultrasound

The use of abdominal sonography has been proposed for the screening of malrotation, based on the position of mesenteric vessels. Normally the superior mesenteric vein (SMV) is located to the right and anterior to the mesenteric superior artery (SMA) in axial plane, and the two vessels course approximately parallel to one another as the artery descends from its origin and courses inferiorly. An association between an intestinal malrotation and a reversal of the relationship between the SMA and SMV (with the vein located anterior and to the left of the artery) (Fig. 2.15) has been observed for decades but remains controversial (Anupindi et al. 2014). Initially it was assumed that if SMV is not to the right of SMA, at the level of SMV's junction with the portal vein, the finding will be suggestive for malrotation.

However, recent studies demonstrated that the relative positions of mesenteric vessels are reverted only in 60 % of children with malrotation and anatomic variations with reversal of the vessel position exist in children with no intestinal abnormality (Dufour et al. 1992; Ashley et al. 2001). At present most authors believe that US cannot exclude malrotation (Ashley et al. 2001; Orzech et al. 2006; Yousefzadeh 2009).

A fluoroscopic upper gastrointestinal series must always be performed in suspect cases, as it remains the reference standard in the evaluation of malrotation.

Recently, evaluation of the position of the third portion of the duodenum (D3) by using a graded compression ultrasonography has been proposed as a screening tool for malrotation. The statement was that a normal retromesenteric course of D3 between the SMA and the abdominal aorta excludes malrotation (Yousefzadeh et al. 2010; Menten et al. 2012). However, subsequent studies on patients with surgically proven malrotation who underwent abdominal CT examinations showed the presence of D3 in a normal retromesenteric location in patients with malrotation, demonstrating that the retromesenteric position of D3 may not be a reliable landmark of normal rotation (Taylor 2011; Menten et al. 2013).

Ultrasound (US) is an inexpensive, noninvasive imaging modality. Performed with high-frequency (6–10 MHz) linear transducers, using warmed gel for the comfort of the baby. US is

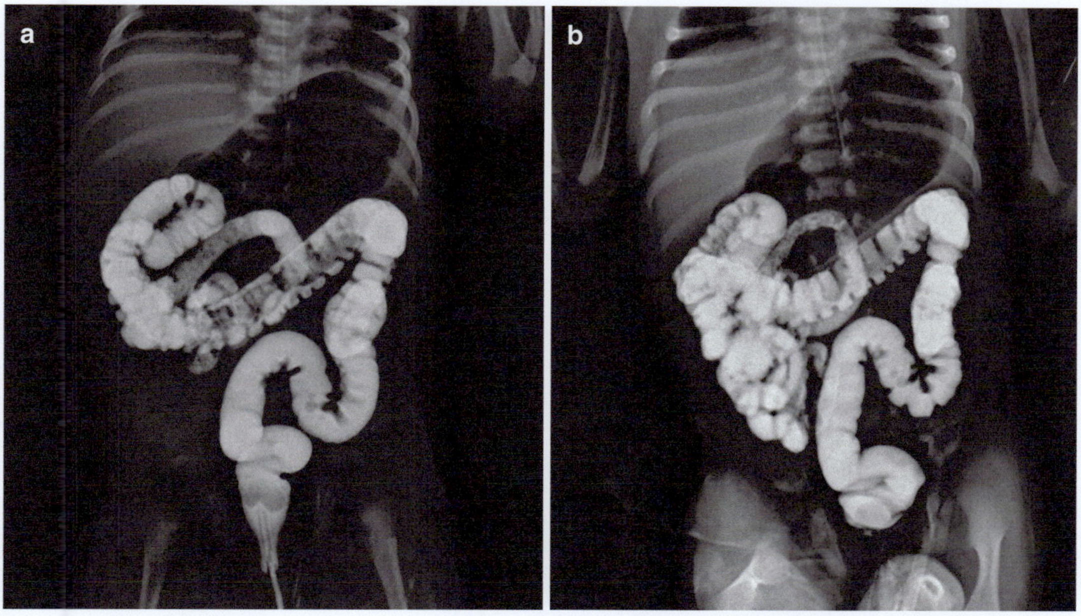

Fig. 2.11 Contrast enema shows abnormal position of the cecum (**a**) and, with reflux of the contrast through the ileocecal valve, small bowel located in the right abdomen (**b**) on anteroposterior views in a 15-day-old newborn with incomplete rotation

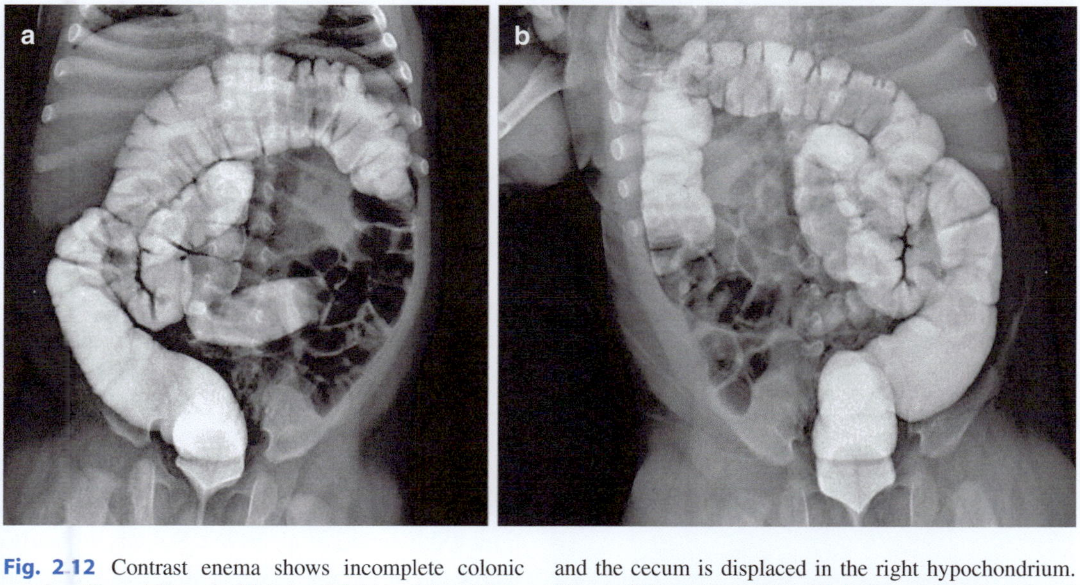

Fig. 2.12 Contrast enema shows incomplete colonic rotation. Sigmoid loop is dilated and right positioned. The ascending colon is located in the middle upper quadrant and the cecum is displaced in the right hypochondrium. The small bowel is not opacified. Anteroposterior (**a**) and posteroanterior (**b**) views

suitable for the small body size of neonates and young children (Di Giacomo et al. 2015). It needs no special preparation and can be performed at the bedside, even at the presence of the parents. Although ultrasound diagnosis of malrotation is challenging, US may be the first examination in which volvulus is discovered. Findings of acute volvulus on conventional US are the following (Hyden et al. 1984; Chao et al. 2000): distended proximal duodenum; tapering of the duodenum

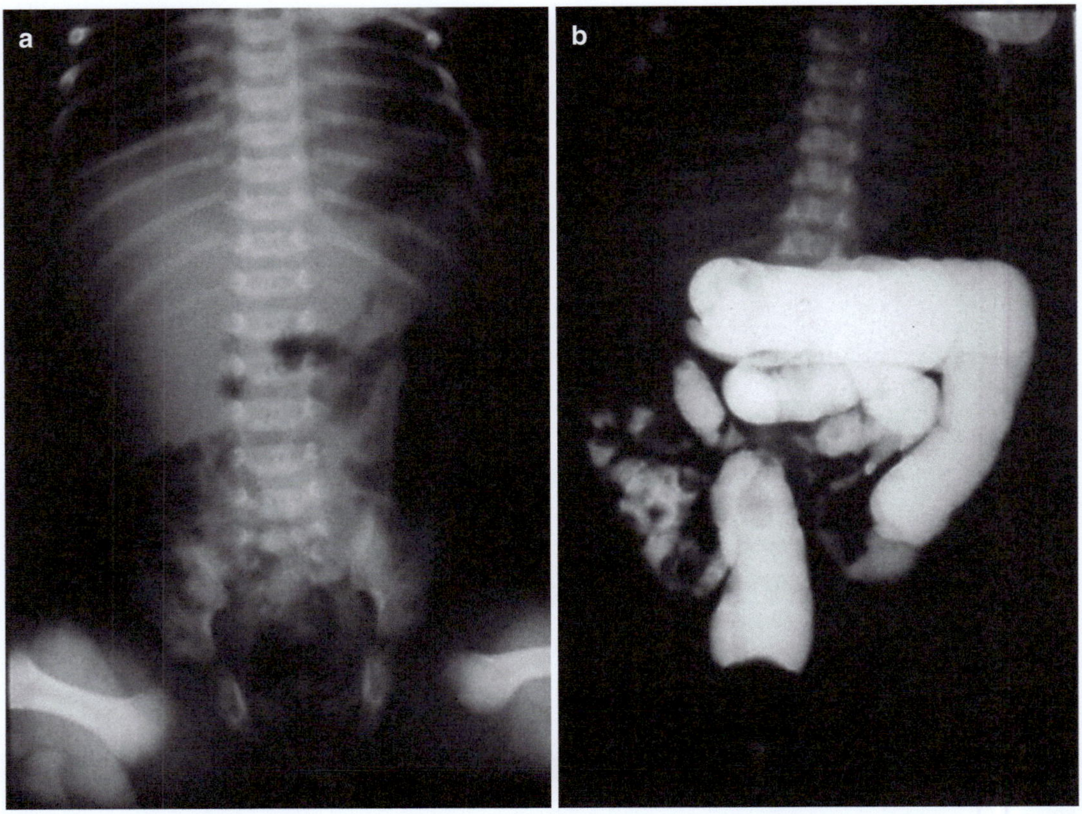

Fig. 2.13 (**a**, **b**) Intestinal malrotation with the cecum and ascending colon in the left abdomen

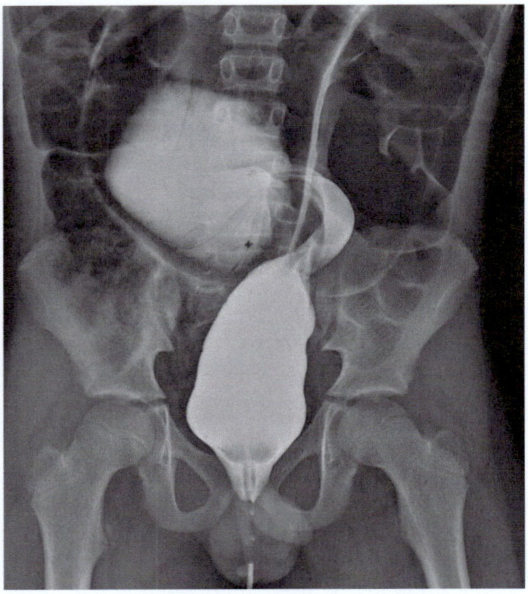

Fig. 2.14 Intestinal obstruction from sigmoid volvulus in a 10-year-old boy. Contrast enema on anteroposterior view clearly shows sigmoid torsion and dilated large bowel loops

over the spine, suggesting an extrinsic compression; thick-walled bowel loops; and the presence of peritoneal fluid.

In midgut volvulus, not only the intestinal tract but also the mesenteric vessels are volvulated. The SMV wraps clockwise around the SMA (Fig. 2.16). A swirling or twisting or a whirlpool relationship between the vessels on color Doppler ("whirlpool sign") is characteristic of a volvulus. It consists of a side-by-side arrangement of vessels with opposing flow directions (Shimanuki et al. 1996). Solitary hyperdynamic pulsating SMA (Sze et al. 2002), truncated appearance of the SMA, and a dilated SMV are other important ancillary vascular signs.

2.5.2.4 CT and MRI

Like other cross-sectional modalities, computed tomography (CT) and magnetic resonance imaging (MRI) can be used to evaluate the position of D3, the location of the DJJ, and the anatomical

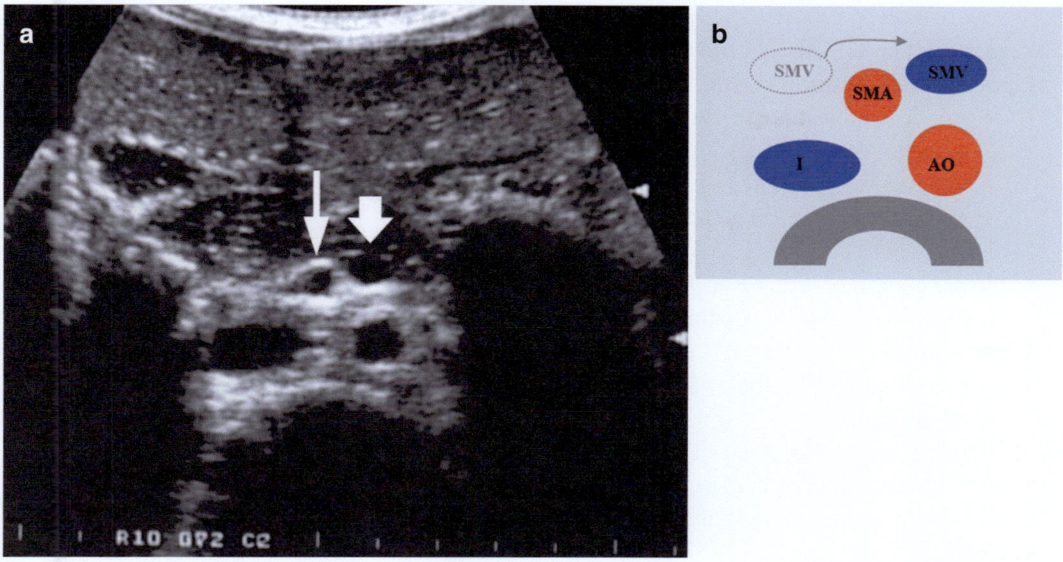

Fig. 2.15 (**a**) Sonogram showing inverted position of mesenteric vessels in malrotation. The superior mesenteric vein (*thick arrow*) is positioned to the left of the superior mesenteric artery (*thin arrow*) on an axial plane. (**b**) Scheme showing the inversion of the anatomic relationship between the SMA and the SMV. *AO* aorta, *I* inferior vena cava

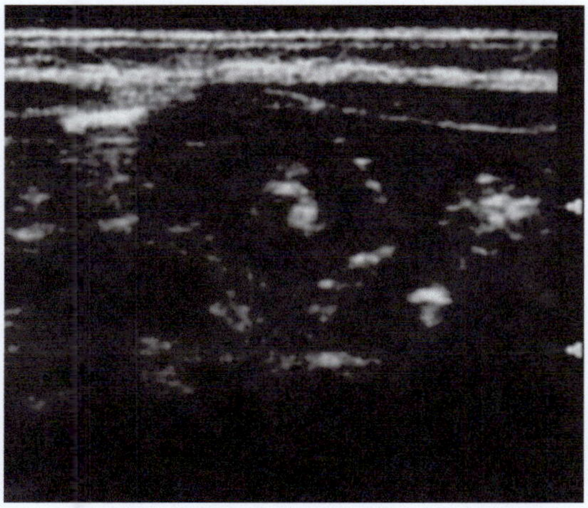

Fig. 2.16 Whirlpool sign. The SMV and the mesentery wrap around the SMA on an axial-oblique plane sonogram in malrotation with volvulus

relationship between the SMA and SMV (Miele and Di Giampietro 2014).

CT imaging of abnormal D3 position has high sensitivity and specificity of diagnosing malrotation (97.3 % and 99 %, respectively) (Taylor 2011). Due to the variation in normal SMA/SMV anatomy as previously discussed, the accuracy of identifying "abnormal" SMA/SMV relation in making the diagnosis of malrotation is about 77 % (Taylor 2011). If volvulus is present, CT scans can identify a central mass composed of mesentery with vessels and bowel twisting around the SMA axis in a whirl pattern ("whirlpool sign").

CT is a quick and complete examination, which can be performed with extremely minimal invasiveness, but is infrequently performed when the clinical suspect of malrotation is high, as it does subject the child to a significant dose of radiation when compared to an UGI. When performed with IV contrast media, CT can detect edema of the mesentery and perfusion abnormalities of the bowel (Aidlen et al. 2005).

Magnetic resonance imaging (MRI), as well as CT, can identify findings of malrotation, including dilation of the proximal duodenum, non-retroperitoneal positioning of the duodenum, bowel malpositioning, and inversion of the SMA/SMV relationship (Strouse 2008). The MRI is the most expensive imaging modality available to aid in diagnosing malrotation; it avoids radiation but relies on suspended respiration or needs the patient to be sedated.

Take Home Points in Midgut Malrotation

Upper gastrointestinal series:
- Abnormal position of duodenojejunal junction
- Corkscrew appearance of the duodenum and proximal jejunum if volvulus is present

Contrast enema:
- Cecum abnormally positioned

Ultrasound:
- Inversion of the SMA/SMV relationship
- Intraperitoneal course of D3
- Whirlpool pattern in mesenteric vessels if volvulus is present

CT/MR
- Non-retroperitoneal positioning of the duodenum
- Inversion of the SMA/SMV relationship
- Bowel malpositioning
- Whirlpool pattern in mesenteric vessels if volvulus is present
- Ischemic impairment of the bowel wall if volvulus is present

References

Aidlen J, Anupindi SA, Jaramillo D, Doody DP (2005) Malrotation with midgut volvulus: CT findings of bowel infarction. Pediatr Radiol 35:529–531

Anupindi SA, Halverson M, Khwaja A, Wang X, Bellah RD (2014) Common and uncommon applications of bowel ultrasound with pathologic correlation in children. AJR 202:946–959

Applegate K, MS, Anderson J, Klatte E (2006) Intestinal malrotation in children: a problem solving approach to the upper gastro-intestinal series. Radiographics 26:1485–1500

Ashley LM, Allen S, Teele RL (2001) A normal sonogram does not exclude malrotation. Pediatr Radiol 31:354–356

Chao HC, Kong MS, Chen JY, Lin SJ, Lin JN (2000) Sonographic features related to volvulus in neonatal intestinal malrotation. J Ultrasound Med 19: 371–376

Di Giacomo V, Trinci M, Van der Byl G, Catania VD, Calisti A, Miele V (2015) Ultrasound in newborns and children suffering from non-traumatic acute abdominal pain: imaging with clinical and surgical correlation. J Ultrasound 18:385–393. doi:10.1007/s40477-014-0087-4, Epub 2014 Apr 9

Dufour D, Delaet MH, Dassonville M, Cadranel S, Perlmutter N (1992) Midgut malrotation: the reliability of sonographic diagnosis. Pediatr Radiol 22:21–23

Hyden CK, Thomes FB, Swischuk LE et al (1984) Sonographic demonstration of duodenal obstruction with midgut volvulus. AJR 143:9–10

Katz ME, Siegel MJ, Shackelford GD et al (1987) The position and mobility of the duodenum in children. AJR 148:947–951

Koch C, Taghavi K, Hamill J, Mirjalli SA (2016) Redefining the projectional and clinical anatomy of the duodenojejunal flexure in children. Clin Anat 29(2):175–182

Long K, Markowitz T (1996) Radiographic patterns of intestinal malrotation in children. Radiographics 16:547–556

Menten R, Reding R, Godding V, Dumitriu D, Clapuyt P (2012) Sonographic assessment of the retroperitoneal position of the third portion of the duodenum: an indicator of normal intestinal rotation. Pediatr Radiol 42:941–945

Menten R, Dumitriu D, Calpuyt P, Yousefzadeh DK (2013) Duodenum between the aorta and the SMA does not exclude malrotation. Pediatr Radiol 43:123 (letter)

Miele V, Di Giampietro I (2014) Diagnostic imaging in emergency. Salute Soc (2EN):127–138. doi:10.3280/SES2014-002010EN

Ortiz-Neira C (2007) The corkscrew sign: midgut volvulus. Radiology 242:315–316

Orzech N, Navarro OM, Langer JC (2006) Is ultrasonography a good screening test for intestinal malrotation? J Pediatr Surg 41:1005–1009

Shimanuki Y, Aihara T, Takano H et al (1996) Clockwise whirlpool sign at color Doppler US: an objective and definite sign of midgut volvulus. Radiology 199:261–264

Sizemore A, Rabbani K, Ladd A, Applegate K (2008) Diagnostic performance of the upper gastrointestinal series in the evaluation of children with clinically suspected malrotation. Pediatr Radiol 38:518–528

Slovis TL, Strouse PJ (2009) Malrotation: some answers but more questions. Pediatr Radiol 39:315–316

Snider WH, Chaffin L (1954) Embryology and pathology of the intestinal tract: presentation of 40 cases of malrotation. Ann Surg 140:368–380

Strouse PJ (2004) Disorders of intestinal rotation and fixation ("malrotation"). Pediatr Radiol 34:837–851

Strouse PJ (2008) Malrotation. Semin Roentgenol 43:7–14

Sze RW, Guillerman RP, Krauter D, Evans AS (2002) Possible new ancillary sign for diagnosing midgut volvulus: the truncated superior mesenteric artery. J Ultrasound Med 21:477–480

Taylor GA (2011) CT appearance of the duodenum and mesenteric vessels in children with normal and abnormal bowel rotation. Pediatr Radiol 41:1378–1383
Torres AM, Ziegler MM (1993) Malrotation of the intestine. World J Surg 17:326–331
Yousefzadeh DK (2009) The position of the duodenojejunal junction: the wrong horse to bet on in diagnosing or excluding malrotation. Pediatr Radiol 39(suppl 2):S172–S177
Yousefzadeh DK, Kang L, Tessicini L (2010) Assessment of retromesenteric position of the third portion of the duodenum: an US feasibility study in 33 newborns. Pediatr Radiol 40:1476–1484
Zissin R, Rathaus V, Oscadchy A et al (1999) Intestinal malrotation as an incidental finding on CT in adults. Abdom Imaging 24:550–555

3 Meconium Ileus

Margerita Trinci, Antonio Alessandro Pallottino, Claudia Lucia Piccolo, Francesca De Narda, Cinzia Orazi, and Vittorio Miele

3.1 Introduction

Meconium is produced after the 13 weeks of gestation; it is the materials that during the fetal life accumulate in the bowel; it is formed of lanugo, bile, mucus, desquamated intestinal cells, desiccated amniotic fluid, and bowel secretion. Meconium goes distally from the small bowel and accumulates in the distal colon and rectum after the 20 weeks of gestation. In normal fetus there is significant evacuation of meconium in utero unless there is a fetal distress.

Meconium ileus represents 9–33 % of all cases of neonatal intestinal obstruction (300 new cases each year in Italy), with an incidence of 1:2,500 newborns; it is the third most common cause of intestinal obstruction of the small intestine after intestinal atresia and malrotation.

Meconium ileus represents the first clinical manifestation of cystic fibrosis (CF) and occurs in 8–15 % of patients with CF at birth. Ninety percent of patients with meconium ileus are affected by CF.

The meconium plug syndrome is a common cause of neonatal intestinal obstruction of the distal colon or rectal portion. The term meconium plug syndrome was introduced in 1956 by Clatworthy; it refers to a neonatal condition with a transient immaturity of neonatal peristalsis of the colon, which causes a colonic obstruction with the presence of inspissated meconium. The incidence of this syndrome is estimated to range from 1 case in 500 to 1 case in 1,000 newborns; its etiology is unclear, but an increase of this pathology is found in infants of diabetic mothers who are treated during pregnancy with magnesium sulfate for preeclampsia. Usually this condition is resolved with the enema that helps to evacuate the meconium; in fact, after the plug is passed, intestinal movements are normal, and the symptomatology resolves. If it does not happen, the most important differential diagnosis is with Hirschsprung disease.

3.2 Epidemiology and Pathogenesis

Cystic fibrosis is more widespread in the North Europe Caucasian population, North American population, and Australian and New Zealand population. The incidence varies according to the different studies and is approximated to 1/3,500

M. Trinci • A.A. Pallottino • F. De Narda (✉)
V. Miele
Department of Emergency Radiology, S. Camillo Hospital, Rome, Italy
e-mail: fra.in@icloud.com

C.L. Piccolo
Department of Medicine and Health Sciences, University of Molise, Campobasso, Italy

C. Orazi
Department of Diagnostic Imaging, Children's Hospital Bambino Gesù, Rome, Italy

V. Miele, M. Trinci (eds.), *Imaging Non-traumatic Abdominal Emergencies in Pediatric Patients*,
DOI 10.1007/978-3-319-41866-7_3

live births. Cystic fibrosis is less common in the African American population (1/17,000 live births) and in the Asian population (1/90,000). The data about the incidence on neonatal screening of this pathology in Italy is between 1/2,730 and 1/3,170 births.

Cystic fibrosis is a genetic disease, with autosomal recessive transmission; it is characterized by a systemic involvement, affecting mainly the respiratory and intestinal tract, and it is the most common autosomal recessive disorder in white people.

The mutated gene responsible for cystic fibrosis, discovered in 1989, is located on the long arm of chromosome 7 and is named "cystic fibrosis transmembrane conductance regulator" (CFTR); this gene encodes a defective chloride channel in epithelial cells. In these patients the chloride channel is locked because the CFTR protein is not functional; the sodium channel also depends on the abnormal CFTR protein as a result much sodium enters inside of the cell; from this it follows that little water comes out from the cell, and thus the periciliary liquid is very little and the ciliary beat is therefore ineffective.

Similar events even occur in the pancreatic, biliary, and deferens ducts leading to dehydration, protein secretions, and the consequent obstruction of the lumen.

The occlusion of pancreatic ducts that already occurs during the second trimester of pregnancy leads to the formation of voluminous, translucent, and malodorous feces.

The absence of normal pancreatic enzymes is responsible to the physical characteristics of the abnormal meconium.

Nowadays gene replacement therapy is not yet used because of the difficulties of targeting the proper cells. The better knowledge of this pathology and the new therapies have improved life expectancy of these patients.

3.3 Clinical Presentation

Concerning to the gastrointestinal tract, the clinical presentation in the case of neonatal bowel obstruction will be the failure to pass meconium during the first 24 h of typical abdominal tenderness; vomit bile-stained material and pancreatic failure are present. The doctor at the clinical evaluation can palpate a mass, in the right flank due to the inspissated meconium located in the lower portion of the ileus, and in the right colon, the mass is often visible through the abdominal wall. Rectal examination is often difficult due to the small caliber of the rectum. The pathologic meconium is related to the presence of an abnormal intestinal mucus, slimy and adherent meconium is very viscous for the increasing of protein content and reducing of carbohydrate content, and this results in dehydration of the consistency of meconium with grayish gummy balls that occlude the loop. The compacted meconium, adherent to the intestinal walls, determines an intraluminal obstruction that occurs in the intermediate section of the distal ileum and colon, which leads to a progressive abdominal distension. A condition of meconium ileus cannot be excluded if the stool has been passed after birth.

Regarding the neonatal occlusions, the differential diagnoses that we have to consider are intestinal atresia, malrotation, volvulus, peritoneal band, duplication of the intestinal tract, and Hirschsprung disease. These conditions are associated with normal meconium, and there is no pancreatic insufficiency. Volvulus of the midgut is often associated with meconium ileus (50 % of cases).

Meconium peritonitis (in about 40–50 % of cases) occurs in the case of perforation of the intestinal tube, with meconium passing into the peritoneal cavity. Meconium peritonitis can happen both during the prenatal time and after birth.

If the peritonitis occurs during the prenatal life or within the first 3 days of life, it will be a chemistry peritonitis because the meconium is sterile; after that period it will be bacterial peritonitis because the meconium will no longer be sterile. Gangrene of the intestinal wall secondary to parietal stretching that results from the accumulation of large amounts of meconium in the loop may be one of the causes of peritonitis.

3.4 Diagnostic Imaging

The imaging plays an important role in the diagnosis of meconium ileus being able to put the suspect since the prenatal exams. In fact, the ultrasound exam performed during the second trimester, after the 18–20 weeks of pregnancy, is already able to visualize the normal meconium in the intestinal loops; nevertheless, it is difficult with ultrasound to differentiate the small bowel from the large one.

In the case of meconium ileus, the ultrasound exam reveals some no specific signs or more suggestive of the pathology as dilated bowel loop immediately preceding the point of obstruction; abdominal circumference disproportionately increased. The hyperechogenicity of the loops, denser than adjacent bone, and the distension of the bowel loops are suggestive of meconium ileus but not specific; also the content of the loops may be hyperechoic; a persistent hyperechogenic bowel in the third trimester of pregnancy can be considered a soft pathological marker of meconium ileus.

In the newborn the ultrasound sign will be almost the same but will be more evident in the distension of the intestinal loops that shows internal diameter >7 mm in combination with strong peristaltic movements.

In complicated cases it is possible to find fluid between the loops. In the case of chemistry peritonitis, we found the presence of abdominal calcification, seen as hyperechoic endoabdominal areas; the calcifications occur rapidly in utero in as little as 12–24 h after the peritonitis. The gallbladder is often absent. Nowadays if it is requested, a more detailed study during the fetal life and magnetic resonance may be considered.

In the case of suspected intestinal obstruction, abdomen plain film radiographs are the first imaging study performed after birth. If the exam is carried out in the first 6 h of life, it may be not diagnostic because of few amount of gas that could be passed through the gastrointestinal tract.

In fact, to be able to make a diagnosis of bowel obstruction at the abdomen, plain film is necessary to know the timing at which the air reaches the different intestinal tracts. In a healthy newborn, the air reaches the stomach in few minutes of birth, within 3 h the small bowel is completely filled of gas, and air takes about 8–9 h to reach the sigmoid tract. The radiological diagnostic suspect of obstruction at the beginning is founded on an irregular or interrupted distribution of the air.

It's important to remember that even clinical causes, such as a brain damage, difficult childbirth, septicemia, severe respiratory distress, or severe hypoglycemia, can cause an altered airflow in the abdomen.

Even if the abdomen plain film in the case of meconium ileus also overlaps with other causes of distal occlusion, radiography is important to confirm the diagnosis and will show nonspecific and suggestive signs of the obstruction. The difference between meconium ileus and meconium plug syndrome is in the site of the obstruction, typically in the distal portion of the colon or in the rectum in meconium plug syndrome, and in the severity of the obstruction:

- Signs in the case of meconium ileus in abdomen plain film and in enema.
- Distended gas-filled proximal loops of varying caliber, above the meconial obstruction, that cause the abdominal tenderness and absence or slight presence of gas in the distal bowel to the level of the obstruction (Figs. 3.1 and 3.2).
- Relative lack of air-fluid levels due to the abnormally thick meconium (Fig. 3.1); however it is possible to find air-fluid levels in complicated forms (Fig. 3.3). In the presence of clinical symptoms and the absence or slight presence of fluid levels in dilated loops of obstructed small bowel, the diagnosis of meconium ileus is strongly suspected.
- "Neuhauser" sign that is a mottled appearance of the affected loops, more frequent in the right lower quadrant and "soap bubble" sign: it is due to the mixture of swallowed air with meconium seen in the distal ileum or colon (Fig. 3.1). This sign is nonspecific of meconium ileus and may be seen in various conditions, including Hirschsprung disease, ileal atresia, and necrotizing enterocolitis.

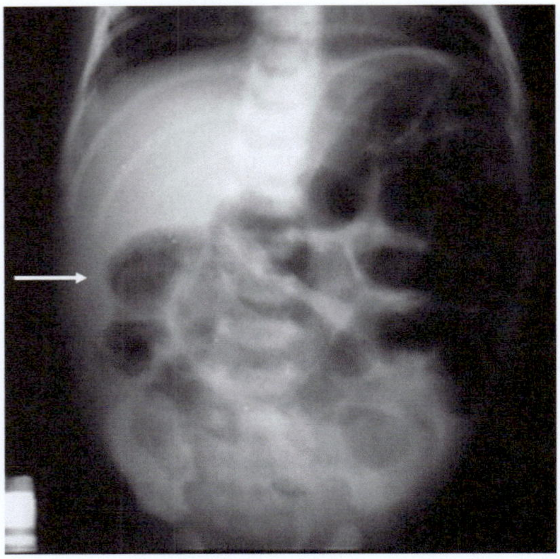

Fig. 3.1 Plain film in newborn with meconium ileus. Note the abnormal distribution of the intraluminal air with proximal distended loops and the absence of gas in distal loops. There are no air-fluid levels. Note the "soap bubbles" and ground-glass aspects on the right flank

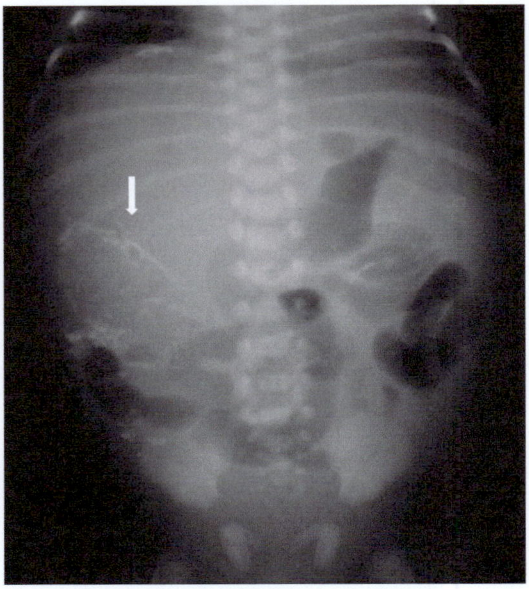

Fig. 3.2 Plain film in newborn with meconium ileus peritonitis shows the presence of distended loops and the absence of gas in distal loops. Note the linear calcification (*white arrow*)

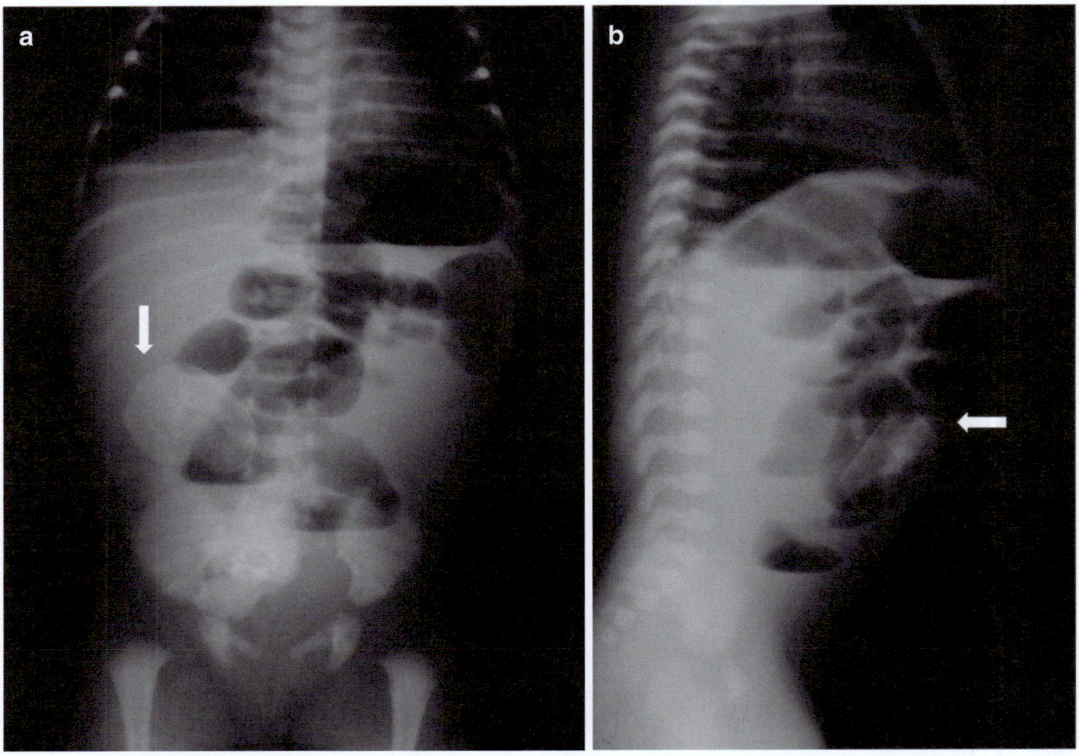

Fig. 3.3 (**a**, **b**) Plain film in newborn with meconium ileus peritonitis shows the presence of distended loops. Note the calcific pseudocyst (*white arrow*). There are air-fluid levels due to the peritonitis

- "Ground-glass" aspect in the loops.
- Calcification: linear, curvilinear, and amorphous within the loops or free in the abdomen; in this case they are the expression of a chemistry peritonitis (Fig. 3.2). In the case of patency of the peritoneovaginal duct, it is possible to find the calcifications even in the scrotum. The calcifications can form cystic or pseudocyst masses (Fig. 3.3).
- It is possible to find a condition of pneumoperitoneum.
- At the enema it is common to find multiple dried meconium pellets within the loops (Figs. 3.4, 3.5, and 3.6).
- The enema often shows functional microcolon due to the failure to pass the small bowel content into the colon during the gestational time (Figs. 3.6 and 3.7).

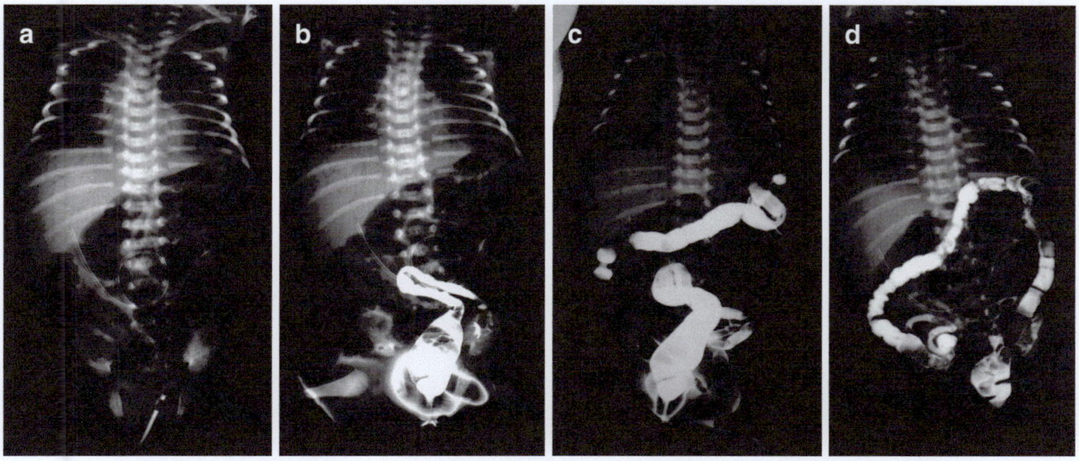

Fig. 3.4 (**a**–**d**) Enema in infant with meconium plug syndrome. Note the typical filling defect in the sigma and colonic tract

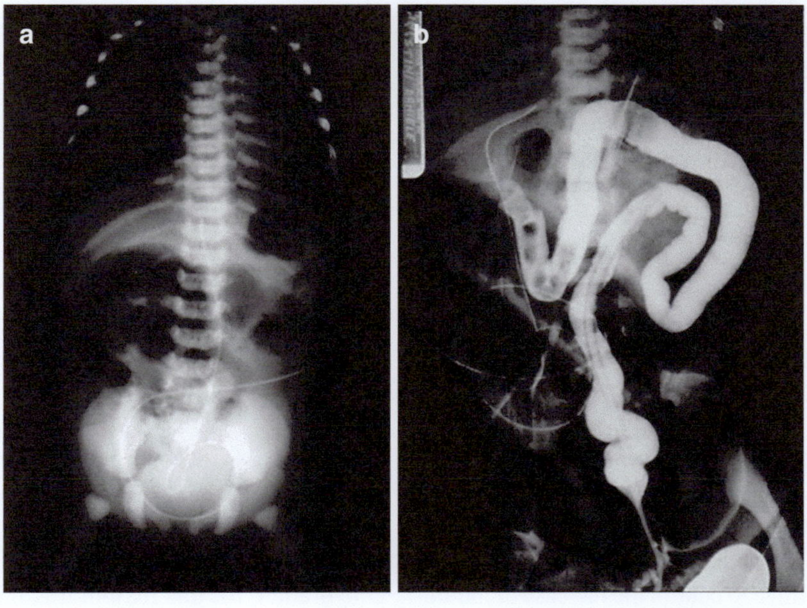

Fig. 3.5 (**a**, **b**) Plain film (**a**) and enema (**b**) in infant with meconium ileus; note the proximal distended loops at the plain film with no air in the lower abdomen. The enema shows typical filling defect in the colonic tract

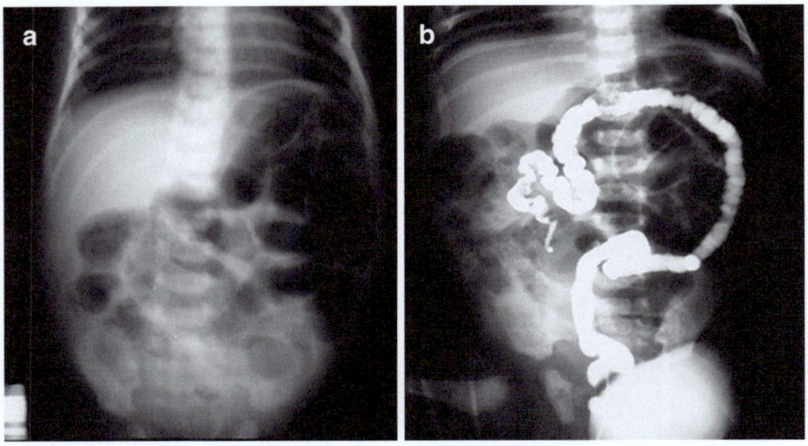

Fig. 3.6 (**a**, **b**) Plain film (**a**) and enema (**b**) in infant with meconium ileus. Note the proximal distended loops at the plain film with no air in the lower abdomen. In this film, it is possible to observe some typical preterm intestinal aspects: the high position of the cecum and a short left colon. The enema shows a disuse microcolon with a typical filling defect

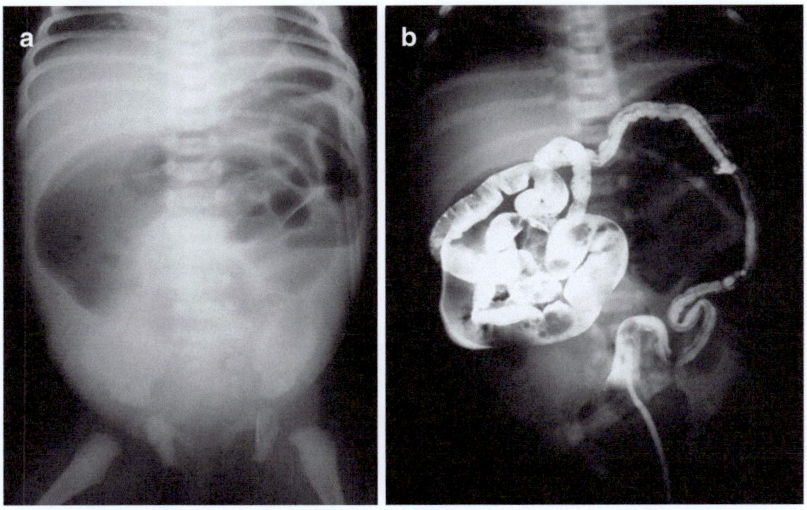

Fig. 3.7 (**a**, **b**) Plain film (**a**) and enema (**b**) in infant with meconium ileus; note at the plain film the proximal distended loops with no air in the lower abdomen. The enema shows a condition on disuse microcolon within typical filling defect

Once suspected of the meconium ileus, it is necessary to perform an RX enema using water-soluble contrast medium. This is important specially in case it is suspected that a perforation can occur. It is needed to place the catheter without balloon inflation to avoid that the intraluminal pressure increases too much. The administration of contrast medium must be carried out under fluoroscopic guidance by hand with syringe to control the increase of intraluminal pressure. The enema can relieve obstruction (at least in 50–60 % of cases).

The enema with about 100 of water-soluble iodinated contrast medium, diluted 1:3–1:5, has also a therapeutic effect because of the high osmolality of contrast medium (about 2,000 mOsm/l), which can draw excess fluid into the lumen, and moisturizes favoring the expulsion of meconium. This procedure is repeatable after 12–24 h; we do not forget the risk of dehydration; for this reason, it is fundamental to monitor vital parameters and a proper hydration of the patients with intravenous fluid.

3.5 Therapy

The therapy regarding the management of meconium ileus includes the administration of laxatives the administration of pancreatic enzymes during meals, a mucolytic drug as acetylcysteine, and the enemas with water-soluble iodinated diluted contrast medium enemas. In more recent studies, it was shown that even the oral administration of water-soluble iodinated contrast medium used once and diluted four times in the volume of water or fruit juice with half doses given on days 2 and 3 was followed by relief of obstruction.

If the enema does not work to resolve the obstruction, an operative evacuation of the obstructing meconium by irrigation will be necessary; in the case of complications such as atresia, perforation, and meconium peritonitis, the therapy is always surgical including resection, intestinal anastomosis, and ileostomy.

References

Berrocal T, Lamas M, Gutieérrez J, Torres I, Prieto C, del Hoyo ML (1999) Congenital anomalies of the small intestine colon and rectum. Radiographics 19 1219–1236

Cuenca AG, Ali AS, Kays DW (2012) "Pulling the plug" – management of meconium plug syndrome in neonates. J Surg Res 175:43–46

De Backer AI, De Schepper AM, Deprettere A, Van Reempts P, Vaneerdeweg W (1999) Radiographic manifestations of intestinal obstruction in the newborn. JBR-BTR 82:159–166

Di Giacomo V, Trinci M, Van der Byl G, Catania VD, Calisti A, Miele V (2015) Ultrasound in newborns and children suffering from non-traumatic acute abdominal pain: imaging with clinical and surgical correlation. J Ultrasound 18:385–393. doi:10.1007/s40477-014-0087-4, Epub 2014 Apr 9

Dimmitt RA, Moss RL (2000) Meconium diseases in infants with very low birth weight. Semin Pediatr Surg 9:79–83

Herson RE (1957) Meconium ileus. Radiology 68:568–571

Jerdee T, Newman B, Rubesova E (2015) Meconium in perinatal imaging: associations and clinical significance. Semin Ultrasound CT MR 36:161–177

Kao SC, Franken EA Jr (1995) Nonoperative treatment of simple meconium ileus: a survey of the Society for Pediatric Radiology. Pediatr Radiol 25:97–100

Keckler SJ, Peter SDS, Spidle TL, Tsao KJ, Ostile DJ, Holcomb GO, Snyder CL (2008) Current significance of meconium plug syndrome. J Pediatr Surg 43:896–898

Kiely EM (1996) Meconium ileus. In: Puri P (ed) Newborn surgery. Butterworth-Heinemann, Oxford, pp 324–327

Loening-Baucke V, Kimura K (1999) Failure to pass meconium: diagnosis neonatal intestinal obstruction. Am Fam Physician 60:2043–2050

McAlister WH, Kronemer KA (1996) Emergency gastrointestinal radiology of the newborn. Radiol Clin N Am 34:819–844

Miele V, Di Giampietro I (2014) Diagnostic imaging in emergency. Salute Soc (2EN):127–138. doi:10.3280/SES2014-002010EN

Miller JP, Smith SD, Newman B (1988) Neonatal abdominal calcification: is it always meconium peritonitis? J Pediatr Surg 23:555–556

Ratien F, Doring G (2003) Cystic fibrosis. Lancet 361:681–689

Shah U, Shafiq Y, Khan MA (2007) Gastrografin use in distal intestinal obstruction syndrome of cystic fibrosis. J Ayub Med Coll Abbottabad 19:58–60

Vinocur DN, Lee EY, Eisenberg RL (2012) Neonatal intestinal obstruction. AJR Am J Roentgenol 198:W1–W10. doi:10.2214/AJR.11.6931

Ziegler MM (1994) Meconium ileus. Curr Probl Surg 31:731–777

Necrotizing Enterocolitis

4

Margherita Trinci, Claudia Lucia Piccolo, Antonio Alessandro Pallottino, Francesco Esposito, Massimo Zeccolini, and Vittorio Miele

4.1 Definition

Necrotizing enterocolitis (NEC) is an acute disorder of gastrointestinal district which could affect every part of bowel but more frequently affects the small intestine, especially the distal part of the ileum and the ascending colon, with a partial or diffuse intestinal necrosis. The duodenum is not usually involved because it has its own vascularization. NEC is characterized by a wide variability of clinical manifestations, because of its quick and sudden onset in the space for a few hours or because it may be preceded by the appearance, in the days before, of the subtle signs of food intolerance (Bohnhorst 2013). The precise etiology is already unknown; however, actually, NEC is considered a multifactorial disease, including genetic components, environmental factors, intestinal microbial flora, immune system, asphyxia, and hypoxia. These factors lead to an inflammatory status and a vascular injury which play an important role in the damage and destruction of bowel mucosa from pathogenic microorganism and endotoxins.

4.2 Epidemiology

NEC primarily afflicts premature infants and is the most common life-threatening gastrointestinal disease in neonatal intensive care. It is less common in term and late preterm infants.

NEC mainly affects preterm infant (about 90 %), but it can even be observed in the newborn at term and "late preterm," and it is characterized by spontaneous intestinal perforations in a third of cases.

The classic form of necrotizing enterocolitis affects mostly infants at birth that have a weight of less than 1,500 g and gestational age less than 32 weeks. In this category the disease in Western countries affects around 6–7 %, but with wide variations between different hospitals and a mortality rate of 20–30 %.

In the years 2007–2013, the prevalence of the disease reported by the Vermont Oxford Network (VON) that collects the admissions of infants with birth weight ≤1,500 g from 900 neonatal units was 6.8 %. In VON Italy (INN) for the same period was 4.3 %. These percentages increase if we take into account the infants with gestational

M. Trinci (✉) • A.A. Pallottino • V. Miele
Department of Emergency Radiology, S. Camillo Hospital, Rome, Italy
e-mail: margherita.trinci@libero.it

C.L. Piccolo
Department of Medicine and Health Sciences, University of Molise, Campobasso, Italy

F. Esposito
Department of Radiology, Santobono Pediatric Hospital, Naples, Italy

M. Zeccolini
Department of Radiology, Pausilipon Pediatric Oncologic Hospital, Naples, Italy

V. Miele, M. Trinci (eds.), *Imaging Non-traumatic Abdominal Emergencies in Pediatric Patients*, DOI 10.1007/978-3-319-41866-7_4

age <26 weeks where the incidence exceeds 10 % (Buonomo 1999).

As regards the mortality, the overall mortality for NEC ranges from 20 to 40 % but approaches 100 % in infants with the most severe form of the disease; males have a higher risk of death than females.

Early diagnosis leads to a prompt therapy, with bowel rest, antibiotics, and hydration, and reduces morbidity and mortality.

4.3 Etiology/Pathophysiology

4.3.1 Environmental Factors

- Breastfeeding is important for several reasons. It plays an important role for the infant in recognition and awareness to external antigens. Breastfeeding permits to get oral tolerance to bacterial microflora and food antigens. Infant formula lacks lactoferrin, which is found in breast milk; it has antibacterial and antiviral effects, as well as anti-inflammatory properties:
  In premature infants there is an immature gastrointestinal system (GIT), which isn't able to have a regular peristalsis. An aggressive way to feed the premature infant may cause stasis of milk substrate in the lumen of the GIT due to dysmotility.
  Residual milk substrate's stasis can advantage an intestinal dilatation with fluid and development of gas and possibly to impairment of the intestinal epithelial barrier (IEB). The increase of toxic particles in the blood in stable premature infants after feeding and attestation from other studies sustain that the IEB of the premature infant is "leakier" compared to that of a more mature one.
  The presence of abnormal microbial colonization (dysbiosis) with an intestinal dilatation can change normal signal transduction across the intestinal epithelial barrier and modify the normal input of growth and repair of enterocytes to one that instead produces excessive inflammatory response and develops apoptosis and necrosis (Chavhan and Parra 2008).
- The normal response of enterocytes of gastrointestinal mucosal and submucosal could be dysregulated against microbial ligand, and it develops an inflammatory destructive response instead of a protective one.
- An important role in NEC may depend on the relationship between the gastrointestinal system and its bacterial microflora; interfering with this relationship and changing this balance, antibiotics might contribute to their etiology. Antibiotics can clearly alter at least temporarily the bacterial microflora changing natural balance and are therefore worth considering as a potential risk factor for developing NEC.
- Cross talk mechanism may lead a relative ischemic state due to an alternated balance between vasoconstriction and vasodilatation caused by different mediators involved in inflammation development.

4.4 Clinical Findings

NEC most commonly manifests within the first 15 days of life.

The clinical manifestation of NEC can change within time from specific evidences that improve insidiously over several days to a rapid onset of gastrointestinal signs, multiorgan system failure (MOF), and systemic shock over a few hours. Clinical presentation depends on the stage of the illness, from the gastrointestinal involvement or systemic involvement, and it's important if the infant has born on term or is premature.

As regards the stage of the pathology, in the early stage, clinical presentation is characterized by feeding intolerance, prefeeding gastric residuals, abdominal pain, vomiting, hematochezia, tender abdomen, and erythematous abdomen; in advanced condition, the patient generally presents abdominal tenderness (Fig. 4.1) associated to frog-leg position, hyporesponsivity, intestinal hemorrhage, perforation, sepsis, multiorgan failure, and shock.

As regards the gastrointestinal side, signs as abdominal pain, feeding intolerance, the presence

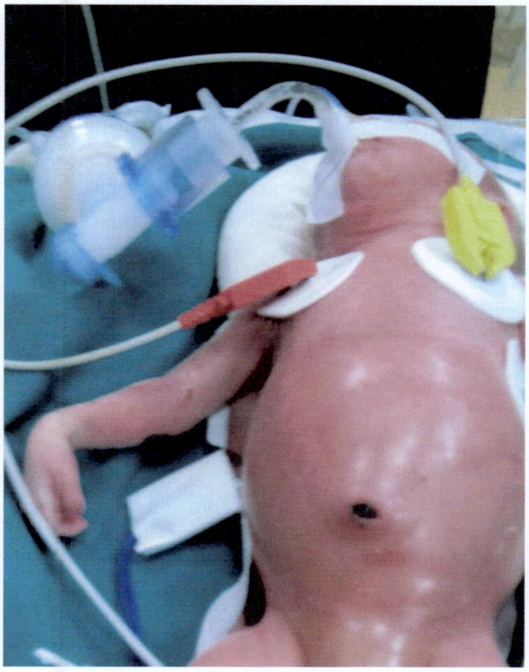

Fig. 4.1 A newborn male in intensive care due to an advanced condition of NEC. Note the abdominal tenderness

of prefeeding gastric residuals, emesis, vomiting, and abdominal distension are typical of jejunum and small bowel ileus initial involvement; instead signs as hematochezia, passage of blood and mucus per rectum, without any other initial signs, are suggestive of initial colic involvement (Chavhan and Parra 2008).

These signs represent also, with a wide variability, the presentation of the NEC disease in the infant born on term; typically, very premature infants do not manifest tenderness and guarding except for the advanced state of NEC.

Pneumoperitoneum is more frequent in extremely premature infants than late term or term infants.

The lab tests could show a condition of metabolic acidosis, occult blood in stool, and an increase of the fatty acid-binding protein (marker of epithelial cell damage), of the PAF (platelet-activating factor), of the TNF (tumor necrosis factor), and of the interleukin. Paracentesis is positive when the sample contains 0.5 ml of brown liquid or bacteria.

Clinical signs		
	Early	Advanced
Time depending	Feeding intolerance, prefeeding gastric residuals, abdominal pain, vomiting, hematochezia, tender abdomen, erythematous abdomen	Abdominal tenderness associated to frog-leg position, hyporesponsivity, intestinal hemorrhage, perforation, sepsis, multiorgan failure, shock
	Specific	Systemic
Anatomic location	Feeding intolerance, tender abdomen, abdominal pain, vomiting, diarrhea, hematochezia, perforation, intestinal hemorrhage	Lethargy, hypotension, poor perfusion and pallor, increased episodes of apnea and bradycardia, worsening of respiratory function, temperature instability, tachycardia, hyperglycemia or hypoglycemia

4.5 Imaging Modalities

The imaging modalities that are used in neonates during the active phase of NEC include plain abdominal radiography and abdominal sonography. Contrast enema is contraindicated in NEC even if with nonionic contrast, but can be useful in case of complications.

4.5.1 Abdominal Radiography

Plain film of the abdomen is the current modality of choice in the study of a patient with suspect of NEC (Coursey et al. 2008) which can also be performed every 6 h for the rapid evolution that may occur in the patients with NEC.

To understand what signs to look for in a radiogram made in a patient with clinically suspected NEC, remember quickly the pathophysiological steps of the disease; this is thought to be associated with a combination of factors including hypoxia, the onset of enteral feeding, and the bacterial colonization of the intestines. Ischemia or hypoperfusion can cause paralysis of the intestines, dilatation of bowel loops with abdominal distention, the loss of normal mucosal integrity, and pathologically coagulative and hemorrhagic necrosis (Rampton 2004; Rigler 1941). The gas produced by overgrowth of intestinal flora leads to further distention of the intestines and allows the entrance of bacteria into the bowel wall by way of mucosal tears, thereby leading to intramural bacterial proliferation and the formation of gas in the intestinal wall, the so-called pneumatosis intestinalis.

The proper way to get a good radiographic examination is to acquire images in two projections, obtained with vertical and horizontal beam, with the patient lying supine; the examination carried out in this way must be performed both at the time of the suspected onset of the disease that is at 48h away in the follow-up (Coursey et al. 2009).

The evaluation of several benefits of radiographic signs can help distinguish if the disease is in a more or less advanced stage.

In 1978, Bell and colleagues proposed a system for the uniform clinical staging of infants with NEC. They classified infants as having stage I (suspect), stage II (definite), or stage III (advanced) disease, on the basis of visible radiographic findings (Epelman et al. 2007).

Guidelines for management of NEC are based on diagnosis according to these criteria.

4.6 Bell's Criteria

Stage	Clinical signs	Radiologic findings
Suspected	Abdominal distension and poor feeding vomiting	Ileus
Definite	Abdominal distension, poor feeding vomiting, and gastrointestinal bleeding	Intestinal pneumatosis and portal venous gas
Advanced	Abdominal distension, poor feeding vomiting, gastrointestinal bleeding, and septic shock	Intestinal pneumatosis and portal venous gas and pneumoperitoneum

4.7 Modified Bell's Criteria

Stage	Systemic signs	Intestinal signs	Radiologic signs	Treatment
Suspected A	Temperature instability, apnea, bradycardia	Elevated pregavage residuals, mild abdominal distension, occult blood in stool	Normal or mild ileus	NPO, antibiotics × 3 days
Suspected B	Same as suspected A	Same as suspected A, plus gross blood in stool	Same as suspected A	Same as suspected A
Definite mildly	Same as suspected A	Same as suspected A, B plus absent bowel sound and abdominal tenderness	Ileus, pneumatosis intestinalis	NPO, antibiotics × 7–10 days
Definite moderately	Same as suspected A, B plus metabolic acidosis and thrombocytopenia	Same as suspected A, B plus absent bowel sound and abdominal tenderness, abdominal cellulitis, right lower abdominal mass	Ileus, pneumatosis intestinalis, portal vein gas with or without ascites	NPO, antibiotics × 14 days

Stage	Systemic signs	Intestinal signs	Radiologic signs	Treatment
Advanced A	Same as definite moderately stage, plus hypotension, bradycardia, respiratory and metabolic acidosis, disseminated intravascular coagulation, neutropenia	Same as suspected and definite plus signs of generalized peritonitis, marked tenderness and distension of abdomen	Same as definite moderately, plus definite ascites	NPO, antibiotics ×14 days, fluid resuscitation, inotropic support, ventilator therapy, paracentesis
Advanced B	Same as advanced A	Same as advanced A	Same as definite moderately plus pneumoperitoneum	Same as definite mildly A plus surgery

Table modified from Prevention and Treatment of Necrotizing Enterocolitis Byong Sop Lee, M.D. Hanyang Med Rev. 2009

There are some signs to look for in radiographic NEC suspect, which mainly deal with the gas available in the abdomen. We must remember that in a healthy baby, gas is distributed throughout the small and the large bowel which are difficult to differentiate between them.

The normal arrangement of the gas inside the loops is small that the large intestine tends to stretch the loops and compress them to one another making it impossible to recognize and developing a characteristic morphology that is called morphology "mosaic" (Fig. 4.2).

The first signs that the radiologist should be suspicious of is the lost of the mosaic pattern with the focal or diffuse dilatation of some loops that take form rounded or elongated or are disposed horizontally in the abdomen (Fig. 4.3).

Dilatation of bowel is an early not specific sign and may even precede the clinical features of NEC by several hours. Moreover, the degree of dilatation generally corresponds well with the clinical severity of the disease, and the distribution of the dilated loops in serial examinations is related to clinical progression; this of course also applies to the remission of the disease, in the sense that if the disease is properly treated, with the passage of time a return to normality of the loop that before had swelled is observed. If, however, the focal dilatation persists even in the follow-up radiographs, it is a telling sign that bends that is going full-thickness necrosis before peritonitis. In fact the evidence of a fixed distended bowel loop that does not alter in size, shape, and position on the subsequent two or three X-ray films "fixed loop sign" is suggestive for NEC (Fig. 4.4).

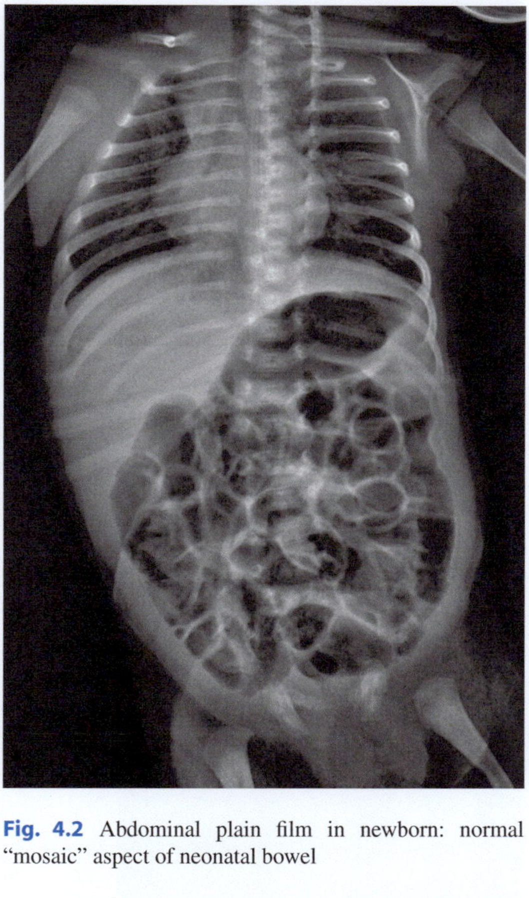

Fig. 4.2 Abdominal plain film in newborn: normal "mosaic" aspect of neonatal bowel

More easily in cross-table lateral abdominal radiograph, it is possible to see free fluid levels in the distended bowel loops (Fig. 4.5) (Stage I: "Suspected" of Bell classification). The second sign that you have to look at is the presence of intramural gas (Stage II: "Definite" of Bell classification) that is also an early pathognomonic sign of NEC. This sign is generally localized in the right lower quadrant of the radiogram, interestingly the distal small bowel, and large bowel, but rarely could be seen interesting the stomach or rectum (Fig. 4.6).

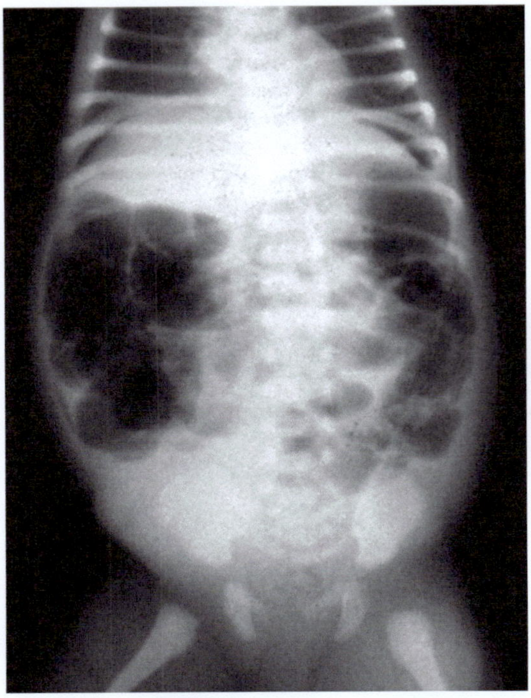

Fig. 4.3 Abdominal plain film in newborn with NEC: pathological aspect of neonatal bowel, loss of "mosaic" aspect and focal distension of the loop

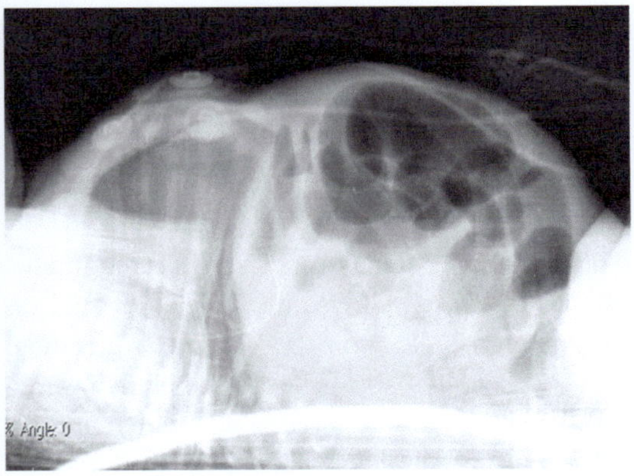

Fig. 4.5 Cross-table abdominal plain film in newborn with NEC shows the condition of intestinal bowel occlusion with air fluid levels in the distended bowel loops

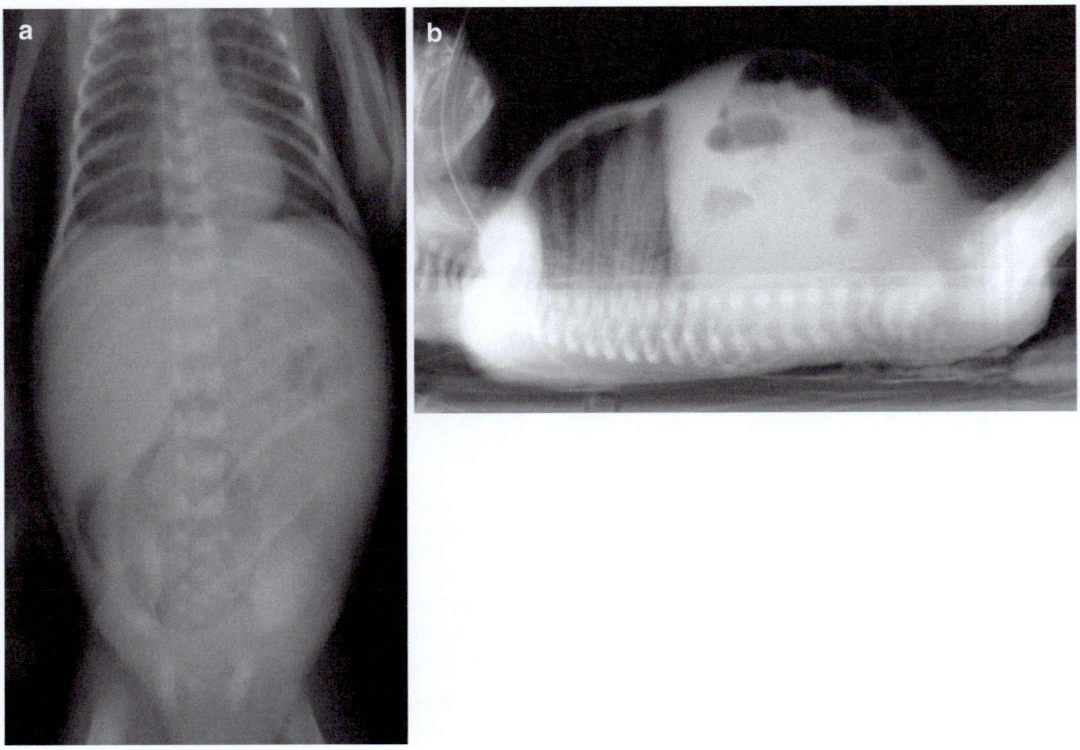

Fig. 4.4 Abdominal plain film in newborn with NEC: (**a**) loss of mosaic aspect of the loops that are dilated and have a horizontal position that maintain over the time "fixed loops sign." (**b**) There is also a condition of pneumoperitoneum

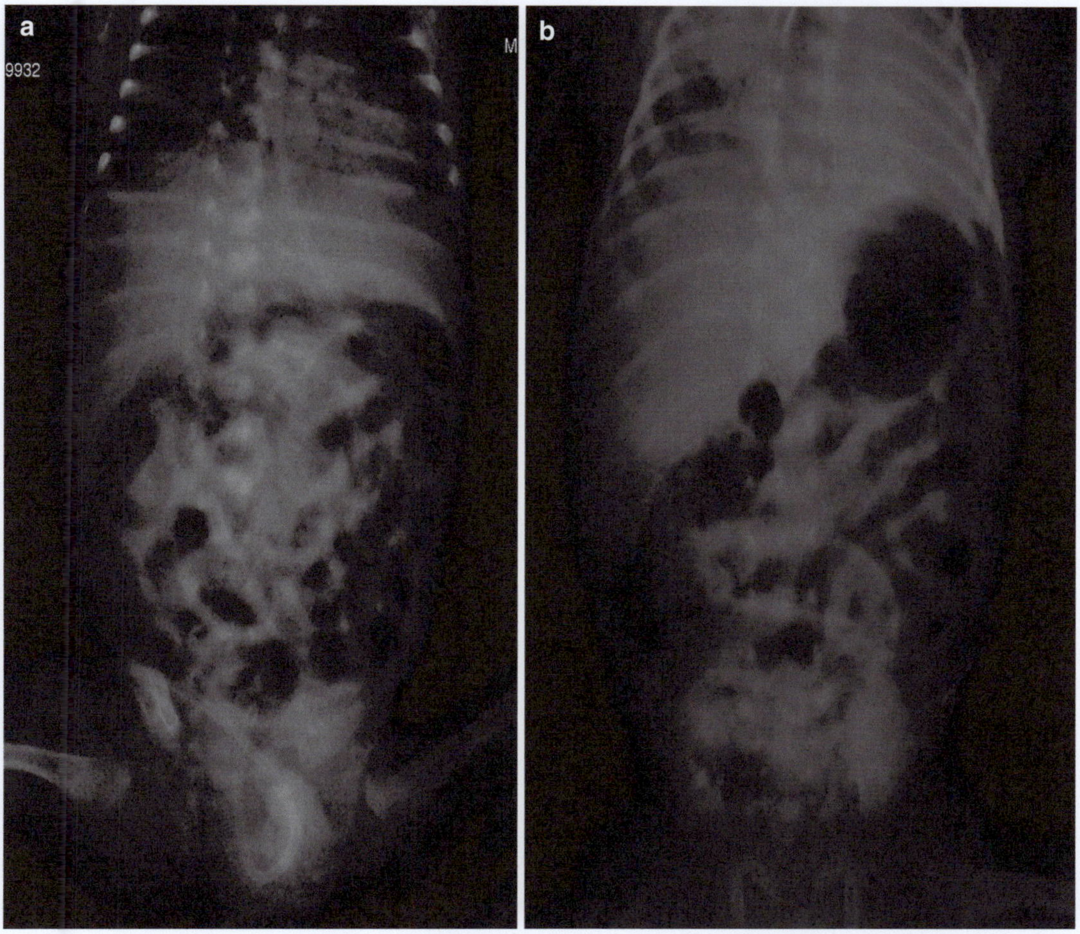

Fig. 4.6 (**a**, **b**) Abdominal plain film of the same patients after few hours with advanced stage of NEC and diffuse pneumatosis

The radiographic aspect of intramural gas depends on the position of the loop in the radiograph. In fact if the X-ray beam hits the profile of the loop, we have the linear pattern of intramural gas. In this case there are two different aspects depending on the filling of the loop. When the loop is filled with gas, the wall of the involved loop has a band of radiolucency called black band in the outer side that is the intramural gas and has an inner soft tissue opacity called white band due to the submucosa and mucosa contrasted on one side to the gas in the serosal layer and on the other side by the gas in the lumen. When the loop is filled with fluid, we don't have the white band. The intramural gas may have two patterns; the first one "cystic/bubbly" pattern is suggestive for the presence of air in mucosal-submucosal layers (Fig. 4.7). The second pattern is the "curvilinear/linear" one, defined by the presence of a thin radiolucent linear morphology located in the outer part and the surface of the bowel, between the tunics serosa and subserosa (Fig. 4.8).

In other way if the X-ray beam hits the face of the loop (Figs. 4.8 and 4.9), the intramural gas mimics a foamy aspect of the loop, and it is important not to mistake the intraluminal stool with the intramural gas.

Hand in hand with the intestinal pneumatosis, we must pay attention to the possible presence of air in the portal vein, clearly visible on the radiograph as radiolucent area feet into the hepatic hilum, or at major venous branching blood vessels of the liver. On a supine plain abdominal

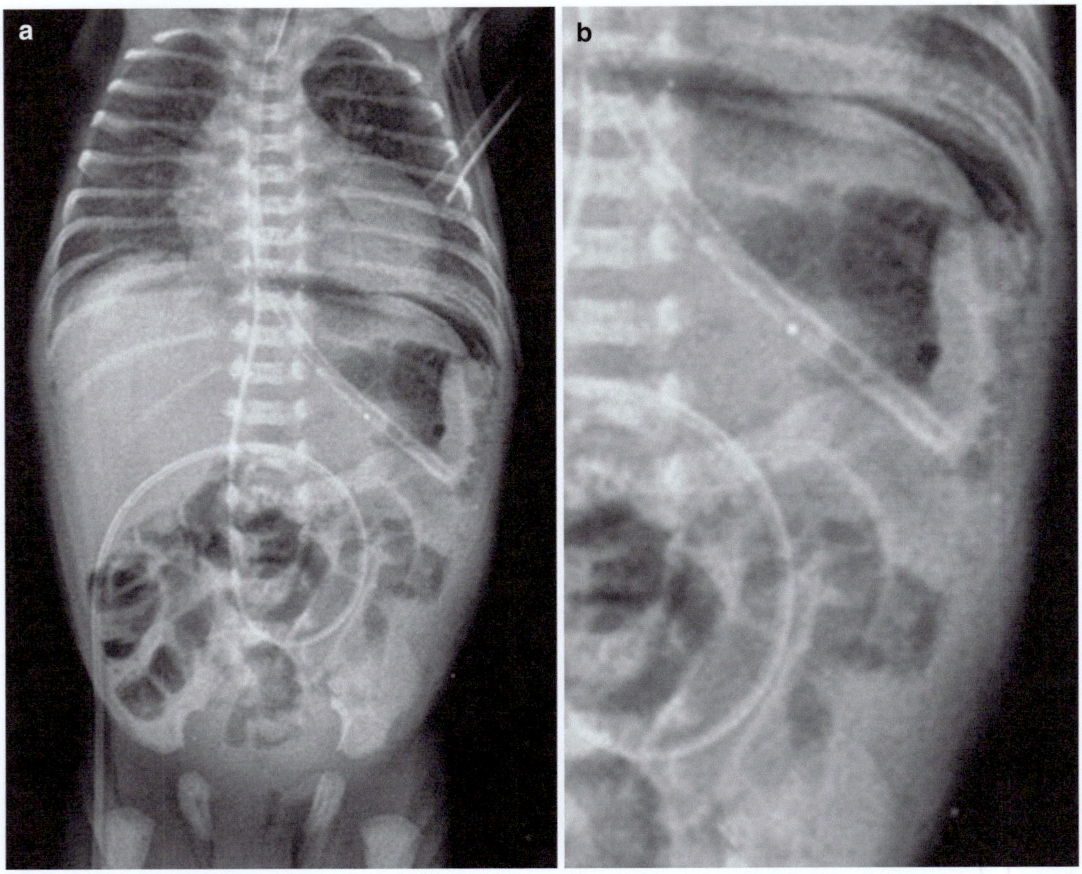

Fig. 4.7 Abdominal plain film in newborn with NEC: (**a**) cystic bubbly pattern of the intramural gas trapped between mucosa and submucosa. There is even a condition of pneumoperitoneum. (**b**) Particular of cystic/bubbly pattern (*black arrows*)

radiograph, portal venous gas appears as branching, linear, radiolucent vessels that may extend from the region of the main portal vein toward the periphery of the hepatic parenchyma (Fig. 4.10). The peripheral extent of the gas pattern is accepted as evidence of its intravascular location as opposed to bile ducts, which are located more centrally; the extent depends on the amount of PVG present. Generally portal venous gas is one of the classic radiologic features of necrotizing enterocolitis and is an uncommon isolated finding because it is most commonly seen in conjunction with pneumatosis intestinalis. In NEC the presence of portal venous gas is considered an advanced stage of the illness, because it's an extension of the process that created intramural gas (Faingold et al. 2005). Anyway we must remember that pneumatosis could be transitory; for this reason in case of pneumatosis, a strict follow-up is requested.

With the separation of the loops between them, there is suspect for free fluid in abdominal cavity and of parietal loop thickening as what happens in peritonitis.

As regards pneumoperitoneum secondary to perforation on a plain radiography, what we should be alarmed is the presence of free air in the abdomen (Stage III: "Advanced" of Bell classification) that can be seen immediately with an air crescent radiolucent below the diaphragm position, right upper quadrant, or easily in lateral X-ray film (Fig. 4.11). Even in the NEC, the pneumoperitoneum is characterized by a lot of radiological signs.

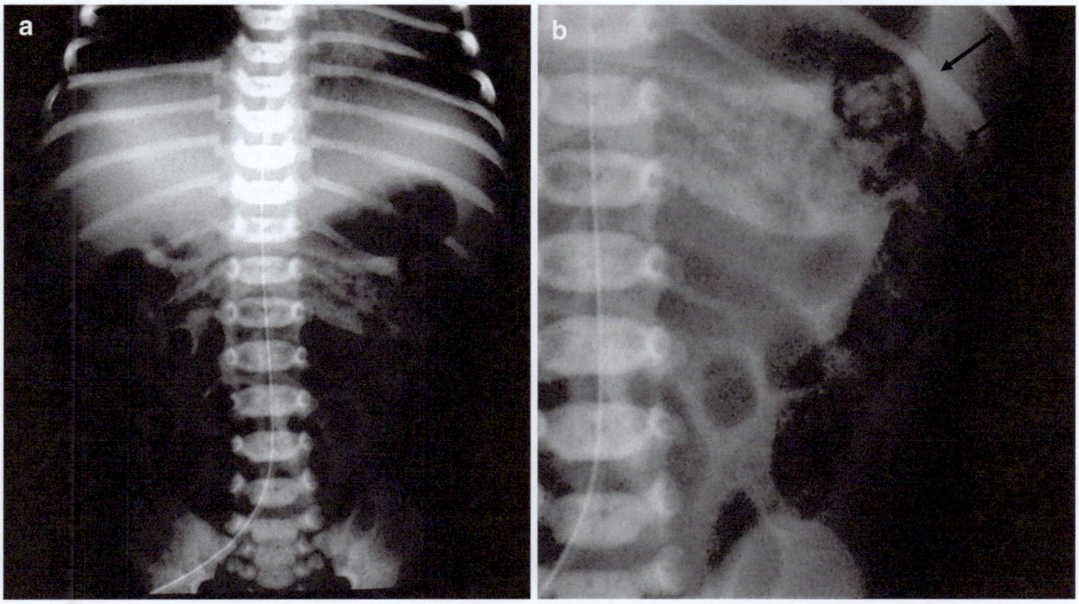

Fig. 4.8 Abdominal plain film (**a**) in newborn with NEC and (**b**) magnification of the left quadrant: the thin radiolucent linear morphology located in the outer part and the surface of the bowel is the *curvilinear/linear* disposition of the gas that is located between the two tunic serosa and subserosa (*black arrows*). This picture also shows the foamy aspect of the intramural gas when the X-ray beam hits the face of the loop

Rigler's sign or double-wall sign (Frey et al. 1987) was first described in 1941 by L G Rigler as a new radiological sign that enables to visualize free air in the peritoneal cavity on supine radiograph. In a healthy patient, it is possible to see the mucosal surface of the intestinal bowel wall as the intraluminal gas. The surface of the serosal layer of the bowel wall is circumscribed by the abdominal tissue and not depicted by air. In case of free peritoneal gas, the bowel wall will be outlined both from the extraluminal and intraluminal air; thus, both sides of the wall, the inner and the outer, will be visible (double-wall sign) (Gire 2014; Goske and Goldblum 1999) (Figs. 4.12 and 4.13).

The football sign was first described by R E Miller in the 1960s, and it describes an oval radiolucency that resembles a rugby ball (Di Giaccomo et al. 2015; Haber and Stern 2000) with the long axis of the football which runs superoinferiorly, with the oval edges formed by the diaphragm and the pelvic floor. The oval shadow seen in the football sign is due to a large pneumoperitoneum, which distends the peritoneal cavity (Figs 4.13, 4.14, and 4.15). The free intraperitoneal air also outlines the falciform ligament (*falciform ligament sign*) which may be seen in the right upper quadrant of the abdomen as a faint linear opacity positioned longitudinally. The vertical opacity of the falciform ligament represents the laces, and the remaining abdomen represents the reaming portion of the rugby ball (Hull et al. 2010).

The presence of the football sign is indicative of an advanced condition of NEC, because of a large quantity of intraperitoneal air relative to the patient size, while Rigler's sign can be seen with a small quantity of free intraperitoneal air and is a more sensitive sign for early pneumoperitoneum and so is a more sensitive sign of perforation in NEC.

The doge's cap sign (Kim and Kim 2005) is represented by the presence of free air in the Morrison's pouch, which is a potential space between the right kidney and the liver. The air that is interposed in this space has a distinctive triangular radiolucent, with the base side down and the apex upward, just like the hat of an ancient Venetian doge (See Fig. 4.13).

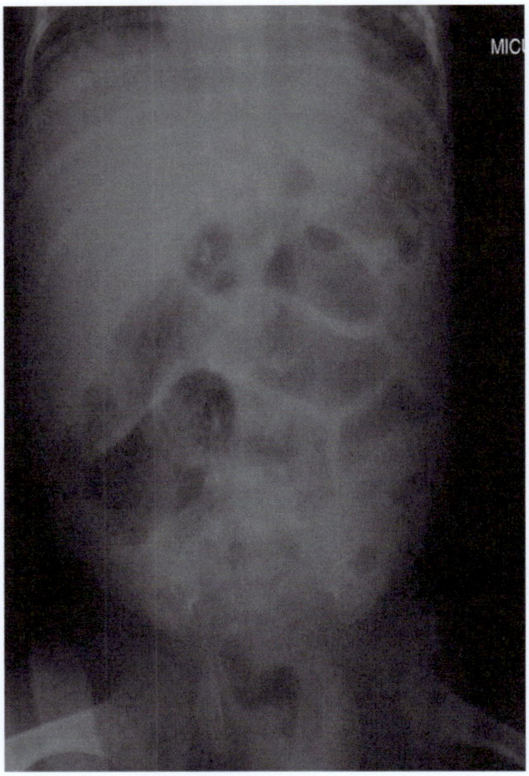

Fig. 4.9 Abdominal plain film in newborn with NEC: stage II of Bell classification: in the left abdominal quadrant, there is a distended loop with intramural gas with foamy aspect

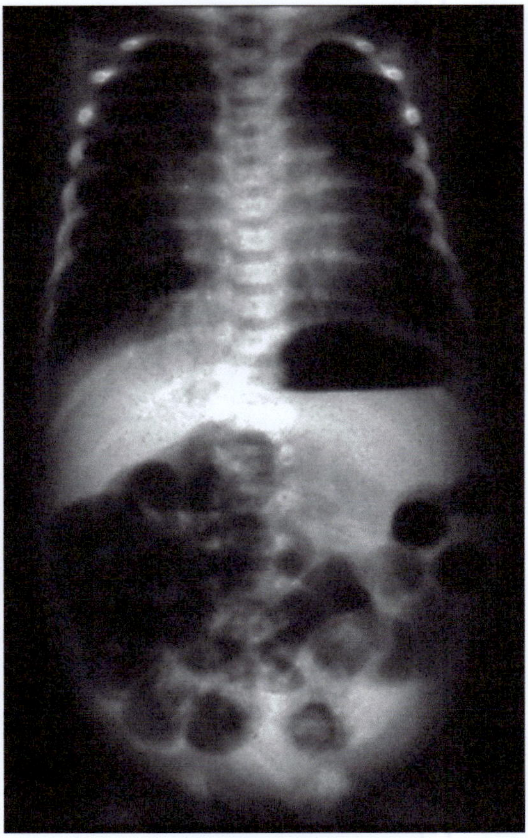

Fig. 4.10 Abdominal plain film in newborn with NEC: portal venous gas seen as a radiolucency linear band in the right hypochondrium on the opacity

The relief of *air anterior to ventral surface of the liver* represents another sign of pneumoperitoneum; consists of the vision of a radiolucent air flap which is localized at the level of the anterior inferior margin of the liver in a different nuance of gray.

Continuous diaphragm sign is visible in case of massive pneumoperitoneum and consists in the presence of abundant air that makes visible the entire diaphragm as a thin radiopaque strip, because it is highly contrasted compared to the air that surrounds it in the abdomen (below) and in the lungs (above) (Figs. 4.13, 4.14, 4.15, and 4.16).

Similar situations can be appreciated in the *sign of the double bubble* (Fig. 4.13), visible in the left upper quadrant for the presence of free subdiaphragmatic air that enhances the radiopaque contour of the diaphragm and of the underlying stomach wall, which is also opposed by the normal presence of air in the stomach. Further situation with similar characteristics is the *sign of the dome* so called for the presence of radiolucent air in correspondence of the tendon at the center of the diaphragm, which is raised appearing just like a dome.

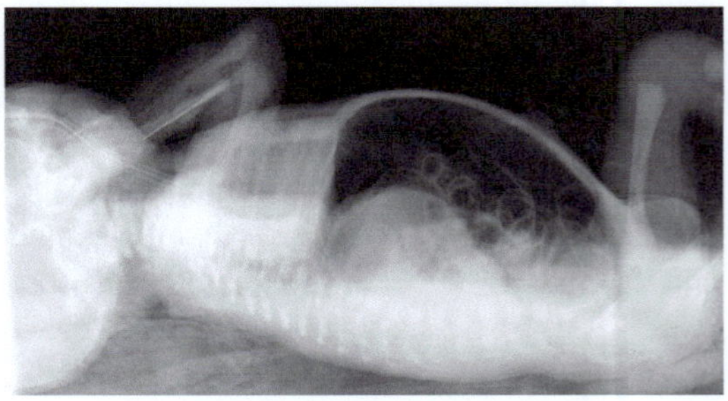

Fig. 4.11 Abdominal plain film in newborn with NEC: latero-lateral view shows a severe pneumoperitoneum

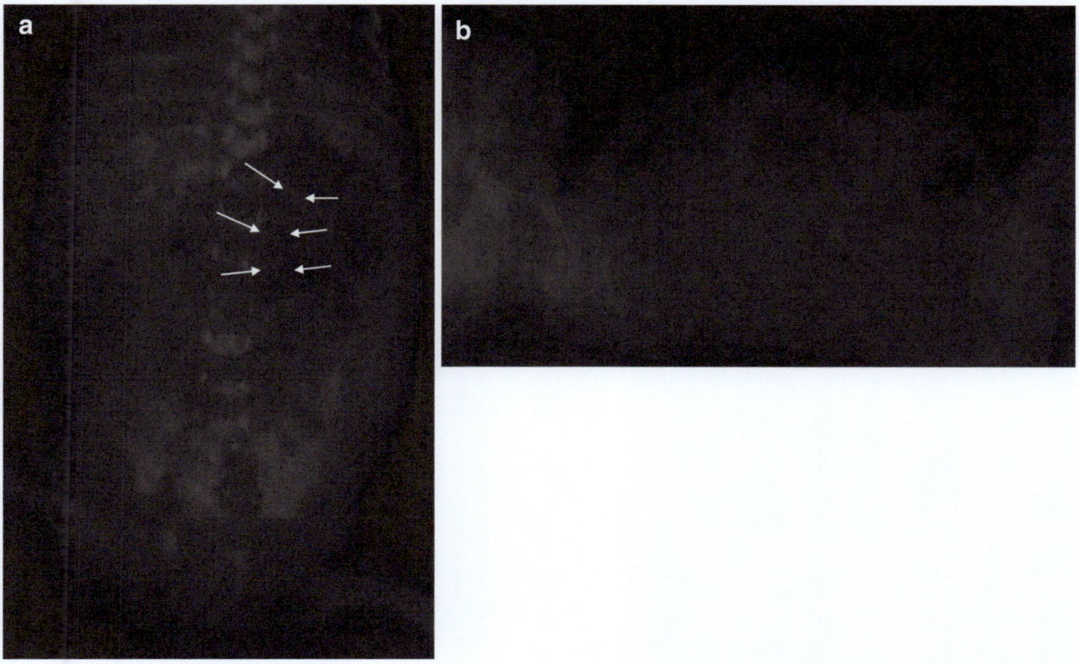

Fig. 4.12 Abdominal supine and latero-lateral plain films in newborn with NEC (**a**–**b**): massive pneumoperitoneum. In this picture on supine film (**a**) it is possible to visualize the "Rigler's sign" bowel wall outlined by extraluminal air due to a pneumoperitoneum and intraluminal air; both sides of the bowel are visible

4.7.1 Ultrasound

While remaining the plain abdominal radiographs, the main mode, and the most used in the evaluation and monitoring of the NEC, sonography represents a valid choice of examination in the study of a patient with suspect of NEC. This is possible because this method is able to visualize intestinal walls, gastrointestinal lumen, and neighboring structures of gastrointestinal tract and intestines, and all these parameters are necessary to have a complementary approach when the diagnosis is uncertain, and abdominal radiography is not exhaustive. However, any findings we are looking for are the same as of the abdominal radiography, because sonography, in a direct or indirect way, is able to visualize the changes due to the presence of air quote in the bowel and in the abdomen; over that it makes possible an optimal evaluation of other parameters as the thickness of the bowel wall, the edema of the bowel wall, the intestinal peristalsis, the presence of free fluid with or without echogenic debris (perforation), the presence of portal venous gas, and the alteration of vascular pattern.

During follow-up of these patients, assessing when is the best time to perform an ultrasound is not yet standardized; however, greater results can occur in patients who while presenting a worsening of the clinical data show no obvious signs of intestinal pneumatosis and/or pneumoperitoneum on X-ray.

In these patients the skill of the ultrasound to evaluate findings related with patient outcomes as to assess the vitality of the intestinal wall using color Doppler, to determine the damage to the wall by identifying the early signs of pneumatosis, and to recognize the presence of free fluid in the abdomen can provide valuable help to guide clinical management.

4.7.1.1 The Normal Bowel Wall in the Newborn

As reported from several studies about NEC, normal bowel wall echogenicity is defined as a

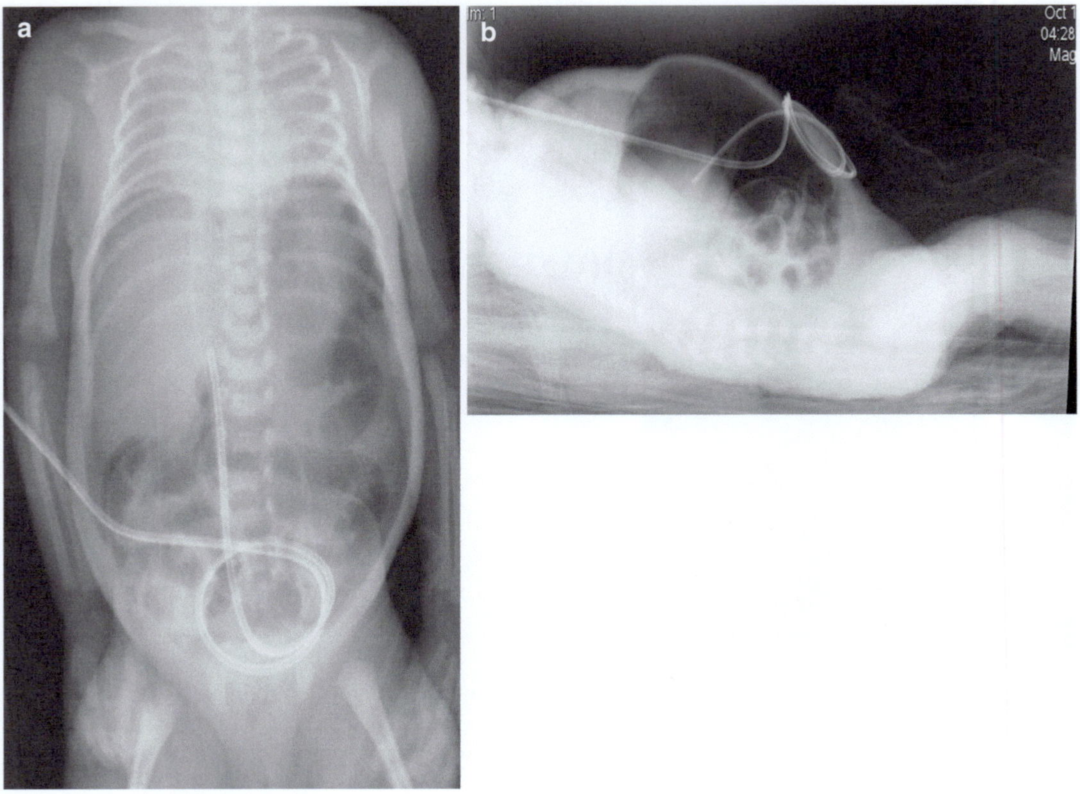

Fig. 4.13 Abdominal supine and latero-lateral plain films in newborn with NEC (**a–b**) and massive pneumoperitoneum. On supine film (**a**) is possible to visualize in the frontal view the football sign and the continuous diaphragm sign,the doge's cap sign, and the football sign

homogeneously hypoechoic wall within no surrounding echogenic intraluminal air.

Normal bowel wall in the newborn has a thickness comprised between 0.7 and 1.1 mm (Sharma and Lawrence 2013). A wall thickness greater than 2.6 mm is generally considered pathological; the use of the power Doppler is important, because for parietal thickness values <1 mm in patients clinically positive for abdominal suffering, a low power Doppler signal could be suggestive of ischemia (Siegel et al. 1997; Silva et al. 2007).

Bowel perfusion in normal neonates, as demonstrated at color Doppler US by using a velocity setting of 8.6 cm/s, ranged from one to nine color dots per square centimeter (Santulli et al. 1975).

4.7.1.2 Ultrasound Signs Suggestive for NEC

As we have already seen for abdominal radiography signs, and according to Bell's criteria, there are some typical sonographic patterns according to the illness stage; sonography is very useful in the early stage because it could be very sensible in the detection of the early changes that occur in the loop; moreover, it can see even the later changes as the detection of the air in the bowel wall that represents the step which is premised to the perforation. The first sign that the operator has to look for is the bowel wall thickness and the relative perfusion at the color Doppler. These early signs are already visible at the ultrasound exam when at traditional radiology only a generic intestinal dis-

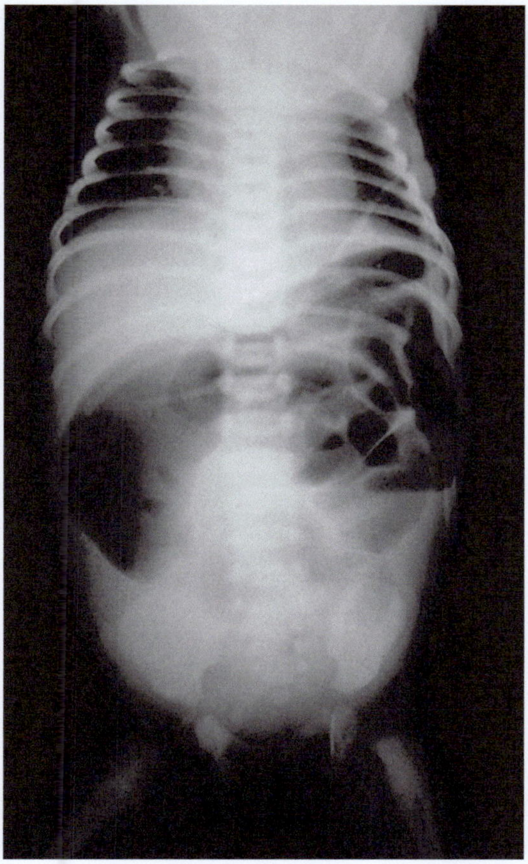

Fig. 4.14 Abdominal plain film in newborn with NEC: massive pneumoperitoneum in this picture is possible to visualize in the frontal view the "football" sign

tention is detectable. Suffering bowel generally presents itself as thickened, with a diameter of the wall that's more than 2.6 due to a congested and edematous condition. The intestinal wall became slightly hyperechoic; this is due to the lack of the normal parietal stratification (Fig. 4.17).

Other signs that we can see during the early stage with color Doppler are an increase in vascularity of the intestinal wall and of the mesenteric perivisceral tissues. A variety of patterns of increased bowel wall perfusion were seen in the patients with Bell stage I and II NEC. We believe that these patterns of hyperemia reflect increased perfusion to the bowel wall due to vasodilatation of mural vessels, including capillary congestion of the serosal surface. These patterns include a "circular or rim" flow pattern completely around the bowel wall, a "Y" pattern of distal mesenteric and subserosal vessel flow (Fig. 4.18), and multiple, parallel color Doppler lines or a "zebra" pattern due to flow in hyperemic mucosal folds (due to hyperemia of the valvulae conniventes) (Haber and Stern 2000).

During the progression of the disease, it is important to look for the presence of intramural gas (Kosloske et al. 1980; Lin and Stoll 2006). This finding represents the sign of the air passage from the intestinal lumen, as a result of the damage of the mucosal barrier. It appears as hyperechoic focus in a layered, thickened bowel wall and has a typical granular pattern (Fig. 4.19) with posterior reverberation artifacts, which, sometimes, don't make possible the correct establishment of the thickening of the wall (Fig. 4.20). The hyperechoic foci could be single or scattered in the wall to complete circumferential involvement of a single or more bowel loops.

It should be emphasized that, at the beginning, the small amount of air detected by ultrasound is not appreciable on radiographic examination.

Radiologic sonographic signs typical for the presence of intramural gas are the "circle sign" (Fig. 4.21) (Miele 2014) that's indicative of bubbles of gas within the circumference of the bowel, which produce an appearance of a continuous echogenic ring on ultrasound, and the "aurora or ring-down sign" (Miller et al. 1993), when the ultrasound beam reaches the gas bubbles, is capable of exciting the liquid trapped between the bubbles, which causes the liquid resonates; these vibrations create a continuous sound wave which is transmitted back to the receiver, so this phenomenon is shown as a line or series of bands extending parallel after the image corresponding to gas.

In the later stage, when radiographic examination shows signs of pneumoperitoneum, at the

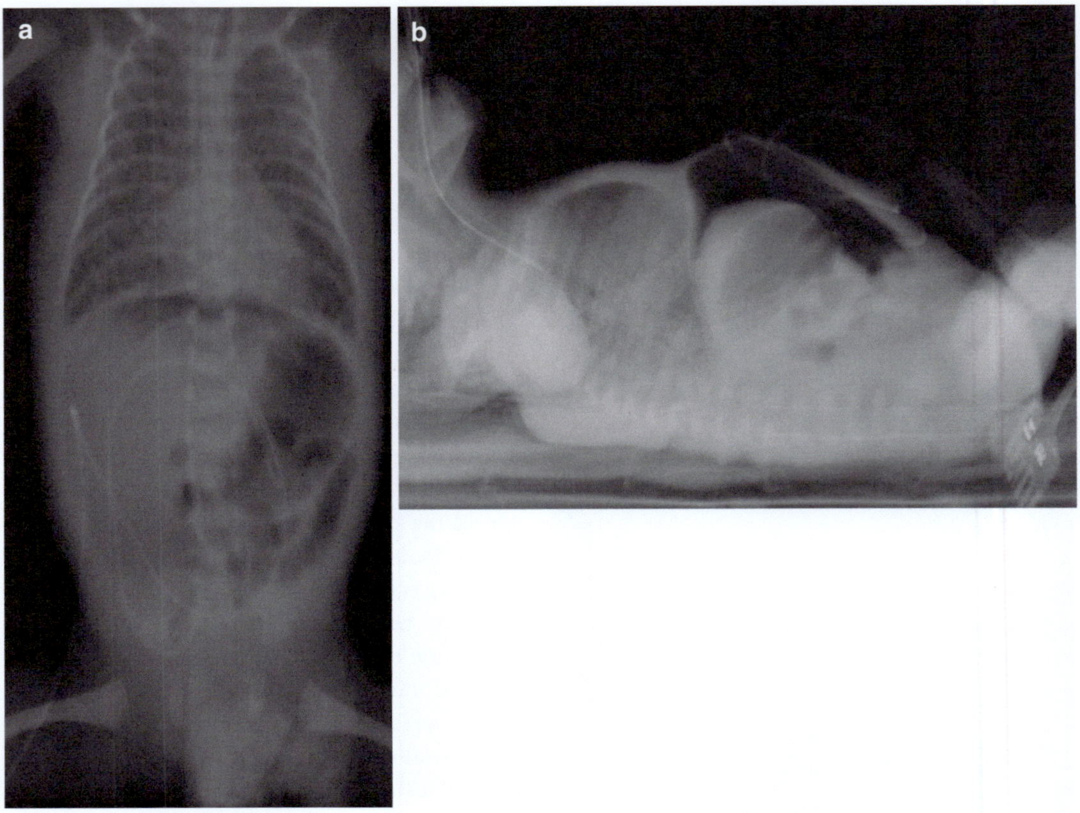

Fig. 4.15 Abdominal plain film in newborn with NEC: massive pneumoperitoneum (**a–b**). In the frontal view (**a**) see the football sign and the continuous diaphragm sign

ultrasound exam, we can find the signs of wall ischemia: in this condition the wall of the loop will be thinning (thickness <1 mm). The thickness reduction should be distinguished from an apparent thinning due to "stretching" of the loop caused by the fluid stagnation in the lumen in patients with or without NEC (Fig. 4.22). The pathologic loop will also hypoperfused at color Doppler exam. Color Doppler flow was determined to be absent when no color Doppler signals were identified in the bowel wall (Haber and Stern 2000). The absence of bowel wall perfusion at color Doppler US is more sensitive and specific than the presence of free air at abdominal radiography in the detection of necrotic bowel in NEC. Generally, the absence of color Doppler signals correlated well with transmural bowel necrosis and so with advanced stage of illness (stage III Bell's criteria), but it's not a rule because color Doppler US also enabled us to differentiate neonates with a single necrotic loop from those with multiple necrotic loops or diffuse bowel necrosis, and this is the difference between an intermediate-advanced stage and an advanced stage.

The use of color Doppler helps in the assessment of the degree of hyperemia and necrosis and therefore leads the team of doctors to the most appropriate treatment choice.

In the intermediate-advanced stage during the abdominal exam, it's also necessary to take attention to the presence of portal venous gas which appears as punctate and linear, branching areas of echogenicity in the portal branches within the liver. The typical appearance is represented by intraluminal echogenic foci moving with the blood flow in the main portal vein and its principal vessels (Figs. 4.23 and 4.24).

Performing the ultrasound exam, some free fluid localized between the loops or in the pelvis, with or without echogenic debris (the presence of which is suggestive of perforation), could be seen. We must remember that with ultrasonography, it is possible to visualize very small amount

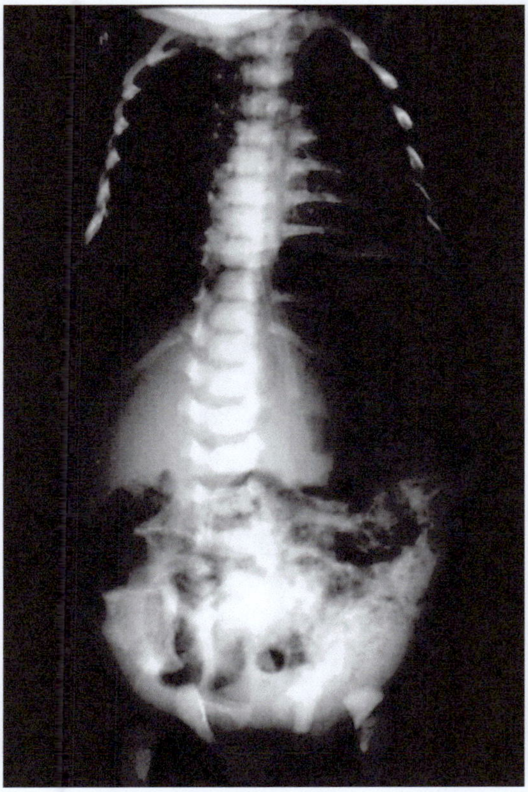

Fig. 4.16 Abdominal plain film in newborn with NEC: massive pneumoperitoneum in this picture is possible to visualize the continuous diaphragm sign

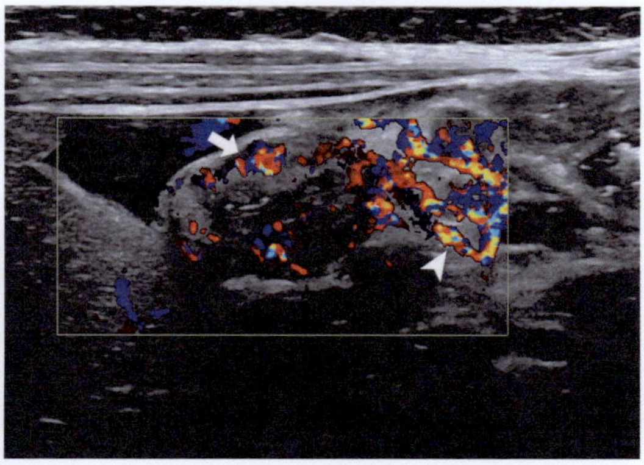

Fig. 4.18 Color Doppler exam in newborn, with early state of NEC, shows the thickened and hypervascular wall bowel (*arrow*); note the hypervascularization of the mesenteric perivisceral tissues (*arrowhead*)

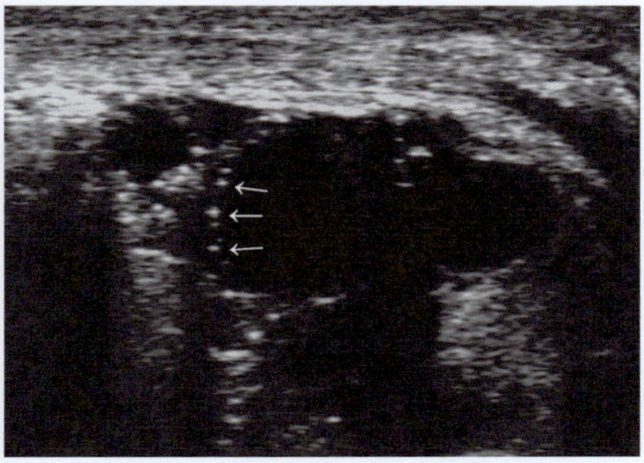

Fig. 4.19 Ultrasound exam in newborn with NEC shows parietal pneumatosis in distended loops with small bubble of air in parietal loop seen as hyperechoic imaging along the wall (*white arrows*)

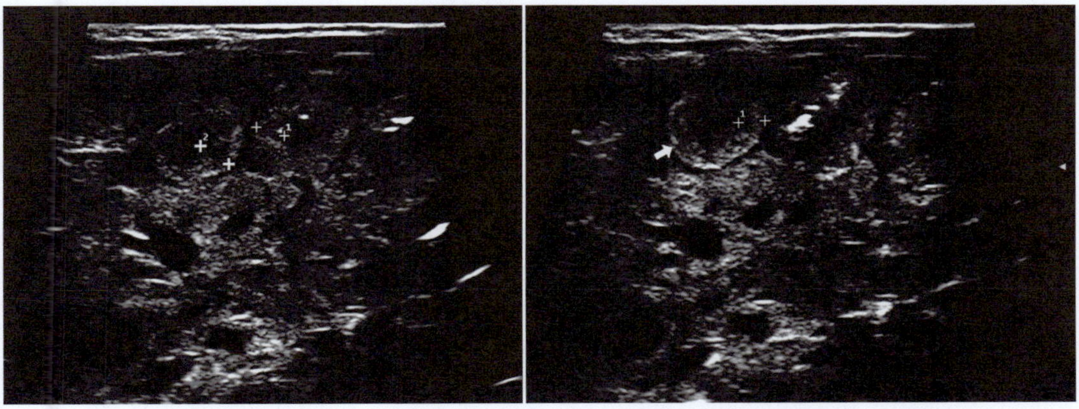

Fig. 4.17 Ultrasound in newborn, with early state of NEC, shows the thickened wall bowel; note the slight hyperechogenicity of the intestinal wall (*white arrow*)

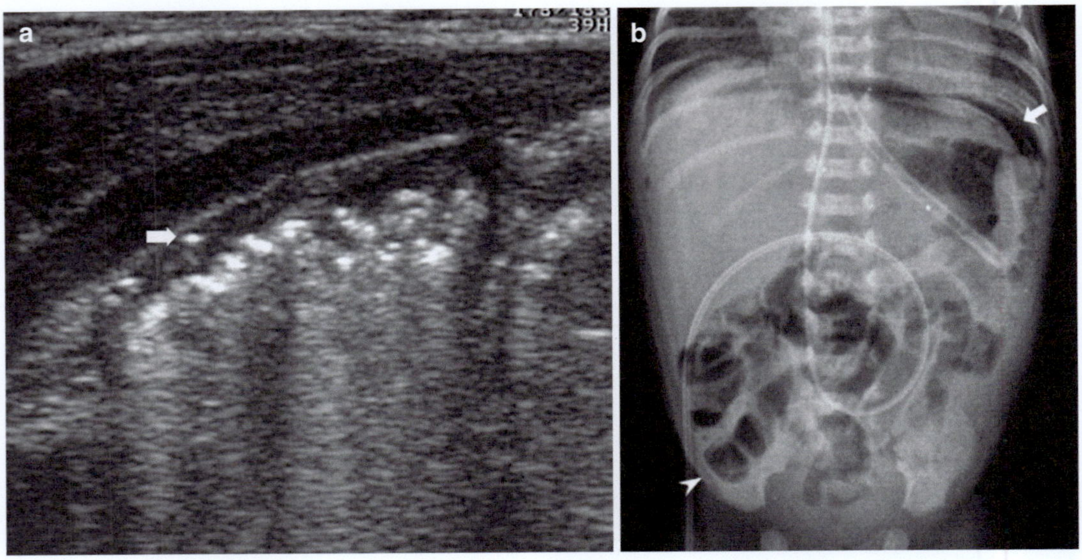

Fig. 4.20 (**a**) Ultrasound exam in newborn with NEC with parietal pneumatosis (*white arrow*); note the posterior reverberation artifacts. (**b**) Plain film shows the pneumatosis (*arrowhead*) and pneumoperitoneum (*arrow*)

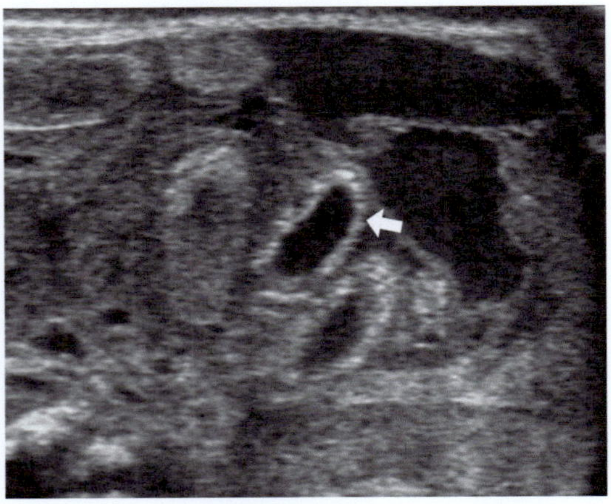

Fig. 4.21 Ultrasound exam in newborn with NEC with parietal pneumatosis in distended loops shows the "circle" sign (*white arrow*)

of free fluid. We must point out that in healthy newborn, there is a small amount of physiological fluid film between the loops. It is fundamental to evaluate the amount and echostructural aspect of the liquid; in fact, in the NEC, the presence of abundant amount of liquid that shows inhomogeneous hypoechoic with echoes and contextual septa is suggestive of perforation (Palleri et al. 2016) (Fig. 4.25).

The presence of reverberation artifacts during abdominal investigation, visible around the bowel loops and suggestive of big quote or free air in the abdomen, is evocative for pneumoperitoneum which is the only sign that has been universally agreed on as an indication for surgery or other interventions; however, this is not present in all babies with bowel necrosis and perforation (Muchantef et al. 2013).

4.7.2 Complications

The complications that can occur in NEC are perforations in 12–30 % of cases, stenosis, and enteroenteric fistulas. Complications result in a worsening of the prognosis net, and mortality can reach 20–30 % of cases.

With the exception of the diagnosis of pneumoperitoneum, abdominal plain film is not sufficient to do the diagnosis, but a contrastographic study, usually an enema but sometimes also completed by an upper gastrointestinal tract, must be carried out. The stenosis is more frequent after 4–12 weeks in 10–30 % of cases; if the stenosis is not severe, surgical treatment is not always requested. Descending colon is involved in 80 %

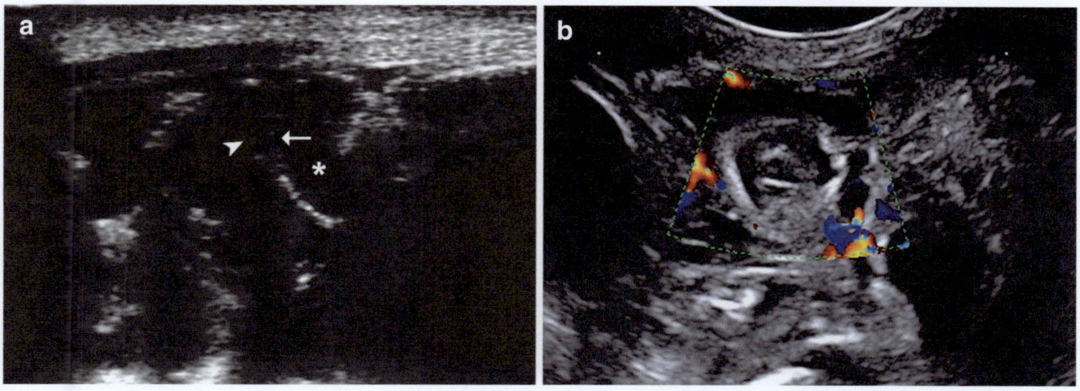

Fig. 4.22 Ultrasound in newborn with NEC. (**a**) Wall ischemia with wall thinning (*white arrow*), perivisceral fluid (*white arrowhead*), and endoluminal fluid (*asterisk*). (**b**) A wall thinning due to distention of the loop by intraluminal content

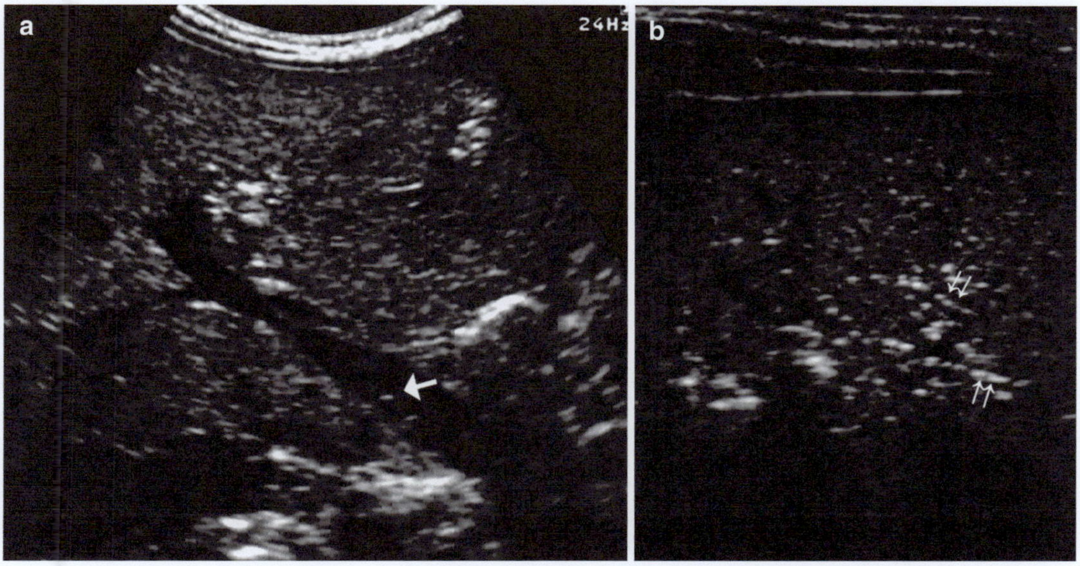

Fig. 4.23 Ultrasound in newborn with NEC. (a) Portal venous gas which appears as punctate and linear, branching areas of echogenicity in the main portal vein (*white arrow*) and (b) in the parenchymal branches within the liver (*small white arrows*)

of cases (Figs. 4.26 and 4.27), and in 30% of cases, the stenosis is multiple.

The enteric fistulization is an uncommon late complication; it happens from a month to 4–5 months and is due to a healing process after a severe bowel ischemia. The symptoms depending on the tract of bowel involved but often include general illness, vomiting, and diarrhea. The plain film findings are not specific for diagnosing enteric fistula, and the investigation of choice is a nonionic water-soluble contrast enema or distal loopogram; barium suspensions are contraindicated. Even if a proximal pathology is less frequent, an upper gastrointestinal tract contrast studies may be required.

Other complications could be related to surgery as anastomotic leakage, abdominal abscess, and short bowel syndrome. Abdominal abscess is

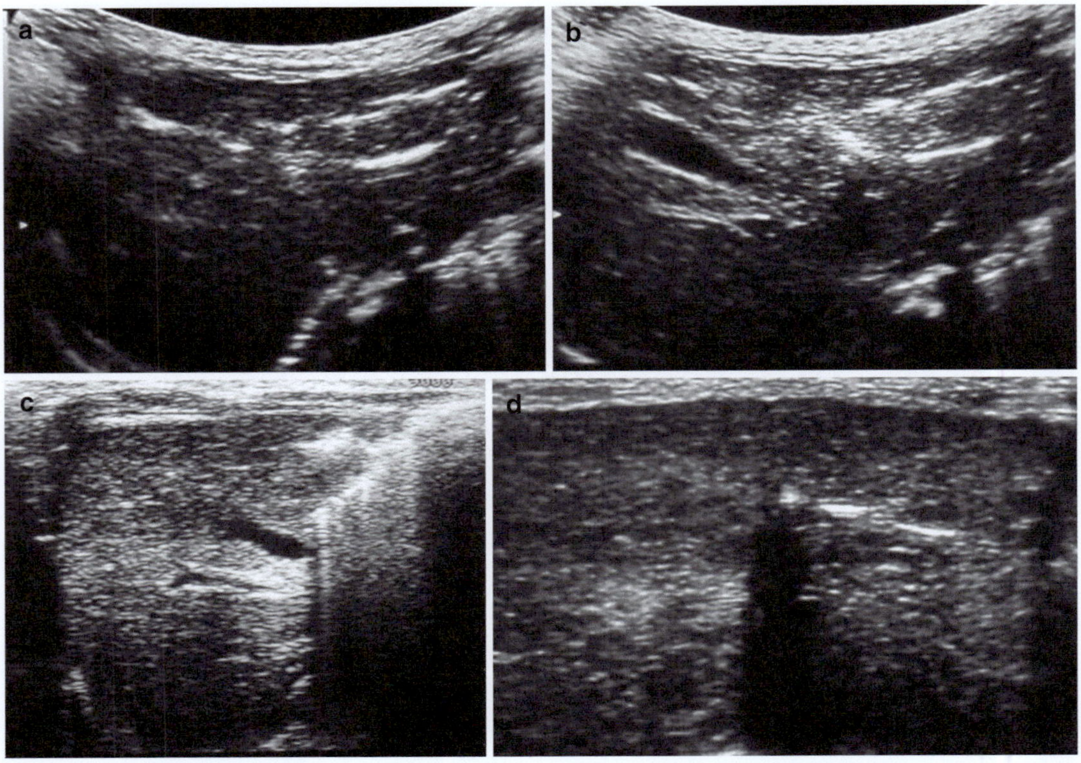

Fig. 4.24 (**a–d**) Ultrasound exam in newborn with NEC shows portal pneumatosis as hyperechoic linear imaging in portal spaces

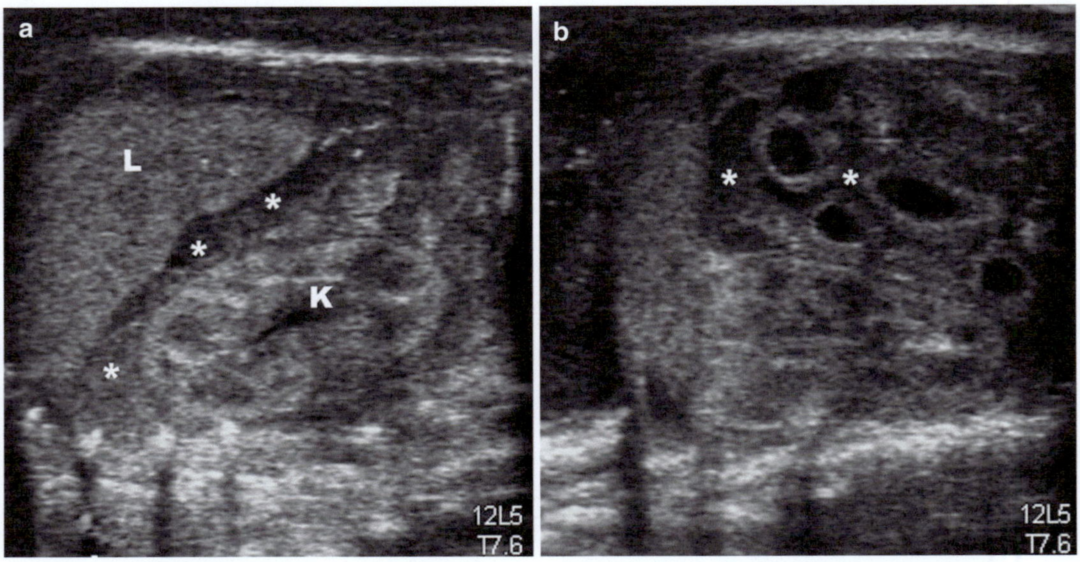

Fig. 4.25 Ultrasound in newborn with NEC. In picture a and b note the inhomogeneous fluid plenty of echoes and contextual septa; this is suggestive for perforation. *L* liver, *K* left kidney, *asterisk* = fluid

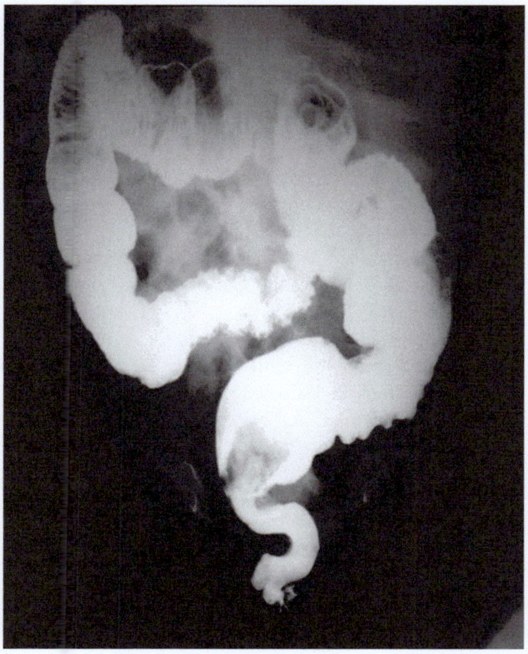

Fig. 4.26 Frontal view barium enema in newborn with severe stenosis of sigma post NEC and distention of the intestinal loop above the stenosis

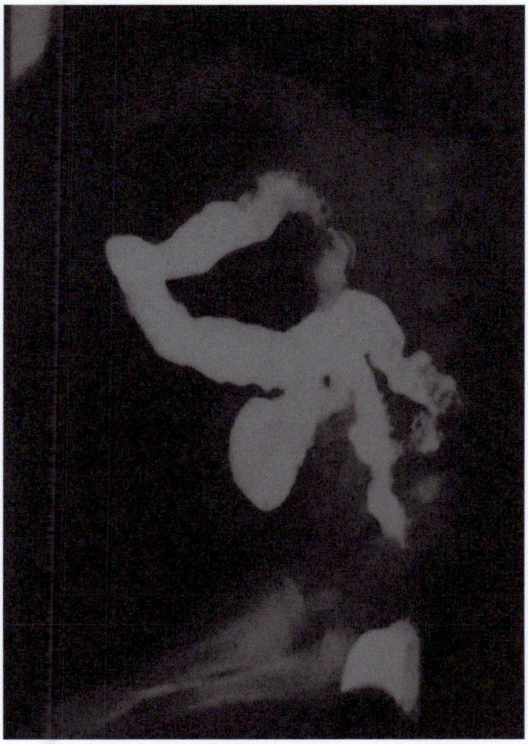

Fig. 4.27 Lateral view barium enema in newborn with a very severe stenosis "threadlike" of sigma post NEC

a rare complication maybe because of the incomplete bacterial colonization of the gut at the time of the NEC.

Fistula, severe stenosis, perforation, and anastomotic leakage are treated with surgery.

References

Bohnhorst B (2013) Usefulness of abdominal ultrasound in diagnosing necrotizing enterocolitis. Arch Dis Child Fetal Neonatal Ed 98:F445–F450. doi:10.1136/archdischild-2012-302848

Buonomo C (1999) The radiology of necrotizing enterocolitis. Radiol Clin North Am 37:1187–1198

Chavhan G, Parra D (2008) Normal doppler spectral waveforms of major pediatric vessels: specific patterns. Radiographics 28:691–706

Coursey CA, Hollingsworth CL, Gaca AM et al (2008) Radiologists' agreement when using a 10-point scale to report abdominal radiographic findings of necrotizing enterocolitis in neonates and infants. AJR Am J Roentgenol 191:190–197. doi:10.2214/AJR.07.3558

Coursey CA, Hollingsworth CL, Wriston C et al (2009) Radiographic predictors of disease severity in neonates and infants with necrotizing enterocolitis. AJR Am J Roentgenol 193:1408–1413

Di Giacomo V, Trinci M, Van der Byl G, Catania VD, Calisti A, Miele V (2015) Ultrasound in newborns and children suffering from nontraumatic acute abdominal pain: imaging with clinical and surgical correlation. J Ultrasound 18:385–393. doi:10.1007/s40477-014-0087-4, Epub 2014 Apr 9

Epelman M, Daneman A, Navarro OG (2007) Necrotizing enterocolitis: review of the state of the art imaging findings with pathologic correlation. Radiographics 27:285–305

Faingold R, Daneman A, Tomlinson G (2005) Necrotizing enterocolitis: assessment of bowel viability with color doppler US. Radiology 235:587–594. doi:10.1148/radiol.2352031718

Frey EE, Smith W, Franken EA Jr, Wintermeyer KA (1987) Analysis of bowel perforation in necrotizing enterocolitis. Pediatr Radiol 17:380–382

Gire C (2014) Prognostic value of abdominal sonography in necrotizing enterocolitis of premature infants born before 33 weeks gestational age. J Pediatr Surg 49:508–513

Goske MJ, Goldblum JL (1999) The "circle sign": a new sonographic sign of pneumatosis intestinalis–clinical, pathologic and experimental findings. Pediatr Radiol 29:535–539

Haber HP, Stern M (2000) Intestinal ultrasonography in children and young adults: bowel wall thickness is age dependent. J Ultrasound Med 19:315–321

Hull A, Buckley P, Wills B (2010) Massive pneumoperitoneum. West J Emerg Med 11:91–92

Kim WY, Kim WS (2005) Sonographic evaluation of neonates with early stage necrotizing enterocolitis. Pediatr Radiol 35:1056–1061

Kosloske AM, Papile L, Burnstein J (1980) Indications for operation in acute necrotizing enterocolitis of the neonate. Surgery 87:502–508

Lin PW, Stoll B (2006) Necrotizing enterocolitis. Lancet 368:1271–1283

Miele V, Di Giampietro I (2014) Diagnostic imaging in emergency. Salute e Società, (2EN):127–138. doi: 10.3280/SES2014-002010EN

Miller SF, Seibert JJ, Kinder DL, Wilson AR (1993) Use of ultrasound in detection of occult bowel perforation in neonates. J Ultrasound Med 12:531–535

Muchantef K, Epelman M, Darge K et al (2013) Sonographic and radiographic imaging features of the neonate with necrotizing enterocolitis: correlating findings with outcomes. Pediatr Radiol 43:1444–1452

Palleri E, Kaiser S, Wester T et al (2016) Complex fluid collection on abdominal ultrasound indicates need for surgery in neonates with necrotizing enterocolitis. Eur J Pediatr Surg. 28 Mar 2016 [Epub ahead of print]

Rampton JW (2004) The football sign. Radiology 231:81–82

Rigler L (1941) Spontaneous pneumoperitoneum. A roentgenologic sign found in the supine position. Radiology 37:604–607

Santulli TV, Schullinger JN, Heird WC et al (1975) Acute necrotizing enterocolitis in infancy: a review of 64 cases. Pediatrics 55:376–387

Sharma R, Lawrence M (2013) A clinical perspective of necrotizing enterocolitis: past, present, and future. Clin Perinatol 40:27–51

Siegel MJ, Friedland JA, Hildebolt CF (1997) Bowel wall thickening in children: differentiation with US. Radiology 203:631–635

Silva CT, Daneman A, Navarro OM et al (2007) Correlation of sonographic findings and outcome in necrotizing enterocolitis. Pediatr Radiol 37:274–282. doi:10.1007/s00247-006-0393-x

5 Hirschsprung's Disease

Domenico Barbuti

5.1 Definition

Hirschsprung's disease (HD), first described by Ruysch in 1691 and Hirschsprung in 1886, is a functional obstruction of the lower intestine due to lack of intrinsic enteric innervations, caused by failed migration of colonic ganglion cells during gestation. The absence of ganglion cells results in the failure of relaxation and non-transmission of peristalsis with dilatation of the intestinal tract upstream from the altered section. HD is also called colonic aganglionosis or congenital megacolon also if the last term should be abandoned because it refers to the effect, the enlarged intestine is the healthy section, while the pathological tract is the restricted one (Inserra et al. 1984). HD causes 15–20% of neonatal bowel obstruction, varies in length but always extends proximally from the anal canal, and most commonly involves the rectosigmoid region of the colon (80%) but can affect the entire colon and, rarely, the small intestine. Ultrashort segment disease, limited to the region of the internal sphincter, is very rare (Berrocal et al. 1999; Buonomo 1997; Kleinhaaus et al. 1979).

D. Barbuti
Diagnostic Imaging Department,
Children's Hospital Bambino Gesù,
S. Onofrio Square, Rome 00165, Italy
e-mail: domenico.barbuti@opbg.net

5.2 Epidemiology

In 90% HD is diagnosed in newborn, 10% later, rarely in adolescent or adults. Males are four times more affected, while there is no gender difference in the total form. The cause of HD is multifactorial, and the disease can be familial or isolated. 1/5,500–7,000 live births in the USA are affected and about 1/5,000 in Italy. In siblings, when one twin is affected, there is a chance that the other is affected especially if male, and the possibility is even higher in total aganglionosis (Coran and Teitelbaum 2000). Congenital type is the most common. Acquired forms derive by vascular causes (ischemia) or nonvascular such as infection by *Trypanosoma* (Chagas disease) or tuberculosis chronic infection or vitamin B1 deficiency. Eight genomes have been associated with HD, but most cases are considered not familial (Amiel and Lyonnet 2001; Parisi and Kapur 2000). HD is usually a solitary anomaly in a full term, otherwise healthy infant. Prematurity is reported in 10%. Associated anomalies occur in nearly 20–25% of cases. Down syndrome (trisomy 21) is the most common chromosomal abnormality associated with the disease, accounting for 10–15% of patients. HD is sporadic in most cases, but it is familial in 8–10%, associated with several genetic mutations of variable penetrance mostly in total form: the gene RET proto-oncogene on chromosome 10q11.2.2,7 has been linked to multiple endo-

V. Miele, M. Trinci (eds.), *Imaging Non-traumatic Abdominal Emergencies in Pediatric Patients*,
DOI 10.1007/978-3-319-41866-7_5

crine neoplasia (MEN) type IIA (Eng 1996). Others reported are ZFHX1B (SIP1) gene mutation, long segment HD-RET, glial cell line-derived neurotrophic growth factor (GNDF), endothelin receptor gene (EDNRB), endothelin 3 (EDN3), and SRY-related transcription factor SOX10 (Donnelly 2005). HD can be associated with urologic (11 %: bladder's diverticulum, renal agenesis, cryptorchidism), cardiovascular (6 %: ventricular septal defect), gastrointestinal (6 %: Meckel's diverticulum, imperforate anus), and neurological (hydrocephalus) abnormalities with 8 % having congenital deafness, Waardenburg syndrome, neuroblastomas, and Ondine's syndrome (Feldmen et al. 2002; Stewart and von Allmen 2003).

5.3 Pathology

The pathologic basis of HD is the absence of ganglion cells in the submucous Meissner's and myenteric Auerbach's plexus and is associated with an increase of the nerve fibers in the affected segment. The neurenteric ganglion cells migrate from the neural crest to the upper end of the alimentary tract and then follow the vagal fibers caudally, so a delay or arrest in this migration results in the neural crest cells failing to reach the distal bowel. Without ganglion cells, the colon spasms cause a functional obstruction. The aganglionic segment is thus smaller than normal in caliber, and the bowel proximal to the affected segment becomes dilated.

The disease affects the rectum and a variable amount of the more proximal colon and may include the entire large bowel and even the small bowel and duodenum, but occurs without skip lesions. It is a unique case in the pathology wherein the distal pathological part of the intestine appears normal and the normal proximal part seems abnormal (Ehrenpreis 1970). The gross pathologic feature of HD is a dilated proximal intestine with a transition zone to normal calibrated distal intestine that is typically funnel like or cone shaped or, less frequently, abrupt (Fig. 5.1). The colon proximal to the aganglionic segment, in an effort to overcome the partial obstruction, becomes distended, and its wall markedly thickened because of muscle hypertrophy; the degree of hypertrophy and dilatation depends upon the duration and degree of obstruction and thus indirectly to the age of the patient.

Grading (Fig. 5.2):

- Short segment, rectosigmoid transition zone (TZ): 70–80 %
- Long segment, TZ above descending colon: 15–20 %
- Ultrashort segment, anorectal TZ, very rare
- Total colonic, distal ileus TZ: 1–4 %
- Total intestinal, very rare

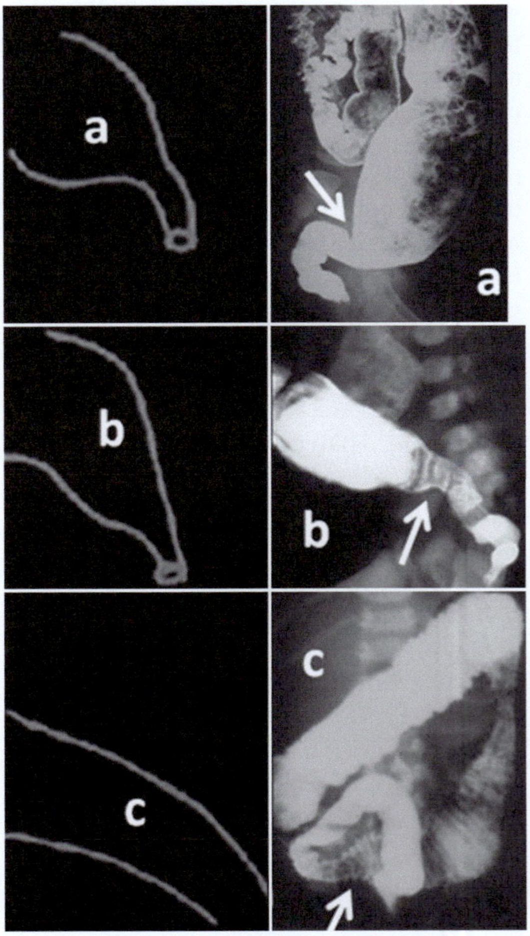

Fig. 5.1 Type of transition zones: (**a**) abrupt, (**b**) conical, and (**c**) funnel. Drawing on the *left*, contrast enema on the *right*

While HD is a common cause of bowel obstruction in neonates, congenital colonic atresia is an uncommon cause of neonatal bowel obstruction. However, coexistence of HD and colonic atresia is a rare phenomenon, and only a few cases have been reported. The association of the two diseases provides a difficult diagnostic and therapeutic challenge. Given the rarity, the coexistence may simply be a random event; however, a possible common etiology may be an impairment to the blood supply of the large intestine. Because clinical and radiological presentation is similar in the two forms, a rectal biopsy specimen will clarify the diagnosis avoiding multiple surgeries causing complications (Kim et al. 1995).

5.4 Clinical Presentation

Eighty percent of patients present in the first few months of life with difficult bowel movements, poor feeding, and progressive abdominal distention. About 90 % of infants with HD fail to pass meconium in the first 24 h of life; however, other causes of this delay also should be considered (see later Sect. 5.7). In other cases HD is manifested by reversible subocclusions where meconium is excreted, even if late, either spontaneously or with stimulus (digital rectal examination, suppositories, enemas), and so the diagnosis is often made only in childhood. In other cases alternating subocclusions and crisis of enterocolitis, viral or bacterial, serious complication is favored by intestinal stasis which can also be fatal if not properly diagnosed; in such cases the baby has severe general condition, abdominal distension (100 %), diarrhea (100 %), dehydration (96 %), bilious vomiting (81 %), and shock (34 %). HD must therefore be suspected in newborns or young infants with fever, abdominal distension, or diarrhea especially with repeated episodes. In fact enterocolitis occurs in about one-third of patients with HD and is burdened by high mortality rate. In about 3 % the disease is manifested by intestinal perforation, especially in total form. During rectal examination or during introduction of a rectal catheter, patient may demonstrate a tight anal sphincter and explosive discharge of stool and gas which are very suggestive findings of HD. Some patients may not have symptoms until later in life; these common symptoms are chronic progressive constipation, recurrent fecal impaction, failure to thrive, and malnutrition (Tomita et al. 2003; Khan et al. 2003).

5.5 Instrumental Diagnosis

1. Imaging
   - Plain film: Direct radiographic examination must be obtained in two "gravitational" images that you can get better view than in the upright position, with consideration for protectionist reasons, in the left lateral decubitus and lateral projection in the prone position "cross table" with horizontal beam incident (Fig. 5.3). There can be an occlusive or subocclusive picture with air-fluid levels both in the small intestine and in the colon; the rectum is small and there are signs of fecal impaction in the colon but always above the rectum. In total forms there is air distension of the small intestine but the colon is not dilated. In infants it is not always easy to distinguish between the colon and the small intestine at direct plain-film examination for reduced haustra of the colon, but generally the colon is disposed more laterally. In the rare case of perforation, an air collection can be seen between the liver and the abdominal walls.
   - Barium or water-soluble enema: As in all intestinal obstructions, it is avoided bowel cleansing. An isosmotic water-soluble contrast is generally preferred in newborn and small infant. The rectal probe is slowly introduced with lubricant without inflating the balloon that could mask a transition zone (TZ). The liquid is manually introduced at low pressure interrupting the introduction when it has shown a TZ with upstream bowel dilatation where you can observe the filling defects from fecal impaction. A late plain film to 8–12 ore can help. The most important sign is rectosigmoid

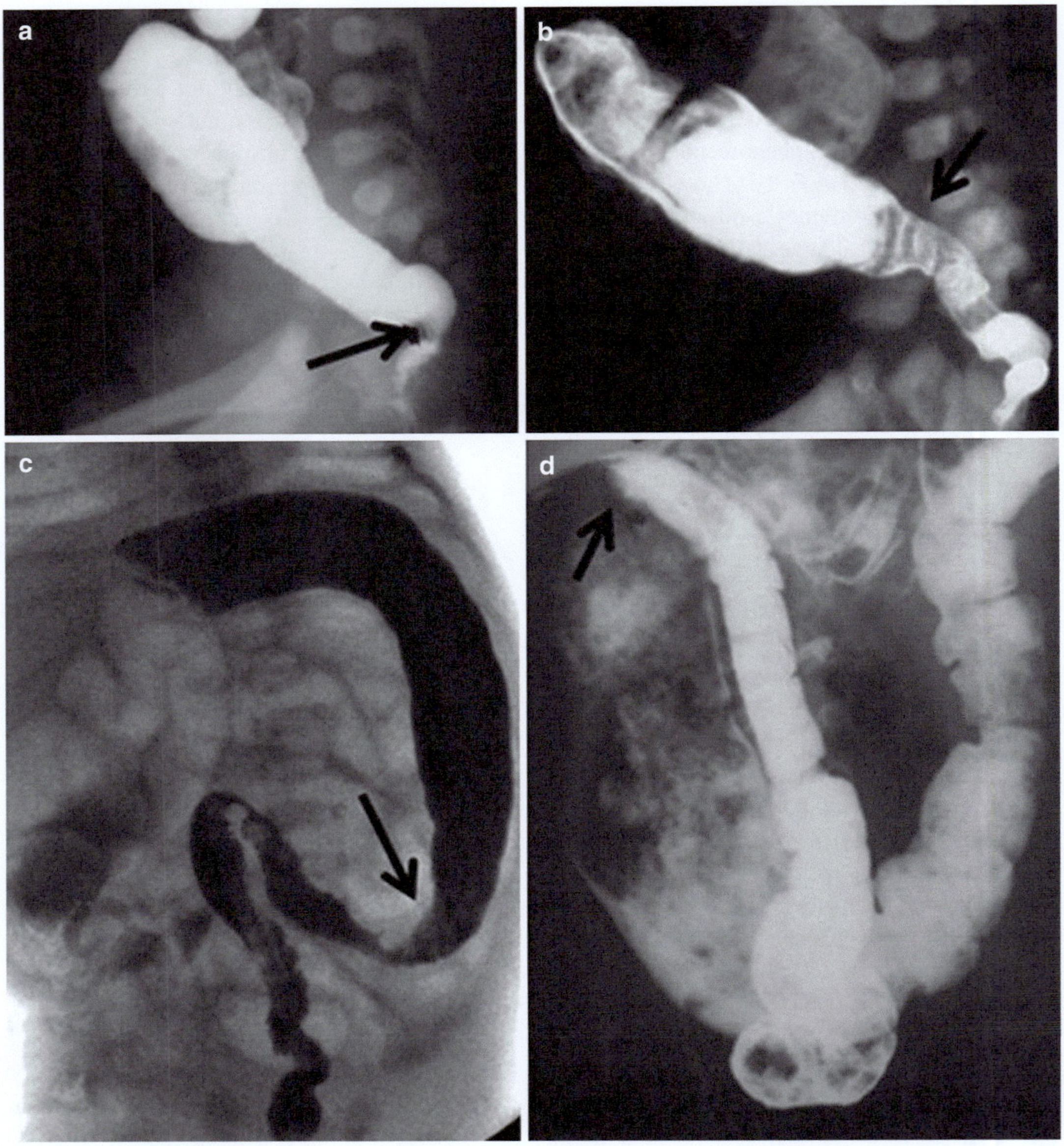

Fig. 5.2 Aganglionic tract (*arrows* sign TZ): (**a**) short, (**b**, **c**) middle, and (**d**) long

ratio <1. The diagnosis is not always easy because sometimes in the first 2 weeks of life, a distended intestinal tract has not yet formed or spontaneously or for "nursing" treatment or in "ultrashort" HD. Other useful signs to the enema may be "fasciculation" or irregular contractions that confer a "sawtooth" aspect of the denervated intestinal tract (Fig. 5.4); unfortunately this sign is not always present and it is not pathognomonic, also seen in colitis. The distance between the rectum and the sacrum may increase for parietal hypertrophy, but generally only in older children. The elimination of the contrast at delayed plain films is reduced with the persistence of TZ and upstream bowel dilatation. In total form of HD, the plain film shows multiple loops of dilated bowel. At contrast enema the findings range from a picture of microcolon

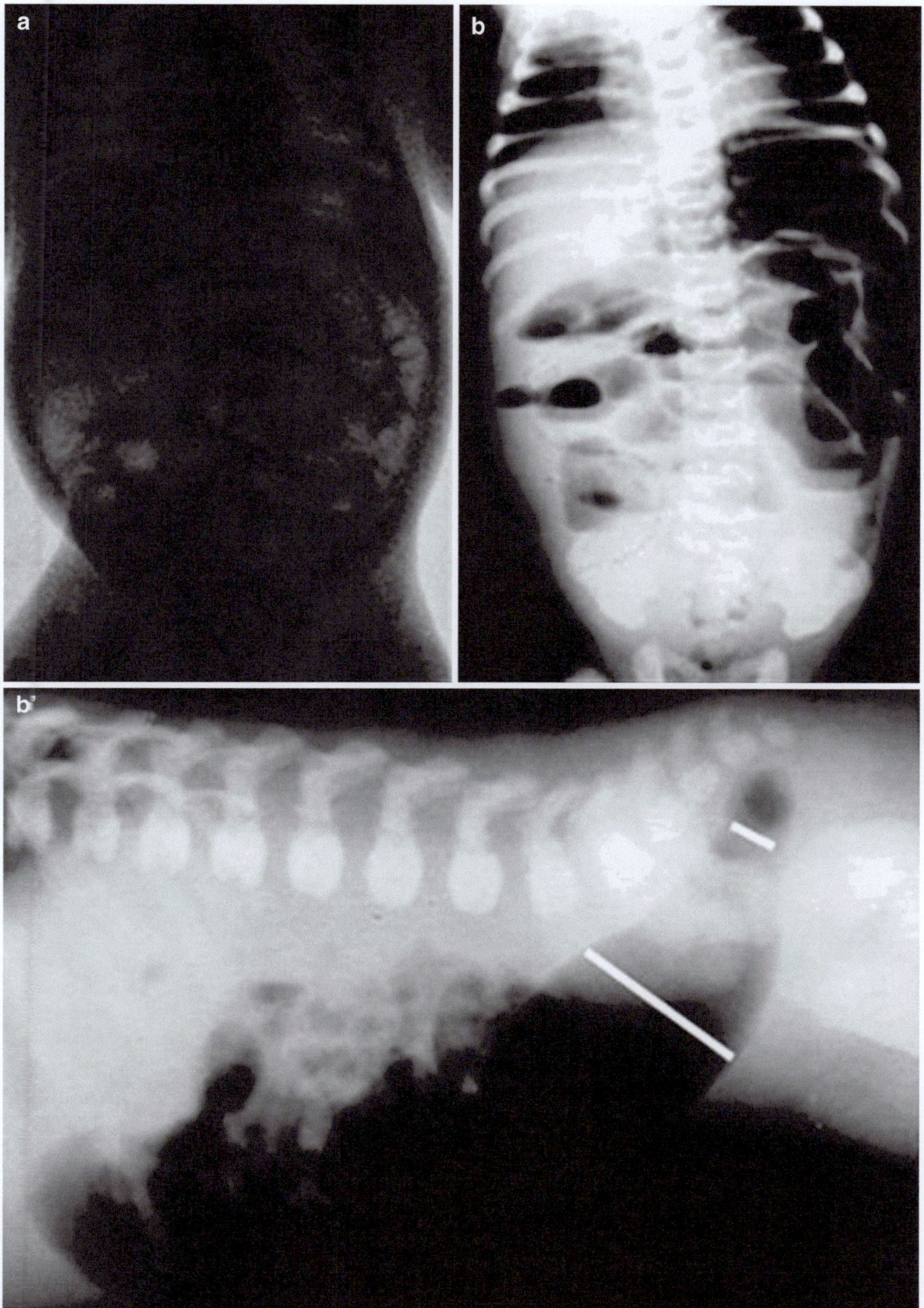

Fig. 5.3 Plain film in HD: (**a**) widespread intestinal dilatation in HD. (**b-b'**) Another case of HD. (**b**) A-P plain film: intestinal dilatation but with little bloating in the rectosigmoid region; (**b'**) the lateral view in prone position "cross table" in the same patient of (b) shows air filling of the rectum and the sigmoid colon with reduced R/S ratio (*white lines*)

without rectosigmoid ratio with dilated small intestine (Fig. 5.5) to a quite regular caliber colon but of simplified form in which the redundancy of the infant colon is reduced with less elongated flexures, with "question mark"-like aspect (Fig. 5.6).
  - Ultrasound (US) shows normal or increased size of the colon, which contains normal hypoechogenic meconium punctuated with gas bubbles (Veyrac et al. 2012). Along the colon, a transition zone may be detected in some cases by US. US is also useful in detecting associated anomaly.
2. Electromanometry: In HD there is absence of the rectoanal inhibitory reflex (RAIR) during rectal distension. While it is an excellent screening in infants and children, RAIR is less useful in neonate: when the RAIR is present, HD can be excluded reliably around 90%, whereas if RAIR is absent, it is not conclusive for the diagnosis of HD.
3. Rectal suction biopsy: HD is diagnosed by the absence of ganglion cells and the presence of hypertrophic nerve trunks (de Lorijn et al. 2005). The biopsy site should be at 1.5 cm above the dentate line because normally there are no ganglion cells in the distal rectum (Ricciardi et al. 1999). If no hypertrophic nerve trunks are found, a full-thickness biopsy may be indicated.

5.6 Treatment

Management of HD varies according to presentation form. In early acute intestinal obstruction, the child needs resuscitation, nasogastric tube, rectal tube, fluid therapy, antibiotics, and rectal irrigations. After multiple seromuscular biopsies of the colon wall to determine the exact extend of the aganglionosis, a colostomy is made and placed above the transition zone, and when the

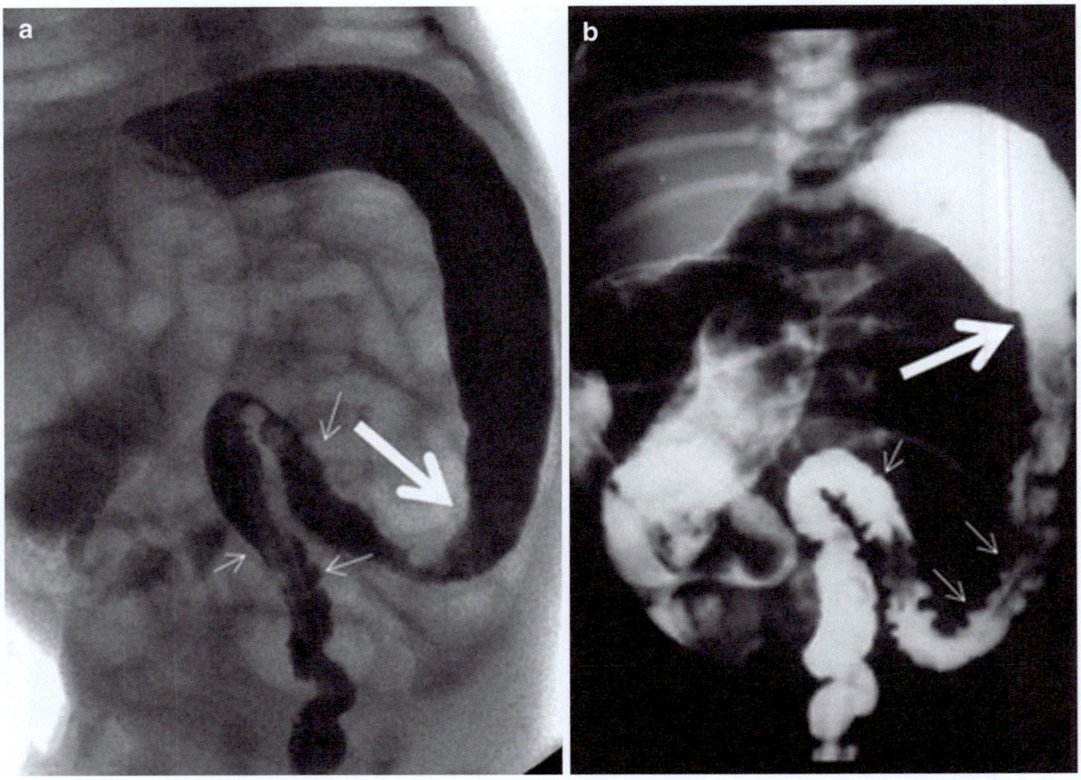

Fig. 5.4 Two cases of HD. The *large white arrow* indicates the transition zone between the descending and sigmoid colon (**a**) and below the splenic flexure (**b**). Both cases in aganglionic intestinal tract are visible anarchic contractions with "sawteeth" appearance (*small white arrows*)

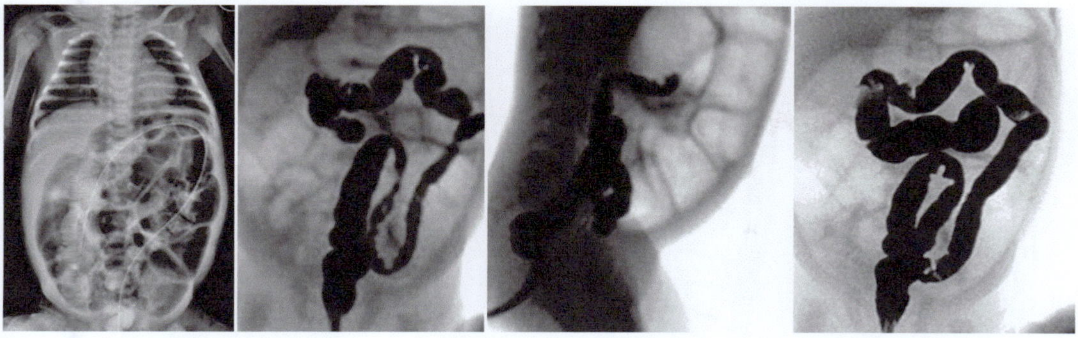

Fig. 5.5 Total HD (histologically proven). Diffuse microcolon, the small intestine is dilated

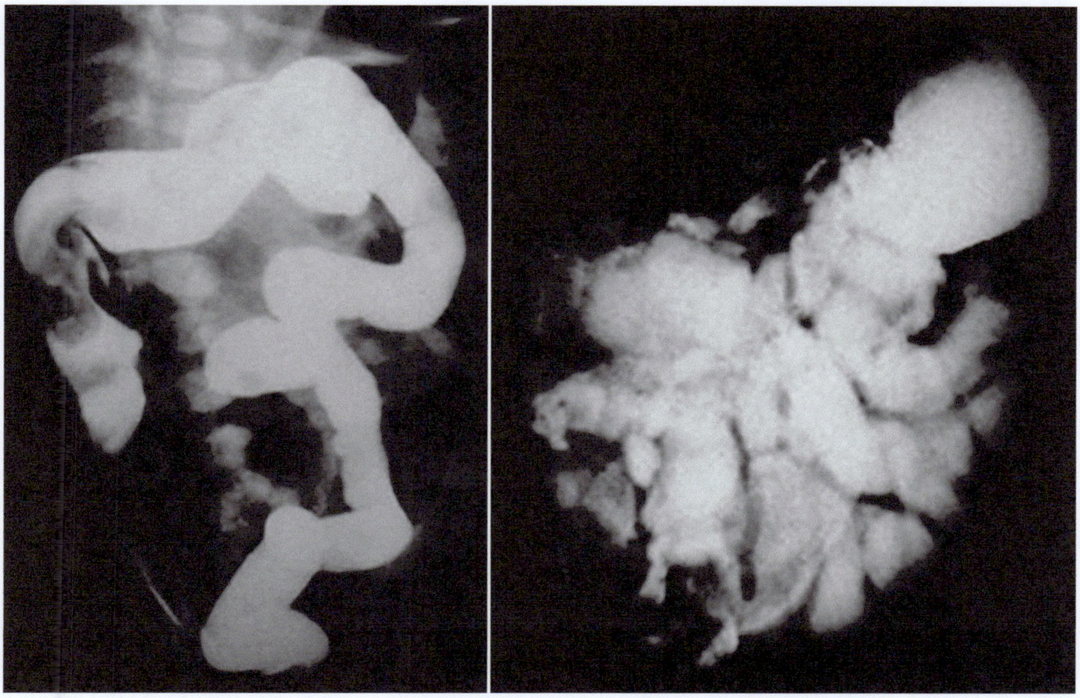

Fig. 5.6 Total HD surgical proven. No microcolon but simplified ("?" symbol) colon at contrast enema; the small intestine is dilated at barium upper gastrointestinal study

patient becomes stable, then the definitive treatment will be planned. If the disease is manifested by chronic constipation, after certain diagnosis, the patient is subjected to saline laxatives and enemas (nursing) until it reaches the age of 6–12 months, or the weight of 9–10 kg, when he can undergo definitive surgery. The treatment is only surgical: removal of intestinal aganglionic segment and subsequent recanalization by colo-anal anastomosis. There are several pull-through techniques, with complication rates ranging from 4–16%. The first operation was Swenson's (2002) one removing the rectum, pulling the healthy innervated colon through, and connecting it to the anus with end-to-end anastomosis between the prolapsed rectum and regularly innervated colon externalized from the anus (Fig. 5.7a). The Duhamel technique, described in 1956 (Vrsansky et al. 1998), means allowing the native rectum in situ, lower "pull-through" the ganglionic colon behind it, in the retrorectal space, and package the end-to-side anastomosis

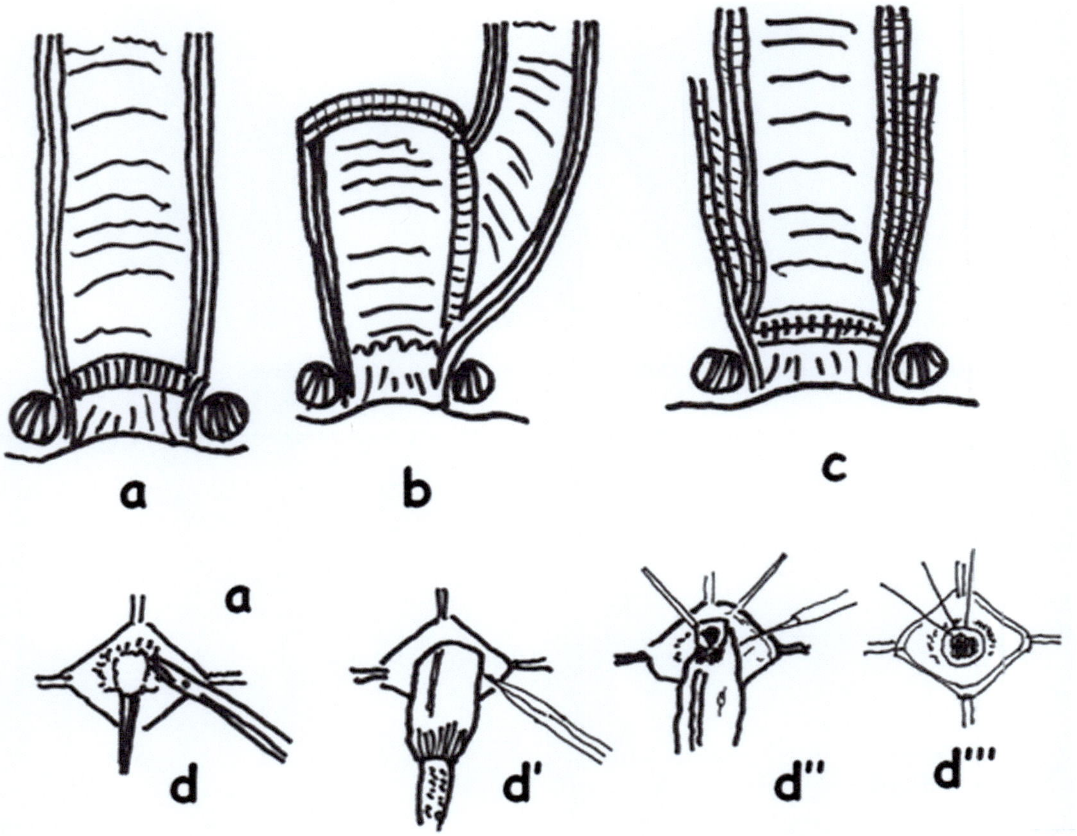

Fig. 5.7 Drawing of surgical treatment of HD: (**a**) Swenson operation, (**b**) Duhamel operation, (**c**) Soave operation, (**d-d'''**) De La Torre transanal pull-through (see text)

(using linear stapler) (Fig. 5.7b). Duhamel operation was now almost abandoned for frequent dilatation of pocket with stagnated stools (Fig. 5.8). Soave's operation in 1960, endorectal pull-through (Soave 1964), consists in mucosectomy of the rectum with preservation of the rectal muscle cylinder, lowering of regularly innervated colon through the cylinder itself, and packaging of anastomosis termino-terminal just above the dentate line (Fig. 5.7c). In recent years the Soave operation is performed in one transanal time: De la Torre operation, also mostly used in our institute in the last years (De la Torre-Mondragon and Ortega-Salgado 1998) as for the procedure for abdominal route, consists in removing all the cylinder of the mucosa of the aganglionic intestinal tract and lowering the intestinal regularly innervated within the cylinder of the residue muscle (Figs. 5.7d-d''' and 5.9). The minimally invasive approach of this technique has many advantages: the average duration of the intervention of about 2 h, ready recanalization intestinal allowing rapid power recovery, reduction of average hospitalization time (an average of 4 days), and the absence of skin scarring with a definite aesthetic advantage. Most patients can achieve good continence, and life expectancy is normal although they are often required repeated dilations in the first year after the operation (Höllwarth et al. 2002).

5.7 Differential Diagnosis

1. Meconium plug/small left colon syndrome. Predisposing factors: maternal diabetes, cesarean section, and prematurity. Symptoms: vomiting, abdominal distention, and delay of the meconium emission. Plain film: low intes-

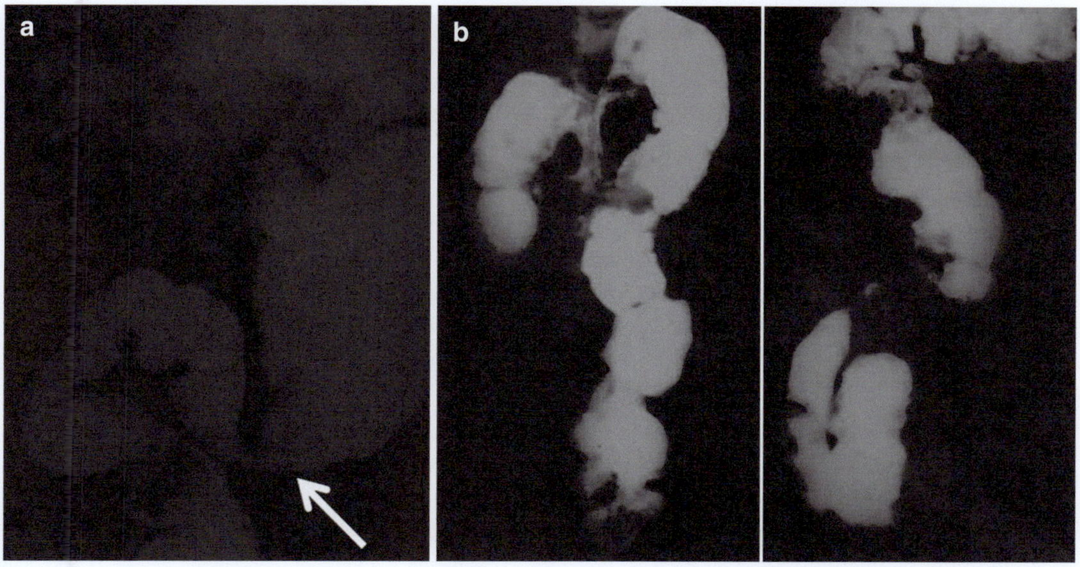

Fig. 5.8 (**a**) Preoperative enema in HD shows TZ (*white arrow*); (**b**) after Duhamel operation the barium enema shows anterior slightly dilated pocket with fecal stagnation (*black arrow*)

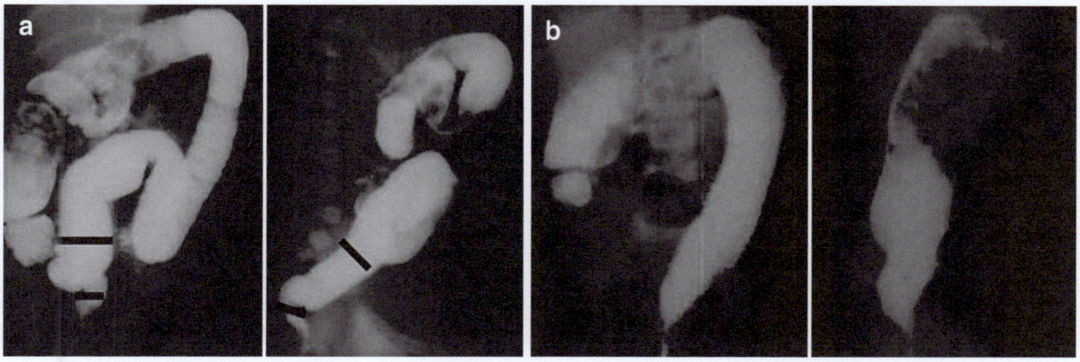

Fig. 5.9 HD (**a**) preoperative enema shows R/S <1; (**b**) barium enema after De La Torre operation

tinal obstruction and bullous appearance for thickened meconium. Contrast enema: left colon reduced caliber with multiple filling defects from meconium plugs, rectum/sigmoid ratio >1. Resolution after contrast enema or anyway in a few days.

2. Meconium ileus. Present in 15 % of cystic fibrosis. Symptoms: vomiting, abdominal distension, and lack of meconium emission. Plain film: dilatation of distal ileum, air-fluid levels scarce or absent, and mottled appearance of the right side due to the thickened meconium. Enema with water-soluble contrast medium: microcolon and dilated ileum with filling defects by thickened meconium plugs. It solves the framework in 50–60 %. Risk of perforation is from 2.7 % to 5 %.
3. Ileal atresia: 1/750 born. Prenatal ultrasound diagnosis. Caused by intrauterine intestinal ischemia. Rare associations. Plain films: three or more air bubbles no air downstream. Contrast enema: microcolon ex non usu, filling defects from meconium bubbles.
4. Colonic atresia (CA), rare, 1/40,000 births, caused by an intrauterine vascular defect. The proximal colon is most affected. Symptoms: abdominal distension and vomiting even after a few days. Plain film: low obstruction. US

examination: CA is suspected in dilated right colon. Contrast enema: microcolon, the liquid stops clubbed or "wind sock" aspect usually in the transverse colon.

5. Allergic colitis. It begins in the first week of life associated with the composition of milk. Contrast enema: no microcolon, R/S ratio can be <1. At rectal biopsy ganglion cells are normally represented and there is eosinophilia.
6. Colic stenosis. It is a late complication of necrotizing enterocolitis that affects very premature babies (prematurity is reported in only 10 % of HD). The restricted tract is often short, sometimes multiple, and the tract upstream and downstream from the stenosis has a higher caliber.
7. Functional constipation (90 %, 10 % is organic). The onset is in the postneonatal age after a long period of normality, normal meconium elimination. The defecation is painful with episodes of abdominal pain, increased meteorism, blood in the stool, episodes of diarrhea, family history of constipation, difficulty evacuating outside the home, fullness of feces at digital rectal examination, encopresis (soiling), and generally the absence of abdominal distension or occlusive disease

5.8 Follow-Up

After diagnosis and surgery, physicians should counsel the patient's family about the importance of a high-fiber diet because constipation and bowel stasis are thought to increase the risk of enterocolitis, and a long-term follow-up is necessary for monitoring the complications: up to 10 % may have constipation, and less than 1 % may have fecal incontinence (Coran and Teitelbaum 2000). Enterocolitis and colonic rupture are the most serious complications and are the most common causes of deaths associated with the HD. Enterocolitis occurs in 17–50 % of infants with HD and most commonly is caused by intestinal obstruction and residual aganglionic bowel, and it has been reported to occur up to 10 years later (Holschneider and Puri 2000).

References

Amiel J, Lyonnet S (2001) Hirschsprung disease, associated syndromes, and genetics: a review. J Med Genet 38:729–739

Berrocal T, Lamas M, Gutiérrez J, Torres I, Prieto C, del Hoyo ML (1999) Congenital anomalies of the small intestine, colon and rectum. Radiographics 19:1219–1236

Buonomo C (1997) Neonatal gastrointestinal emergencies. Radiol Clin N Am 35:845–864

Coran AG, Teitelbaum DH (2000) Recent advances in the management of Hirschsprung's disease. Am J Surg 180:382–387

De la Torre-Mondragon L, Ortega-Salgado JA (1998) Transanal endorectal pull-through for Hirschsprung's disease. J Pediatr Surg 33:1283–1286

de Lorijn F, Reitsma JB, Voskuijl WP, Aronson DC, Ten Kate FJ, Smets AM et al (2005) Diagnosis of Hirschsprung's disease: a prospective, comparative accuracy study of common tests. J Pediatr 146:787–792

Donnelly LF (2005) Diagnostic imaging pediatrics AMYRS Ed

Ehrenpreis TH (1970) Hirschsprung disease. Year Book Publisher, Chicago

Eng C (1996) Seminars in medicine of the Beth Israel Hospital, Boston The RET proto-oncogene in multiple endocrine neoplasia type 2 and Hirschsprung's disease. N Engl J Med 335:943–951

Feldmen M, Friedman LS, Sleisenger MH (2002) Hirschsprung's disease. In: Sleisenger & Fordtran's gastrointestinal and liver disease: pathophysiology, diagnosis, management, 7th ed. Saunders, Philadelphia pp 2131–2315

Höllwarth ME, Rivosecchi M, Schleef J, Ceriati E, Ciprandi G, DePeppo F (2002) The role of transanal endorectal pull-through in the treatment of Hirschsprung's disease – a multicenter experience. Pediatr Surg Int 18:344–348

Holschneider AM, Puri P (2000) Hirschsprung's disease and allied disorders, 2nd edn. Harwood Academic Publishers, Amsterdam

Inserra A, Ponticelli A, Barbuti D, Bergami G, Rivosecchi M (1984) Il megacolon neonatale: aspetti diagnostici e terapeutici. Aggiornamento Pediatrico XXXV:107–122

Khan AR, Vujanic GM, Huddart S (2003) The constipated child: how likely is Hirschsprung's disease? Pediatr Surg Int 19:439–442

Kim PCW, Superina RA, Ein S (1995) A colonic atresia combined with Hirschsprung's disease: diagnostic and therapeutic challenge by Toronto. J Pediatr Surg 30(8):1216–1217

Kleinhaaus S, Boley S, Sherair M et al (1979) Hirschsprung's disease: a survey of the members of the surgical section of the American Academy of Pediatrics. J Pediatr Surg 14:588–597

Parisi MA, Kapur RP (2000) Genetics of Hirschsprung disease. Curr Opin Pediatr 12:610–617

Ricciardi R, Counihan TC, Banner BF, Sweeney WB (1999) What is the normal aganglionic segment of anorectum in adults? Dis Colon Rectum 42:380–382

Soave F (1964) A new surgical technique for treatment of Hirschsprung's disease. Surgery 56:1007–1014

Stewart DR, von Allmen D (2003) The genetics of Hirschsprung disease. Gastroenterol Clin N Am 32:819–837

Swenson O (2002) Hirschsprung's disease a review. Pediatrics 109:914–918

Tomita R, Ikeda T, Fujisaki S, Tanjoh K, Munakata K (2003) Hirschsprung's disease and its allied disorders in adults' histological and clinical studies. Hepatogastroenterology 50:1050–1053

Veyrac C, Baud C, Prodhomme O, Saguintaah M, Couture A (2012) US assessment of neonatal bowel (necrotizing enterocolitis excluded). Pediatr Radiol 42(Suppl 1):S107–S114

Vrsansky P, Bourdelat D, Pagés R (1998) Principal modifications of the Duhamel procedure in the treatment of Hirschsprung's disease. Analysis based on results of an international retrospective study of 2,430 patients. Pediatr Surg Int 13:25–32

6 Complications of Neonatal Abdominal Devices in Emergency

Riccardo Ferrari, Antonio Alessandro Pallottino, Claudia Lucia Piccolo, Maria Napoletano, Margherita Trinci, and Vittorio Miele

6.1 Introduction

Pediatric abdominal devices are mandatory for life support of newborn and pediatric patient.

Umbilical catheters, nasojejunal catheters, and percutaneous enteral alimentation by means of gastrostomy or gastrojejunostomy are the most useful and frequent abdominal devices used in pediatric patients during emergency care. The use of intraperitoneal Foley catheter is limited to reduce peritoneal pressions in severe burned patients.

The modern role of radiologists is crucial in the evaluation of complications caused by these devices; in particular, it is very important to understand and recognize the incorrect positioning of umbilical catheters or nasogastric/nasojejunal catheters; it is otherwise important to evaluate the presence of thrombosis at the top of the tip in venous catheters and the radiology signs of infection.

R. Ferrari (✉) • A.A. Pallottino • M. Trinci • V. Miele
Department of Emergency Radiology, S. Camillo Hospital, Rome, Italy
e-mail: ferrariboard@gmail.com

C.L. Piccolo
Department of Medicine and Health Sciences, University of Molise, Campobasso, Italy

M. Napoletano
Division of Radiology, Department of Surgical and Biomedical Sciences, S. Maria della Misericordia Hospital, Perugia, Italy

Less important is the impact of the radiologist in the evaluation of gastrostomy and gastrojejunostomy device complications that have an evident and immediate clinical impact on patients.

Multimodality Radiology is the right approach choosing US, CT, MR, or plain X-ray with the right protocol to obtain the right answers to the clinician's questions. Radiologists should be aware of patient's exposure to diagnostic radiations in particular in pediatric patient.

6.2 Gastroenteric Feeding Accesses

The enteric feeding access could be allowed by positioning nasoduodenal or nasojejunal tubes as well as gastrostomy or jejunostomy.

The recent literature established that the use of nasojejunal feeding catheter is a better choice comparing it to nasogastric feeding catheter because it reduces gastric and pancreatic secretion reflux and the possibility to develop pancreatitis or inspiration pneumonia (Itkin et al. 2011).

The use of nasojejunal tube is to be considered when limited enteric feeding time is needed. If a longer enteric feeding time is required, gastrostomy or jejunostomy is the mandatory choice.

Jejunostomy and gastrostomy are placed surgically or endoscopically guided, less frequent radiologically guided.

V. Miele, M. Trinci (eds.), *Imaging Non-traumatic Abdominal Emergencies in Pediatric Patients*,
DOI 10.1007/978-3-319-41866-7_6

6.2.1 Normal and Radiological Anatomy

The duodenum is derived from the embryonic foregut and proximal midgut. It develops its loop-like morphology to the rapid elongation and the asymmetric growth of the stomach.

The duodenum developed a mature path and position in the third gestational month and becomes relatively fixed in position by a series of mesenteric fusions during the next 30 days.

The mobile intraperitoneal stomach and pyloric channel are oriented along a longitudinal axis: the stomach in the infant is most frequently horizontal but may occasionally rotate into a more vertical (adult) orientation when patients are in supine position.

The proximal duodenum and the superior flexure is intraperitoneal and freely movable. At the apex of the superior flexure, the anterior and posterior peritoneal layers join together on the superior border to form the hepatoduodenal ligament.

Just distal to the superior flexure, the descending duodenum is crossed by the mesenteric fixation colon and becomes completely retroperitoneal which continues into the inferior flexure.

The retroperitoneal descending duodenum and inferior flexure have a medial fibrous attachment to the head of the pancreas which tends to secure it more rigidly.

The third or transverse portion begins at the inferior flexure, to the right of the inferior vena cava, and courses across the midline to the lateral border of the aorta, where the fourth portion ascends to the duodenojejunal junction.

The distal duodenal loop is gradually surrounded by the peritoneum, so that it is once again completely intraperitoneal at the duodenojejunal junction. The position of the duodenojejunal junction is normally maintained by the ligament of Treitz, a flat fibromuscular band arising from the diaphragm.

Nasoenteric tube could be placed manually or guided by endoscopy or radiology. Several recent prospective randomized clinical trials that compared endoscopy-guided and image-guided placement of postpyloric tubes demonstrated no differences in tube positioning success rate that is usually very high, greater than 90 %. The catheter should be at least 8 French and 140, 200 cm length with the tip placed 20 cm after the Treitz ligament (Foote et al. 2004; Ott et al. 1991; Fang et al. 2005).

In this paper Merten et al. (1980) suggested to take only a radiogram after aspiration of alkaline pH secretion and advancing the tube for 5–7 cm. Pobiel et al. (1994), in a more recent paper, described a different positioning method, using fluoroscopy guide: inserting the catheter with patient in supine position, rotating him in oblique position if the progression through the pylorus would be difficult, monitoring with fluoroscopy when necessary, especially in the first part, and avoiding the dislocation of the catheter inside the airways.

6.2.2 Mean Complications and Role of the Radiologist

Nasojejunal tube positioning mean complications are misplacing it inside the airways, nasal bleeding, recoiling of the tube in the stomach, and duodenal perforation. Itkin et al. report that 40–80 % of nasogastric tubes become dislodged in a long period (Johnston et al. 2008), that is the reason why it is mandatory to use nasojejunal feeding tube for a short time.

The radiologist should evaluate the misplacing of the catheter inside the airway or its looping inside the stomach. The presence of the high radiotransparent air and the radiopaque catheter tip helps the evaluation of the anatomic position. Placing the tube during fluoroscopy could help avoid positioning of the catheter in the airway (Fig. 6.1).

6.3 Arterial and Venous Umbilical Catheters

Umbilical vessel catheterization is a very common technique for treating neonatal and perinatal severe complications in intensive care perinatal units. Umbilical catheters are used during resuscitations, exchange transfusions, and critical care

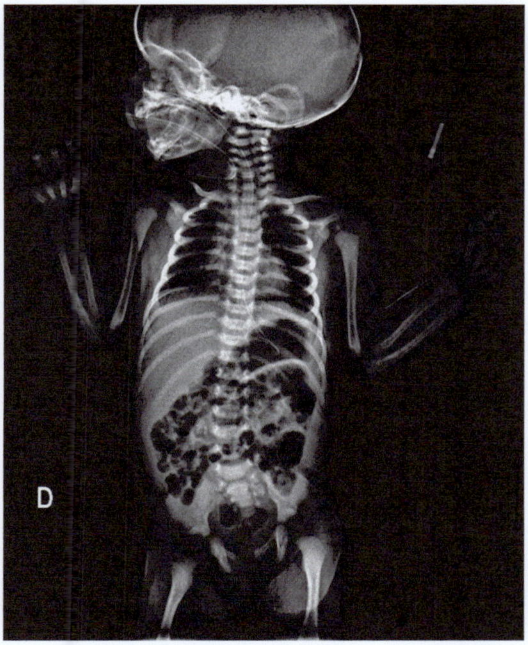

Fig. 6.1 Nasogastric catheter, normal positioning

monitoring or for prolonged nutritional and medication support performing blood sampling, blood pressure monitoring, and infusion of intravenous fluids or medications.

Catheterization could be performed using arterial umbilical vessels or venous umbilical vessels (Hermansen and Hermansen 2005a); arterial catheterization is less used with a more frequent possibility of adverse reaction especially if for prolonged time.

Primary contraindications are omphalitis, omphalocele, necrotizing enterocolitis, and peritonitis.

The catheter positioning is a relatively easy technique but should lead to severe complications; radiology helps positioning and monitoring umbilical catheters during treatment avoiding the mispositioning and the common adverse reactions.

6.3.1 Normal and Radiological Anatomy of Umbilical Artery

The umbilical artery originates from the anterior division of the internal iliac artery, and it is the communication between the placenta and maternal circulation during pregnancy. At birth it usually obliterates with its remnant developing the medial umbilical ligament, which courses superomedially to the umbilicus, within a fold of peritoneum called "the medial umbilical fold" in the posterior wall of anterior abdominal wall. It is a paired structure and lies lateral to the medial umbilical ligament (the urachal remnant) and medial to the lateral umbilical fold, which contains the inferior epigastric vessels. In the adult, the superior bladder artery originates as a branch from umbilical arteries and remains during the life-giving vascular supply to the superior bladder, the portion of the ureter next to this, and the ductus deferens (Dalley and Agur 2011).

6.3.1.1 Radiologic Positioning

The tip of the umbilical arterial catheter should be placed in the aorta in high (T6 to T10) or low (L3 to L5) position away from major aorta's branches, to avoid vessel ischemia or avoid instilling high-concentration solutions directly into an organ-feeding vessel. There is a recent meta-analysis that prefers the high position for its capability to reduce the rate of complications. Intermediate position should be avoided (Hermansen and Hermansen 2005b; Hunter and Taljanovic 2005) (Figs. 6.2 and 6.3).

6.3.2 Normal and Radiological Anatomy of the Umbilical Vein

The umbilical vein is 2–3 cm long with a diameter of 5–6 mm. It arises from the umbilical scar to the left main portal vein; it continues in the umbilical duct (Aranzio's vein) that is 2–3-cm long with a diameter of 4–5 mm. Aranzio's vein is a continuation of the umbilical vein, which originates from left branch of the portal vein, in front of the outlet of the umbilical vein. Aranzio's vein is localized between the right and left hepatic lobe in the sagittal median plane of the body. It ends with the hepatic veins, in the inferior cava vein. The umbilical vein and ductus venosus do not enter the liver parenchyma but pass along the visceral surface (Fig. 6.4).

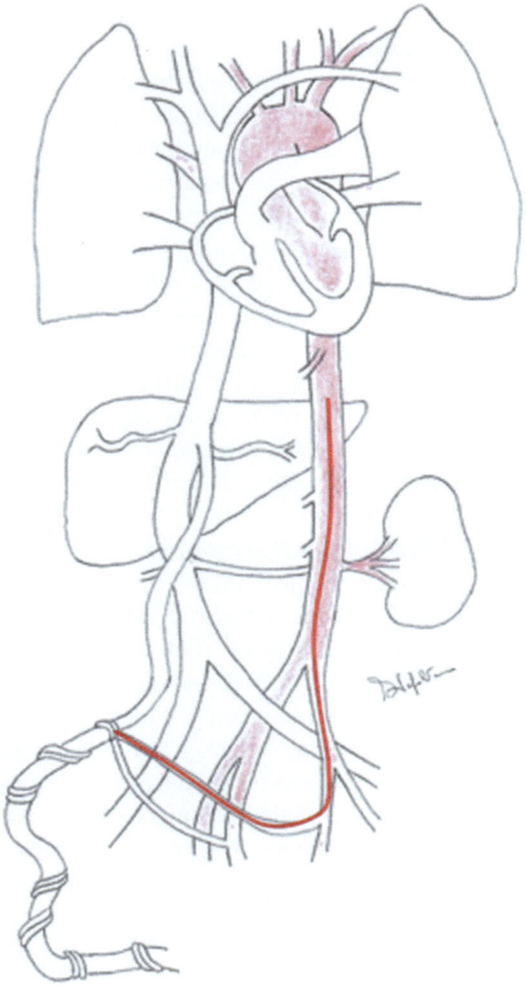

Fig. 6.2 Schematic anatomical representation of the course of arterial umbilical catheter

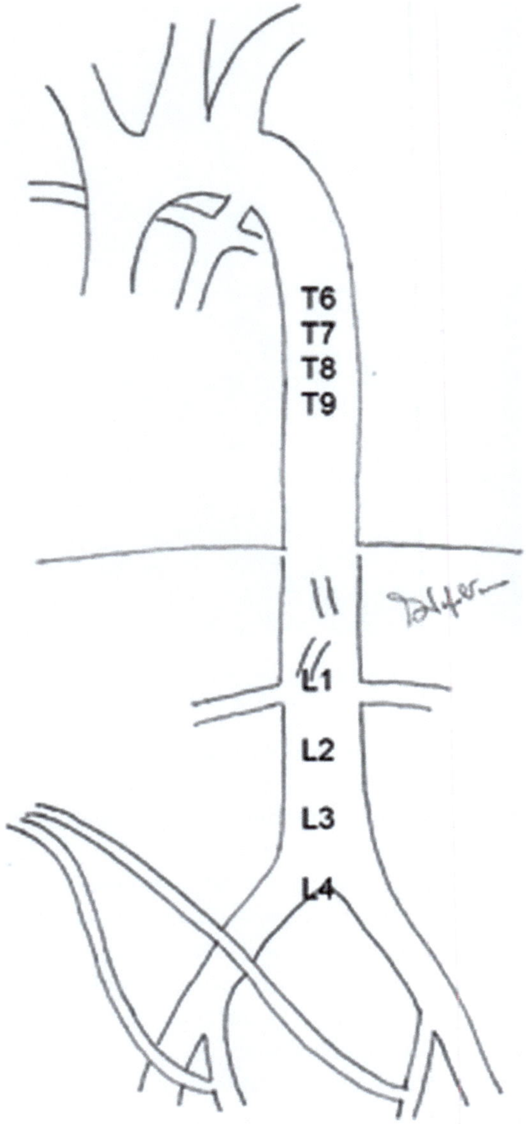

Fig. 6.3 Schematic representation of high and low positions of umbilical arterial catheter

After the birth the exclusion of Aranzio's vein is caused by the ligation of the umbilical vein, and it obliterates between the 30 and 90° day of life with the transformation in the venous ligament. The intra-abdominal portion of the umbilical vein will transform in the hepatic round ligament for an obliteration process which completes itself within the third month of life (Rosen and Reich 1970; Horn 1991).

6.3.2.1 Radiologic Positioning

Radiologic positioning of the umbilical vein catheter results quite simple when the umbilical vein and Aranzio's duct are perfectly aligned on opposite side of the left portal vein. However Aranzio's inlet is often located slightly to the right of the umbilical vein outlet. This may result in coiling of the catheter or misdirection into the left portal vein (Figs. 6.5 and 6.6).

The correct position of umbilical venous catheter tip must project radiologically at the level of the right diaphragm and/or between the T8 and T9 vertebral body, corresponding to the superior part of the IVC, below the right atrium (Fig. 6.7).

If the umbilical venous catheter is not in a proper position, it could be a cause of severe complication; despite this, a recent analysis estimated that only 73 % of all umbilical venous catheters are positioned at an appropriate level (Grizelj et al. 2014). Some papers suggest to use ultrasound control in case of doubt to be sure about the exact location of the umbilical venous catheter's tip.

6.3.3 Mean Complications and Role of the Radiologist

6.3.3.1 Malpositioning

Arterial Umbilical Catheter

There is still debate on the right arterial umbilical catheter position between high (T6 to T10) and low (L3 to L5) position.

A recent Cochrane Database Review of six controlled trials found that "high" catheters were associated with a decreased incidence of "clinical vascular complications" without a statistically significant difference in the incidence of intraventricular hemorrhage, hypertension, hematuria, or death between the two groups.

The duration time of use for functional catheter was greater with the "high" catheters.

The Cochrane Review concluded that "there appears to be no evidence to support the use of low-placed umbilical artery catheters. High catheters should be used exclusively."

What we know quite well is that UACs that are located between the "high" and "low" positions are never appropriate.

Mean complication caused by catheters in these positions are:

- Refractory hypoglycemia (infusion into the celiac axis)
- Paraplegia (infusion into the artery of Adamkiewicz)
- Thromboses that affect the kidneys (infusion into the renal arteries) or the gut (infusion into the mesenteric arteries)

A catheter that is found in this intermediate position should be pulled to a "low" position or removed. For the same reason, catheters should not be placed below the level of L5 because of the risk of gluteal skin necrosis and sciatic nerve damage. Catheters that are placed below the level of L5 should be removed promptly (Miele et al. 2002a).

Venous Umbilical Catheter

Malpositioning of the venous umbilical catheter causes severe complications.

UVC could be pushed too far, entering inside the heart in the right atrium (Fig. 6.8). Going further the more frequent way is not straight inside the superior vena cava but more often the catheter passes through the foramen ovale into the left atrium; from there, the catheter may enter the left ventricle or in a pulmonary vein. The catheter inside the heart could cause cardiac arrhythmia; if pushed too far inside the pulmonary parenchyma, it could cause pleural effusion. More rare is the atrial perforation and the pericardial effusion.

Quite often Aranzio's duct is not well aligned with the umbilical vein outlet so it is quite simple that the catheter enters in the left portal vein and continues into the right portal vein (Figs. 6.9, 6.10, 6.11, and 6.12). In this case the catheter tip could cause direct injury to the liver parenchyma, portal vein thrombosis, or lacerations. Indirect damages should be caused by hypertonic or irritant solution administration inside the liver parenchyma causing portal thrombosis or sterile abscesses which can progress to infection or hepatic necrosis (Grizelj et al. 2014; Miele et al. 2002a, b).

6.3.3.2 Infection, Liver Abscess, and Hematoma

The presence of a foreign body inside the central venous system like central venous catheter could cause infections, as pathogenic microorganisms can gain direct access to the bloodstream, directly by contaminated catheter or infusion of contaminated solution.

Several studies demonstrated that 22–59 % of umbilical venous catheters are colonized, and 3–8 % are having intravenous catheter-related bloodstream

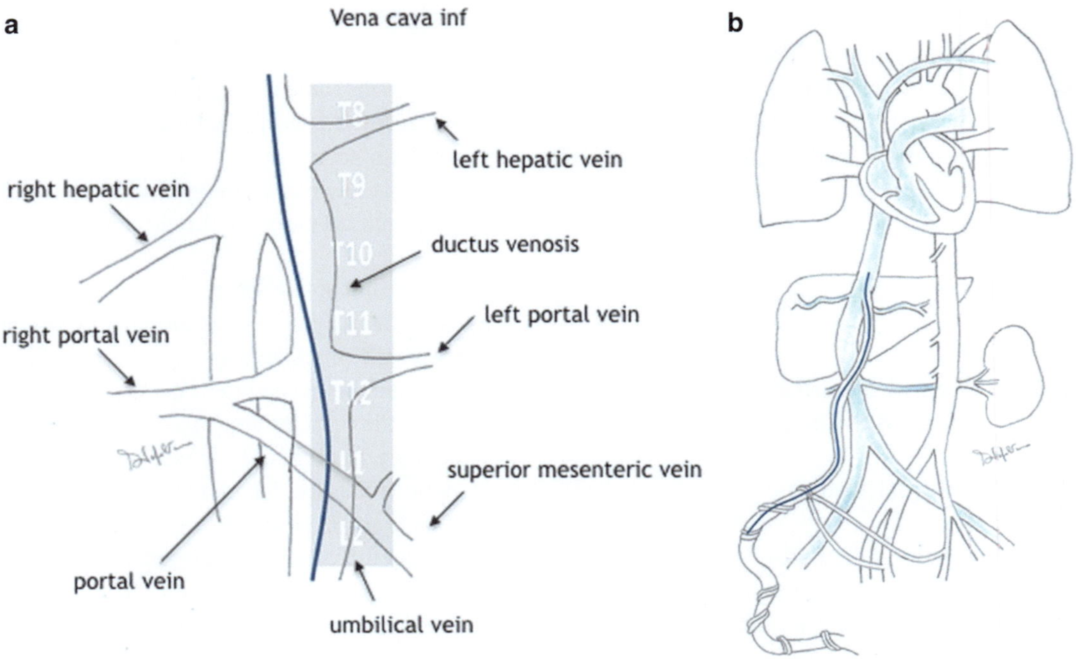

Fig. 6.4 (**a**, **b**) Schematic anatomy of venous umbilical vein and *right* position of the umbilical venous catheter

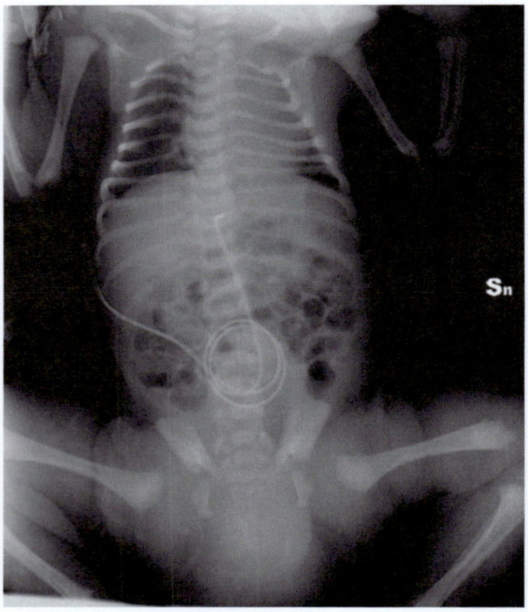

Fig. 6.5 Umbilical venous catheter: wrong position with the tip in the *left* main portal vein

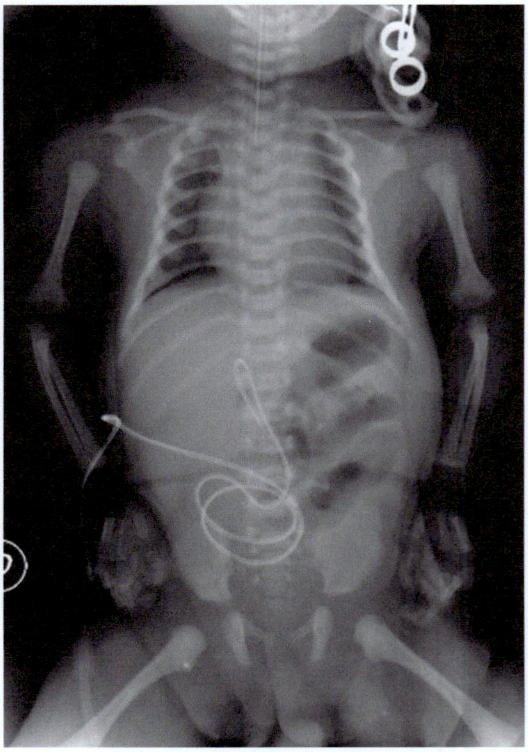

Fig. 6.6 Umbilical venous catheter: wrong position, coiling inside the inferior vena cava

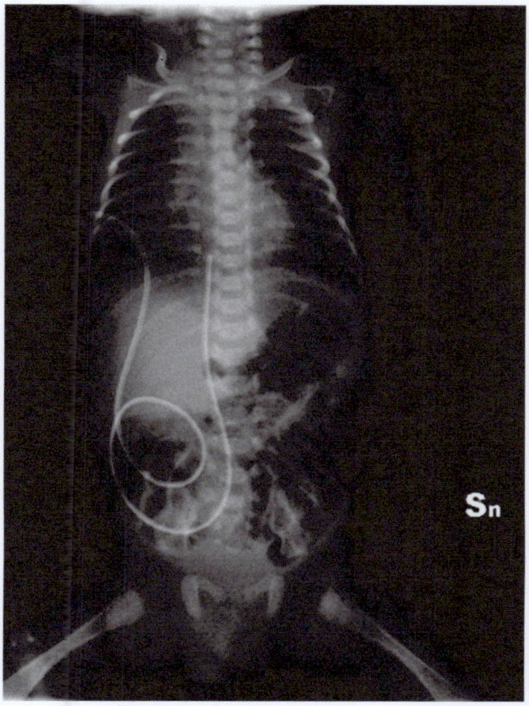

Fig. 6.7 Umbilical venous catheter: *right* position inside the inferior cava vein, radiologically projecting at the diaphragm

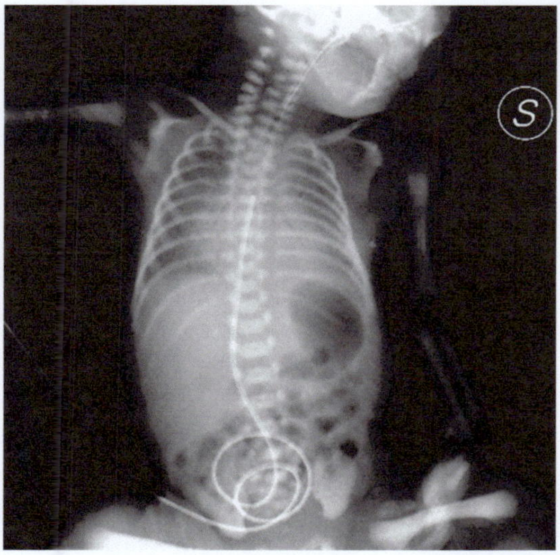

Fig. 6.8 Umbilical venous catheter: wrong position with the tip inside the heart

infections. Gram-positive organisms were the prominent organisms found, with coagulase-negative *Staphylococcus* being the most common.

We just discussed previously as a misplaced catheter could cause traumatic hematoma with

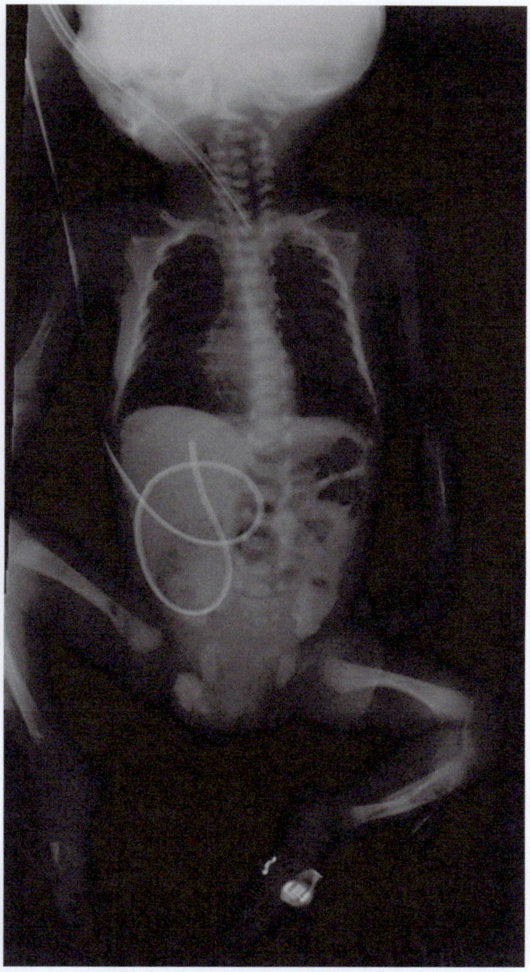

Fig. 6.9 Umbilical venous catheter: wrong position inside the right portal vein

the further possibility of infection. It is important to perform abdominal ultrasound when there is the suspect of intrahepatic hematoma or abscess; if the diagnosis is not clear, CT or MR with endogenous contrast should be performed to obtain a correct diagnosis and localization of the lesion (Miele et al. 2002a, b). Liver hematomas should be treated with removal of the UVC and with a wait and watch approach, monitoring the natural resolution, which usually results in calcification and resolution of the hematoma within 2–18 months. An infectious process including a liver abscess should be observed after removal of the catheter and performed antibiotic therapy (Fuchs and Sweeney 2014) (Figs. 6.13 and 6.14).

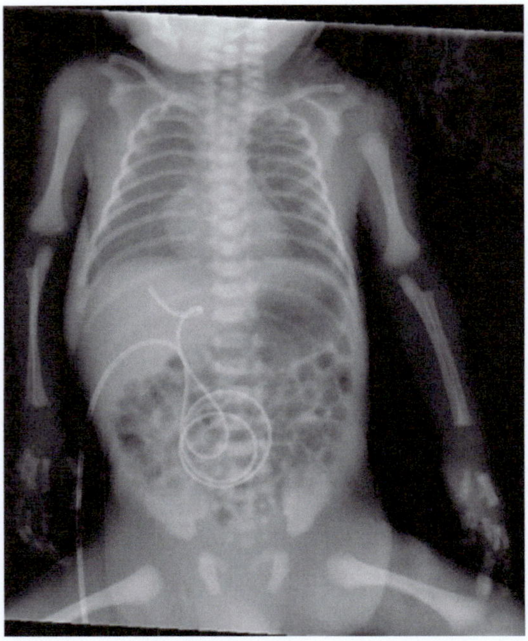

Fig. 6.10 Umbilical venous catheter: wrong position inside the right portal vein

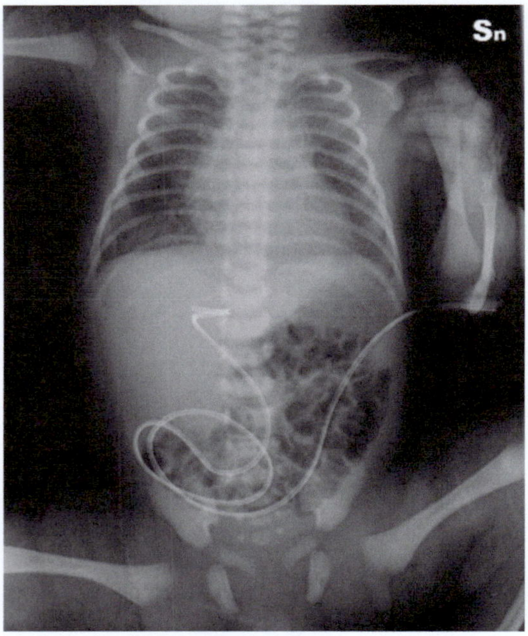

Fig. 6.11 Umbilical venous catheter: wrong position inside the right portal vein

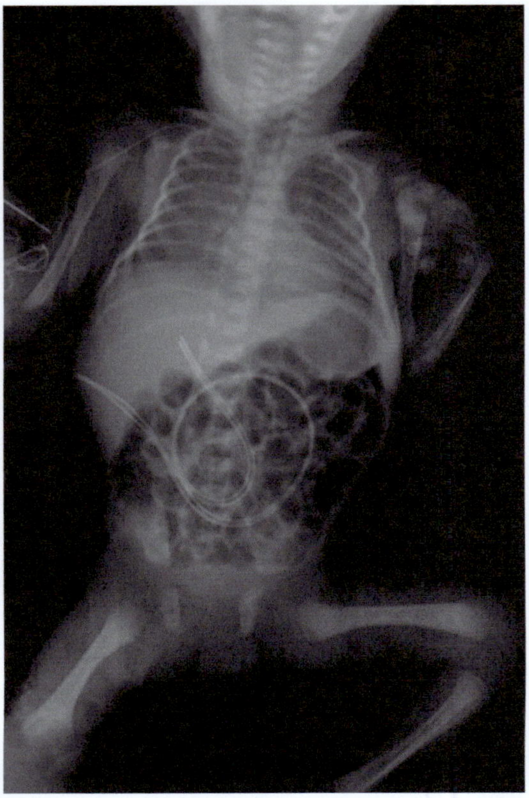

Fig. 6.12 Umbilical venous catheter: wrong position inside the right portal vein

6.3.3.3 Embolic Complications

Embolic complications are strictly linked to vascular endothelial lesions, reduction of hematic flow, and hypercoagulability.

If the complication is limited to the portal system, there are direct consequences for the liver, in terms of vascularization and parenchymal suffering.

If the problem occurs in the venous duct, there should be complication for the pulmonary circle and for all the organs, due to embolism. There is a higher mortality if thrombosis occurs in the right atrium or in the superior cava vein. Prognosis is generally good with a rapid diagnosis if the catheter is removed quickly.

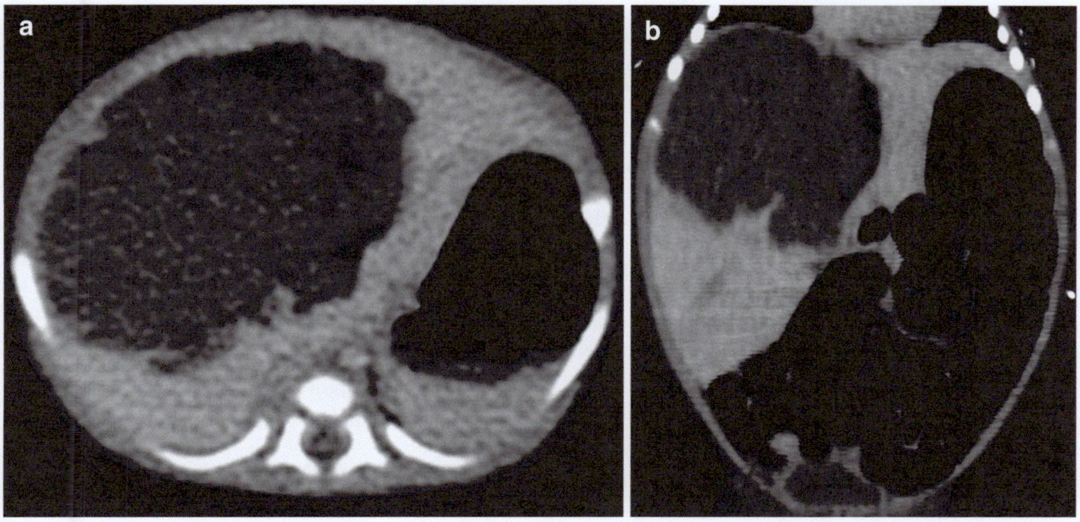

Fig. 6.13 (**a**, **b**) CT imaging of the liver of a neonatal with voluminous abscess (axial and coronal MPR reconstruction)

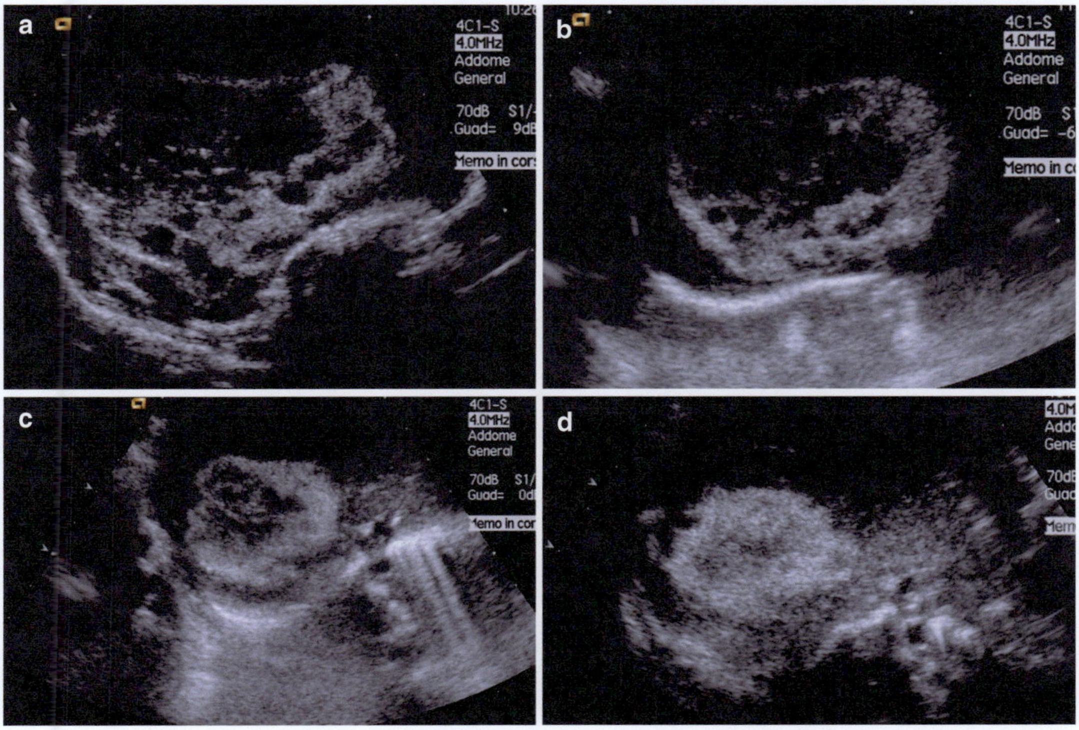

Fig. 6.14 (**a–d**) US imaging of the liver of a neonatal with voluminous abscess: different follow-up exams demonstrating the reduction of the mass and its progressive calcification

References

Dalley AF, Agur AM (2011) Clinically oriented anatomy, 6th edn. Lippincott Williams & Wilkins, Churchill Livingstone

Fang JC, Hilden K, Holubkov R, DiSario JA (2005) Transnasal endoscopy vs. fluoroscopy for the placement of nasoenteric feeding tubes in critically ill patients. Gastrointest Endosc 62:661–666

Foote JA, Kemmeter PR, Prichard PA et al (2004) A randomized trial of endoscopic and fluoroscopic placement of postpyloric feeding tubes in critically ill patients. JPEN J Parenter Enteral Nutr 28:154–157

Fuchs EM, Sweeney AG (2014) Umbilical venous catheter-induced hepatic hematoma. J Neonatal Perinatal Med 7:137–142

Grizelj R, Vukovic J, Bojanic K, Loncarevic D, Stern-Padovan R, Filipovic-Grcic B et al (2014) Severe liver injury while using umbilical venous catheter: case series and literature review. Am J Perinatol 31:965–974

Hermansen MC, Hermansen MG (2005a) Pitfalls in neonatal resuscitation. Clin Perinatol 32:77–95

Hermansen MC, Hermansen GM (2005b) Intravascular catheter complications in the neonatal intensive care unit. Clin Perinatol 32:141–156

Horn LM (1991) Evaluation of umbilical catheter and tube placement in premature infants. Radiographics 11:849–863

Hunter TB, Taljanovic MS (2005) Medical devices of the abdomen and pelvis. Radiographics 25:503–523

Itkin M, Delegge MH, Fang JC, Mc Clave SA, Kundu S, Janne B, et al (2011) Multidisciplinary practical guidelines for gastrointestinal access for enteral nutrition and decompression from the society of interventional radiology and American Gastroenterological Association (AGA) Institute, with endorsement by Canadian Interventional Radiological Association (CIRA) and Cardiovascular and Interventional Radiological Society of Europe (CIRSE) oral or nasal enteric tubes. JVIR [Internet]. Elsevier Inc 22(8):1089–1106

Johnston RD, O'Dell L, Patrick M, Cole AT, Cunliffe RN (2008) Outcome of patients fed via nasogastric tube retained with bridle loop. Do bridle loops reduce the requirement for percutaneous endoscopic gastrostomy insertion and 30-day mortality. Proc Nutr Soc 67:E116

Merten DF, Mumford L, Fliston HC, Brumley GW Jr, Effmann EL (1980) Radiological observations during transpyloric tube feeding in infants of low birth weight. Radiology 136:67–75

Miele V, Andreoli C, De Cicco ML, Adami L, David V (2002a) Hemoretroperitoneum associated with liver bare area injuries: CT evaluation. Eur Radiol 12:765–769

Miele V, Andreoli C, Cortese A, De Cicco ML, Luzietti M, Stasolla A, David V (2002b) Hemoperitoneum following ovarian cyst rupture: CT usefulness in the diagnosis. Radiol Med 104:122–126

Ott DJ, Mattox HE, Gelfand DW, Chen MY, Wu WC (1991) Enteral feeding tubes: placement by using fluoroscopy and endoscopy. AJR Am J Roentgenol 157:769–771

Pobiel RS, Bisset GS, Pobiel MS (1994) Nasojejunal feeding tube placement in children: four-year cumulative experience. Radiology 190:127–129

Rosen MS, Reich SB (1970) Umbilical venous catheterization in the newborn: identification of correct positioning. Radiology 95:335–340

7 Biliary Atresia and Choledochal Cyst

Lidia Monti, Amato Infante, and Marco Salsano

7.1 Introduction

Biliary atresia (BA) and choledochal cyst (CC) are two well-known causes of obstructive jaundice in neonates and young infants and have similar clinical presentation.

BA is a progressive obstructive cholangiopathy diagnosed in the newborn period and characterized by partial or complete lack of the extrahepatic bile ducts.

CC is a dilatation of the biliary tract due to congenital anomaly of the bile duct; it is usually present prior to the age of 2 years and can be antenatally diagnosed.

Patients with BA or CC usually have jaundice and acholic stools in the neonatal or young infantile period.

However, BA and CC are two entities with dramatically different approaches and prognosis. While BA requires portoenterostomy, CC is usually treated by cyst excision with hepaticojejunostomy or choledochojejunostomy. Children with BA usually have poor long-term prognoses even after Kasai portoenterostomy.

L. Monti (✉)
Department of Diagnostic Imaging, Children's Hospital Bambino Gesù, Rome, Italy
e-mail: lidia.monti@opbg.net

A. Infante • M. Salsano
Department of Radiological Sciences, Institute of Radiology, Catholic University of Sacred Heart, Rome, Italy

Although most patients who undergo surgery before 60 days of age show good bile excretion, ultimately many of them develop cirrhosis and liver failure.

Conversely, patients with CC have good outcomes with early surgical management. Because of the difference in management and prognosis between BA and CC, radiologic, particularly ultrasonographic (US), differentiation of the two entities is important.

In almost 10 % of BA cases, there is a cyst at the porta hepatis. For this reason BA with cystic component is likely to be mistaken for CC.

This short review attempts to summarize the imaging modalities of the two entities, in order to differentiate them. This is of paramount relevance in the differential diagnosis between cystic BA and CC.

7.2 Biliary Atresia

BA is an inflammatory cholangiopathy that results in progressive fibrosis and obliteration of extrahepatic and intrahepatic bile ducts and is the most frequent and severe cause of neonatal cholestasis affecting approximately 1 on 10,000–20,000 births.

The inflammatory process of the biliary tree leads to progressive obliterative scarring of the bile ducts. In BA the extrahepatic biliary system is disrupted. Progressive damage of extrahepatic

V. Miele, M. Trinci (eds.), *Imaging Non-traumatic Abdominal Emergencies in Pediatric Patients*,
DOI 10.1007/978-3-319-41866-7_7

and intrahepatic bile ducts secondary to inflammation occurs, leading to fibrosis, biliary cirrhosis, and liver failure. Although the exact etiology remains unknown, the primary therapy is surgical. Only early surgical treatment can stall biliary cirrhosis, which is why rapid identification of BA is crucial.

Previously, the disease was described as occurring in two distinct clinical forms: the fetal-embryonic form (or syndromic) and the perinatal (or acquired) disease. The fetal-embryonic form is characterized by early cholestasis; it appears in the first 2 weeks of life and accounts for 10–35 % of all cases. In this form, the bile ducts are discontinuous at birth, and 10–20 % of affected neonates have associated congenital malformations, such as polysplenia (100 %), situs inversus (50 %), or cardiac anomalies (50 %), and/or vascular malformations, e.g., preduodenal portal vein (60 %). The perinatal form of BA accounts for the remaining 65–90 % cases. This form is typically found in neonates and infants aged 2–8 weeks. Progressive inflammation and obliteration of the extrahepatic bile ducts occur after birth. This form is not associated with congenital anomalies, and infants may have a short jaundice-free interval.

Cases of BA can be stratified (Kasai classification system) according to their location of the involvement and degree of pathology. *Three main types* of biliary atresia are defined. Type I is characterized by the obliteration of the common bile duct, while the proximal bile ducts are patent. In type II, atresia of the hepatic duct is seen, with cystic bile ducts found at the porta hepatis. In type IIa, the cystic and common bile ducts are patent, whereas in type IIb, the cystic, common bile duct, and hepatic ducts are obliterated. Type III atresia refers to discontinuity of the right and left hepatic ducts to the level of the porta hepatis. This form of BA is common, accounting for more than 90 % of cases.

Diagnosis of BA and performance of a hepatoportoenterostomy (HPE; Kasai procedure) by 8–10 weeks of age are optimal for transplant-free survival beyond early childhood. It is thought that approximately 80–90 % of currently affected infants will survive to adolescence following Kasai procedure.

Only 16 % of children with BA survive up to 2 years with their native liver if the total serum bilirubin measured 3 months after Kasai procedure is over 6 mg/dL, compared to 84 % for those with a total bilirubin less than 2 mg/dL.

Hepatobiliary scintigraphy has been used in the diagnosis of BA for many years, but actually only in controversial cases because of the introduction of other diagnostic imaging modalities.

7.3 Diagnostic Imaging

In 2004, the Cholestasis Guideline Committee of the North American Society for Pediatric Gastroenterology, Hepatology, and Nutrition (NASPGHAN) examined the value of diagnostic tests in neonatal cholestasis. About hepatobiliary scintigraphy, these guidelines stated, "Although the high sensitivity for biliary atresia makes this a fairly good single test for detecting disease, it is time consuming and expensive and does have significant false positive and false-negative results. The Cholestasis Guideline Committee concludes that hepatobiliary scintigraphy generally adds little to the routine evaluation of the cholestatic infant but may be of value if other means for excluding biliary obstruction are not available."

In BA patients, although some imaging findings are highly suggestive of the disease, none is pathognomonic, and reliance on more than one test is common. Well-coordinated multidisciplinary approach is required in the assessment of suspected cases of BA.

A detailed abdominal *ultrasonography* (*US*) is generally the initial investigation in neonates with cholestatic disease.

It is used to evaluate the neonatal parenchyma and the hepatobiliary system and may exclude other anatomic anomalies.

US performed by operators with specific experience in the pediatric setting represents the first step. In BA the hepatic parenchyma is often inhomogeneous, with a marked increase in periportal echoes due to fibrosis (Fig. 7.1). Although dilatation of the intrahepatic bile duct occurs infrequently, it suggests BA when present.

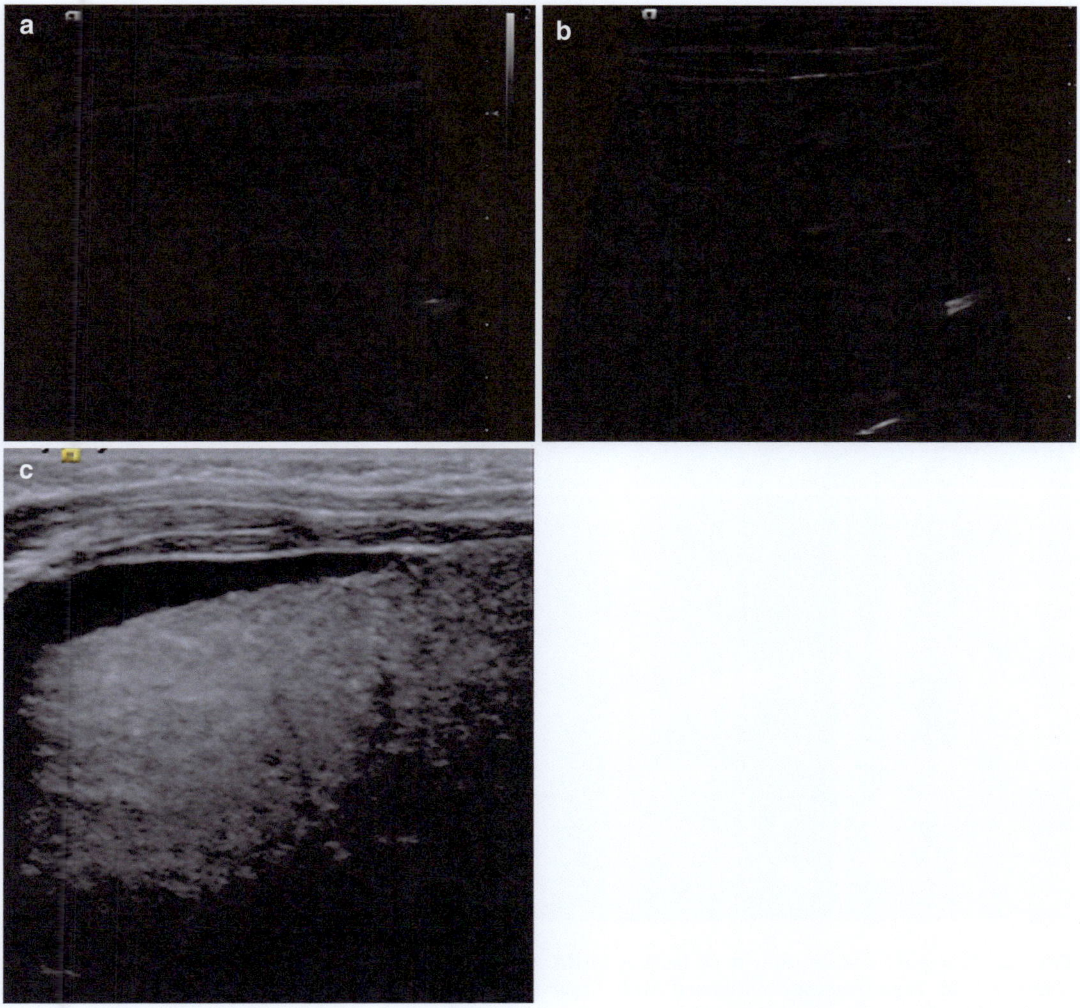

Fig. 7.1 High-frequency sonographic scans show normal glissonian profile and liver echogenicity in (**a**, **b**) and a micronodular glissonian profile and a hepatic inhomogeneous parenchyma due to fibrosis in BA. Note a small amount of perihepatic ascites in (**c**)

US shows the absence or the reduction in size of the gallbladder and the presence of a triangular cord (TC) sign (Fig. 7.2). The TC sign is defined as the thickness of 4 mm or more of the anterior wall of the right portal vein, seen near the portal bifurcation. It corresponds to the fibrosis of the extrahepatic biliary system. The identification of a TC sign results in a sensitivity of 80 %, a specificity of 98 %, a positive predictive value of 94 %, a negative predictive value of 94 %, and an accuracy of 94 % for diagnosing BA.

Numerous *other US features* have been used in the diagnosis of BA. In particular, abnormalities in the shape and wall of the gallbladder, enlargement of the hepatic artery diameter (a prominent hepatic artery is often seen in cirrhotic changes), measurement of portal vein diameter (Fig. 7.3), and enlargement of the liver and spleen are also helpful in diagnosis. The portal vein in children with BA is often hypoplastic and diseased, having intramural thrombi or intimal inflammation. Portal vein velocity also is often diminished in this group of children with BA due to steal effect from collateral shunts. In addition, assessing the hepatic arterial subcapsular flow by color Doppler US has recently been reported to

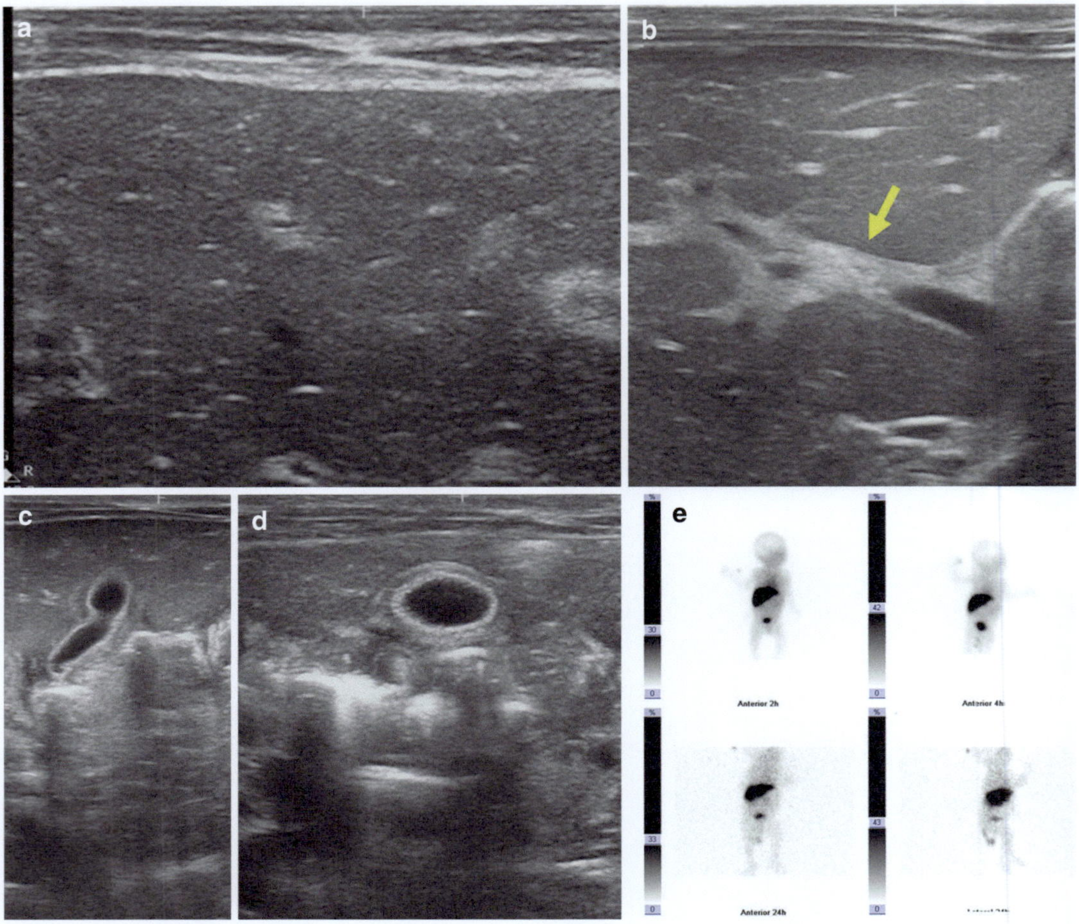

Fig. 7.2 Sonographic scans show main features of BA diagnosis. (**a**) High-frequency ultrasound with linear probe is used to evaluate the hepatic parenchyma. Transverse scan shows the hepatic parenchyma inhomogeneous, with a marked increase in periportal echoes due to fibrosis. (**b**) TC sign. Triangular- or tube-shaped echogenic focus at the porta hepatis that follows the portal veins more than 4 mm in thickness (*arrow*) that anatomically corresponds to the extrahepatic bile ducts replaced by a dense fibrous tissue. (**c**) Longitudinal ultrasound scan shows a normal gallbladder length >2 cm. (**d**) Transverse ultrasound scan depicts an irregular lining and wall of the gallbladder. (**e**) Hepatobiliary scintigraphy. Delayed static images performed at 2, 4, and 24 h confirm the absence of tracer passage in the bowel. Lateral projection is useful when a faint abdominal activity is evident

enable the discrimination of BA from other causes of cholestasis (Fig. 7.4). However, the correct weighting among these features remains unknown. Recently, high-frequency US has been shown to provide improved sensitivity, specificity, and accuracy for the diagnosis of BA.

Findings in BA typically include an atretic gallbladder and a thin, indistinct gallbladder wall (lack of smooth/complete echogenic mucosal lining with an indistinct wall) with an irregular or lobulated contour. Although a normal (1.5 cm) or long (>4 cm) gallbladder may be seen in up to 10 % of patients with BA, a length of less than 1.9 cm is most common. The constellation of findings constituting the gallbladder ghost triad are a gallbladder length less than 1.9 cm, a thin or indistinct gallbladder wall, and an irregular and lobulated contour (Fig. 7.5).

The triad is up to 97 % sensitive and up to 100 % specific for BA. We should note that the absence of gallbladder contraction is only suggestive of BA, as many as 20 % of BA neonates have normal gallbladder contraction. Furthermore, the

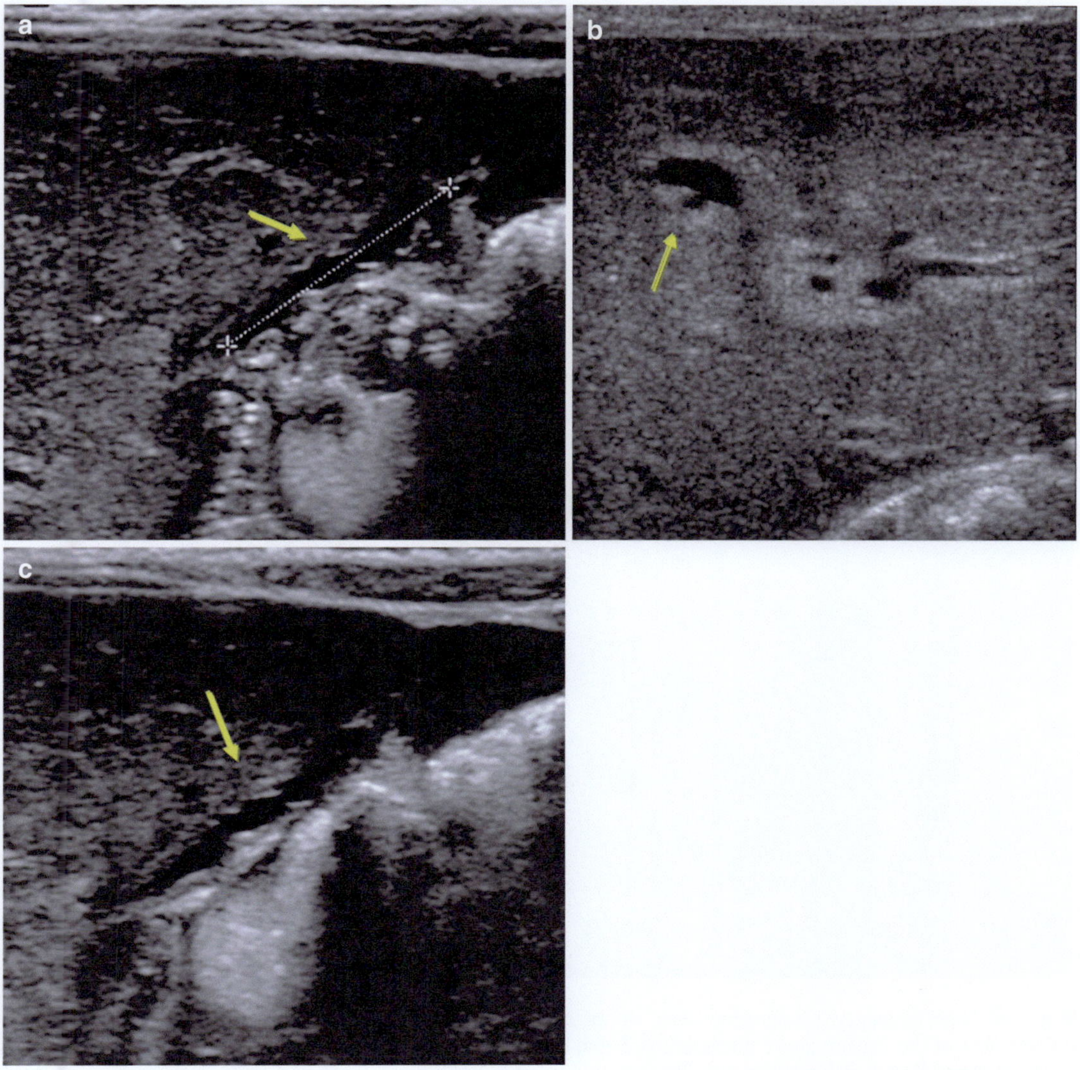

Fig. 7.3 Sonographic scans show the "gallbladder ghost triad." (**a**) Atretic gallbladder less than 1.9 cm in length; (**b**, **c**) thinned or lack of a smooth, complete echogenic mucosal lining with indistinct walls; knobbly, irregular, or lobular contour (*arrow* in **b**)

absence of gallbladder contraction is seen in children with cholestasis due to other causes.

An absent common bile duct is thought to be 93 % sensitive and 92 % specific for the diagnosis of BA.

Congenital anomalies may be present in BA. In particular, situs inversus and polysplenia are among the associated congenital anomalies that may be seen on sonograms.

Central biliary cysts and choledochal cysts may be associated with BA and are well depicted by US.

Shear-wave elastography (SWE) is the newest ultrasound-based technique and offers a noninvasive, nonionizing, low-cost, and well-tolerated approach to quantifying liver stiffness and presumably fibrosis. Although data are limited in children, SWE can be likely used to establish the presence of fibrosis as well as to assess the progression of liver fibrosis in BA over time (Fig. 7.6).

Magnetic resonance cholangiopancreatography (MRCP) is a noninvasive technique for

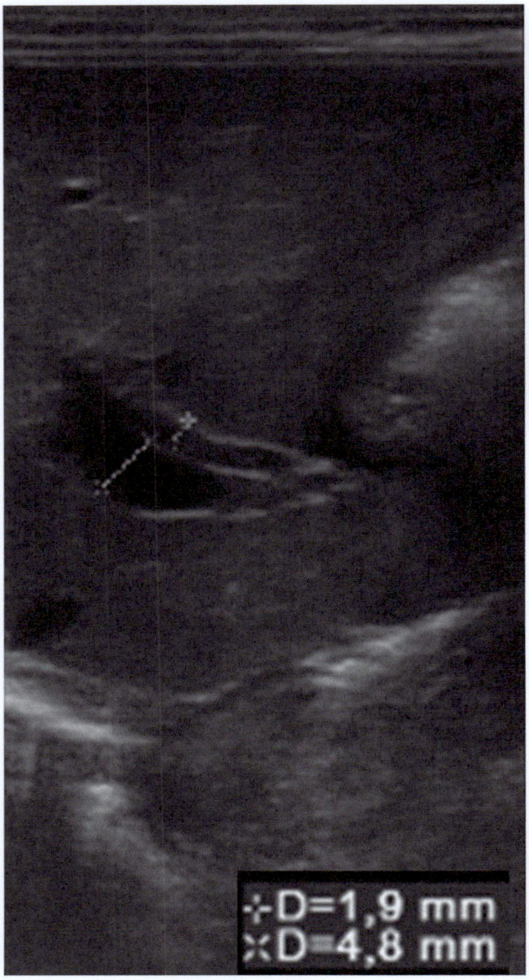

Fig. 7.4 High-frequency sonographic scan shows an enlargement of the hepatic artery diameter (>1.5 mm at the level of proximal right hepatic artery). This sign, combined with other US findings, can be highly suggestive of BA. The hepatic artery and portal vein are easily detectable structures in the porta hepatis as shown in this figure. In BA the ratio HA/PV is higher because of artery hypertrophy

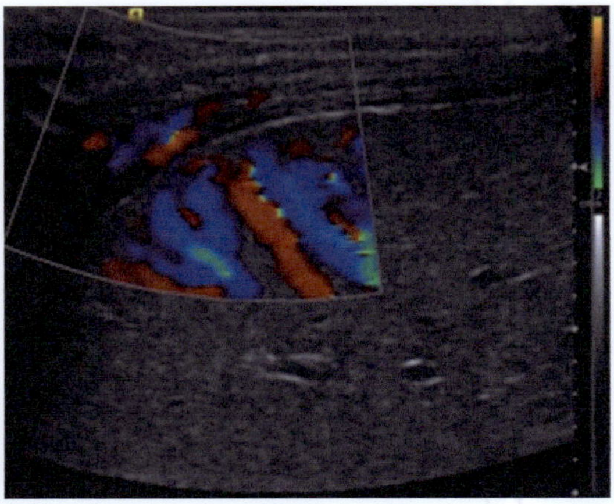

Fig. 7.5 Sonographic scan shows the increment of subcapsular flow in BA. It is a consequence of dilatation and hypertrophy of hepatic vessels in the subcapsular area, secondary to portal hypertension

neonatal imaging. Findings in infants with BA include incomplete visualization of the extrahepatic biliary system and periportal high signal intensity on T2-weighted magnetic resonance imaging (MRI) scans. These findings suggest cystic dilatation(s) of fetal bile ducts with surrounding fibrosis. Complete visualization of the extrahepatic biliary system excludes BA, whereas nonvisualization of the common or hepatic bile ducts suggests the disease. MRCP has not proved to be useful to exclude BA as the normal biliary tree is not consistently seen under the age of 3 months.

Endoscopic retrograde cholangiopancreatography (*ERCP*) is a diagnostic imaging modality in the young child. Although it is a rarely used invasive technique, results from a study by Petersen et al. led the investigators to recommend the ERCP to be performed before explorative laparotomy in all patients suspected of having BA. In the study, ERCP was performed in cholestatic patients younger than 6 months who were suspected of an extrahepatic cause of cholestasis, particularly BA. In this series, the sensitivity of ERCP for diagnosing BA was 92 % and the specificity was 73 %. The authors concluded that in preselected patients, ERCP, while not an alternative to noninvasive imaging, can be used to avoid surgery in approximately 25 % of cases. ERCP allows direct visualization of the extrahepatic biliary tree with the injection of radiologic contrast agent into the extrahepatic biliary system through the papilla of Vater. It requires a general anesthetic, substantial expertise, and the availability of sufficiently small endoscopes. This technique can show the obstruction in the common bile duct and enables visualization of the extrahepatic biliary system distal to the common hepatic duct and of the extrahepatic biliary system with bile lakes at the porta hepatis.

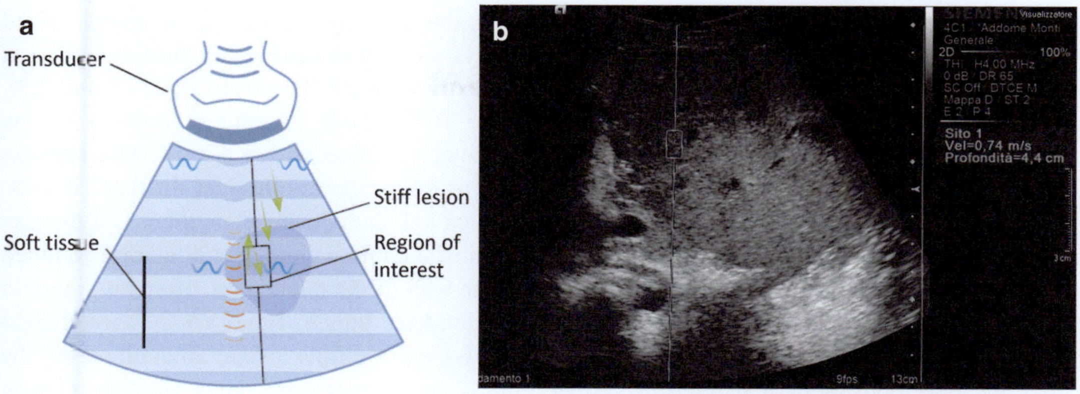

Fig. 7.6 (**a**) Schematic draft of ARFI technique. (**b**) In ARFI examination a preselected region of interest of 10×6 mm visualized in B-mode imaging is mechanically excited using short-duration, high-intensity, acoustic pulses to generate localized tissue displacement. The shear waves originated from the displacement area are tracked using US correlation-based methods. The shear-wave velocity, expressed in meters per second, is an intrinsic and reproducible property of tissue and is proportional to the square root of tissue elasticity, so stiffer tissue will have higher ARFI values. ARFI can be used to establish the presence of fibrosis as well as assess the progression of liver fibrosis in BA over time

Although an extraordinary evolution has been achieved by the noninvasive diagnostic tests, the gold standard in the diagnosis of BA remains the *percutaneous liver biopsy*. Liver biopsy is therefore used to confirm the diagnosis of BA. Pathologic examination remains an integral part of the diagnostic algorithm and, therefore, plays a pivotal role in the diagnostic evaluation of this disease. Liver biopsy leads to the diagnosis in 79–98 % of cases. However, liver histology at the time of HPE is of limited value in prognosis making in BA. We should note that biliary obstructive features obtained by US must be confirmed histologically and distinguished from various nonobstructive etiologies of neonatal cholestasis.

Percutaneous transhepatic cholangiography can be technically challenging, and the results are definitive only if a normal intrahepatic and extrahepatic biliary system is seen.

US-guided *percutaneous cholecystocholangiography* is a relatively new technique in which radiographic contrast material is injected into the gallbladder under US guidance, and the extrahepatic biliary system is viewed with fluoroscopy. Although invasive, the technique is easy to perform, and should be chosen when the preoperative imaging is lacking or inconclusive.

Intraoperative cholangiography is typically performed by injecting contrast material through the gallbladder. The procedure is performed in a preliminary phase at the surgical exploration during the Kasai procedure.

BA is diagnosed if there is no communication between the biliary tree and the gastrointestinal tract.

7.4 Prognosis

BA is universally fatal if untreated and is the single most common cause of liver disease leading to liver transplantation in children representing at least 50 % of all pediatric liver transplantation.

Post-HPE complications include ongoing cholestasis, cholangitis, portal hypertension with or without variceal hemorrhage, poor weight gain, fat-soluble vitamin deficiencies, hepatopulmonary syndrome, portopulmonary hypertension, and rarely hepatocellular carcinoma.

The cases that failed Kasai procedure should be referred for *liver transplantation* (*LT*) and should be transplanted according to their level of liver failure. In specialized institutions, reported overall survival in BA patients who underwent Kasai procedure followed by LT is 100 %.

In summary, US is generally the initial investigation in neonates with cholestatic disease, adds important information, and indicates further steps. Histology remains the gold standard. However, in the clinical practice, intraoperative cholangiogram should be performed in cases with absence of definitive characterization and guide the surgical management.

Ultrasonography is a powerful tool for diagnosis of BA in cholestatic neonates.

Next step for identification of BA should consider the development of a diagnostic system based on the definition of minor and major criteria including clinical, laboratoristic, and ultrasonographic findings, in order to bypass liver biopsy and direct the patient straight to the Kasai procedure.

7.5 Choledochal Cyst

Choledochal cyst (CC) is a rare development anomaly consisting in a *cystic dilatation of the biliary tract*. The incidence of CC in the Western population is 1 in 100,000–150,000 live births, although it is more frequent in Asian populations with a reported incidence of 1 in 1,000, with two-thirds of CC diagnosed in Japan. However, the reason for this geographic distribution is unknown. Although CC may be discovered at any age, the 60 % is diagnosed in children younger than 10 years old. There is a strong female predilection with a M:F ratio of 1:4.

The etiology of CC remains uncertain but Babbitt's *theory* is widely accepted. This theory attributes CC formation to the presence of an abnormally long pancreaticobiliary junction outside the ampulla of Vater (at least longer than 1.5 cm) draining pancreatic and bile duct. The reflux of pancreatic juice into the bile duct activates pancreatic enzymes, causing inflammation, cholangitis, and bile duct wall destruction, with subsequent distal stenosis due to scarring and ductal dilatation.

The *Todani classification system* is widely accepted and currently used (Fig. 7.7). Type I CCs, the most common type, are characterized by cystic-focal or fusiform-diffuse dilatation of the extrahepatic biliary tree (Figs. 7.8 and 7.9). Type II CCs are discrete diverticula of the extrahepatic ducts with a narrow stalk connection to the common bile duct. In type III CCs, also called choledochoceles, there is a distinctive distal common bile duct dilatation confined to the wall of the duodenum, often bulging into the duodenal lumen. Type IVA CCs are characterized by multiple cystic dilatations of the intra- and extrahepatic ducts with stricture at the junction. Type IVB CCs involve multiple dilatations of the extrahepatic ducts only. In type V CCs, there are multiple saccular or cystic dilatations of the intrahepatic bile ducts. This condition is also known as Caroli disease (Fig. 7.10). This is an autosomal recessive inherited disorder characterized by congenital ductal plate malformation. Some patients develop hepatic fibrosis, and when associated with renal abnormalities, such as medullary sponge kidney or autosomal dominant polycystic kidney disease, some refer to this entity as Caroli syndrome.

7.6 Clinical Findings

The clinical findings of congenital hepatic fibrosis are portal hypertension, predominant splenomegaly, and varices with spontaneous gastrointestinal hemorrhage. MRI is the most sensitive method for evaluating the biliary tree and the renal anomalies associated to congenital hepatic fibrosis. MRCP does not show any shrinking of the intrahepatic biliary ducts, which remain enlarged throughout the liver parenchyma, often forming cyst-like areas (ductal ectasia).

In addition, central biliary cysts and CC may be associated with BA and are well depicted on sonograms (Fig. 7.11). However, cystic BA and CC are two entities with radically different approach and prognosis. While

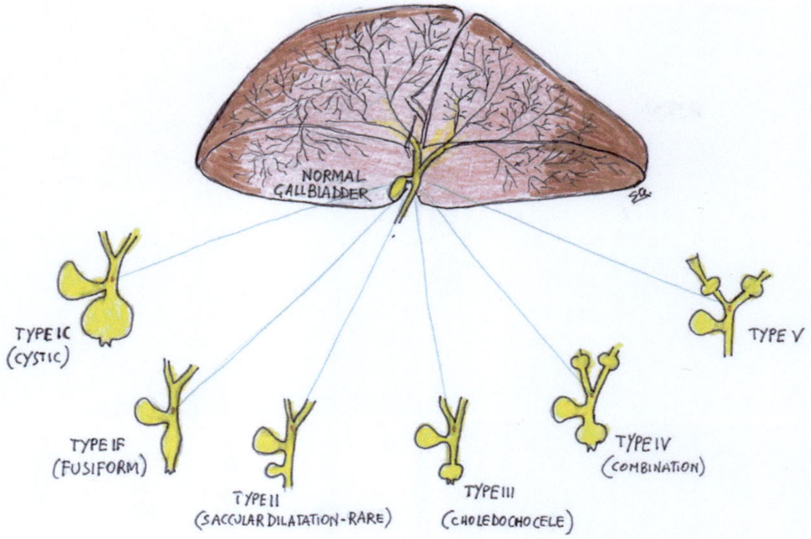

Fig. 7.7 Types of CC according to the Todani classification. Type I CC makes up the majority, approximately 70–90 %, of CC. They are characterized by cystic (c) or fusiform (f) dilatation of the extrahepatic bile ducts – subtypes: IA is a cystic dilatation with associated anomalous pancreaticobiliary junction (APBJ), IB is a segmental dilatation without APBJ, and IC is diffuse, fusiform dilatation with associated anomalous pancreaticobiliary junction (APBJ). *Type II* CC are rare, comprising only 2–3 % of all CC. They manifest as an extrahepatic biliary diverticulum without APBJ. *Type III* CC (or choledochoceles) is also uncommon, making up 1–5 % of all CC, and is characterized by dilatation of the intraduodenal part of the common bile duct and is not associated with APBJ. *Type IV* CC is the second most common type, making up 10–20 % of all CC, the majority of which are type IVA. They are characterized by intra- and extrahepatic fusiform or cystic dilatation of the bile ducts. Type IVA choledochal cysts have intra- and extrahepatic biliary ductal dilatation and are usually associated with APBJ. Type IVB CC is rare and appears as multiple extrahepatic cysts. *Type V* CC, otherwise known as Caroli disease, are characterized by multifocal segmental intrahepatic biliary ductal dilatation

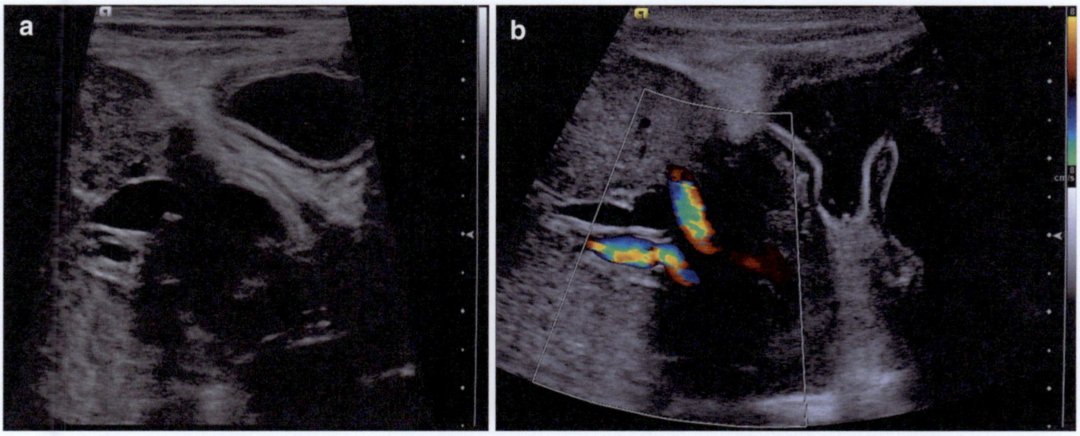

Fig. 7.8 Choledochal cyst: US scans. Type IC cysts are smooth fusiform dilations of the entire extrahepatic bile duct (**a**) usually extending from the pancreaticobiliary junction to the intrahepatic biliary tree. (**b**) Color Doppler US identifies vascular structures

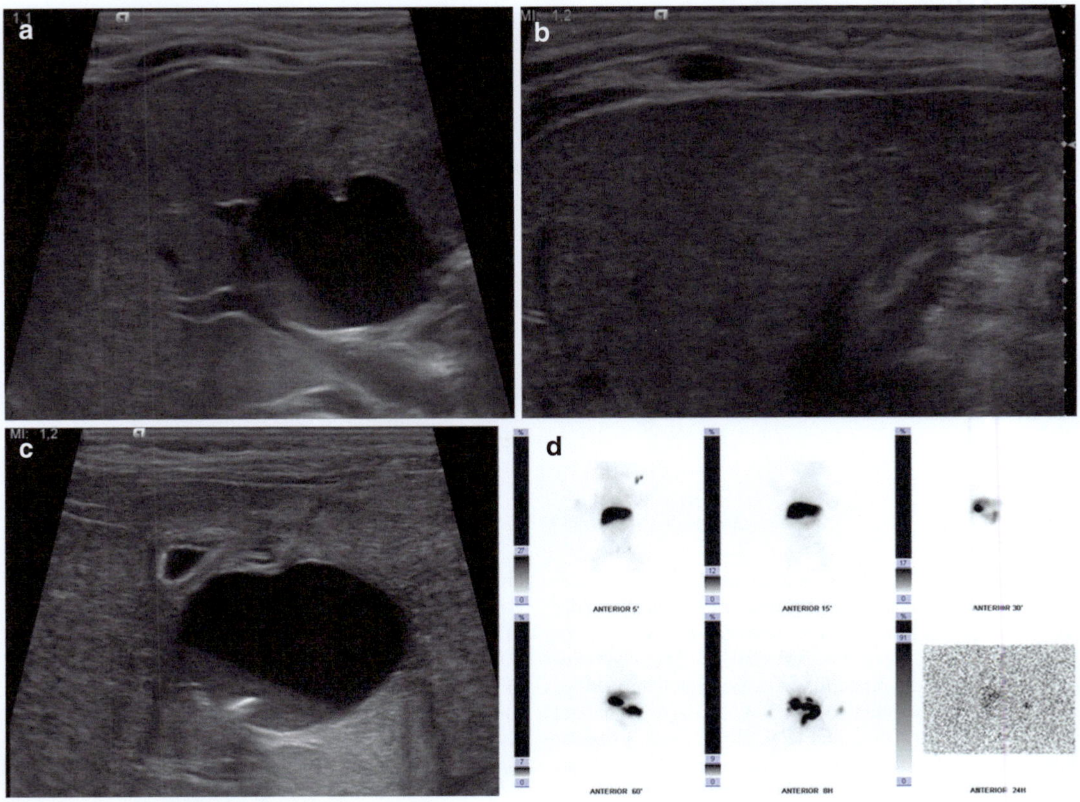

Fig. 7.9 (**a**–**d**) CC type I: US scans. Dilated intrahepatic ducts and normal gallbladder above the cyst demonstrates the continuity with the bile duct. Cyst is associated with sludge deposits. Treatment of choice is complete excision of the involved portion of the extrahepatic bile duct; a Roux-en-Y hepaticojejunostomy is performed to restore biliary-enteric continuity. (**d**) Hepatobiliary scintigraphy: time-sequential static images are performed up to 4 h after tracer administration showing intense and homogeneous hepatic uptake of tracer with normal heart/liver ratio at 5 min. By visual imaging evaluation, a photon-deficient area in the porta hepatis is detected with progressive biliary tracer filling up to the late image (performed at 8 h) and subsequent decreased activity at 24 h. Tracer transit in the bowel is observed at 30 min after tracer administration, whereas gallbladder was not clearly seen, probably due to the compression of the large choledochal cysts. Physiological urinary excretion is observed. According to the ultrasound scan, the nuclear medicine finding is compatible with choledochal cysts

portoenterostomy is required for cystic BA, cyst excision with hepaticojejunostomy or choledochojejunostomy is usually performed for CC. Because of the different management, radiologic, particularly ultrasonographic (US), differentiation of the two entities is important (Fig 7.12). We should note there is no difference in age between cystic BA and CC, but in both conditions, there is a female preponderance. All patients with cystic BA have jaundice and acholic stools at presentation.

7.7 Diagnostic Imaging

US criteria for differentiating the two diseases are the presence of a focal cystic dilatation and the measurement of gallbladder length. US shows abnormally small gallbladders in BA patients, whereas the gallbladder is normal or slightly distended in the CC. Cystic dilatation is usually small and focal in patients with cystic BA as it occurs at the residual portion of the common bile duct. Intrahepatic bile ducts are

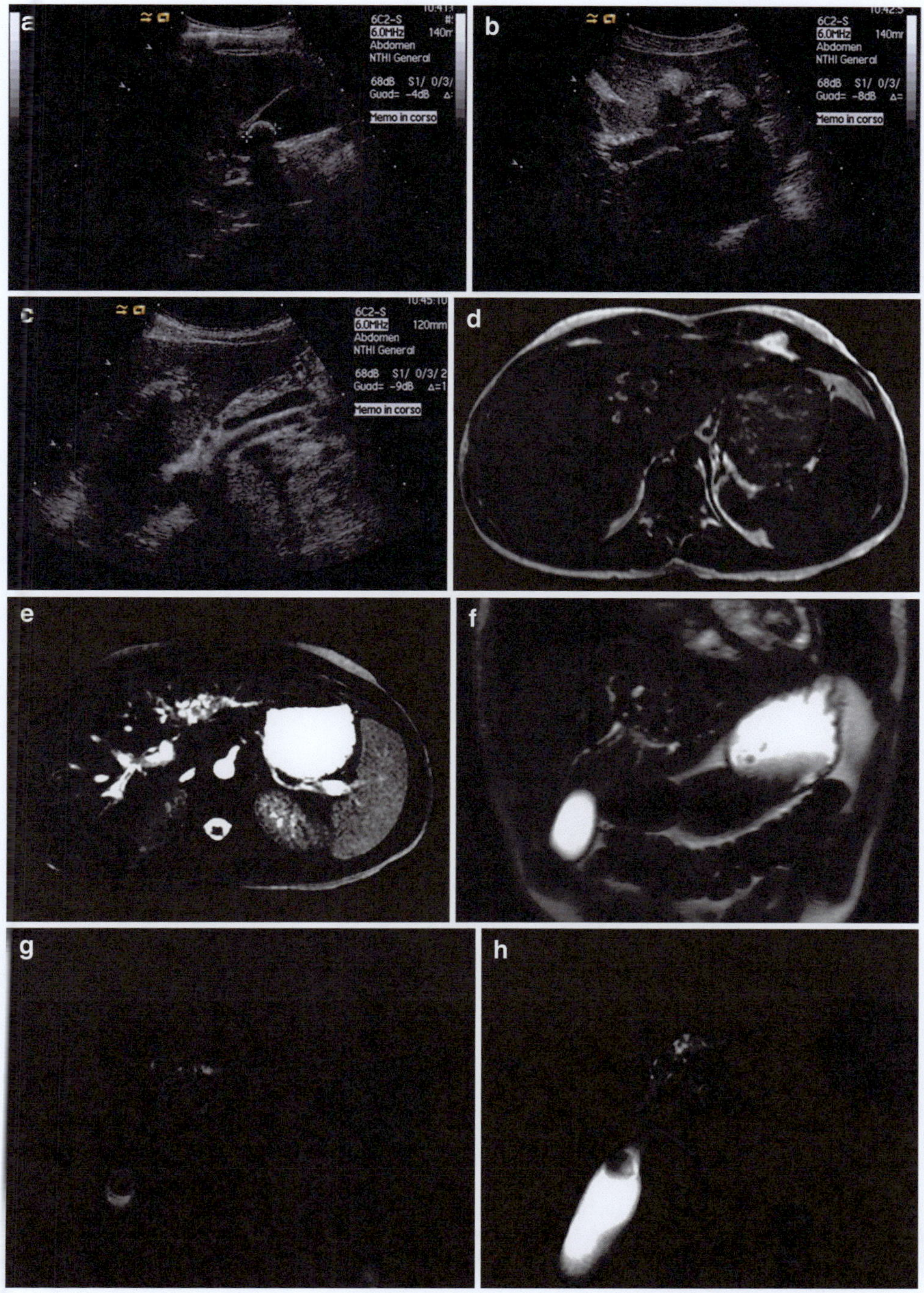

Fig. 7.10 Caroli disease. US scans (**a–c**) demonstrate intrahepatic saccular dilatation with no underlying obstruction or extrahepatic biliary tree involvement and cholelithiasis. MRI (**d–f**): axial and coronal T2-weighted images demonstrate intrahepatic biliary ductal dilation isolated to the left lobe of the liver, with rounded hypointense filling defects in the bile ducts consistent with stones. The liver parenchyma in the left lobe is asymmetrically T2 hyperintense. MR cholangiopancreatography (**g-i**) shows multiple saccular or cystic dilatations of the intrahepatic bilie ducts. See also cholelithiasis

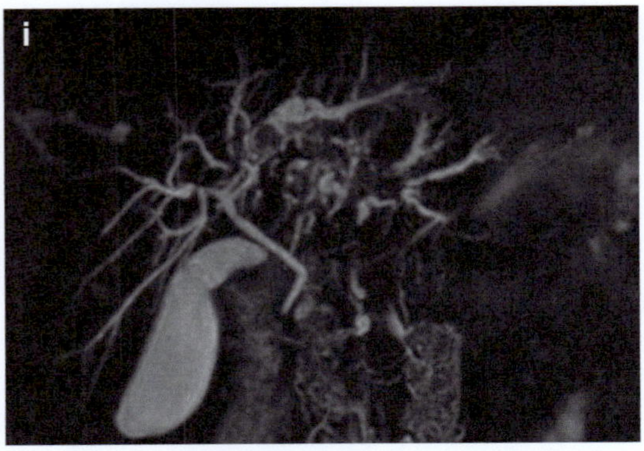

Fig. 7.10 (continued)

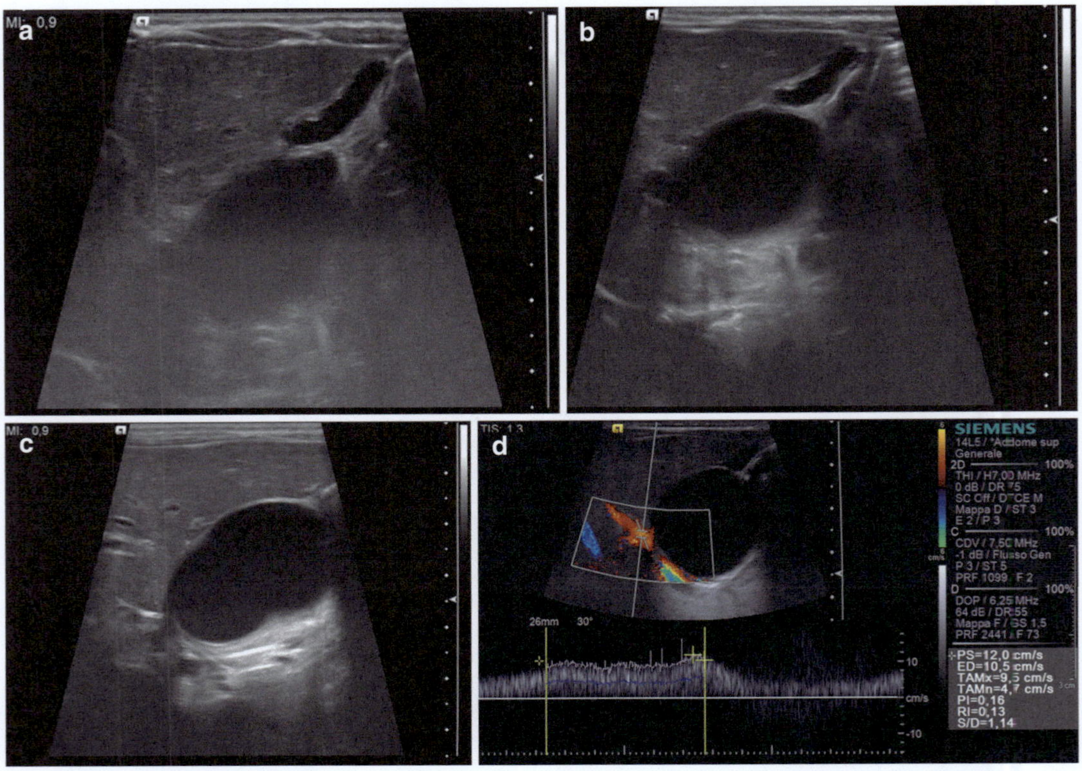

Fig. 7.11 Cystic biliary atresia (CBA). (**a**, **b**) US shows a cystic structure in the *right* upper quadrant at the site of CBD apart from the gallbladder, irregularly elongated. The cystic dilation of the common bile duct doesn't involve the intrahepatic bile ducts. The cystic duct and gallbladder arise from the dilated common bile duct. (**c**, **d**) US shows the presence of a triangular cord sign in the porta hepatis and the enlargement of the hepatic artery diameter. The portal flow is reduced. CC in the neonate may be associated with atresia of the distal common bile duct; CBA is an uncommon variant of BA in which prognosis may be relatively favorable but liable to misdiagnosis as CDC. It is classified into three types according to the Japanese classification system based on the atretic segment of bile duct into type 1 (distal atresia), type 2 (proximal atresia), and type 3 (complete atresia). The cyst can occur anywhere along the atretic segment and is proximal to atresia in types 1 and 2 and distal to it in type 3

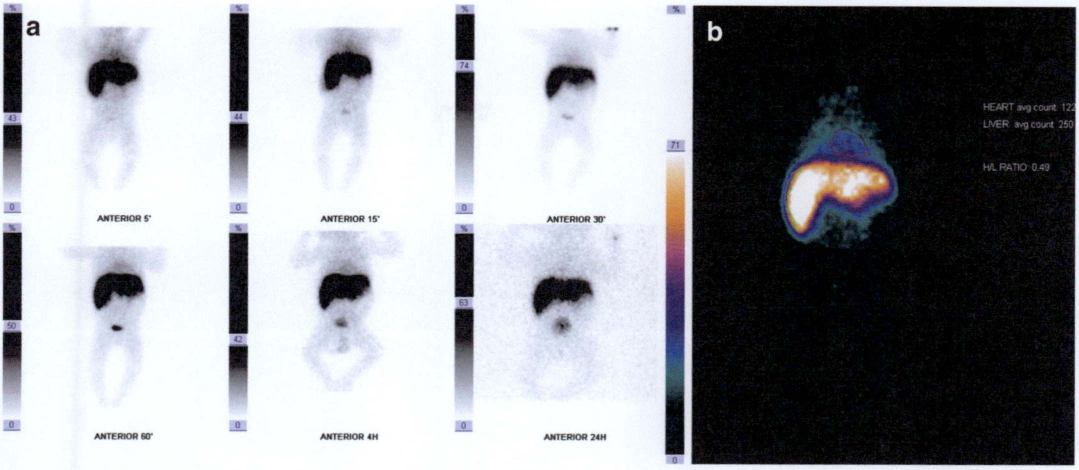

Fig. 7.12 Cystic biliary atresia (CBA). (**a**, **b**) Time-sequential static images are performed up to 24 h after tracer administration showing intense and homogeneous hepatic uptake of tracer with normal heart/liver ratio at 5 min. By visual imaging evaluation, an area devoid of tracer corresponding to CC (detected by US) is appreciable without biliary activity up to the study end. No evidence of tracer in the intestine up to 24 h is also detectable. Physiological urinary excretion is observed. Ultrasound scan of the abdomen showed evidence of a CC and sonographic signs suspicious of BA. Therefore, hepatobiliary scintigraphy was performed, and "no draining" of the radiolabeled tracer in the small bowel within 24 h was seen as in keeping with extrahepatic BA

instead typically dilated markedly and diffusely in patients with CC. Dilatation of the intrahepatic ducts is usually absent in patients with cystic BA because of the panductular or panductal sclerosis of the biliary tree. An early diagnosis is very important to ensure the effectiveness of the operation (Kasai procedure in BA patients and hepaticojejunostomy or choledochojejunostomy in CC patients).

The clinical presentation of CC includes sign related to abdominal mass often with abdominal pain. These features have been summarized in a specific triad (jaundice, abdominal mass, and abdominal pain). Although this triad is present in ~40 % (range 19–60 %) of cases, palpable mass is the least common manifestation.

Multiple imaging modalities can be used to diagnose CC including US, computed tomography (CT), magnetic resonance cholangiopancreatography (MRCP), endoscopic retrograde cholangiopancreatography (ERCP), and percutaneous transhepatic cholangiography (PTC) for exact measurements of size and ductal involvement allowing direct visualization of the pancreaticobiliary junction. In addition to its diagnostic yield, ERCP can be therapeutic by allowing biliary drainage and endoscopic sphincterotomy.

Abdominal US is the cornerstone of diagnostic tools for initial evaluation of children with suspected hepatobiliary disease.

It is a patient-friendly and radiation-free imaging modality.

The relative small size of the child and the fat-free intra-abdominal content results in improved penetration of the sound waves compared to adults, increasing the image quality. Furthermore, the ubiquitous availability of high-frequency transducers allows a better tissue differentiation and real-time evaluation. Optimal use of sonographic equipment is mandatory; the frequency of the emitted sound waves should be as high as possible to optimize imaging.

US can detect dilatation of the intrahepatic bile ducts in all patients with CC and can reach a correct diagnosis in up to 70 % of the patients, leading to an appropriate CC classification (Fig. 7.13).

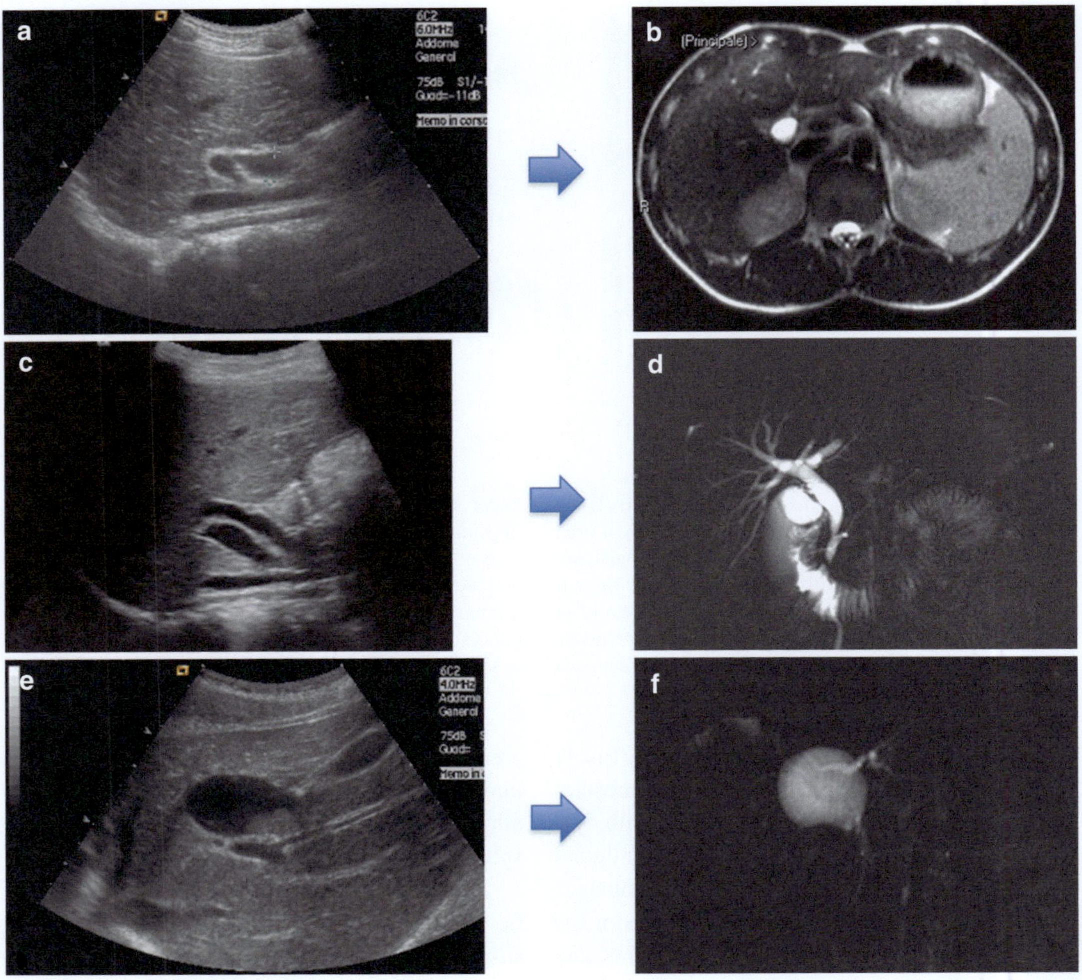

Fig. 7.13 US (**a**, **c**, **e**) and MRCP features (**b**, **d**, **f**). Anomalous pancreaticobiliary junction in a 1-year-old with elevated pancreatic enzymes and US findings of biliary dilatation (a, c). (b) axial T2-weighted half-Fourier acquisition single-shot turbo spin echo (HASTE), MRI reveals fusiform dilatation of the common bile duct, with a filling defect representing a stone distal to the pancreaticobiliary junction. (**d**) In coronal T2-weighted 3-D maximum-intensity projection, MRI shows a long common channel of 15 mm; the stone is lodged distal to the anomalous pancreaticobiliary junction, causing secondary pancreatitis with a dilated upstream pancreatic duct. (e) US shows a cystic biliary dilatation with sludge (f) MRCP appearance

CT is only used to assess other causes of biliary ductal dilatation (trauma and staging of malignancies). Furthermore, if CT is required (Fig. 7.14), it should be optimized in order to keep the radiation dose as low as reasonably achievable (ALARA).

The initial imaging modality of choice is US followed by MRCP. MRCP is a reliable and safe technique and *provides accurate evaluation of* the anatomy of the biliary tract (70–100 % sensitivity and 90–100 % specificity). MRCP has the advantage of simultaneously delineating both the biliary and pancreatic duct.

It can be helpful to demonstrate signs of associated chronic pancreatitis and, accordingly to the cholangiography morphology, to classify the images with high diagnostic accuracy for CC (Fig. 7.15).

MRCP can be used as an alternative modality for ERCP.

Because pediatric ducts are slim, their delineation is difficult and sometimes diagnosis is

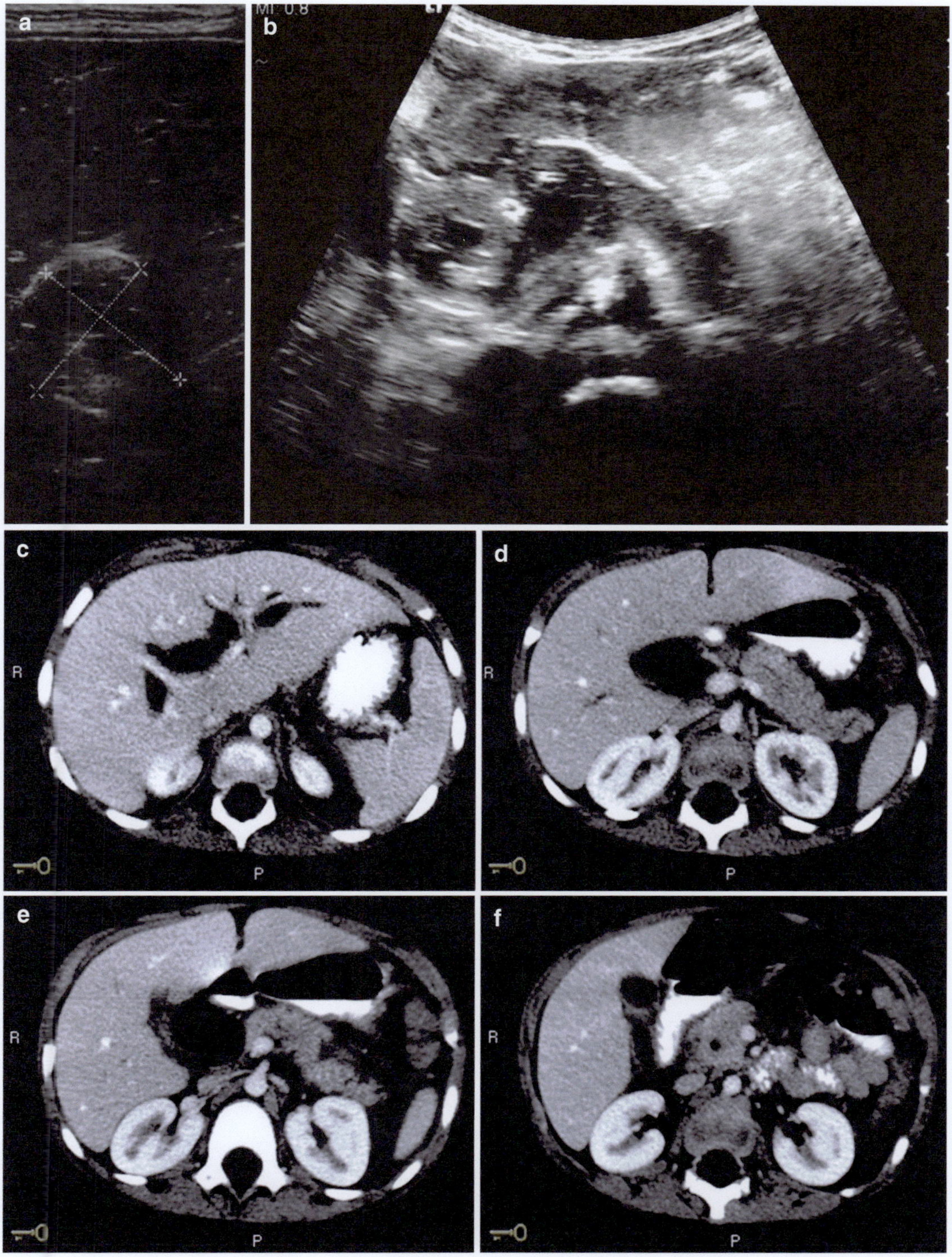

Fig. 7.14 Biliary rhabdomyosarcoma. US scans (**a**, **b**) show a rounded heterogeneous cystic lesion at the liver hilum arising from the common bile duct. CT scans of the abdomen (**c**–**f**) show a noncalcified heterogeneously enhancing mass (cystic-like) centered at the liver hilum. This intraductal mass causes marked intrahepatic ductal dilatation and dilatation of the common bile duct. There is no evidence of metastasis

challenging. To improve the diagnostic power of MRCP, we use secretin injection during the exam that stimulates the pancreatic exocrine activity, enhancing the visualization of both biliary and pancreatic ducts.

MR of the liver and pancreas in children have to be planned individually and tailored to the clinical question as well as the age, size, and cooperation of the child. Head or body phased-array coils are usually employed depending on the size of the child.

The standard protocol consists of T1- and T2-weighted (turbo) spin echo (TSE) sequences in the axial plane with breath-hold or respiratory gating. Other planes can be helpful, but it is seldom necessary to image in all three orthogonal planes. MRCP is typically acquired with both 2-D and 3-D techniques. Two-dimensional MRCP technique is performed using a heavily T2-weighted fat-suppressed single-shot turbo spin echo (TSE) with 40-mm slice thickness. Multiple thin slices can be obtained with half-Fourier acquisition single-shot turbo spin echo (HASTE) sequences, the most frequently used pulse sequences to obtain MRCP images demonstrating the pancreaticobiliary anatomy because of their rapid acquisition time, which enables MR image acquisition during breath-hold, virtually eliminating motion artifacts. MRCP images can be obtained during breath-hold and can be repeated frequently in order to obtain dynamic images. Breath-hold techniques, including single thick-slab and multiple thin-slab sequences, are faster and more suitable for the older children.

Two-dimensional MRCP images have the advantage of rapid acquisition. Three-dimensional MRCP images are acquired in the coronal plane using a 3-D TSE technique,

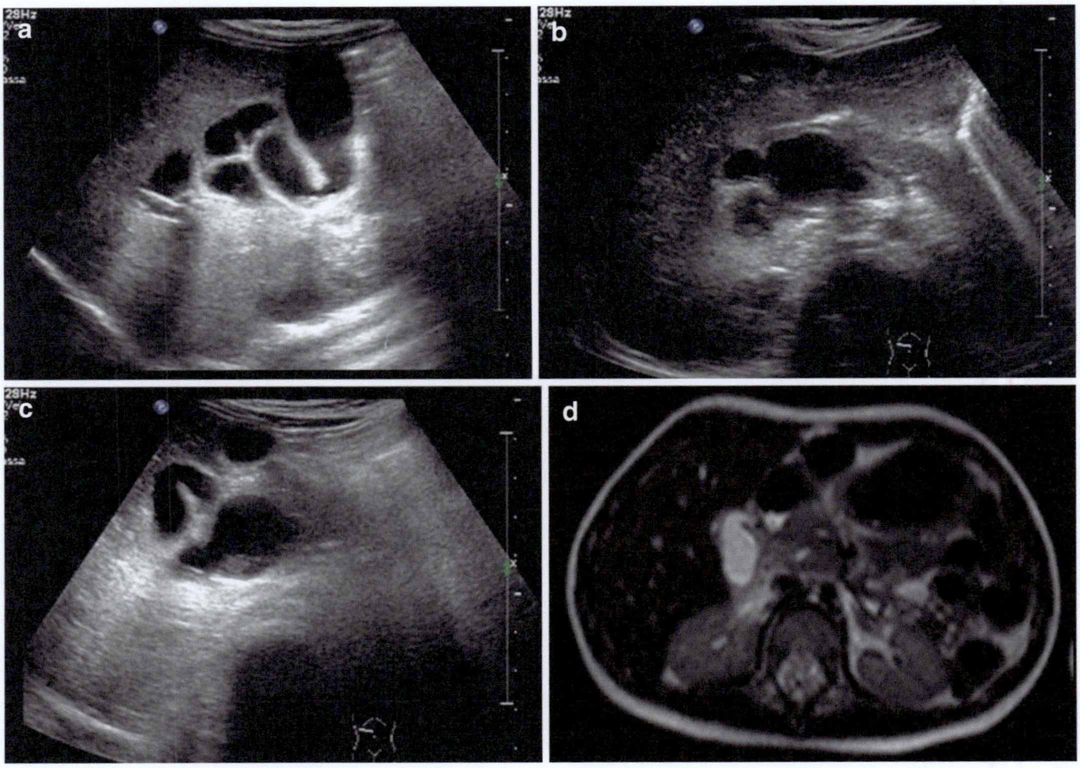

Fig. 7.15 US scans (**a**–**c**) and MRI (**d**–**h**) reveal a fusiform swelling of the common bile duct extending into the common hepatic duct with hydrops of the gallbladder involvement of the common bile duct and extension into the common hepatic duct, with dilatation of the cystic duct. The intrahepatic biliary ducts were slightly dilated, and a diagnosis of type IC CC was concluded

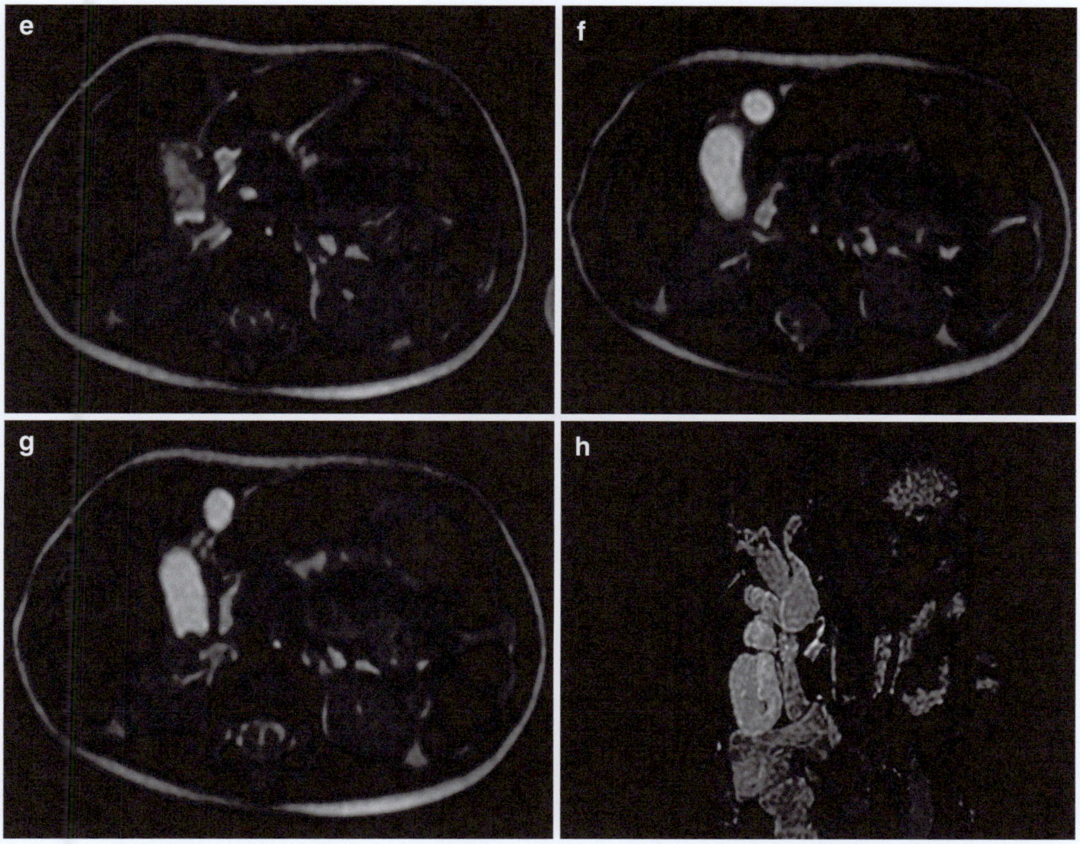

Fig. 7.15 (continued)

allow high-resolution imaging of the biliary tree and have the ability to perform multiplanar reconstructions.

Maximum intensity projection reformats are acquired in the coronal oblique plane.

Different oral contrast agents in the form of manganese-rich juices have been employed to optimize the evaluation of pancreaticobiliary diseases (they make bowel lumen dark on T2-weighted sequences). We use pineapple juice per oral that nullifies the high signal contrast in the duodenum and provides better visualization of the pancreaticobiliary junction. Hepatobiliary MR contrast agents allow a better visualization of the bile ducts than heavily T2-weighted sequences because their elimination through the biliary system improves evaluation of the communication between a cystic lesion and the biliary tract.

In summary, *diagnosis* relies on the exclusion of other conditions (e.g., gallstones, inflammation, pancreatitis) as a cause of biliary duct dilatation. US is generally the initial investigation to assess the hepatobiliary system. MRCP adds important information about anatomy, helps to exclude variants and other anatomic anomalies (duodenal duplication, pancreatic cysts) and indicate further steps.

References

Anupindi S, Chauvin NA, Khwaja A, Biko DM (2016) Magnetic resonance imaging of pancreaticobiliary diseases, in children: from technique to practice. Pediatr Radiol 46:778–790

Babbitt DP, Starshak RJ, Clemett AR (1973) Choledochal cyst: a concept of etiology. Am J Roentgenol Radium Ther Nucl Med 119:57–62

Caponcelli E, Knisely AS, Davenport M (2008) Cystic biliary atresia: an etiologic and prognostic subgroup. J Pediatr Surg 43:1619–1624

Chavhan GB, Babyn PS, Manson D, Vidarsson L (2008) Pediatric MR cholangiopancreatography: principles, technique, and clinical applications. Radiographics 28:1951–1962

Davenport M, Kerkar N, Mieli-Vergani G, Mowat AP, Howard ER (1997) Biliary atresia: the King's College Hospital experience (1974–1995). J Pediatr Surg 32:479–485

Davenport M, Tizzard SA, Underhill J, Mieli-Vergani G, Portmann B, Hadzic N (2006) The biliary atresia splenic malformation syndrome: a 28-year single-center retrospective study. J Pediatr 149(3): 393–400

De Angelis P, Foschia F, Romeo E et al (2012) Role of endoscopic retrograde cholangiopancreatography in diagnosis and management of congenital choledochal cysts: 28 pediatric cases. J Pediatr Surg 47:885–888

Dillman JR, Heider A, Bilhartz JL, Smith EA, Keshavarzi N, Rubin JM, Lopez MJ (2015) Ultrasound shear wave speed measurements correlate with liver fibrosis in children. Pediatr Radiol 45(10):1480–1488

El-Guindi MA, Sira MM, Konsowa HA, El-Abd OL, Salem TA (2013) Value of hepatic subcapsular flow by color doppler ultrasonography in the diagnosis of biliary atresia. J Gastroenterol Hepatol 28(5):867–872

El-Guindi MA, Sira MM, Sira AM, Salem TA, El-Abd OL, Konsowa HA, El-Azab DS, Allam AA (2014) Design and validation of a diagnostic score for biliary atresia. J Hepatol Jul 61(1):116–123

Fitoz S, Erden A, Boruban S (2007) Magnetic resonance cholangiopancreatography of biliary system abnormalities in children. Clin Imaging 31:93–101

Hartley JL, Davenport M, Kelly DA (2009) Biliary atresia. Lancet 374:1704–1713

Huang FC, Hwang KP (2006) Differential diagnosis of infantile choledochal cyst with or without biliary atresia. Acta Paediatr Taiwan 47:175–180

Jiexiong F, Minju L, Hongfeng T, Weizhong G et al (2003) Clinical and pathological characteristics of cystic lesions of extrahepatic bile duct in neonates. Acta Paediatr 92:1183–1189

Kasai M, Sawaguchi S, Akiyama H, Saito S, Suruga K, Yura J et al (1976) A proposal of new classification of biliary atresia (in Japanese with English abstract). J Jpn Soc Pediatr Surg 12:327–331

Keil R, Snajdauf J, Rygl M, Pycha K, Kotalova' R, Dra'bek J et al (2010) Diagnostic efficacy of ERCP in cholestatic infants and neonates—a retrospective study on a large series. Endoscopy 42:121–126

Kim WS, Kim IO, Yeon KM et al (1998) Choledochal cyst with or without biliary atresia in neonates and young infants: US differentiation. Radiology 209:465–469

Kim MJ, Park YN, Han SJ, Yoon CS, Yoo HS, Hwang EH et al (2000) Biliary atresia in neonates and infants: triangular area of high signal intensity in the porta hepatis at T2-weighted MR cholangiography with US and histopathologic correlation. Radiology 215:395–401

Kim WS, Cheon JE, Youn BJ, Yoo SY, Kim WY, Kim IO, Yeon KM, Seo JK, Park KW (2007) Hepatic arterial diameter measured with US: adjunct for US diagnosis of biliary atresia. Radiology 245:549–555

Lee HJ1, Lee SM, Park WH, Choi SO (2003) Objective criteria of triangular cord sign in biliary atresia on US scans. Radiology 229(2):395–400

Manco M, Lo Zupone C, Latini A, Lucidi V, Monti L (2011) Noninvasive assessment of cystic fibrosis-associated liver disease with acoustic radiation force impulse imaging. Hepatology 53(5):1779–1780; author reply 1780-1

Moreira RK, Cabral R, Cowles RA, Lobritto SJ (2012) Biliary atresia: a multidisciplinary approach to diagnosis and management. Arch Pathol Lab Med 136(7): 746–760

Moyer V, Freese DK, Whitington PF et al (2004) Guideline for the evaluation of cholestatic jaundice in infants: recommendations of the North American Society for Pediatric Gastroenterology, Hepatology and Nutrition. J Pediatr Gastroenterol Nutr 39:115–128

Murphy AJ, Axt JR, Crapp SJ et al (2012) Concordance of imaging modalities and cost minimization in the diagnosis of pediatric choledochal cysts. Pediatr Surg Int 28:615–621

Pakarinen MP, Rintala RJ (2011) Surgery of biliary atresia. Scand J Surg 100:49–53

Park WH, Choi SO, Lee HJ et al (1997) A new diagnostic approach to biliary atresia with emphasis on the ultrasonographic triangular cord sign: comparison of ultrasonography, hepatobiliary scintigraphy, and liver needle biopsy in the evaluation of infantile cholestasis. J Pediatr Surg 32:1555–1559

Park WH, Choi SO, Lee HJ (1999) The ultrasonographic 'triangular cord' coupled with gallbladder images in the diagnostic prediction of biliary atresia from infantile intrahepatic cholestasis. J Pediatr Surg 34(11): 1706–1710

Park DH, Kim MH, Lee SK et al (2005) Can MRCP replace the diagnostic role of ERCP for patients with choledochal cysts? Gastrointest Endosc 62:360–366

Poddar U, Thapa BR, Das A et al (2009) Neonatal cholestasis: differentiation of biliary atresia from neonatal hepatitis in a developing country. Acta Paediatr 98:1260–1264

Rasekhi AR, Gheisari F (2010) Triangular cord sign in detection of biliary atresia: is it a valuable sign? Dig Dis Sci 175(1):172–175

Scottoni F1, De Angelis P, Dall'Oglio L et al (2013) ERCP with intracholedocal biopsy for the diagnosis of biliary tract rhabdomyosarcoma in children. Pediatr Surg Int 29(6):659–662

Serinet MO, Wildhaber BE, Broue P, Lachaux A, Sarles J, Jacquemin E, Gauthier F, Chardot C (2009) Impact of age at kasai operation on its results in late childhood and adolescence: a rational basis for biliary atresia screening. Pediatrics (2009) 123(5):1280–1286

Siles P, Aschero A, Gorincour G, Bourliere-Najean B, Roquelaure B, Delarue A, Petit P (2014) A prospective pilot study: can the biliary tree be visualized in children younger than 3 months on magnetic resonance cholangiopancreatography? Pediatr Radiol 44(9): 1077–1084

Singhavejsakul J, Ukarapol N (2008) Choledochal cysts in children: epidemiology and outcomes. World J Surg 32(7):1385–1388

Sokol RJ, Mack C, Narkewicz MR et al (2003) Pathogenesis and outcome of biliary atresia: current concepts. J Pediatr Gastroenterol Nutr 37:4–21

Suita S, Shono K, Kinugasa Y, Kubota M, Matsuo S (1999) Influence of age on the presentation and outcome of choledochal cyst. J Pediatr Surg 34:1765–1768

Suzuki M, Shimizu T, Kudo T et al (2006) Usefulness of nonbreath-hold 1-shot magnetic resonance cholangiopancreatography for the evaluation of choledochal cyst in children. J Pediatr Gastroenterol Nutr 42:539–544

Takamizawa S, Zaima A, Muraji T, Kanegawa K, Akasaka Y, Satoh S et al (2007) Can biliary atresia be diagnosed by ultrasonography alone? J PediatrSurg) 42(12):2093–2096

Tipnis NA, Werlin SL (2007) The use of magnetic resonance cholangiopancreatography in children. Curr Gastroenterol Rep 9:225–229

Todani T, Watanabe Y, Narusue M et al (1977) Congenital bile duct cysts: classification, operative procedures, and review of thirty-seven cases including cancer arising from choledochal cyst. Am J Surg 134:263–269

Tsuchiya H, Kaneko K, Itoh A et al (2013) Endoscopic biliary drainage for children with persistent or exacerbated symptoms of choledochal cysts. J Hepatobiliary Pancreat Sci 20:303–306

Vegting IL, Tabbers MM, Taminiau JA et al (2009) Is endoscopic retrograde cholangiopancreatography valuable and safe in children of all ages? J Pediatr Gastroenterol Nutr 48:66–71

Yang J-G, Ma D-Q, Peng Y et al (2009) Comparison of different diagnostic methods for differentiating biliary atresia from idiopathic neonatal hepatitis. Clin Imaging 33:439–446

Yonem O, Bayraktar Y (2007) Clinical characteristics of Caroli's syndrome. World J Gastroenterol 13: 1934–1937

Zhou LY, Guan BY, Li L, Xu ZF, Dai CP, Wang W et al (2012) Objective differential characteristics of cystic biliary atresia and choledochal cysts in neonates and young infants: sonographic findings. J Ultrasound Med 31:833–841

Zhou LY, Wang W, Shan QY, Liu BX, Zheng YL, Xu ZF, Xu M, Pan FS, Lu MD, Xie XY (2015) Optimizing the US diagnosis of biliary atresia with a modified triangular cord thickness and gallbladder classification. Radiology 277(1):181–191

Part II

Pediatric Acute Abdomen

Hypertrophic Pyloric Stenosis (HPS)

8

Margherita Trinci, Claudia Lucia Piccolo, Antonio Alessandro Pallottino, Michele Galluzzo, Eugenio Rossi, Massimo Zeccolini, and Vittorio Miele

8.1 Introduction

The hypertrophic pyloric stenosis (HPS) is an incomplete high bowel obstruction. It is a common condition due to a hypertrophy and hyperplasia of the antropyloric muscular ring that causes gastric outlet obstruction; the typical aspect is the narrowing and elongation of the pyloric canal (Fig. 8.1). Even a variable degree of thickening of the pyloric canal mucosa contributes to obstruction of the lumen. A defect of muscular layer innervation is also thought responsible of the failure of relaxation of the pyloric muscle.

The pylorus is the terminal portion of the stomach situated to the right side of the incisura angularis. The pylorus is divided from the sulcus intermedius in two zones, the pyloric vestibule and the pyloric antrum or canal; this is the portion that ends in the pyloric sphincter, responsible for opening of the stomach in the duodenum. The pyloric muscle is composed by two circular muscular loops connected by longitudinal muscle fiber tracts; in patients with HPS, the antrum and the muscular pyloric ring are no longer distinguishable but are fused in a rigid canal. The pyloric muscle's function is to prevent large undigested food particles to enter the small intestine as well as the food reentering the stomach when the small bowel contracts (Hernanz-Schulman 2003).

HPS is the most common surgical cause of vomiting in infants, because hypertrophy of the pyloric muscle progressively leads to almost complete obstruction of the gastric outlet. It occurs between the 3° and the 10° weeks of life, in a healthy infant, with peak between the 4° and the 7° weeks; rarely it happens after the 12° weeks of life (Peters et al. 2014). The incidence of HPS is approximately 2–5 per 1,000 births per year, more frequently in white populations; although wide variations have been found related to geographic location, season and ethnic origin. In fact, while as we have said, in the Western world, the incidence of HPS is 2–5:1,000 live births, it is four times lower in the Southeast Asian and Chinese populations. A decline in its incidence has been reported in the northern European countries related to the change in babies' sleeping position, along with a decrease in incidence of the sudden infant death syndrome. Nevertheless, a population-based study in the USA showed that these two syndromes share some risk factors, but other factors are involved

M. Trinci (✉) • C.L. Piccolo • M. Galluzzo • V. Miele
Department of Emergency Radiology, S. Camillo Hospital, Rome, Italy
e-mail: margherita.trinci@libero.it

A.A. Pallottino
Department of Emergency Radiology, S. Camillo Hospital, Rome, Italy

E. Rossi • M. Zeccolini
Department of Radiology, Pausilipon Pediatric Oncologic Hospital, Naples, Italy

V. Miele, M. Trinci (eds.), *Imaging Non-traumatic Abdominal Emergencies in Pediatric Patients*,
DOI 10.1007/978-3-319-41866-7_8

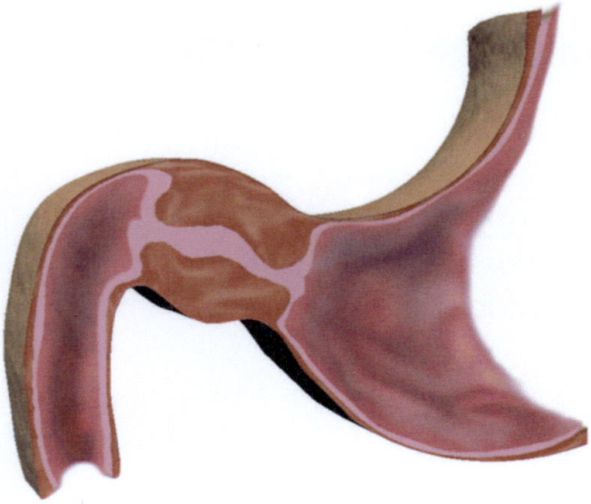

Fig. 8.1 The drawing shows the hypertrophic pyloric stenosis (HPS), with the typical aspect of narrowing and elongation of the pyloric canal due to a variable degree of thickening of the pyloric muscle. (Thanks to Edoardo Sarperi for the drawing)

in their genesis with different effects on the two conditions (MacMahon 2006; Lisonkova and Joseph 2014).

8.2 Pathogenesis

The etiology remains unknown: the HPS is considered an acquired pathology due to a long spasm with pylorus ischemic suffering during the neonatal period, which led to hypertrophy of antrum muscle fibers. Between the hypotheses, there are abnormalities of hormonal control, an abnormal innervation of the pylorus, and abnormalities of smooth muscle cells. It also postulated a genetic predisposition (McKeown et al. 1951). HPS is more frequent in male than in female with male to female ratio 5:1 (Hernanz-Schulman 2003).

Up to now a possible explanation for this prevalence may only be hypothesized by the theory of the x-linked transmission or with the theory of sex hormone influence. It has been hypothesized that the testosterone can be involved, although those disorders characterized by an alteration in the levels of sexual hormones do not show an increase in HPS incidence, arguing against such an influence (Krogh et al. 2011).

HPS typically affects the firstborn children. Typically the presence in the family history of a first-degree relative affected by HPS increases the risk more than fivefold (Frković et al. 2001).

Several studies defined this condition as complex disorder involving both genetic and environmental factors, such as maternal smoking and alcohol addiction.

Exposure to medications, such as macrolide antibiotics, especially erythromycin, has been studied as an important determinant of HPS. In fact, erythromycin is a motilin agonist which induces contraction of the gastrointestinal tract; so high levels of this drug may lead to a continuous contraction of the pyloric muscle (Panteli 2009).

A young mother's age (<20 years) has also been indicated as risk factor, but this association could not be demonstrated in other study populations (Pedersen et al. 2008). Breastfeeding has been indicated as one of the main protective factors.

8.3 Clinical Presentation and Diagnosis

Usually, at birth, infants with HPS are clinically normal. The symptoms develop during the first weeks of postnatal life, including nonbilious vomiting, because the obstruction is previous to the Vater ampulla. Vomiting is often violent, described as "projectile" after feeding. Initially the vomiting of gastric contents is intermittent, but the frequency increases during the time with the feedings.

A bilious vomiting should be presumed to be from a malrotation or Hirschsprung's disease (Aspelund and Langer 2007).

If the condition lasts for a long time, the vomiting might be blood tinged because of a concurrent gastritis.

At the beginning there is a voracious appetite; despite distention of the stomach, the infant is nervous with crisis of inconsolable crying. As the days pass, the infant does not grow and there is a weight loss; these patients often show a characteristic facies, wrinkled appearance. As time goes vomiting leads to dehydration condition and to emaciation. In emaciated infants, the distended stomach may be identifiable in the hypochondrium, with active peristaltic activity visible through the abdominal wall. Affected children usually show the classic electrolyte abnormalities of hypochloremia, hypokalemia, and metabolic alkalosis. Laboratory tests are required to evaluate serum sodium, chloride, potassium, and bicarbonate values. If the situation remains untreated, it may result in death. Surgical treatment is necessary for the cure.

The clinical diagnosis is based on abdominal palpation of the thickened pylorus, called "olive," which has a 99 % positive predictive value (White et al. 1998; Taylor et al. 2013; Senquiz 1991).

As usual for many medical tests, the outcome of the abdominal palpation is not always successful because it is depending on a lot of factors such as the experience of the examiner, if the infant is calm or not, and the presence of gastric distention. In some cases there is an absence of mandibular frenulum.

The differential diagnosis includes overfeeding, milk protein allergy, intestinal rotation anomalies, gastroesophageal reflux, and other forms of obstructions.

Gastroesophageal reflux is usually the first hypothesis to think about in the presence of a vomiting infant, and it is treated with thickened feeds and histamine blockers or proton pump inhibitors. When the little patient does not respond to this therapy, one may think about milk protein allergy, managed by changing the infant's formula. The persistence of symptoms leads the clinician to consider other conditions (Ricketts 1984).

When the clinical examination and the symptoms are not enough to find the pathology of the infant, imaging techniques are necessary in confirming the diagnosis (Hernanz-Schulman 2003; Lisonkova and Joseph 2014; McKeown et al. 1951).

8.4 Imaging

Imaging plays a key role in the diagnosis of HPS especially when the clinical exam is not sufficient. The imaging techniques used in Emergency Radiology in children are conventional radiology and ultrasound (Miele et al. 2006; Miele and Di Giampietro 2014).

8.4.1 Radiology

The radiographic exam of upper gastrointestinal (UGI) tract has been for a long time the goal standard in the diagnosis of HPS. At present, in agreement with the radioprotection criteria, the ultrasound exam is preferred. However it is necessary to know how to do a study of the GI superior tract and the signs of HPS.

UGI is performed with the infant in the right anterior oblique position to facilitate gastric emptying (Ricketts 1984; Hiorns 2011). We must give the child to drink 30–40 cc of barium meal diluted 1:2 in the baby bottle; the nasogastric tube is not necessary if the baby normally feeds; sometimes it can be useful for emptying an overdistended stomach preventing vomiting. Only in special cases, for example, in preterm and if there is a risk of aspiration, a high density water-soluble nonionic contrast media is safer and preferable. During the exam the patient will change his decubitus from supine position to lateral position usually in left oblique posterior position to facilitate the opacification of the antrum and pylorus canal (Hiorns 2011).

In a healthy newborn, the contrast medium fills the stomach and passes easily from the stomach to the duodenum and in the following intestinal loops (Fig. 8.2).

During the fluoroscopic observation, in an infant with HPS, we will see a vigorous active peristalsis, the "caterpillar sign," of the gastric wall that abruptly stops at the pyloric antrum; the barium outlines the external thickened muscle as an extrinsic impression in the antrum, termed the "shoulder sign" (see later). In HPS there is a typical elongation of the pyloric canal, if the peristaltic wave force pylorus is possible to see a thin line of contrast in the pyloric canal "string sign" (see later); if the contrast remains in the redundant mucosa it can also see the "double-track" sign (see later).

Conventional abdominal film may show nonspecific findings:

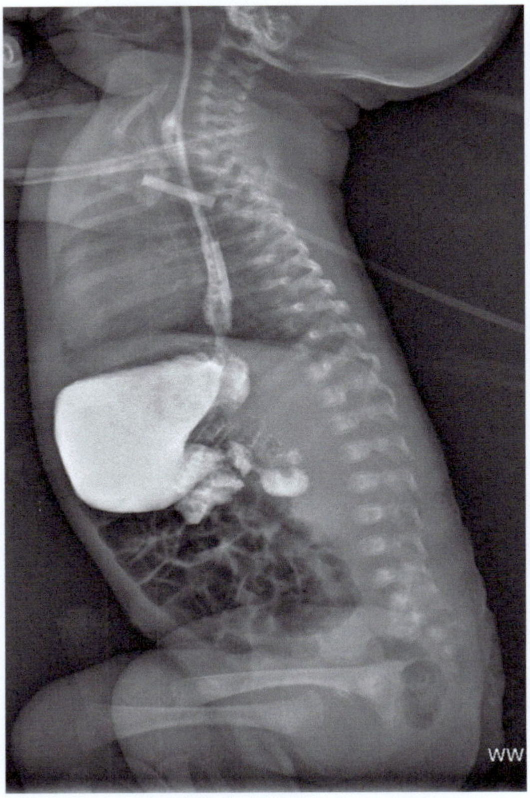

Fig. 8.2 In a healthy infant, UGI radiographic study, lateral view, shows the normal aspect of the antropyloric region and of the duodenal cap

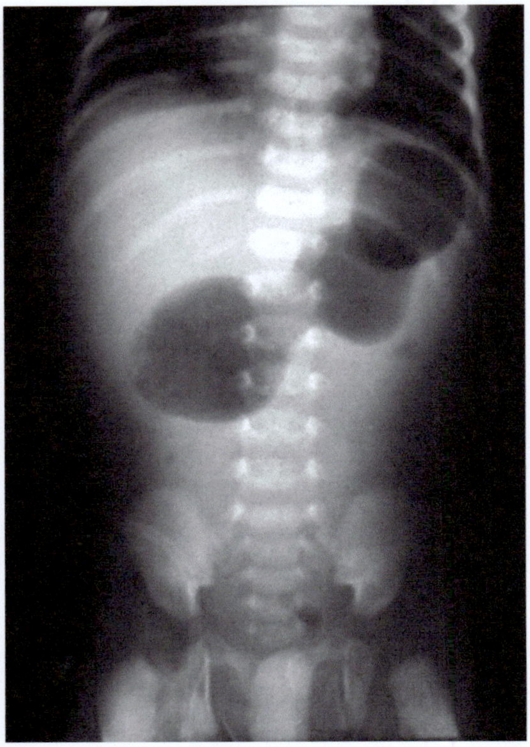

Fig. 8.3 Abdominal plain film in newborn with HPS shows a large distended stomach by air with few amount of distal gas pattern

- Large, distended stomach (>7 cm diameter) (Fig. 8.3) (Frković et al. 2001)
- Abnormal distance between the stomach and the duodenal cap, both distended by air (Fig. 8.4)
- Minimal distal gas pattern in small and large bowel (see Fig. 8.3)

UGI tract shows some indirect and direct signs:

- Contrast in distended stomach because of barium is unable get through the pylorus (Fig. 8.5).
- Delayed gastric emptying (see Figs. 8.5 and 8.6).
- Gastric retroperistalsis and eventually gastroesophageal reflux (see Fig. 8.5).
- Typical elongation and narrowing of the pyloric canal "mouse tail" (Fig. 8.6).
- The "string sign" is characterized by contrast material outlining the canal coursing through the mucosal interstices.
- The "double-track sign" represents several tracts of contrast material separated by the mucosa (Fig. 8.7). This sign was used to demonstrate the intervening redundant mucosa outlined as a filling defect by the contrast material, helping in differentiation from pylorospasm (Haran et al. 1966).
- The "shoulder sign" is seen during barium examination and refers to the bulging of the hypertrophied pyloric muscle into the lumen of the antrum. This bulging causes a flattening of the prepyloric area of the lesser curvature (Fig. 8.8). This sign is closely related to the cervix sign of pyloric stenosis at the ultrasound imaging.
- "Beak sign" is due to the contrast medium that tries to enter in the proximal portion of the pyloric canal with a "beak" shape (Fig. 8.8).

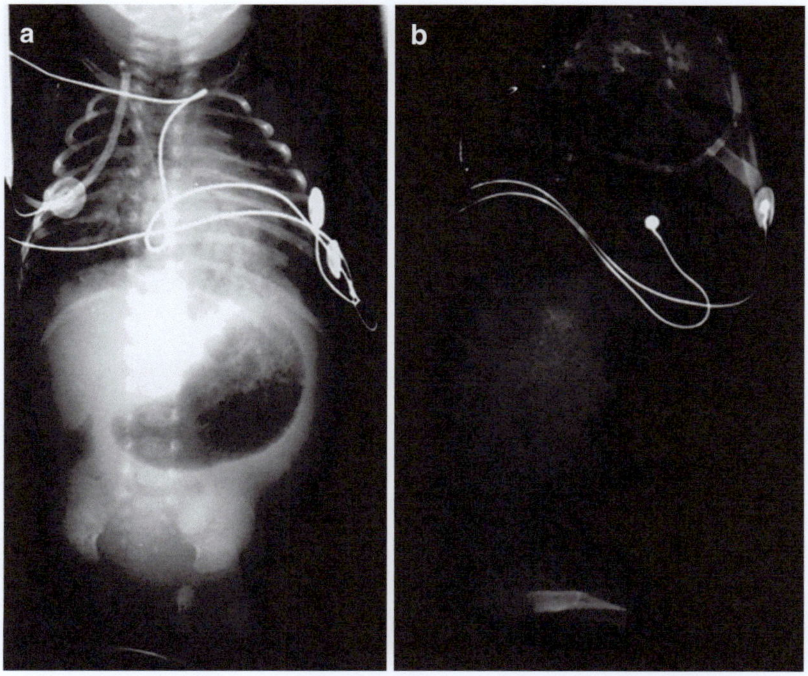

Fig. 8.4 Abdominal plain film in newborn with HPS. (**a**) Frontal and (**b**) lateral views show a large distended stomach, with an abnormal distance between the stomach and the duodenal cap, both distended by air

- The thickened pyloric muscle can indent the base of the duodenal bulb (mushroom sign) (Fig. 8.7) (Frković et al. 2001).

8.4.2 Ultrasound

Ultrasound (US) is the modality of choice for the diagnosis of HPS because it is generally available, and it is low-cost noninvasive technique and does not use radiation, allowing direct observation of the pyloric canal morphology and its dynamism (Di Giacomo et al. 2015; Fonio et al. 2013) (Fig. 8.9).

As usual in newborn, the examination should be performed with high-frequency linear transducers between 6 and 10 MHz. For the comfort of the baby, it is important to have an adequate ambient temperature of the room, gel warmed, and presence of the parents.

Ultrasonography exam of the antrum-pyloric region was performed both with the infant in supine position for axial scanning and with the patient in the lateral decubitus position, right side down, which is an anti-reflux position. In the lateral decubitus, a longitudinal scanning is performed (Fonio et al. 2013). Feeding previous the exam is not requested even because of the possibility that the gastric distention displaces

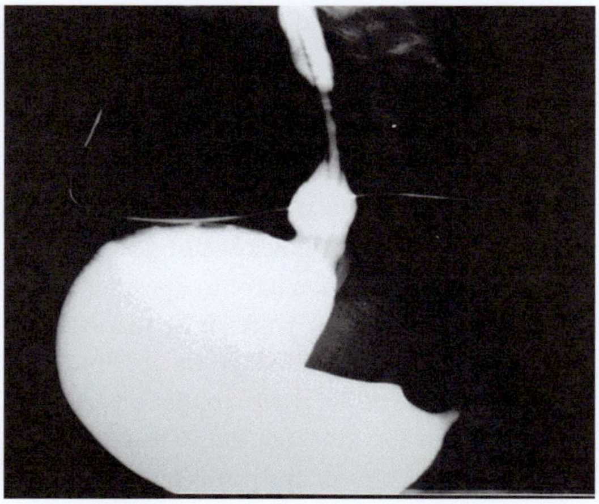

Fig. 8.5 UGI tract film in newborn with HPS. Radiographic oblique view shows a large distended stomach, filled from barium, and delayed gastric emptying. Gastroesophageal reflux is associated

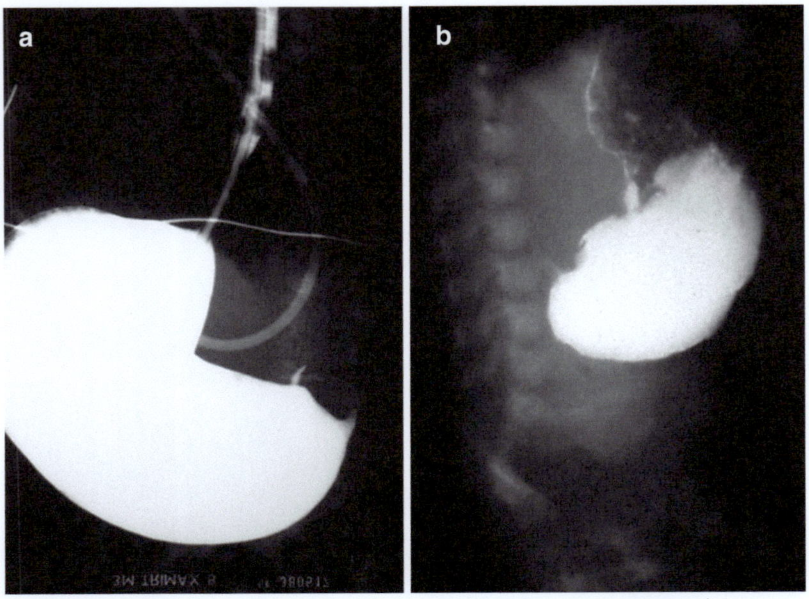

Fig. 8.6 UGI tract radiographic study in newborn with HPS. (**a**) Oblique and (**b**) lateral views show a large distended stomach filled from barium and delayed gastric emptying. Typical elongation and narrowing of the pyloric canal "mouse tail"

the gastroduodenal junction and for the eventuality that the ingestion of air during the feeding hides the pylorus and displaces it dorsally. Changing position during the exam from supine position moving the baby with the left side up moves the fluid toward the antrum, helps to recognize it, and leads the pylorus to rise to an anterior position. The severe stomach distention can be an indirect finding indicative of gastric outlet obstruction. Anyway we have to consider that in many cases of infants with HPS, the stomach remains partially repleted from the previous feeding because of the gastric outlet obstruction. Some fluid in the stomach helps to outline the antrum-pyloric region and to observe real-time passage of gastric content through the pyloric canal into the duodenum. For this reason sometimes the infant was given with a bit of milk or sugar water orally.

There are some landmarks that makes it easier finding the pylorus; in fact it is situated medially and posteriorly to the gallbladder, medially to the liver, anteriorly to the right kidney, caudal to the portal vein, and lateral to the pancreas head (Fig. 8.10).

The ultrasound exam begins with the patient in supine position by placing the transducer in mesogastric space, transversely below the xiphoid process. In this position we can see the esophagus as it enters the abdomen. Caudally moving of the probe, we can identify the gastric fundus and then the gastric body, antrum, and duodenal cap.

In the normal pylorus, the muscular layer is usually a hypoechoic thin layer less than 2 mm in thickness, sometimes too thin to measure, and the longitudinal diameter is really short (Fig. 8.11). Under the muscular layer, there is an inner echogenic layer, which represents the mucosa and submucosa; there is an innermost anechoic center that is fluid in the pyloric canal (Panteli 2009).

Anyway there is a range of dimension of normal pylorus: the transverse diameter is 7–11 mm and the length of pyloric canal is 10–13 cm. In some cases the thickening of the pyloric canal may be transient due to peristalsis or pylorospasm. In these situations it is important to prolong the evaluation and observation of the pylorus to visualize the pyloric opening. In case of pylorospasm, the muscle may appear a little more thick, but usually no more than 3 mm, and the length of the pyloric

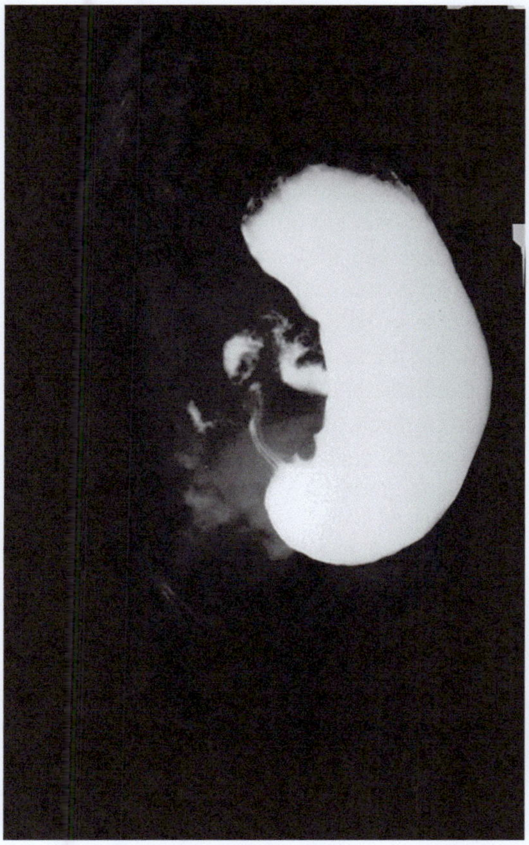

Fig. 8.7 UGI tract radiographic study in newborn with HPS. Oblique view shows a large distended stomach filled by barium. Note the elongated pylorus with "double-track" sign

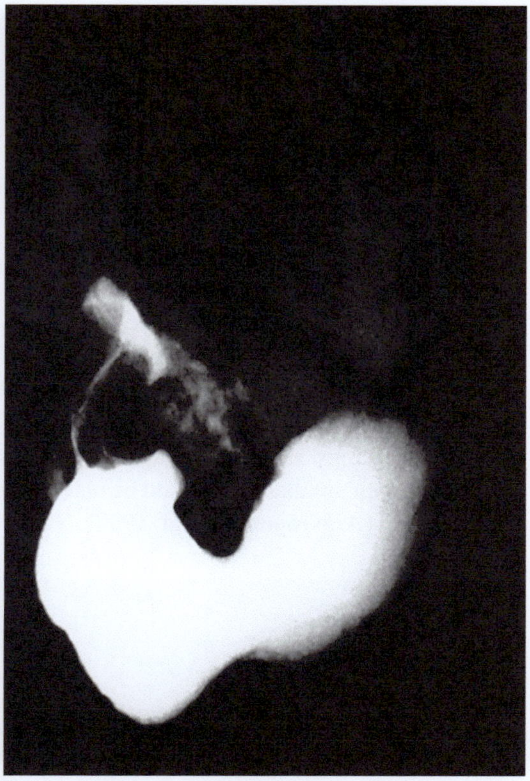

Fig. 8.8 In an infant with HPS, UGI radiographic study, lateral view, shows the typical aspect of narrowing and elongation of the pyloric canal, the shoulder sign, the beak sign, and the deformation of the duodenal cap (mushroom sign) (Compare with Fig. 8.1, normal pylorus)

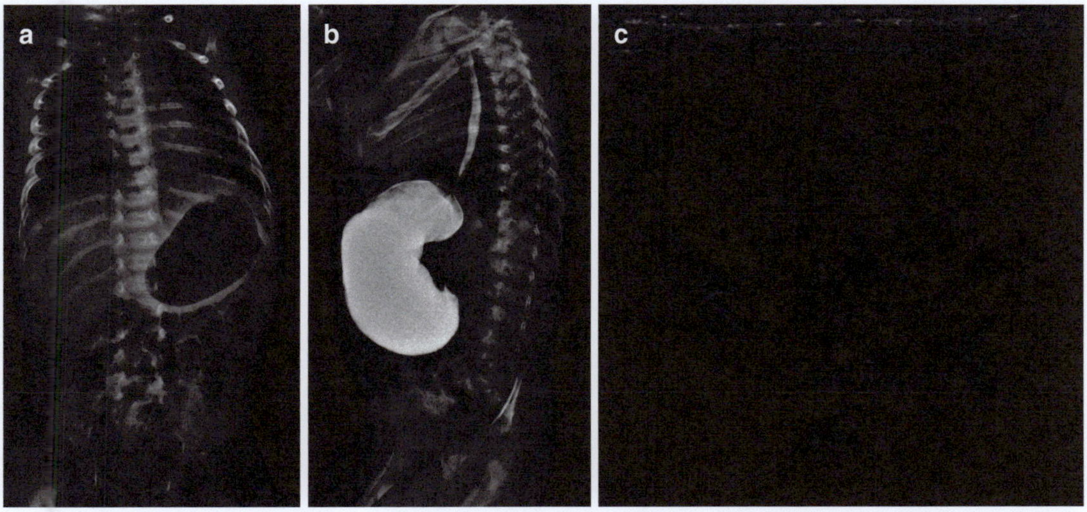

Fig. 8.9 Newborn with HPS. (**a**) Plain film, (**b**) UGI tract and (**c**) ultrasound images show, respectively, nonspecific and specific signs of HPS

canal is <15 mm. In other cases the measures of pylorus are a little bit greater but not clearly pathological, "transitional pylorus"; in these situations it is recommended to have a subsequent control after a few days to view the evolution of the situation.

Studies in preterm infants showed that the pylorus increases its dimensions: muscle thickness, canal length, and canal width according to the gestational age and even documented a stronger correlation with body weight. For those reasons it is important to pay attention at the age of the infant at the time of the exam; in fact in premature infants and in the infants up to 3 weeks old, HPS develops at the same age as in term infants, but their smaller size should be taken into consideration (Argyropoulou et al. 1998).

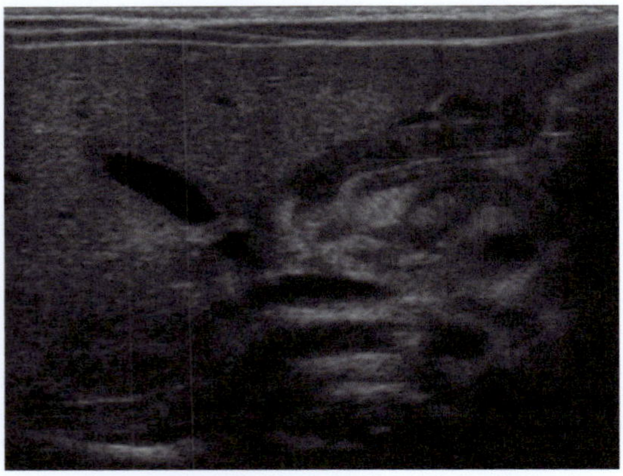

Fig. 8.10 Ultrasound shows the anatomical landmarks to find the pylorus. Here you see the relationship between the pathological pylorus, which is located medially to the gallbladder and the liver

After the pylorus has been found and measured, a fundamental step is to observe if there is the passage of the gastric content through the pylorus, due to the distention of the antropyloric region. This dynamic evaluation is easily possible with sonography and is really important because if we see a wide-open pylorus with normal passage of food, we can exclude HPS (Costa Dias et al. 2012) (Fig. 8.12).

In case of HPS, the sonographic examination shows the thickened prepyloric antrum between the duodenal bulb and a various degrees distended stomach.

As for the conventional radiology and also in ultrasound, there are both indirect and direct signs of HPS.

Ultrasound direct signs of HPS are based on the size of the pylorus (Fig. 8.13):

- The pyloric canal length greater than 15 mm usually >17 mm (range 15–20 mm).
- The muscle wall thickness greater than 3.5 mm usually >0.4–1 cm (Hernanz-Schulman 2009; Malcom et al. 2009; Olson et al. 1998).
- The transverse diameter >12 mm; this diameter includes the lumen and both walls of the pylorus (Frković et al. 2001).
- Pyloric volume: <1.5 cc.

Preference was given to the width measurement in case of mixed finding between length and width.

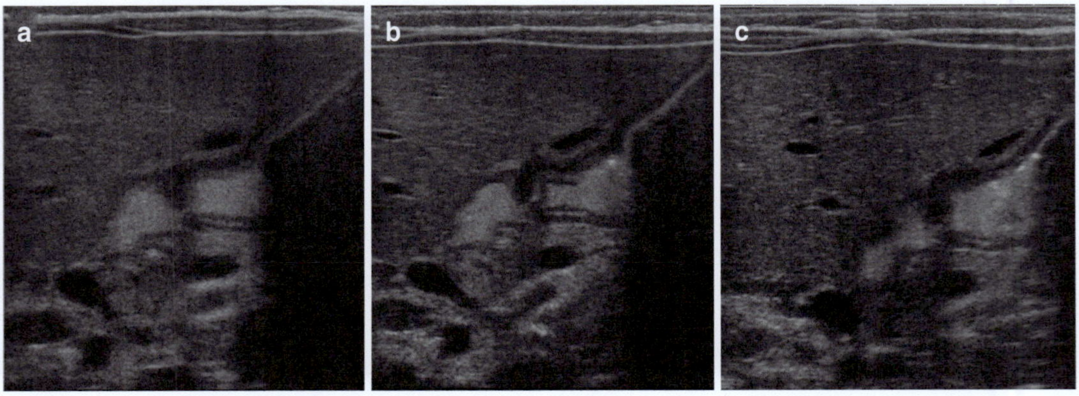

Fig. 8.11 (**a–c**) Dynamic ultrasound longitudinal scans in newborn show the normal aspect of pylorus muscle, between the stomach and the duodenal cap

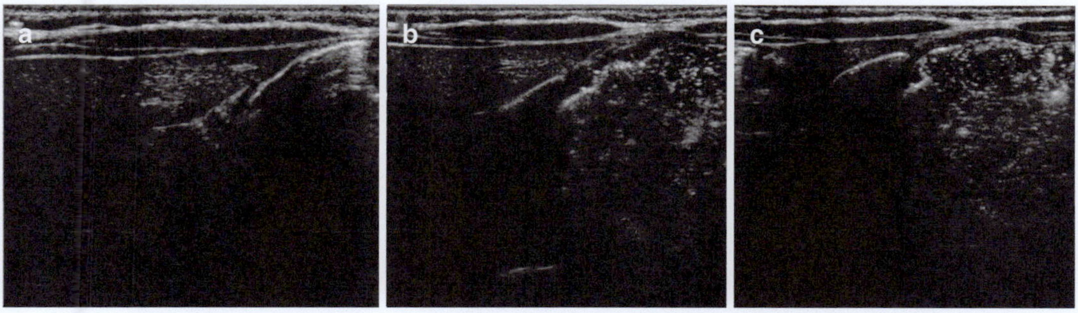

Fig. 8.12 Dynamic ultrasound exam in a child with suspected HPS. The sequence of the images shows (**a**) the profile of the stomach, the gastroduodenal junction and the duodenal cap, (**b**) the gastric peristalsis, and (**c**) the opening of pylorus with the move of gastric contents

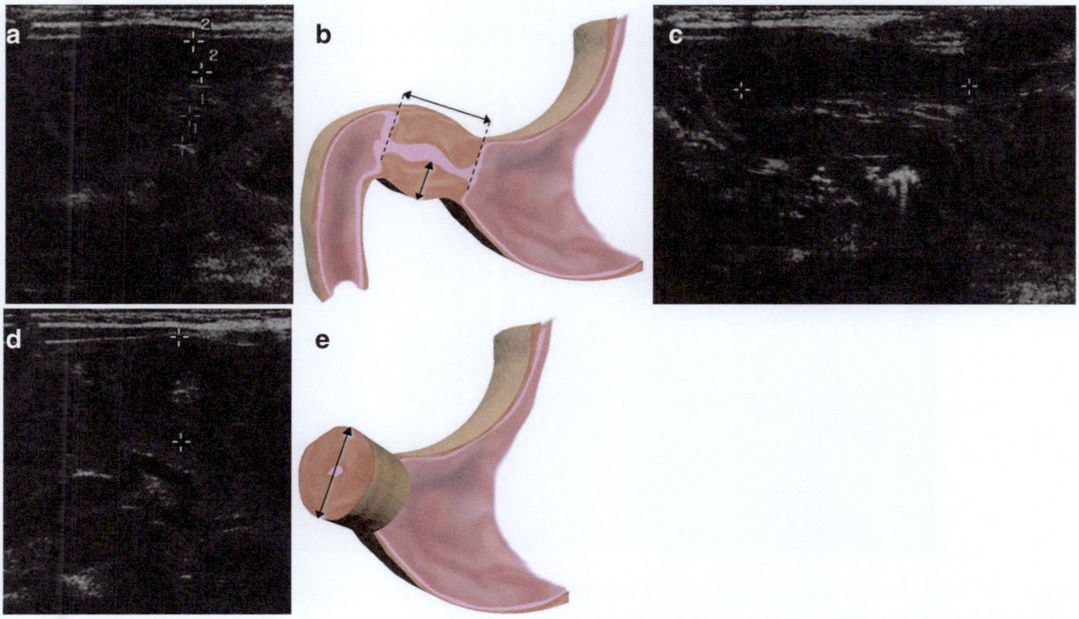

Fig. 8.13 Ultrasound measurements of HPS in newborn. (**a**–**c**) Longitudinal scan and (**d**) transversal scan show the elongation and lumen narrowing of the pyloric canal, the thickening of the pyloric muscle, and the increase of the pyloric transverse diameter B. (**e**) Anatomical diagrams help to understand where the measures are to be taken. (Thanks to Edoardo Sarperi for the drawing)

Related signs of HPS are the following:

- Cervix sign: it is the prolapse of the pyloric canal mucosa into the fluid-filled antrum (Fig. 8.14).
- Fortio sign: it is the protrusion of the pylorus in the duodenum (Fig. 8.15).
- Target sign: it is due to hypertrophied hypoechoic muscle surrounding the echogenic mucosa; it is seen in the transverse axis (Figs. 8.16 and 8.17) (Frković et al. 2001).
- Donut sign: it consists of a prominent anechoic rim of thickened muscle and an echogenic center of the mucosa and submucosa.
- The antral nipple sign refers to redundant pyloric mucosa protruding into the gastric antrum and can be seen filling the lumen on transverse sections.
- "Shoulder sign" as just treated in the UGI direct sign refers to the bulging of the hypertrophied pyloric muscle into the lumen of the antrum; the bulging causes a flattening of the

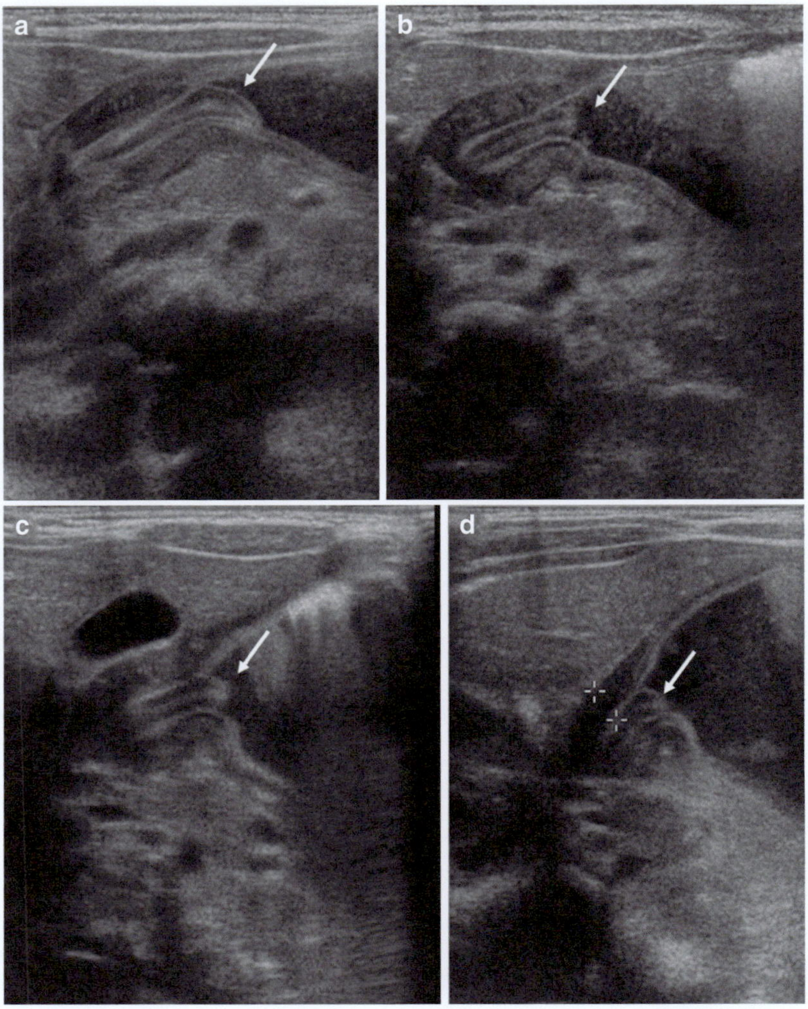

Fig. 8.14 (**a**–**d**) Child, 5 weeks. Ultrasound shows "cervix" sign (*white arrow*): prolapse of the pyloric canal mucosa into the fluid-filled antrum

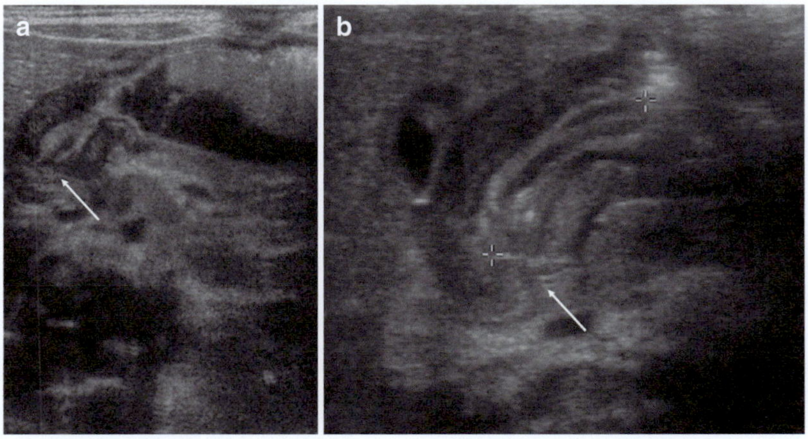

Fig. 8.15 (**a**, **b**) Ultrasound longitudinal scan shows "portio sign" due to the protrusion of the pylorus (*white arrow*) in the duodenal bulb

prepyloric area of the lesser curvature (Fig. 8.18).

Ultrasound indirect signs of HPS are the following:

- Gastric distention with movements of mixing of gastric contents due to an increase of gastric peristalsis which attempts to force the lock caused by pylorus (Fig. 8.19)
- The failure of pyloric sphincter relaxation due to an inefficient peristalsis and the lack of visualization of gastric content passing into the duodenum (Hernanz-Schulman 2009; Malcom et al. 2009; Olson et al. 1998)
- Gastroesophageal reflux due to the overdistention of the stomach

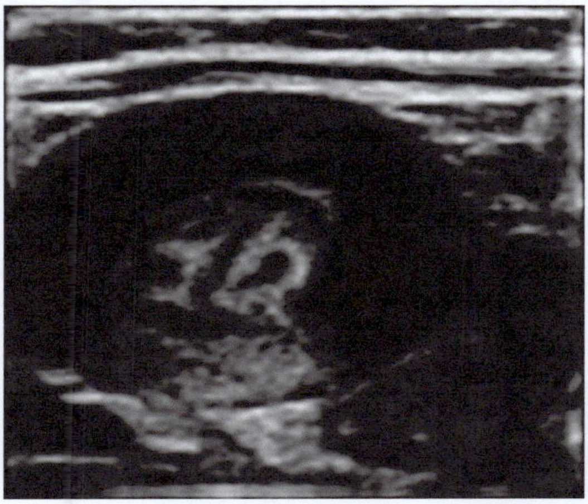

Fig. 8.16 Ultrasound transversal scan shows "target" sign due to hypertrophied hypoechoic muscle surrounding echogenic mucosa

As we have seen, the ultrasound study and the X-ray plain imaging and UGI have some specific or nonspecific signs of HPS in common like gastrectasy, hyperperistalsis, beak sign, shoulder sign, and so on.

The sensitivity and specificity of US to diagnose this condition is 98 % and 100 %, respectively. Nevertheless, in infants younger than 3 weeks, US cannot be useful because of the thin pyloric muscle thickness, so that they should be reevaluated after 2 days when the condition may be more clinically or radiologically evident.

8.5 Differential Diagnosis

The differential diagnoses regard especially gastroesophageal reflux and the spasm of the pyloric muscle.

In case of gastroesophageal reflux the clinic manifestation is different: in fact we don't have a "projectile" vomiting after feeding, the vomiting is not violent, and does not take place immediately after the feeding. Furthermore the clinical symptoms don't get better by putting to bed the baby immediately after the meal and using medical treatment.

However ultrasound allows to make the diagnosis of gastroesophageal reflux, viewing directly the food flowing back from the stomach to the esophagus; moreover, gastrectasy is frequent, and during the exam the pyloric muscle opens, allowing the passage of gastric contents in the duodenum (Figs. 8.20 and 8.21).

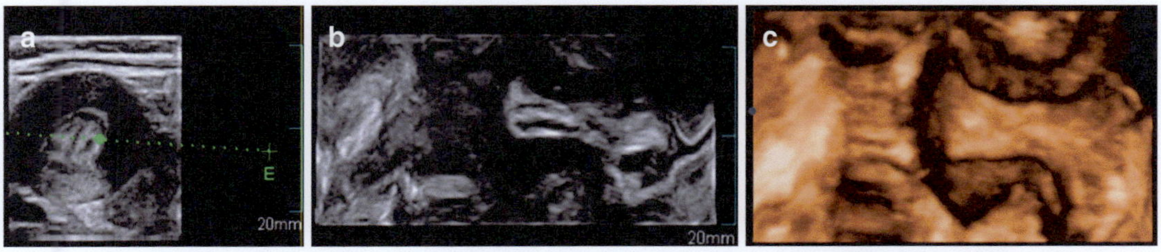

Fig. 8.17 (**a**) Two-dimensional and (**b**, **c**) three-dimensional ultrasound scans demonstrate the hypertrophic pyloric stenosis

Even for the spasm of the pyloric muscle, there are specific signs both with the radiology and with ultrasound; they have been just treated before in the text.

When the muscle layer is 2–3 mm thick and during the real-time ultrasound examination it does not relax, clinical follow-up with repeat US is recommended (Krogh et al. 2011).

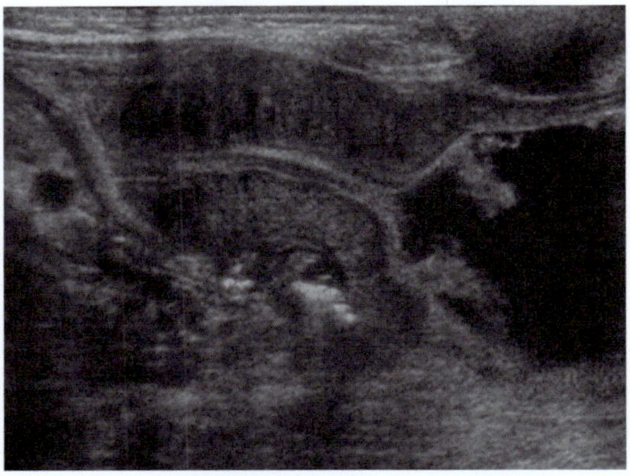

Fig. 8.18 Ultrasound longitudinal scan: "shoulder" sign due to the bulging of the hypertrophied pyloric muscle into the lumen of the antrum. The bulging causes a flattening of the prepyloric area of the lesser curvature

8.6 Treatment

Before performing any surgical intervention, the infant needs to be stabilized by correcting the electrolyte imbalance and dehydration.

The resuscitation period should last 24 h, but in the presence of a severe metabolic imbalance, an aggressive approach should be avoided because of rapid fluid and electrolyte shifts leading to seizures and other complications.

Intravenous administration of 5 % dextrose in 0.45 normal saline containing 20 mEq/l of potassium chloride is an optimal regimen to correct the metabolic imbalance. It is also necessary to control the urine output and serum electrolytes because potassium can be administered only in the presence of diuresis. After correcting serum chloride and serum bicarbonate imbalances, surgery can be performed.

HPS is managed surgically since 1892; at the beginning, the surgical approach consisted of gastroenterotomy; in 1899, Nicoll has been the first to attempt a surgery directed at the pylorus (Hernanz-Schulman 2003).

Nowadays the surgical treatment consists of pyloromyotomy, which is a longitudinal splitting

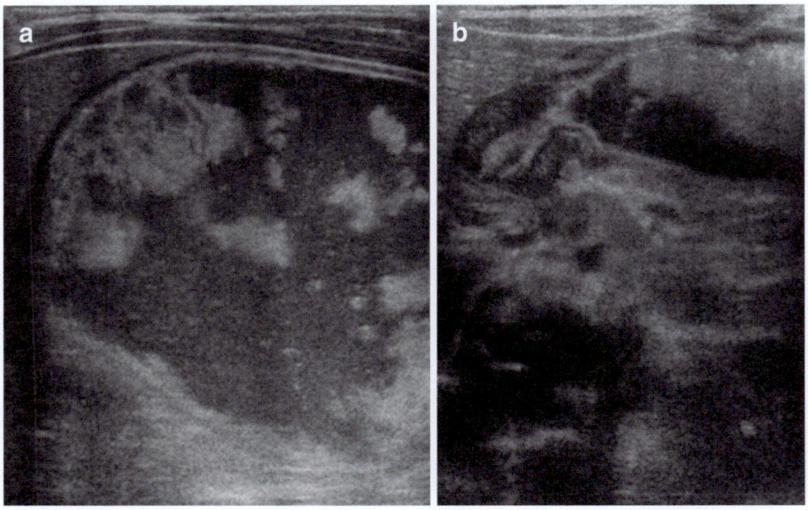

Fig. 8.19 (**a**, **b**) Ultrasound shows indirect signs of HPS: the stomach is distended and gastric peristalsis is increased, causing the "foamy" aspect of the gastric content due to the peristaltic movements which cause mixing of the luminal content

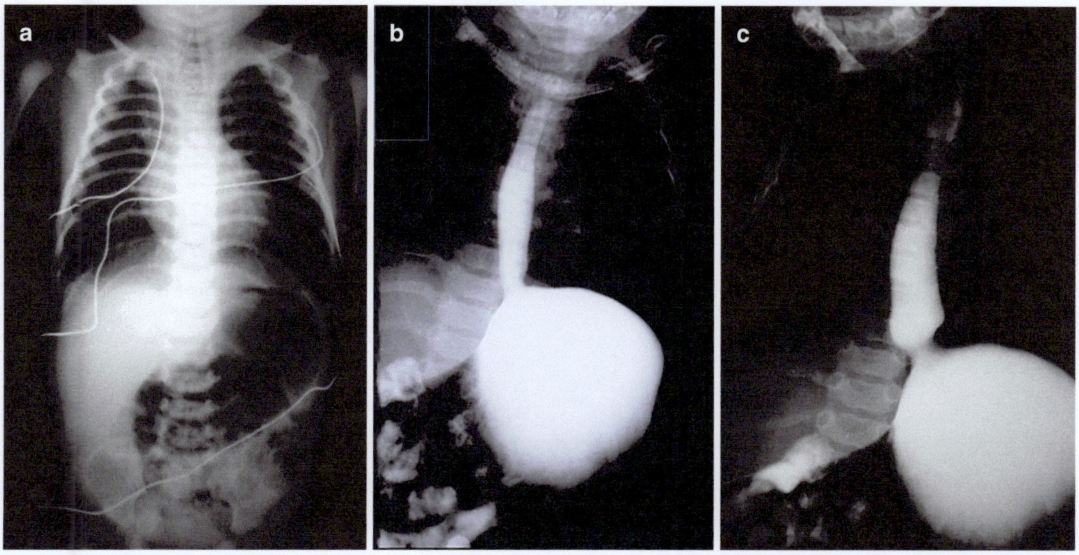

Fig. 8.20 Infant with spasm of the pyloric muscle and gastroesophageal reflux. (**a**) Plain film shows air gastric distention and the air passage in the bowel loops. (**b**, **c**) UGI radiographic examination shows gastrectasy, barium in the distal loops, and gastroesophageal reflux

of the seromuscular layer of the pylorus without suturing, through a right upper quadrant transverse incision.

Other approaches have been introduced, like that of Tan and Bianchi, who performed the pyloromyotomy through a supraumbilical skinfold incision, with an excellent cosmetic outcome.

In 1991, the laparoscopic approach was introduced by Alain, who described several advantages, like a short recovery, improved cosmesis, lower complication rates, and less postoperative pain (Ostlie and St Peter 2010; Alain et al. 1996).

There are also some reports from Asian countries about its nonsurgical management with atropine, whose rationale is that this condition may be due in part of impaired function of acetylcholine and muscarinic receptors. Atropine is an anticholinergic agent with antimuscarinic activity, so it can decrease intestinal peristalsis by relaxing smooth muscles. Nevertheless, this seems to be an alternative when surgery or anesthesia cannot be performed (Mercer and Philips 2013).

8.7 Posttreatment Imaging of HPS

A posttreatment imaging after surgical pyloromyotomy is requested just in case the vomiting is persisting. We have to remember that even after a successful surgery, the pyloric muscle may remain thickened for many weeks; in fact during the first week after surgery, the muscle can be so thick as before surgery or thicker than before surgery (because of edema). Generally after surgery, 6 weeks are enough to return to normal, but it can take up to 5 months for healing.

Related to the anterior surgical approach to the muscle, the anterior part of the muscle tends to normalize first, and the posterior part is the last to normalize.

In case of persistent vomiting, if further controls are necessary after surgery, ultrasound examination is usually performed because it can provide quite detailed information. Nevertheless, in order to evaluate an incomplete pyloromyotomy or gastroesophageal reflux or to exclude a duodenal leak, an upper GI examination is required (Hernanz-Schulman 2003; Costa Dias et al. 2012).

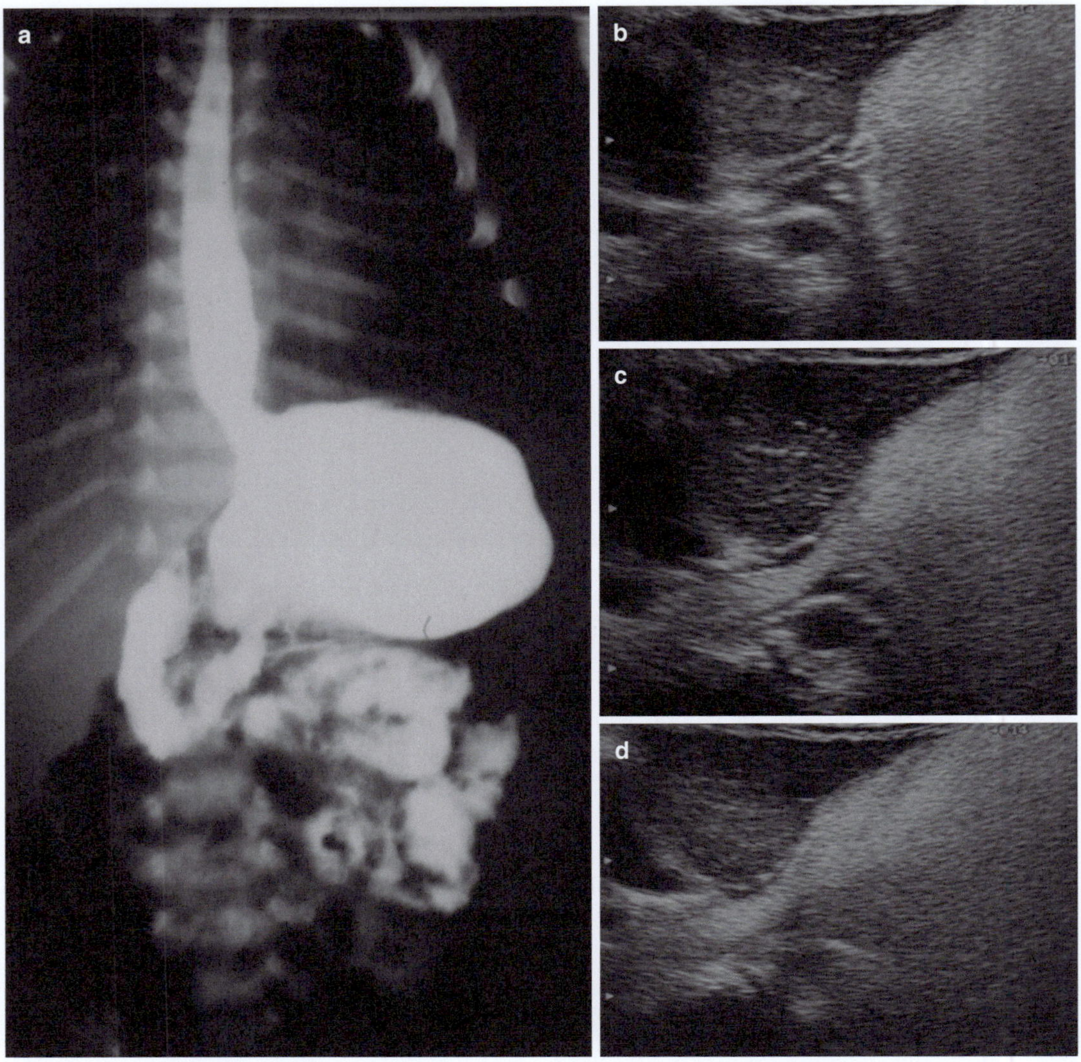

Fig. 8.21 Infant with gastroesophageal reflux. (**a**) UGI radiographic examination shows clearly the reflux of contrast medium in distal esophagus. (**b–d**) Several phases of ultrasound examination of gastroesophageal junction: we see the opening of the cardia and the large reflux of gastric contents into the esophagus. Note the gastrectasy and (**a**) the passage of contrast medium in the intestinal loops

Take-Home Points: Main Messages

- Hypertrophic pyloric stenosis is defined by the thickening of the muscular layer and failure in relaxation of the pyloric canal.
- The main diagnostic criterion is a measurement of more than 3 mm in thickness of the muscular layer.
- Abnormal elongation of the canal is characterized as greater than 12 mm in length.
- It is important to spend time watching for visualization of the passage of gastric contents through the pyloric canal because any visualization of active passage of gastric contents through a dilated, relaxed pylorus was also considered a negative study.
- It is recognized that older infants may have larger pyloric masses than younger infants presenting with HPS but that the minimum abnormal muscle wall measurement is 3 mm.
- In case of spasm of the pyloric muscle, the length of pyloric canal is <15 mm, the thickness of the pyloric muscle is <3 mm, and there is passage of gastric contents in the duodenum.

References

Alain JL, Grousseau D, Longis B, Ugazzi M, Terrier G (1996) Extramucosal pyloromyotomy by laparoscopy. Eur J Pediatr Surg 6:10–12

Argyropoulou MI, Hadjigeorg CG, Kiortsis DN (1998) Antro-pyloric canal values from early prematurity to full-term gestational age: an ultrasound study. Ped Radiol 28:933–936

Aspelund G, Langer JC (2007) Current management of hypertrophic pyloric stenosis. Semin Pediatr Surg 16:27–33

Costa Dias S, Swinson S, Torrão H, Gonçalves L, Kurochka S, Vaz CP, Mendes V (2012) Hypertrophic pyloric stenosis: tips and tricks for ultrasound diagnosis. Insights Imag 3:247–250

Di Giacomo V, Trinci M, Van der Byl G, Catania VD, Calisti A, Miele V (2015) Ultrasound in newborns and children suffering from nontraumatic acute abdominal pain: imaging with clinical and surgical correlation. J Ultrasound 18:385–393. doi:10.1007/s40477-014-0087-4, Epub 2014 Apr 9

Fonio P, Coppolino F, Russo A, D'Andrea A, Giannattasio A, Reginelli A, Grassi R, Genovese EA (2013) Ultrasonography (US) in the assessment of pediatric non traumatic gastrointestinal emergencies. Crit Ultrasound J 5(Suppl 1):S12

Frković M, Kuhar MS, Perhoč Z, Barbarić-Babić V, Molnar M, Vuković J (2001) Diagnostic imaging of hypertrophic pyloric stenosis (HPS). Radiol Oncol 35:11–16

Haran P, Darling D, Sciammas F (1966) The value of the double track sign as a differentiating factor between pylorospasm and hypertrophic pyloric stenosis in infants. Radiology 86:723–725

Hernanz-Schulman M (2003) Infantile hypertrophic pyloric stenosis. Radiology 227:319–331

Hernanz-Schulman M (2009) Pyloric stenosis: role of imaging. Pediatr Radiol 39(Suppl 2):S134–S139. doi:10.1007/s00247-008-1106-4

Hiorns MP (2011) Gastrointestinal tract imaging in children: current techniques. Pediatr Radiol 41:42–54

Krogh C, Cohen AS, Basit S, Hougaard DM, Biggar RJ, Wohlfhart J, Melbye M, Fischer TK (2011) Testosterone levels in umbilical-cord blood and risk of pyloric stenosis. Pediatrics 127:e197–e201. doi:10.1542/peds.2010–2127

Lisonkova S, Joseph KS (2014) Similarities and differences in the epidemiology of pyloric stenosis and SIDS. Matern Child Health J 18:1721–1727

MacMahon B (2006) The continuing enigma of pyloric stenosis of infancy: a review. Epidemiology 17:195–201

Malcom GE 3rd, Raio CC, Del Rios M, Blaivas M, Tsung JW (2009) Feasibility of emergency physician diagnosis of hypertrophic pyloric stenosis using point-of-care ultrasound: a multi-center case series. J Emerg Med 37:283–286

McKeown T, MacMahon B, Record RG (1951) Size of tumor in infantile pyloric stenosis related to age at operation. Lancet 29:556–558

Mercer AE, Philips R (2013) Question 2: can a conservative approach to the treatment of hypertrophic pyloric stenosis with atropine be considered a real alternative to surgical pyloromyotomy? Arch Dis Child 98:474–477

Miele V, Di Giampietro I (2014) Diagnostic imaging in emergency. Salute Soc (2EN):127–138. doi:10.3280/SES2014-002010EN

Miele V, Andreoli C, Grassi R (2006) The management of emergency radiology: key facts. Eur J Radiol 59:311–314, Epub 2006 Jun 27

Olson AD, Hernandez R, Hirschl RB (1998) The role of ultrasonography in the diagnosis of pyloric stenosis: a decision analysis. J Pediatr Surg 33:676–681
Ostlie DJ, St Peter SD (2010) The current state of evidence-based pediatric surgery. J Pediatr Surg 45:1940–1946
Panteli C (2009) New insights into the pathogenesis of infantile pyloric stenosis. Pediatr Surg Int 25: 1043–1052
Pedersen RN, Garne E, Loane M, Korsholm M, Husby S, EUROCAT working group (2008) Infantile hypertrophic pyloric stenosis: a comparative study of incidence and other epidemiological characteristics in seven European regions. J Matern Fetal Neonatal Med 21:599–604
Peters B, Oomen MWN, Bakx R, Benninga MA (2014) Advances in infantile hypertrophic pyloric stenosis. Expert Rev Gastroenterol Hepatol 8:533–541
Ricketts RR (1984) Workup of neonatal intestinal obstruction. Am Surg 50:517–521
Senquiz AL (1991) Use of decubitus position for finding the "olive" of pyloric stenosis. Pediatrics 87:266
Taylor ND, Cass DT, Holland AJ (2013) Infantile hypertrophic pyloric stenosis: has anything changed? J Paediatr Child Health 49:33–37
White MC, Langer JC, Don S, DeBaune MR (1998) Sensitivity and cost minimization analysis of radiology versus olive palpation for the diagnosis of hypertrophic pyloric stenosis. J Pediatr Surg 33:913–917

Intestinal Intussusception

9

Michele Galluzzo, Francesco Gaudino,
Riccardo Palliola, Eugenio Rossi,
Massimo Zeccolini, and Margherita Trinci

9.1 Introduction

Nontraumatic acute abdominal pain is one of the most common causes of access in the pediatric emergency department. Clinical evaluation of the child with abdominal pain is challenging because of the wide range of potential diagnosis. Intussusception is one of the leading causes of acute abdomen in infants and children younger than 1 year (85 % of cases), with a male predominance (M/F 3:1).

The vast majority of intussusceptions (95 %) occur after the first 3 months of life. From an anatomical point of view, invagination is an intestinal hernia, which is determined by the penetration with a telescopic, anterograde mechanism of a section of the bowel.

The characteristic symptomatic triad is represented by intermittent acute colicky abdominal pain, "red currant jelly" or bloody stool, and palpable mass or vomiting.

The role of imaging is crucial not only in confirming the clinical hypothesis, in establishing the grade of severity of the disease, and in the differential diagnosis but also in the therapeutic phase through reduction of intussusception.

Ultrasound examination is considered the technique of choice for the diagnosis, because of its high sensitivity (97.9 %) and specificity (97.8 %) especially if the symptoms are typical or strongly suspected.

9.2 Pathogenesis

Nontraumatic acute abdominal pain is one of the most common causes of access in the pediatric emergency department.

The clinical evaluation of the child with acute abdominal pain is challenging because of the wide range of potential diagnoses, which include congenital and acquired pathologies (Di Giacomo et al. 2014; Babcock 2002).

Intussusception is one of the leading causes of acute abdomen in infants and children younger than 1 year (85 % of cases), with a male predominance (M/F 3:1) (Shiyi et al. 2015; Lochhead et al. 2013; Costantino et al. 2015; Samad et al. 2013; Serayssol et al. 2014; Tarcà et al. 2015).

Based on the age, we have two different groups; in the first group, we have patients from 3 to 9 months old in which the cause is generally idiopathic, while in the second group, the children is older than 2 years and a pathologic lead

M. Galluzzo (✉) • F. Gaudino • R. Palliola • M. Trinci
Department of Emergency Radiology, S. Camillo Hospital, Rome, Italy
e-mail: galluzzom@tiscali.it

E. Rossi • M. Zeccolini
Department of Pediatric Radiology, Pausilipon Oncologic Pediatric Hospital, Naples, Italy

V. Miele, M. Trinci (eds.), *Imaging Non-traumatic Abdominal Emergencies in Pediatric Patients*,
DOI 10.1007/978-3-319-41866-7_9

point could be suspected (Di Giacomo et al. 2014; Shiyi et al. 2015; Tareen et al. 2015; Huppertz et al. 2006; Wong et al. 2015).

The vast majority of intussusceptions (95 %) occur then after the first 3 months of life (Di Giacomo et al. 2014; Esposito et al. 2006; Dinkel et al. 1983). In this age, in which a lead point cannot be identified, invagination in most cases is generally associated with the presence of enlarged lymph nodes as a result of an infection (Costantino et al. 2015; Wong et al. 2015; Bartocci et al. 2014; Hryhorczuk and Lee 2012; Csernia et al. 2007; Sorantin and Lindbichler 2004; Fischer et al. 2004; Okimoto et al. 2011; Cogley et al. 2012). This condition is rare in the first 3 months of life because passive immunity is still paramount.

Seasonal distribution is observed; in fact, the prevalence is more significant in spring and autumn (Huppertz et al. 2006).

The peak of incidence is around 6–8 months of life with the start of weaning, from here the hypothesis of the relationship between invagination and food allergies.

Other pathogenetic hypotheses for the idiopathic form include the hypertrophy of the lymphatic tissue of the gut, often secondary to viral infections; this is still the most accepted pathogenic hypothesis.

Also the greater disproportion between the size of the ileum and the ileocecal valve in young children than in older is discussed.

Another cause could be the absence of the normal bowel rotation and fixation (Waugh's syndrome, association between intussusception and malrotation).

Another hypothesis is the increase of the intestinal peristalsis and the ileocecal valve relaxation due to the increase of the production of nitric oxide caused by inflammatory reactions that usually precede the intussusception.

Also any cause of hyperperistalsis can lead to an intussusception as malabsorption syndrome (celiac disease and so on).

From anatomical point of view, invagination is an intestinal hernia, which is determined by the penetration with a telescopic, anterograde mechanism of a section of the bowel (colonic or ileal loop) into itself (Bartocci et al. 2014; Del-Pozo et al. 1999; Dankoff et al. 2015) (Fig. 9.1).

The "receiving loop" (intussuscipiens) contains the "donor loop" (intussuscepted). In the intussuscipiens, the central entering and the edematous returning limbs are contained. The intussusception is usually composed of three cylinders, in some complex shapes from five or seven (Cogley et al. 2012; Del-Pozo et al. 1999).

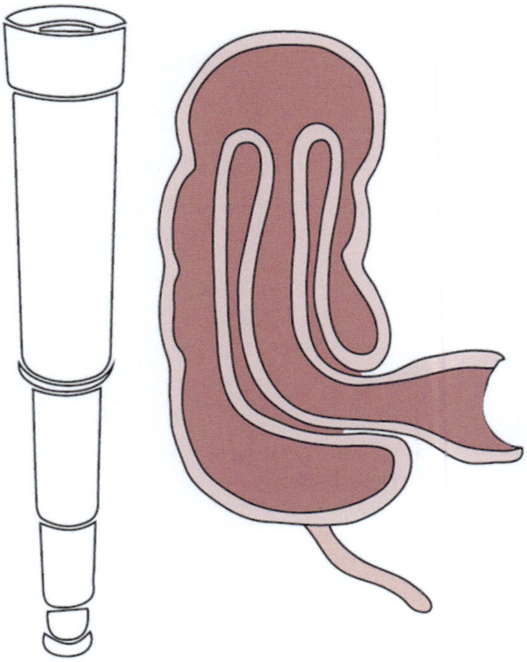

Fig. 9.1 The drawing illustrates that the invagination is determined by the penetration with a telescopic, anterograde mechanism of a section of the bowel into itself. (Thanks to Paola Valori for the drawing)

The most frequent localization is the ileocecal form, where the lead point of the invaginated segment is represented by the valve of Varolio (Tareen et al. 2015; Dankoff et al. 2015; Di Fiore 1999). The intussusception can be ileo-colonic where the head is the ileocecal valve and the ileum is the collar, and rarely it can also be colocolonic or ileoileal (Fig. 9.2).

The stretching and compression of the mesenteric vascular pedicle will cause over time a venous congestion followed by edema of the intestinal wall with a possible wall necrosis and/or perforation (Wong et al. 2015; Di Fiore 1999; Pinto et al. 2016; Sessa et al. 2016).

Strangulation of mesenteric vascular pedicle causes mechanical ileus. The mechanical ileus, if untreated, may progress into a paralytic ileus.

In the idiopathic form, the herniation of intestine in the intestine and the combination of

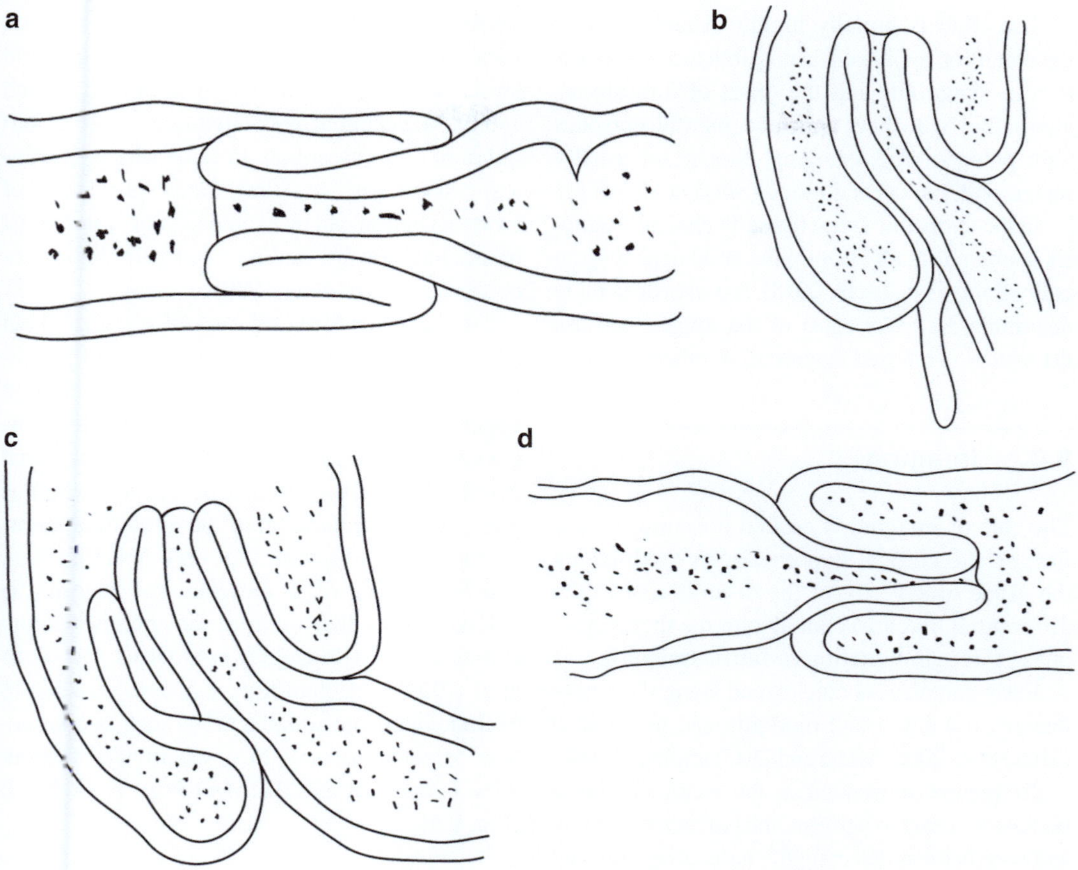

Fig. 9.2 Types of intussusception: (**a**) ileoileal, (**b**) ileocolic, (**c**) ileocecal, and (**d**) colo-colic. (Thanks to Paola Valori for the drawing)

the greater peristalsis and insufficient fixing of the right colon, which prevents progression of intestinal contents, often cause the herniation progression in the stretch downstream.

In the population of older children as in adults, the intussusception is usually secondary; the mechanism is generally caused by the presence of a focal alteration, which works as a lead point, for example, appendicitis, the presence of Meckel diverticulum, polyp, hemangioma, or association with conditions causing hypertrophy of Peyer patches (i.e., Henoch-Schönlein purpura, lymphoma, rotavirus infection) (Di Giacomo et al. 2014; Shiyi et al. 2015; Costantino et al. 2015; Tarcà et al. 2015; Wong et al. 2015; Bartocci et al. 2014; Del-Pozo et al. 1999; Dankoff et al. 2015; Kim et al. 1982; Mandeville et al. 2012; Applegate 2009; Navarro et al. 2000; Rogers and Robb 2010; Miele et al. 2001; Valentini et al. 2015).

9.3 Clinical Findings

The characteristic symptomatic triad represented by intermittent acute colicky abdominal pain, "red currant jelly" or bloody stool, and palpable mass or vomiting is present in a proportion of cases, which varies between 36 % and 68 % (Cogley et al. 2012; Del-Pozo et al. 1999); in fact, many of the young patients do not present the full symptomatic triad, especially in traditional forms (Bartocci et al. 2014).

Some authors describe, especially at an early stage of diagnosis, abdominal pain, vomiting, and indrawing of the legs, whereas "currant jelly stool" is a late sign, expressing wall necrosis (Shiyi et al. 2015).

The abdominal pain is often very intense and violent and may occur suddenly particularly at night. Vomiting is frequent, while the bowel motion may be initially normal.

The child is initially highly irritable, and as the condition evolves, it is possible to see a reduction in symptoms and the onset of drowsiness, alternating with new appeared painful episodes with paleness and sweating. Stools are usually mixed with mucus and blood (Shiyi et al. 2015).

In the idiopathic form, the early clinical diagnosis is often difficult because the child appears generally florid (Tarcà et al. 2015). It is also difficult to determine the exact onset of the disease because the history is referred by parents or other persons.

9.4 Imaging

The role of imaging is crucial not only in confirming the clinical hypothesis, in establishing the grade of severity of the disease, and in the differential diagnosis but also in the therapeutic phase through reduction of intussusception.

Early diagnosis is crucial, and along with early therapy, morbidity and mortality can be reduced (Miele et al. 2006; Miele and Di Giampietro 2014).

At present ultrasound is the exam of choice because it is easy to perform, it has a high sensibility and specificity in detecting the intussusception, and there is no radio exposition for the young patient and the operator. In the past time, X-ray study was performed; anyway it is important to know the limits and advantages of both techniques.

Especially in the past, several authors discussed the residual role of plain abdominal film (Tareen et al. 2015; Cogley et al. 2012; Del-Pozo et al. 1999).

Some authors argue that "Intussusception cannot be reliably ruled out with clinical examination and plain radiograph" (Del-Pozo et al. 1999).

At present days, in our experience, plain radiograph is not the exam of choice in the case of abdominal pain but can be helpful especially when examined by the same radiologist who performs the ultrasound examination and when clinical findings are confusing and the ultrasound exam is unclear.

9.5 Plain Film Semeiotics

The plain radiograph shows no specific signs; it evaluates the position of the blind end of the cecum, the distribution of intestinal gas and stools, and the bowel dilation above the stenosis with stagnation of liquids showing as air-fluid levels. Viewing the normal position of the blind end of the cecum is associated rarely with a condition of intussusception. In cases where the clinical suspicion is low, the presence of intussusception can be excluded, and search must be oriented toward finding other pathologic processes (Del-Pozo et al. 1999).

At the plain film, we can have some direct signs due to the intussuscepted segment, represented as an image of soft tissue mass in the right upper quadrant; it is also possible to see the "target sign," which consists of a soft tissue mass that contains concentric circular of lucency, which is due to the mesenteric fat of the intussusceptions, or the "meniscus sign," a very specific sign, which consists of a crescent gas within the colonic lumen that outlines the intussusceptum (Wong et al. 2015; Cogley et al. 2012; Del-Pozo et al. 1999). On plain film, it is also possible to exclude intestinal complications such as obstruction or perforation, with a sensitivity of about 45 % (Cogley et al. 2012; Del-Pozo et al. 1999) (Fig. 9.3).

9.6 Barium Enema Semeiotics

To perform the examination of the contrast sac, containing barium sulfate at high dilution, it is positioned at a meter in height than the patient's level; a rectal tube is positioned and barium falls by gravity. The retrograde progression of barium column is followed by fluoroscopy (Hryhorczuk and Lee 2012; Burns et al. 2014; Raval et al. 2015; Sadigh et al. 2015; Shiels et al. 1991).

Semiotics of barium enema is a filling defect, which is simply concave, and looks as "nipper" or "gallows" if the barium enters into the sheath and sometimes as a "coiled spring" when the final stretch of invaginated is filled (Fig. 9.4a–d).

In the past, barium was widely used as a contrast medium. This causes a series of possible serious complications; the most severe is the intestinal perforation (1/1,000), which can cause chemistry barium peritonitis and occurs when there is a condition of malacia of the intestinal wall (Fig. 9.5). Chemistry peritonitis can be a

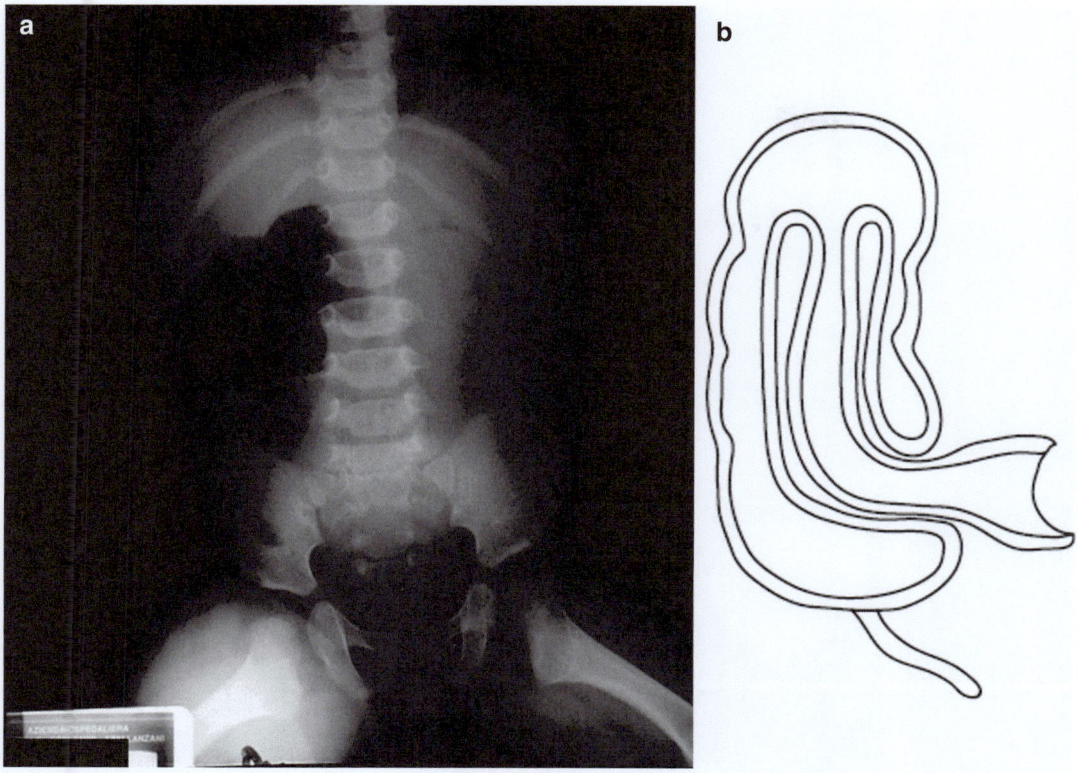

Fig. 9.3 (**a**) Plain film of an infant shows the absence of the blind end of the cecum and the "meniscus sign". (**b**) The drawing illustrates the invagination site. (Thanks to Paola Valori for the drawing)

life-threatening disease, because it determines a further worsening of the general condition. Also in the case of timely surgical intervention, it can cause severe adhesion syndromes.

Actually, enema is performed using a solution of iodinated hydrosoluble contrast medium, diluted at 10 % in 1,000 ml water. This technique will be described extensively later.

9.7 Ultrasound Semeiotic

Ultrasound examination is considered the technique of choice for the diagnosis, because of its high sensitivity (97.9 %) and specificity (97.8 %) especially if the symptoms are typical or strongly suspected (Tareen et al. 2015; Wong et al. 2015; Bartocci et al. 2014; Cogley et al. 2012; Del-Pozo et al. 1999; Kim et al. 1982; Britton and Wilkinson 1999; Flaum et al. 2015).

The components of intussusception produce characteristic appearances like a large structure (>5×2.5 cm) that displaces bowel loops and can be "readily identified," even by "inexperienced operators" (Del-Pozo et al. 1999; Ramsey and Halm 2014).

The majority of intussusceptions (ileocolic type) occur in the right side in subhepatic region (Del-Pozo et al. 1999).

To perform the exam, the child is in supine position; the use of linear probe (5–7.5 Mhz) is preferred in the younger baby, while in the older the convex probe (3.5 Mhz) can add some information and give an important panoramicity.

The examination is performed with axial, longitudinal, and oblique scans that usually start from right lower abdominal quadrant. It is important to complete the exam with a complete exploration of the abdominal cavity to exclude any other cause of pathology.

The sonographic semiotics is based on direct sign and indirect sign; the evaluation of the intestinal loops in real time is even important.

Ultrasound direct signs are represented to the visualization of the intussuscepted loop: in the

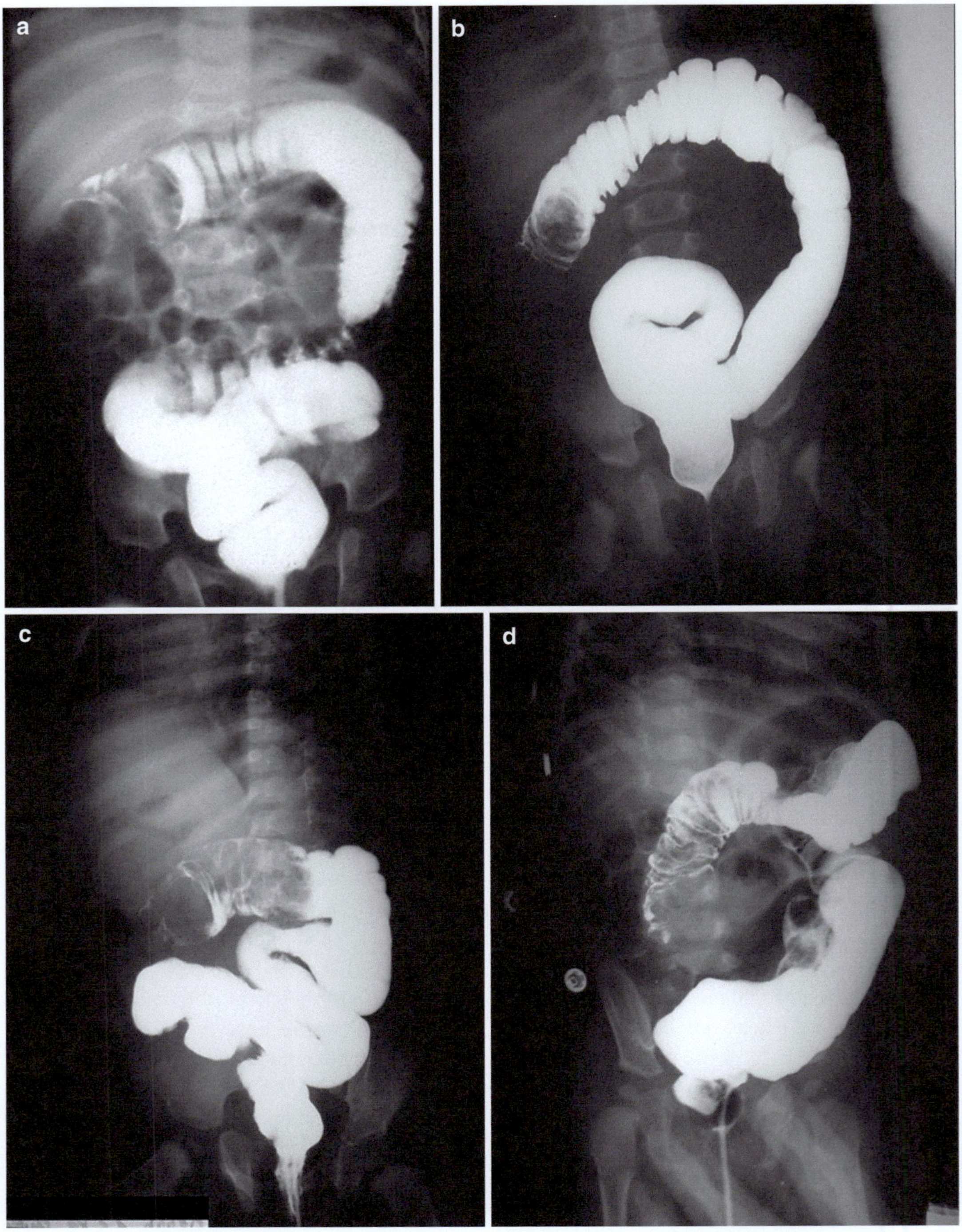

Fig. 9.4 (**a–d**) Semiotics of enema: a filling defect of the right colon, which may be simply concave, as "nipper" or "gallows" and sometimes as a "coiled spring"

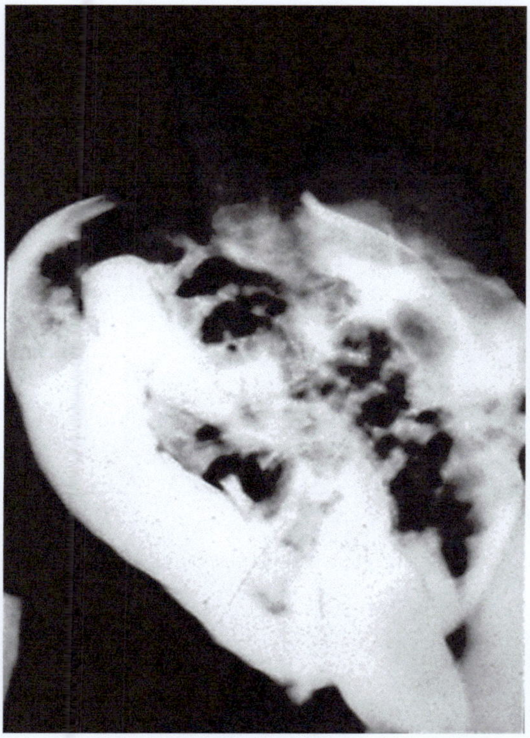

Fig. 9.5 Barium enema: this film shows an infant with intestinal perforation

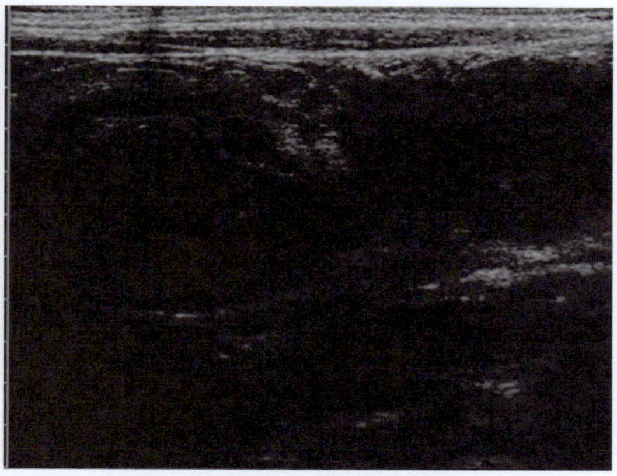

Fig. 9.6 Ultrasound axial scan in an infant with intestinal intussusception shows an inhomogeneous rounded mass due to the herniation of the intussuscepted loop in the receiving one, with the mesenteric fat and lymph nodes in the center

axial scans, we can see an inhomogeneous rounded pseudotumor, because of the presence of the different layers of the intestinal loops, the receiving loop, and the intussuscepted one, with the mesenteric fat and often lymph nodes in the center (Fig. 9.6).

The complex ultrasound aspect is due to these different components; in fact we can see a hyperechoic outer ring separated with a hypoechoic component from another thin hyperechoic layer. The two hyperechoic rings is supposed to be the opposed serous surface of the intussuscepted. The mass also has a hyperechoic center that is the mesenteric fat and inner lymph nodes. This complex and stratified aspect is called "target sign" or "crescent in doughnut" or "pseudokidney aspect" in the oblique scan (Di Giacomo et al. 2014; Babcock 2002; Bartocci et al. 2014; Cogley et al. 2012; Del-Pozo et al. 1999; Kim et al. 1982; Ramsey and Halm 2014; Sanchez et al. 2015; Lioubashevsky et al. 2013; Lam et al. 2014) (Fig. 9.7a, b).

In the longitudinal scans, we can observe the intussuscepted loops that enter in the intussuscipiens loop and the mesentery that is dragged along with the bowel loop; this image is called "sandwich sign" or "bowel-in-bowel" sign. In particular, in longitudinal scan we have an outer parallel hypoechoic band due to the edematous everted portion of the intussuscepted and the thin intussuscipiens, a central parallel hypoechoic band that is the central limb of the intussuscepted. The hypoechoic bands are separated with hyperechoic layers that represent the mesentery fat (Fig. 9.8).

In some cases it is possible to see the loops that push in the receiving loop when the baby cries for the increasing of the intra-abdominal pressure.

A complete exam also includes executing color Doppler: this technique may offer some additional information about the condition of the loop; in fact if the wall of the loop is well perfused, we have a typical double-ring sign (Di Giacomo et al. 2014) (Fig. 9.9a–c).

On the contrary, the absence of hyperemia is a specific index of ischemic wall damage, which increases the risk of perforation (Cogley et al. 2012).

The presence of the signal does not exclude at all, however, the presence of suffering ischemic areas.

The careful research of the presence of free fluid in the abdomen or interposed fluid between bowel loops of the intussuscepted tract, the so-called trapped fluid sign, is also essential (Del-Pozo et al. 1999). This sign is very significant because it is associated with a lower reduction rate and the increased likelihood of the presence of necrotic tracts (Bartocci et al. 2014; Del-Pozo et al. 1999) (Fig. 9.10).

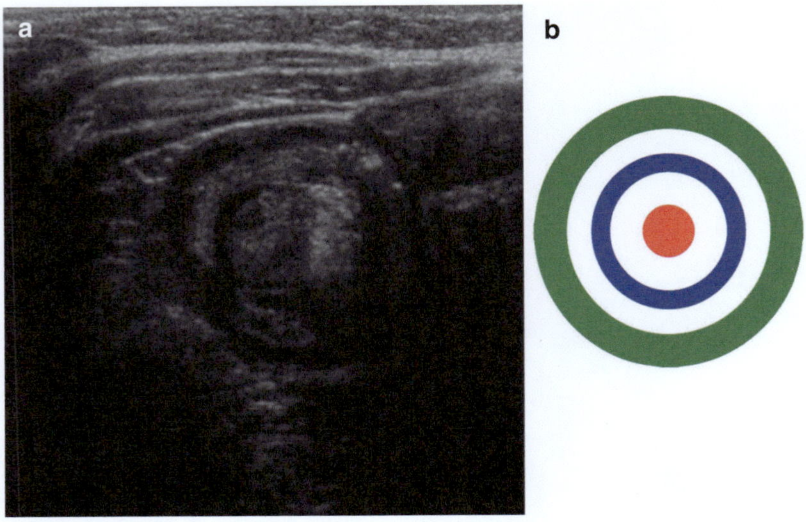

Fig. 9.7 (**a**, **b**) Ultrasound axial scan in an infant with intestinal intussusception and the scheme shows the "target" sign. (Thanks to Paola Valori for the drawing)

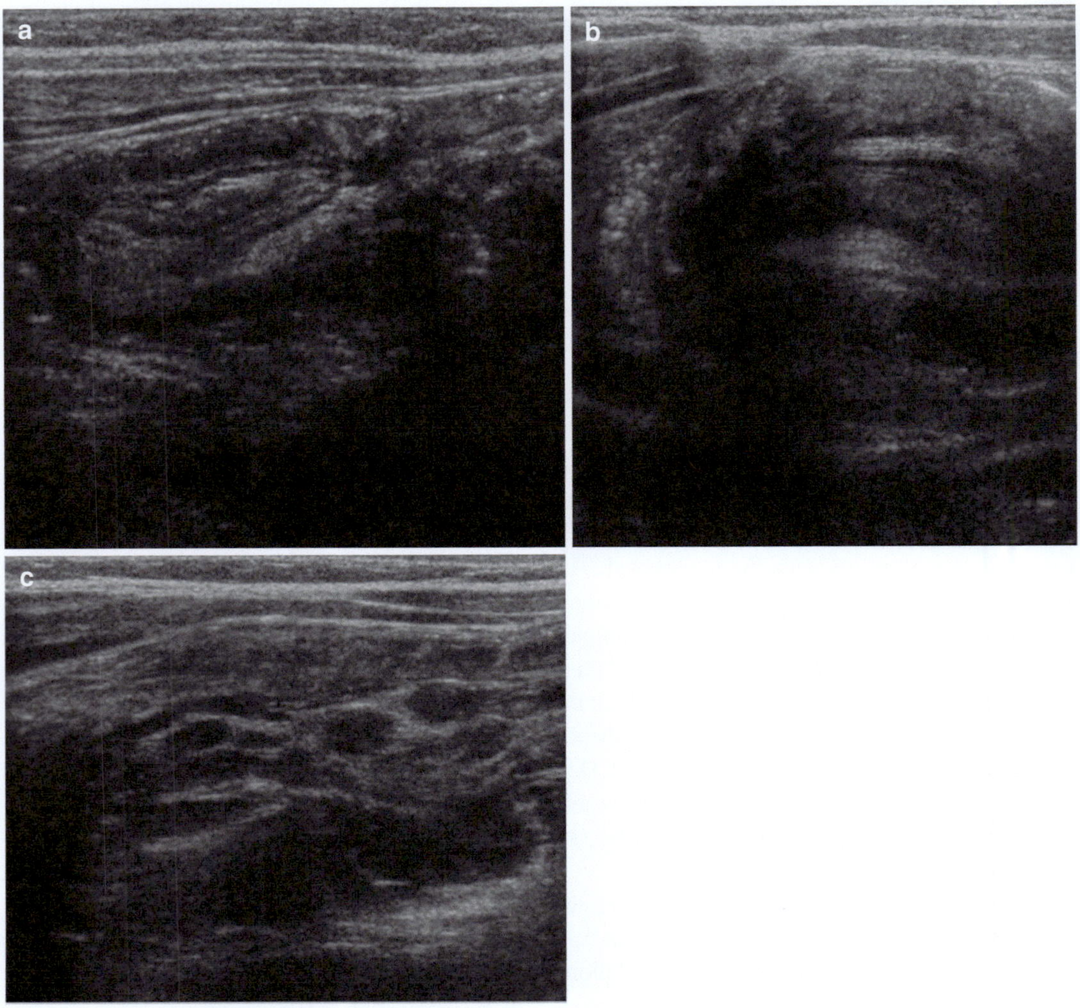

Fig. 9.8 (**a–c**) Ultrasound longitudinal scan in an infant with intestinal intussusception shows the typical aspect "sandwich sign." Note in "**c**" many inflammatory lymph nodes in the mesenteric root

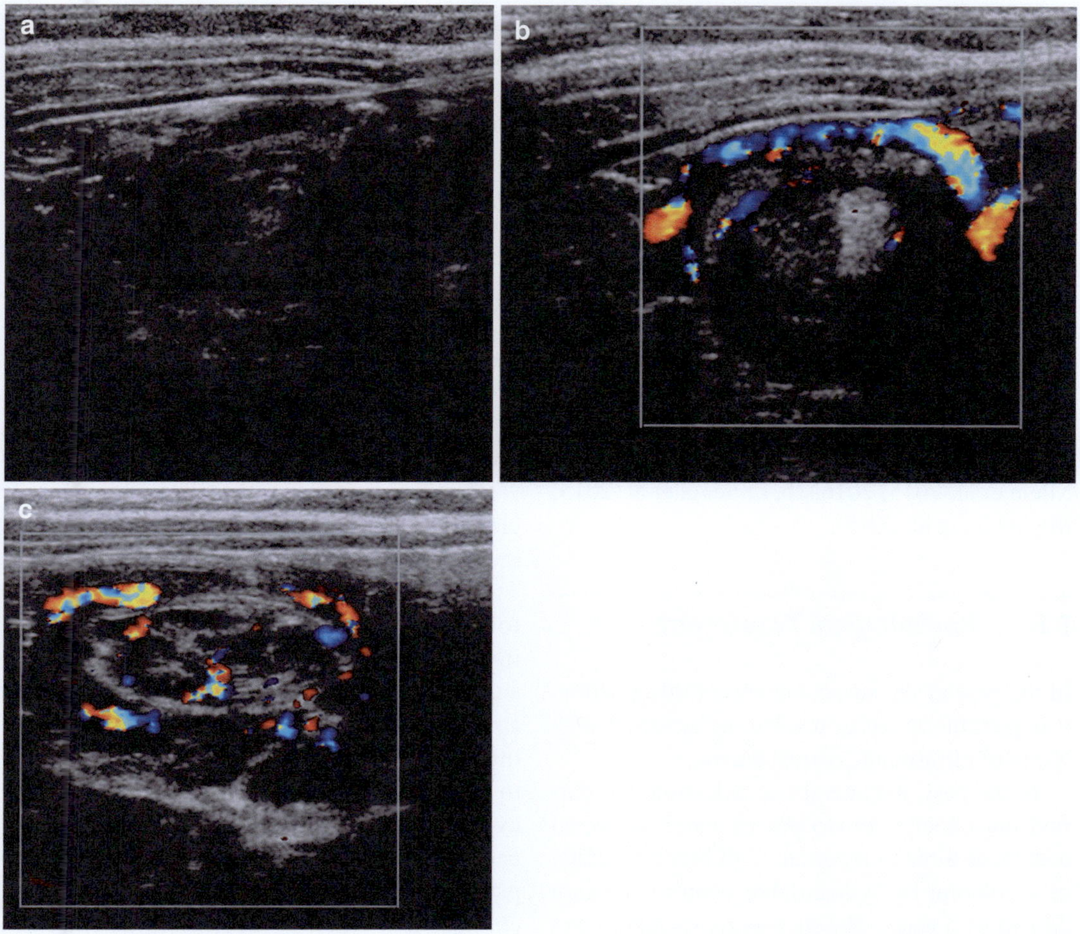

Fig. 9.9 (**a–c**) Ultrasound B-mode and color Doppler scans in an infant with intestinal intussusception show the typical aspect "double-ring" sign in the wall of the perfused loop

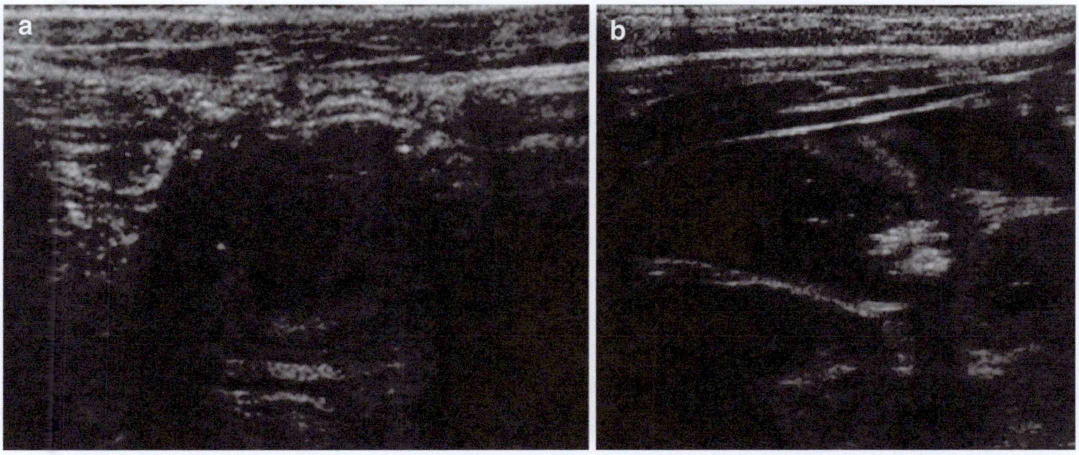

Fig. 9.10 (**a**, **b**) Ultrasound axial and longitudinal scans in teenager with intestinal intussusception due to appendicitis; note the presence of free fluid between the loops

The presence of free fluid, the absence of color Doppler signal in the wall loop, and the indirect sign of intestinal bowel occlusion as fluid-distended loops and hypoperistalsis have a bad prognostic value and are suggestive for a not recent pathology event.

In this case, the surgical approach is recommended as soon as possible to prevent the necrosis of the loop, the perforation, and the peritonitis.

CEUS is frequently used in traumatic acute abdominal emergencies, and it is still not defined the exact role in the nontraumatic acute abdominal pain in pediatric patients (Catalano et al. 2004; Farina et al. 2015; Pinto et al. 2014, 2015; Miele et al. 2015, 2016a, b, c; Sessa et al. 2015; Menichini et al. 2015).

9.8 Radiological Treatment

In the case of the suspect of recent invagination, it is possible to try to resolve the situation with X-ray or ultrasound contrast enema.

In the past, the attempt of reduction was carried out under fluoroscopic guidance, using an enema, as already reported, with barium sulfate, or a solution of hydrosoluble contrast medium diluted with water. The success rate is reported in 72 % and 87 % of cases (Rogers and Robb 2010; Flaum et al. 2015).

Most recent papers describe the attempt of reduction using pneumatic pressure air, always under fluoroscopic guidance (Britton and Wilkinson 1999; Flaum et al. 2015; Munden et al. 2007; Bai et al. 2006).

The main disadvantages of this method are the radiation exposure for both the medical team and the young patient (Shiels et al. 1991; Sanchez et al. 2015).

At present day, the ultrasound technique is a valid alternative and in some centers is preferred to the X-ray method. This method has been described for the first time by Kim et al. (1982).

The procedure takes place after having obtained the informed consent from the parents. In the ultrasound room where a venous access to the infant is placed, the radiologist performs the exam with the presence of a pediatric surgeon, and the operating room has been alerted.

The child is placed on the bed in the ultrasound room in supine position.

A Foley catheter is positioned into the rectum, without inflating the balloon. We prepare a sac for the enema with a 1,000 ml solution of iodinated contrast medium diluted at 10 % with warm water.

The presence of contrast medium in the solution is necessary, because at the end of the ultrasound reduction attempt, an abdomen plain film is carried out, to demonstrate with certainty the success or the failure of the procedure.

The sac containing the enema solution is placed at a meter in height than the patient's level; the solution falls by gravity.

During the ultrasound exam, we have to follow the retrograde progression of the water into the colon to the point of colonic intussusception. Intestinal loops progressively stretch; when the fluid reaches the point of intussusception, we can gently use the probe to force the fluid to penetrate between the cylinders of intussusception. When the procedure is successful, the morphology of the pseudotumor due to the bowel invagination changes gradually. In fact the fluid penetrates between the intestinal rings, which oversteps the point of the stop and goes beyond (Fig. 9.11a–l).

In the case of success of the procedure, the sonographic signs of intussusception are no longer recognizable in the different scans; the pain of the baby stops immediately.

Success rates vary depending on different cases from 76 % to 95 % and are similar to those that involve the use of conventional contrast barium or air under fluoroscopic guidance (Sadigh et al. 2015; Shiels et al. 1991; Britton and Wilkinson 1999).

The final radiographic plain film allows documenting the complete opacification of the colon and the possible passage of contrast in the distal intestinal tract.

In the case of failure of this procedure, the water stops close to the intussuscepted segment, and surgical reduction of the intussusception is needed (Fig. 9.12).

It is recommended to perform the ultrasound-guided reduction attempts no more than three times.

Every time at the end of the procedure, we have to remove the Foley catheter and from the rectum will flow out water mixed with stool; if the color of the water is reddish, it means that there is a suffering of the involved loop. In this case, the exam has to be stopped, and the patients must undergo surgical treatment as soon as possible.

The procedure is not recommended if the history of intussusception is not recent, i.e., >48 h, because it is possible that the intestinal wall has had an ischemic sufferance; in the case of a second episode of intussusception, because it is possible that the cause could be an organic disease, as a polyp or Meckel diverticulum; and/or in older children because usually the intussusception is secondary.

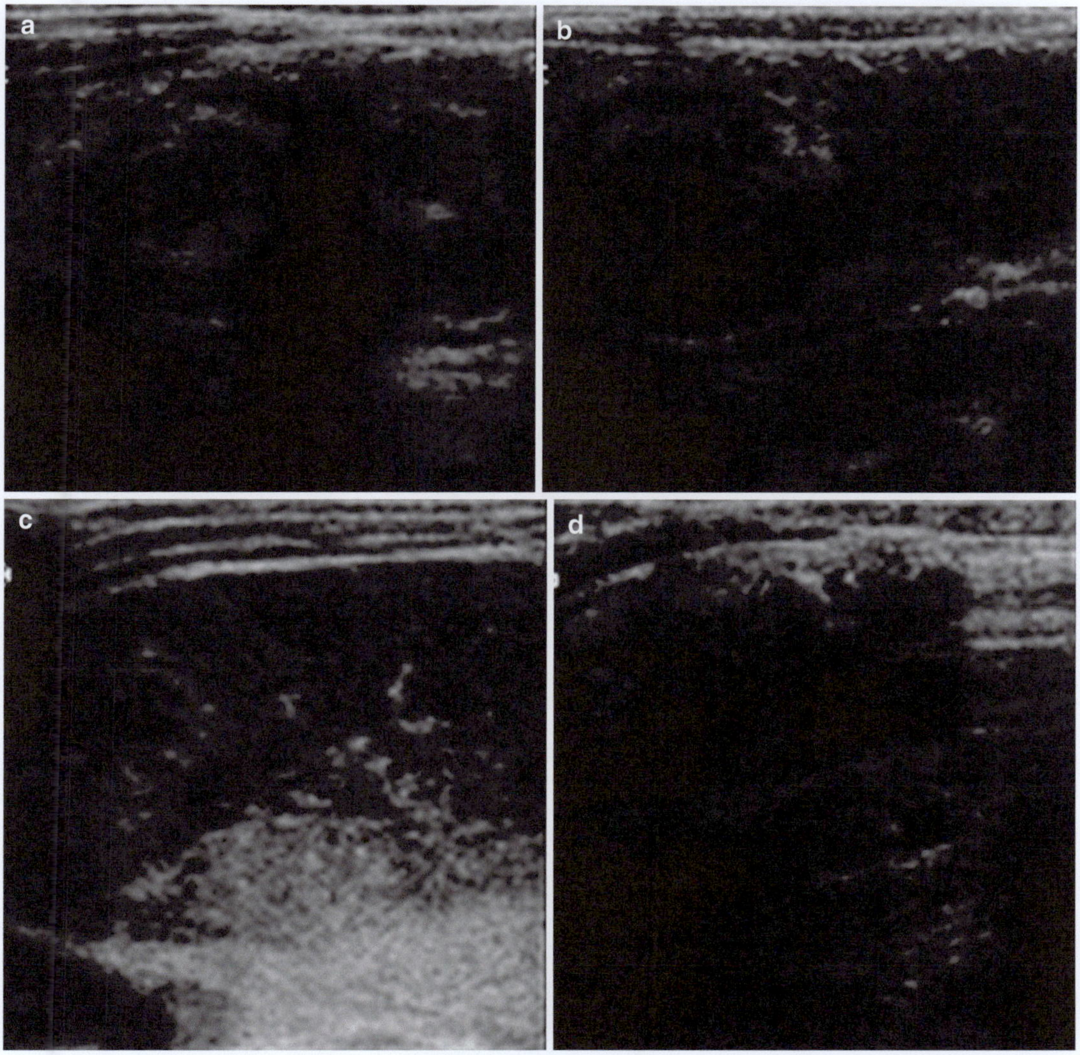

Fig. 9.11 (**a–j**) Ultrasound axial and longitudinal scans in an infant with intestinal intussusception during the enema under ultrasound guidance. X-ray performed at the end of the procedure confirms the success of the procedure

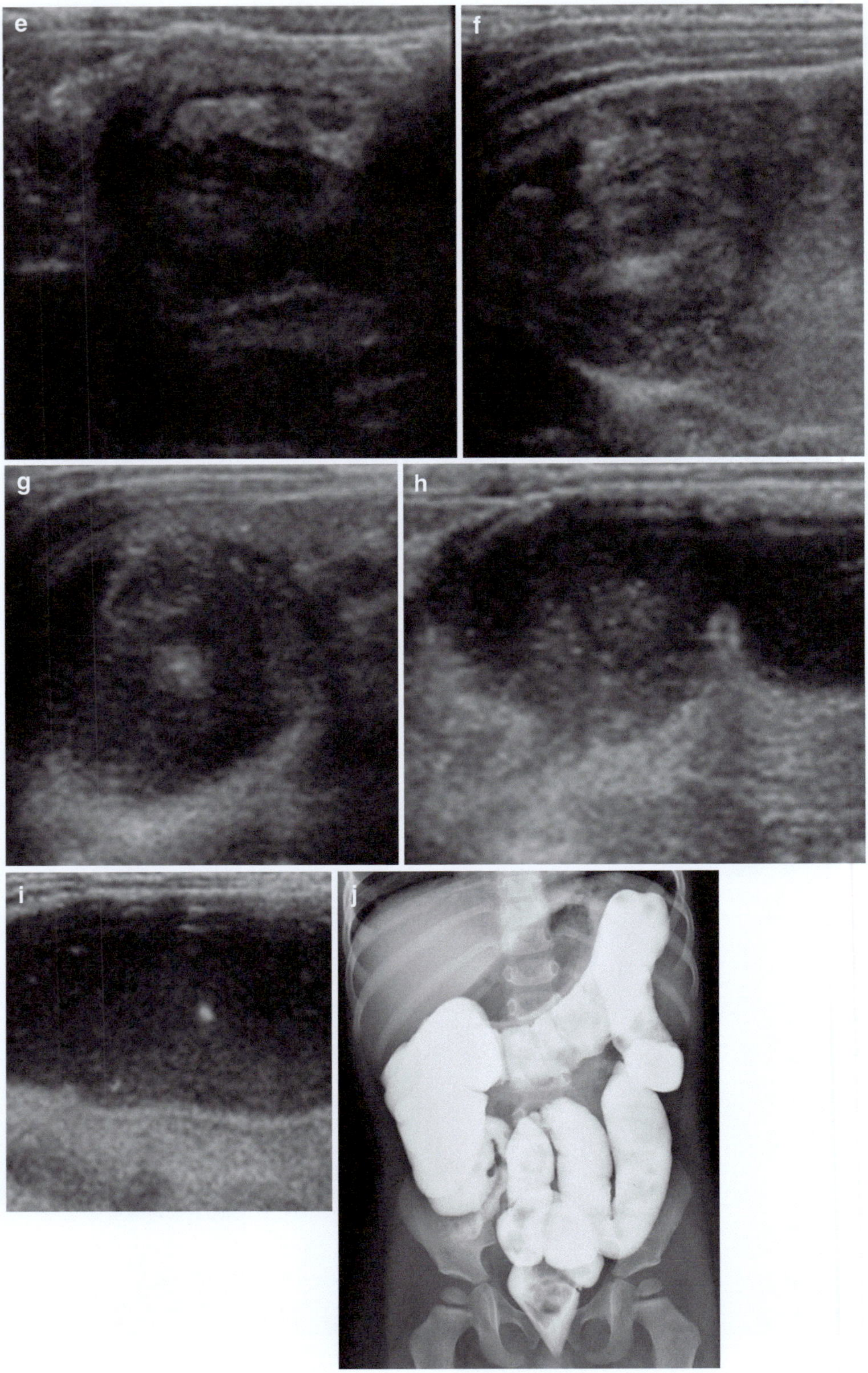

Fig. 9.11 (continued)

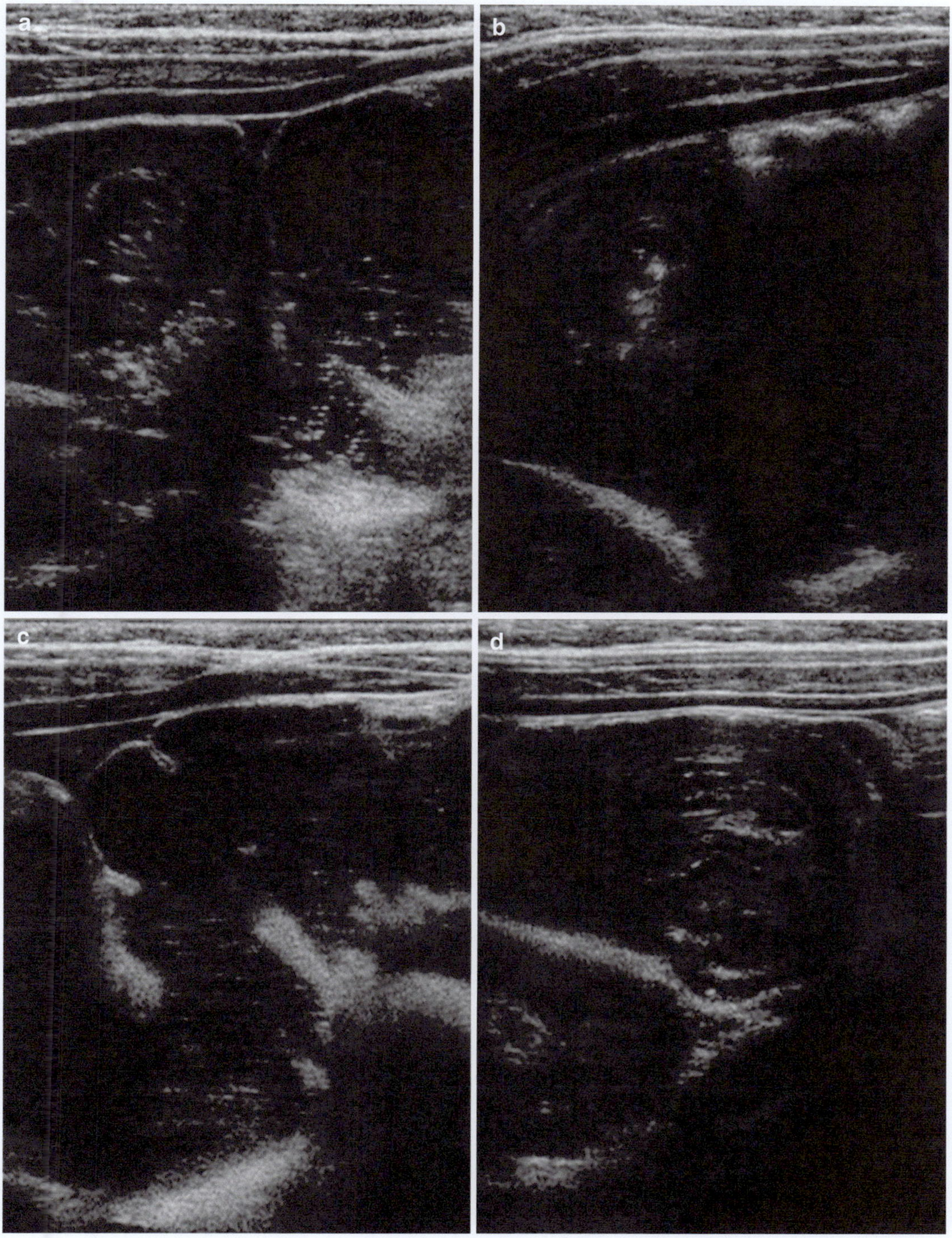

Fig. 9.12 (**a–d**) Ultrasound axial and longitudinal scans in an infant with intestinal intussusception during the enema under ultrasound guidance. The ultrasound enema is unsuccessful: in fact during the ultrasound exam, the water reaches the intussuscepted tract but doesn't go beyond the invaginated tract. Note a small amount of free fluid between the loops

References

Applegate KE (2009) Intussusception in children: evidence-based diagnosis and treatment. Pediatr Radiol 39(Suppl 2):S140–S143

Babcock DS (2002) Sonography of the acute abdomen in the pediatric patient. J Ultrasound Med Off J Am Inst Ultrasound Med 21(8):887–899 (quiz 900–881)

Bai YZ, Qu RB, Wang GD et al (2006) Ultrasound-guided hydrostatic reduction of intussusceptions by saline enema: a review of 5218 cases in 17 years. Am J Surg 192:273–275

Bartocci M, Fabrizi G, Valente (2014) Intussusception in childhood, role of sonography on diagnosis and treatment. J Ultrasound 18:2015–11

Britton I, Wilkinson AG (1999) Ultrasound features of intussusception predicting outcome of air enema. Pediatr Radiol 29:705–710

Burns R, Adler M, Benya E et al (2014) Fluoroscopy screen time during contrast enema for evaluation and treatment of intussusception. Pediatr Emerg Care 30:327–330

Catalano O, Lobianco R, Sandomenico F, Mattace Raso M, Siani A (2004) Real time contrast enhanced sonographic imaging in emergency radiology. Radiol Med 108:454–469

Cogley JR, O'Connor SO, Houshyar et al (2012) Emergent pediatric US: what every radiologist should know. RadioGraphics 32:651–665

Costantino C, Restivo V, Cuccia M et al (2015) Analysis of hospitalizations due to intussusception in Sicily in the pre-rotavirus vaccination era (2003–2012). Ital J Pediatr 10:261–265

Csernia T, Parana S, Puria P (2007) New hypothesis on the pathogenesis of ileocecal intussusceptions. J Pediatr Surg 42(9):1515–1519

Dankoff S, Puligandia P, Beres A et al (2015) An unusual presentation of small bowel intussusception. CJEM 17:318–321

Del-Pozo G, Albillos JC et al (1999) Intussusception in children: current concepts in diagnosis and enema reduction. Radiographics 19:299–319

Di Fiore JW (1999) Intussusception. Semin Pediatr Surg 8(4):214–220

Di Giacomo V, Trinci M, Van der Byl G (2014) Ultrasound in newborns and children suffering from non-traumatic acute abdominal pain: imaging with clinical and surgical correlation. J Ultrasound 18:385–393

Dinkel E, Dittrich M, Pristor G et al (1983) Sonographic diagnosis of intussusception in childhood. Z Kinderchir 38:220–223

Esposito F, Quarantelli M et al (2006) Segni ecografici di irriducibilità dell'invaginazione in età pediatrica. Nostra esperienza e review della letteratura. G Ital Ecografia 9(1):49–54

Farina R, Catalano O, Stavolo C, Sandomenico F, Petrillo RL (2015) Emergency radiology. Radiol Med 120:73–84. doi:10.1007/s11547-014-0480-2121

Fischer TK, Bihrmann K, Perch M et al (2004) Intussusception in early childhood: a cohort study of 1.7 million children. Pediatrics 114(3):782–785

Flaum V, Schneider A, Ferreira CG et al (2015) Twenty years' experience for reduction of ileocolic intussusceptions by saline enema under sonography control. J Pediatr Surg 51:179–182

Hryhorczuk AL, Lee EY (2012) Imaging evaluation of bowel obstruction in children: updates in imaging techniques and review of imaging findings. Semin Roentgenol 47(2):159–170

Huppertz HI, Soriano-Gabarrò M et al (2006) Intussusception among young children in Europe. Pediatr Infect Dis J 25:22–29

Kim YG, Choi BI, Yeon KM et al (1982) Diagnosis and treatment of childhood intussusception using real time ultrasonography and saline enema: preliminary report. J Korean Soc Med Ultrasound 1:66–70

Lam SH, Wise A, Yenter C (2014) Emergency bedside ultrasound for the diagnosis of pediatric intussusception: a retrospective review. World J Emerg Med 5:255–258

Lioubashevsky N, Hiller N, Rozovsky K et al (2013) Ileocolic versus small-bowel intussusception in children: can US enable reliable differentiation. Radiology 269:266–271

Lochhead A, Jamjoom R, Ratnapalan S (2013) Intussusception in children presenting to the emergency department. Clin Pediatr (Phila) 52:1029–1033

Mandeville K, Chien M, Anthony Willyerd F et al (2012) Intussusception: clinical presentations and imaging characteristics. Pediatr Emerg Care 28(9):842–844

Menichini G, Sessa B, Trinci M, Galluzzo M, Miele V (2015) Accuracy of Contrast-Enhanced Ultrasound (CEUS) in the identification and characterization of traumatic solid organ lesions in children: a retrospective comparison with baseline-US and CE-MDCT. Radiol Med 120:989–1001. doi:10.1007/s11547-015-0535-z, Epub 2015 Mar 31

Miele V, Di Giampietro I (2014) Diagnostic imaging in emergency. Salute Soc (2EN):127–138. doi:10.3280/SES2014-002010EN

Miele V, De Cicco ML, Andreoli C, Buffa V, Adami L, David V (2001) US and CT findings in complicated Meckel diverticulum. Radiol Med 101:230–234

Miele V, Andreoli C, Grassi R (2006) The management of emergency radiology: key facts. Eur J Radiol 59:311–314, Epub 2006 Jun 27

Miele V, Di Giampietro I, Ianniello S, Pinto F, Trinci M (2015) Diagnostic imaging in pediatric polytrauma management. Radiol Med 120:33–49. doi:10.1007/s11547-014-0469-x, Epub 2014 Nov 7

Miele V, Piccolo CL, Sessa B, Trinci M, Galluzzo M (2016a) Comparison between MRI and CEUS in the follow-up of patients with blunt abdominal trauma managed conservatively. Radiol Med 121:27–37. doi:10.1007/s11547-015-0578-1Epub2016Jan8

Miele V, Piccolo CL, Galluzzo M, Ianniello S, Sessa B, Trinci M (2016b) Contrast-enhanced ultrasound (CEUS) in blunt abdominal trauma. Br J Radiol 89(1061):20150823. doi:10.1259/bjr.20150823Epub2016Jan8

Miele V, Piccolo CL, Trinci M, Galluzzo M, Ianniello S, Brunese L (2016c) Diagnostic imaging of blunt abdominal trauma in pediatric patients. Radiol Med 121:409–430. doi:10.1007/s11547-016-0637-2, Epub 2016 Apr 13

Munden MM, Bruzzi JF, Coley BD et al (2007) Sonography of pediatric small-bowel intussusception: differentiating surgical from nonsurgical cases. AJR 188:275–279

Navarro O, Dugougeat F, Komecki A et al (2000) The impact of imaging in the management of intussusception owing to pathologic lead points in children. Pediatr Radiol 30(9):594–603

Okimoto S, Hyodo S, Yamamoto M et al (2011) Association of viral isolates from stool samples with intussusception in children. Int J Infect Dis 15(9):e641–e645

Pinto F, Miele V, Scaglione M, Pinto A (2014) The use of contrast-enhanced ultrasound in blunt abdominal trauma: advantages and limitations. Acta Radiol 55:776–784. doi:10.1177/0284185113505517, Epub 2013 Sep 23

Pinto F, Valentino M, Romanini L, Basilico R, Miele V (2015) The role of CEUS in the assessment of haemodynamically stable patients with blunt abdominal trauma. Radiol Med 120:3–11. doi:10.1007/s11547-014-0455-3, Epub 2014 Aug 21

Pinto A, Miele V, Schillirò ML, Nasuto M, Chianese V, Romano L, Guglielmi G (2016) Spectrum of signs of pneumoperitoneum. Sem US CT MRI 37:3–9. doi:10.1053/j.sult.2015.10.008Epub2015Oct28

Ramsey KW, Halm BM (2014) Diagnosis of intussusception using ultrasound by a pediatric resident in the emergency department. Hawaii J Med Publ Health 73:58–60

Raval MV, Minneci PC, Deans KJ et al (2015) Improving quality and efficiency for intussusception management after successful enema reduction. Pediatrics 136:e1345–e1352

Rogers TN, Robb A (2010) Intussusception in infants and young children. Surgery 28:402–405

Sadigh G, Zou KH, Razavi SA et al (2015) Meta-analysis of air vs liquid enema for intussusception reduction in children. AJR 2015:542–549

Samad L, Cortina-Borja M et al (2013) Intussusception incidence among infants in the UK and Republic of Ireland: a pre-rotavirus vaccine prospective surveillance study. Vaccine 31(38):4098–4102

Sanchez TR, Doskocil B, Stein-Wexler R (2015) Nonsurgical management of childhood intussusception. J Ultrasound Med 32:59–63

Serayssol C, Abbo O, Mouttalib S et al (2014) Seasonal pattern of intussusceptions in infants and children: is fall/winter predominance still worth consideration? A 10-year retrospective epidemiological study. Arch Pediatr 21(5):476–482, Article in French

Sessa B, Trinci M, Ianniello S, Menichini G, Galluzzo M, Miele V (2015) Blunt abdominal trauma: role of contrast-enhanced ultrasound in the detection and staging of abdominal traumatic lesions compared with US and CE-MDCT. Radiol Med 120:180–189. doi:10.1007/s11547-014-0425-9, Epub 2014 Jun 25

Sessa B, Galluzzo M, Ianniello S, Pinto A, Trinci M, Miele V (2016) Acute perforated diverticulitis: assessment with multidetector computed tomography. Sem Ultrasound CT MRI 37:37–48. doi:10.1053/j.sult.2015.10.003Epub2015Oct9

Shiels WE, Mayes CK, Hedlund GL et al (1991) Air enema for diagnosis and reduction of intussusception. Radiology 181:169–172

Shiyi EY, Ganapathy S et al (2015) Intussusception in children presenting to the emergency department – an Asian perspective. Pediatr Emerg Care pp. 1–5

Sorantin E, Lindbichler F (2004) Management of intussusception. Eur Radiol 14(Suppl 4):L146–L154

Tarcă E, Savu B, Criscov I et al (2015) Intussusception in infants – storm from a clear sky. Rev Med Chir Soc Med Nat Iasi 119:141–146

Tareen F, McLaugghlin D, Cianci F et al (2015) Abdominal radiography is not necessary in children with intussusception. Pediatr Surg Int 32:89–92

Valentini V, Buquicchio GL, Galluzzo M, Ianniello S, Di Grezia G, Ambrosio R, Trinci M, Miele V (2016) Intussusception in adults: the role of MDCT in the identification of the site and the cause of the obstruction. Gastroenterol Res Pract 2016:5623718. doi:10.1155/2016/5623718, Epub 2015 Dec 27

Wong CWY, Chan IHY, Chung PHY et al (2015) Childhood intussusception: 17-year experience at a tertiary referral centre in Hong Kong. Hong Kong Med J 21:518–523

10 Acute Appendicitis

Grazia Loretta Buquicchio, Gavina Cuneo, Stefano Giannecchini, Caterina Pizzi, Carmelo Rende, and Margherita Trinci

10.1 Introduction

Appendicitis is the most common cause of acute abdominal pain that requires surgical intervention in the pediatric population.

It is one of the major causes of hospitalization in children.

Appendicitis typically develops in older children and young adults; it is rare under the age of 2 years. The peak incidence of appendicitis occurs between 10 and 19 years of age.

Appendicitis occurs with equal frequency in males and in females.

Patients with appendicitis may present with a wide variety of symptoms that can lead to confusion and delay in diagnosis and treatment.

The delayed diagnosis of appendicitis has severe consequences, including perforation, abscess, peritonitis, sepsis, bowel obstruction, wound infection, infertility, adhesions, and death (Klein 2007).

Early diagnosis is essential to reduce morbidity. Morbidity and mortality in acute appendicitis are related to appendiceal perforation.

The prevalence of appendiceal perforations varies from 23 % to 73 % (Tseng et al. 2016).

G.L. Buquicchio (✉) • G. Cuneo • S. Giannecchini
C. Pizzi • C. Rende • M. Trinci
Department of Emergency Radiology, S. Camillo Hospital, Rome, Italy
e-mail: graziabuquicchio@gmail.com

The advent of antibiotics and effective surgical management have substantially reduced appendicitis-related mortality; however, deaths from appendicitis still occur, particularly in the elderly.

The normal appendix is a blind-ended tubular structure (Fig. 10.1) with a diameter of less than 7 mm and a wall thickness of less than 2 mm and arises from the posteromedial wall of the cecum, approximately 3 cm below the ileocecal valve. Except for its proximal part, the remainder portion of the appendix is free and can occupy different positions in the abdominal cavity (Gaitini 2011).

The appendix may lie in a retrocecal, subcecal, retroileal, preileal, or pelvic site, and this variability in location may influence the clinical presentation (Fig. 10.2).

There are a variety of other conditions in childhood that occur with abdominal pain that must be differentiated from acute appendicitis.

The majority of children with acute abdominal pain have self-limited nonsurgical disease, such as viral syndrome, gastroenteritis, and constipation.

Clinical signs and symptoms associated with acute appendicitis include crampy, periumbilical, or right lower quadrant pain, nausea, vomiting, point tenderness in the right lower quadrant, rebound tenderness, and leukocytosis; the pain often radiates to the right leg, causing lameness (Taylor 2004).

V. Miele, M. Trinci (eds.), *Imaging Non-traumatic Abdominal Emergencies in Pediatric Patients*,
DOI 10.1007/978-3-319-41866-7_10

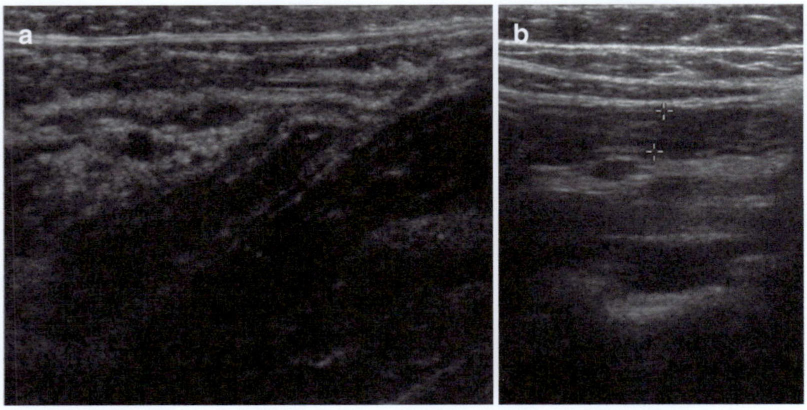

Fig. 10.1 (**a**, **b**) US scan: normal appendix is a blind-ended tubular structure which arises from the posteromedial wall of the cecum

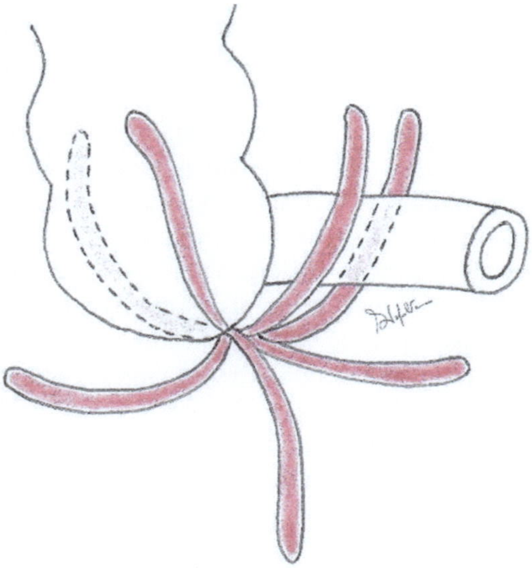

Fig. 10.2 The figure represents the various positions in which the appendix may lie (retrocecal, subcecal, retroileal, preileal, or pelvic site)

Approximately one-third of children with acute appendicitis have atypical clinical findings.

Recurrent and chronic forms of appendicitis occur with an, respectively, incidence of 10 % and 1 % (Koike et al. 2014).

10.2 Pathogenesis

Appendicitis is usually the result of the obstruction of its lumen.

The lumen obstructed becomes distended; the pressure through the walls increases with consequent reduction of the mural perfusion. If appendectomy is not performed, gangrene and perforation occur.

The first pathogenetic event in most patients with acute appendicitis is the obstruction of the lumen that can be caused by fecaliths, lymphoid hyperplasia, foreign bodies, parasites, and tumor. Once the obstruction is verified, the continuous secretion of mucus causes an increase in intraluminal pressure and a distension of the lumen. At this stage abdominal pain is mild, is poorly localized, and disappears in 4–6 h; anorexia, nausea, and vomiting are often associated.

The increased intraluminal pressure exceeds the capillary perfusion pressure causing venous engorgement, arterial compromise, and consequent tissue ischemia.

Such as mucosal barrier is compromised, the bacteria proliferate and invade the wall of the appendix and determine transmural inflammation (Brennan 2006). Continued tissue ischemia results in appendiceal infarction and perforation. Inflammation then may extend to the parietal peritoneum and adjacent structures, which include the terminal ileum, cecum, and pelvic organs.

At this stage the typical migration in the right lower quadrant of pain occurs that is continuous and more severe than the early visceral pain.

Patients with acute appendicitis usually are afebrile or have low-grade fever.

Perforation should be suspected when the patient's temperature exceeds 38.3 °C.

If perforation does occur, periappendiceal phlegmon or abscess will result.

Peritonitis usually develops if there is free perforation into the abdominal cavity.

Clinical findings suggesting possible perforation include progression from localized right lower quadrant to generalized abdominal pain, temperature greater than 38 °C, and signs of peritonitis or a right lower quadrant mass at physical examination.

10.3 Clinical Diagnosis

The clinical diagnosis of acute appendicitis is often not simple because one-third of children with appendicitis have atypical clinical signs and symptoms.

The clinical diagnosis of acute appendicitis is based primarily on typical symptoms that include poorly localized periumbilical pain, followed by nausea and vomiting, with subsequent migration of pain to the right lower quadrant.

This classic presentation occurs in only 50–60 % of patients, and the diagnosis may be missed or delayed when atypical patterns of disease are encountered.

The rate of misdiagnoses at initial presentation is high, as 57 % in children younger than 12 years and as 100 % in children younger than 2 years.

Younger children often present with nonspecific signs and symptoms and are unable to clearly describe their symptoms or localize pain. As a result, delayed or incorrect diagnoses and complications such as appendiceal perforation are common.

Results of laboratory tests, such as white blood cell count and C-reactive protein level, can be helpful but are not specific (Gendel et al. 2011).

The classic presentation is the onset of periumbilical pain that migrates to the right lower quadrant at McBurney's point over a period of 12–24 h, with associated anorexia, leukocytosis, and, often, low-grade fever.

Since younger children are not able to describe their symptoms and up to one-third have atypical clinical findings, the correct diagnosis may delay, and in 30–74 % serious complications occur such as perforation, peritonitis, sepsis, or even death.

10.4 Radiological Findings

When the presentation is typical, most investigators and clinicians agree that imaging is unnecessary; however, the presentation is atypical in approximately 35–45 % of patients, and for these patients imaging plays a key role in the diagnosis of suspected appendicitis (Sivit 2004; Hagendorf et al. 2004).

10.5 US Normal Appendix

The evaluation of the appendix by US should be performed using a high-resolution linear-array transducer (5–12 MHz).

Graded-compression ultrasonography has been proved to be an effective aid in the diagnosis of acute appendicitis (Strouse 2010).

Gradual pressure is applied with the probe to displace bowel loops (Binkovitz et al. 2015).

Graduated compression with the probe helps differentiate between normal compressible intestinal loops and inflamed appendix that is not compressible (Fig. 10.3).

Key anatomic landmarks that must be visualized include the cecum, iliac vessels, and psoas muscle (Fig. 10.4).

The cecum is recognized as an aperistaltic large-caliber bowel that contains gas and fluid and is contiguous with the ascending colon.

The terminal ileum ends into the cecum at the ileocecal valve and is a readily compressible structure that demonstrates active peristalsis. The appendix arises from the posteromedial surface of the cecal base a few centimeters inferior to the ileocecal valve, although its distal tip may have a variable location.

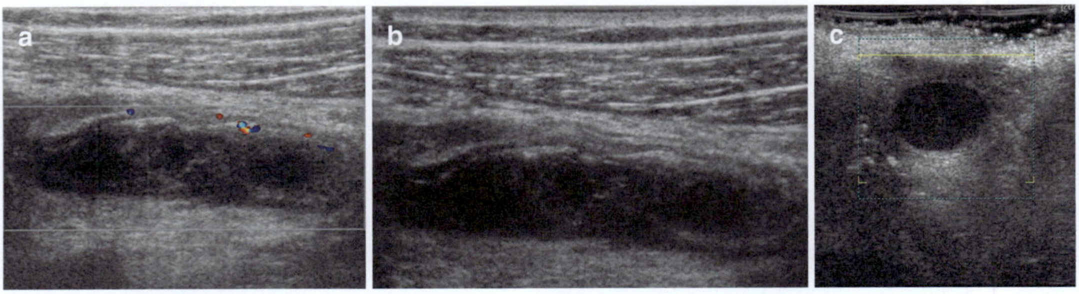

Fig. 10.3 (**a–c**) US: inflamed appendix appears like a blind-ended tubular structure that is not compressible at the graduated compression with the probe

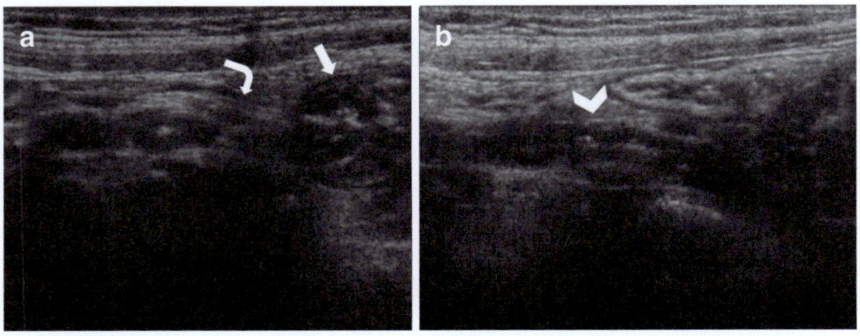

Fig. 10.4 (**a**, **b**) US, key anatomic appendix landmarks: the cecum (*arrow*) is recognized as an aperistaltic large-caliber bowel that contains gas and fluid; the terminal ileum (*curved arrow*) ends into the cecum at the ileocecal valve and is a readily compressible structure that demonstrates active peristalsis; appendix (*arrow head*)

Measurement of the maximal mural thickness (MMT) is one of the most important morphologic criteria used to identify a normal or abnormal appendix (Fig. 10.5a) (Je et al. 2009; Simonovsky 2002).

The mural thickness of the appendix was defined as the distance from the hyperechoic luminal interface to the outer hyperechoic line.

The thickening of the appendiceal walls is due to mucosal edema, as a result of reactive changes.

The mean MMTs in the young children, older children, and adolescent are 1.9 mm ± 0.4, 2.0 mm ± 0.5, and 2.1 mm ± 0.5, respectively.

Although MMT evaluation can be considered a valuable index of the status of the appendix in patients with suspected appendicitis, it should be stressed that the accuracy is higher when there are several US criteria simultaneously, such as the presence or absence of periappendiceal inflamed fat, tenderness at the site of the appendix, and hyperemia at power or color Doppler US.

In children aged 6 years or younger, the appendiceal mural thickness should be regarded as normal only when it is less than 3 mm.

Although MMT measurement is more accurate, it is also using the maximal outer diameter (MOD) (Prendergast et al. 2014), which measures the outer wall to outer wall diameter at the widest point of the appendix during transducer compression (Fig. 10.5b). To measure diameters, the electronic calipers were placed between the outer borders of the hypoechoic tunica muscularis. The outer diameters were measured in the transverse plane of the appendix.

The MOD limits suggested to be positive for appendicitis vary between 6 mm or greater and greater than 7 mm (Goldin et al. 2009).

The normal appendix measures 6 mm or less in maximal outer diameter, is compressible, and lacks adjacent inflammatory changes. In addition, it has no demonstrable flow at color flow Doppler imaging.

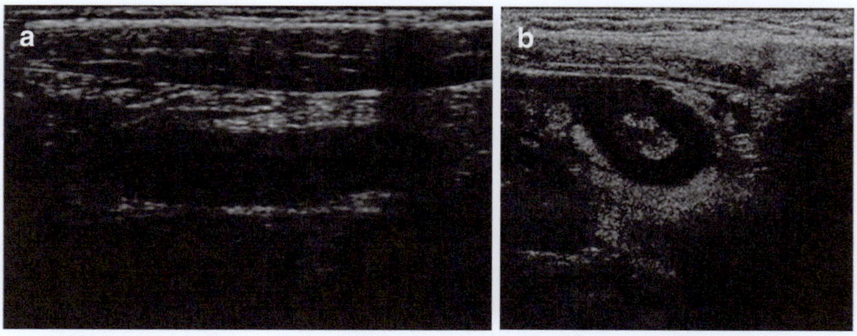

Fig. 10.5 Longitudinal and transverse US scan: the maximal mural thickness (MMT) is the distance from the hyperechoic luminal interface to the outer hyperechoic line (**a**). Cross-sectional image of a distended normal appendix: the maximal outer diameter (MOD) measures the outer wall to outer wall diameter at the widest point of the appendix (**b**)

A normal appendix should have an outer wall diameter of 6 mm or less, and its lumen should at least partially collapse under compression. Occasionally, a normal appendix may be slightly larger than 6 mm in diameter but will remain compressible.

10.6 Imaging of Acute Appendicitis

Although abdominal radiography remains a widely used examination in children with acute abdominal pain, it has been shown to be a relatively insensitive and nonspecific means for evaluating appendicitis, and its use adds unnecessary cost and radiation exposure; furthermore the findings that can be seen in the RX are totally nonspecific and consist of the display of an appendicolith and signs of paralytic ileus (greater evidence of the margin of the psoas and analgesic convexity of the spine) (Doria 2011).

Although magnetic resonance (MR) imaging shows promise in the presurgical assessment of patients who are suspected of having appendicitis, the application of this modality to the pediatric patient is yet undeveloped; furthermore the length of the MR imaging examination may substantially curtail its utility in younger patients who would need sedation (Kearl et al. 2016).

The principal imaging technique for evaluating children with suspected appendicitis is graded-compression US. The clinical utility of US lies primarily in those children with present equivocal clinical findings (Leeson and Leeson 2013; Fonio et al. 2013; Di Giacomo et al. 2015).

Tip appendicitis is a rare condition that occurs when the inflammation is focally confined to the distal portion of the appendix (Mazeh et al. 2009); the pathophysiology in tip appendicitis is much less clear than acute appendicitis. The prevalence of this condition has been reported as high as 5 % (Lim et al. 1996).

10.7 US

Although computed tomography (CT) can help clinicians rapidly and accurately diagnose or exclude acute appendicitis, CT represents potential risks of radiation exposure, need for sedation, risk of contrast medium, and high cost.

Because of the concern over excessive radiation exposure, several institutions have emphasized ultrasonography (US) as the primary initial modality for use in the assessment of possible pediatric appendicitis (Krishnamoorthi et al. 2011).

Although today computed tomography (CT) has become the predominant imaging method used to diagnose appendicitis in children in the United States, outside of the United States, ultrasonography remains the predominant imaging method to diagnose appendicitis in children (Hryhorczuk et al. 2012).

US is in fact an extension of the clinical examination. The sonographer can ask the child where it hurts and directly scan the painful region.

The sensitivity of US in children has ranged from 44 % to 94 %, and the specificity has ranged from 47 % to 95 %. But in experienced hands, US has reported sensitivities of 75–90 %, specificities of 86–100 %, accuracies of 87–96 %, positive predictive values of 91–94 %, and negative predictive values of 89–97 % for the diagnosis of acute appendicitis (Pastore et al. 2014).

Scanning is performed in both longitudinal and transverse planes, and the examination begins with the identification of the ascending colon, which appears as a nonperistaltic structure containing gas and fluid (Fig. 10.4).

The transducer is then moved inferiorly to identify the terminal ileum, which is easily compressible and displays active peristalsis.

The cecal tip where the appendix arises is approximately 1–2 cm below the terminal ileum, and it is located anteriorly to the iliac vessels and psoas muscle.

Gentle, gradual pressure is used to compress the anterior abdominal wall, resulting in displacement and compression of normal bowel loops (Butler et al. 2011).

Normal appendix appears as a blind-ended lamellated structure without peristalsis.

On longitudinal images, the inflamed, nonperforated appendix appears as a fluid-filled, noncompressible, blind-ended tubular structure, and the maximal appendiceal diameter is greater than 6 mm (Fig. 10.6).

If fluid is present within the appendiceal lumen, a target appearance, characterized by a fluid-filled center and surrounded by an echogenic mucosa and submucosa and hypoechoic muscularis, may be seen when imaging in the axial plane.

Other findings of appendicitis include an appendicolith, which appears as echogenic foci with acoustic shadowing (Fig. 10.7); pericecal or periappendiceal fluid (Fig. 10.8); increased periappendiceal echogenicity representing fat infiltration (Figs. 10.8 and 10.9); and enlarged mesenteric lymph nodes (Fig. 10.9).

But the only US sign that is specific for appendicitis is an enlarged, aperistaltic, and noncompressible appendix measuring greater than 6 mm in maximal diameter.

The use of color Doppler US provides a useful adjunct in the evaluation of suspected acute appendicitis; the color Doppler US of nonperforated appendicitis typically demonstrates peripheral wall hyperemia, reflecting inflammatory hyperperfusion (Fig. 10.10).

In early inflammation, color flow may be absent or limited to the appendiceal tip.

Color flow may also be absent in gangrenous appendicitis.

Depending on its location, the appendix can be classified as retrocecal, abdominal, midpelvic, or deep pelvic.

Abdominal appendices were those located in the abdominal cavity above a horizontal line defined by the iliac crests.

Midpelvic appendices were those located above the iliac vessels (external iliac artery and

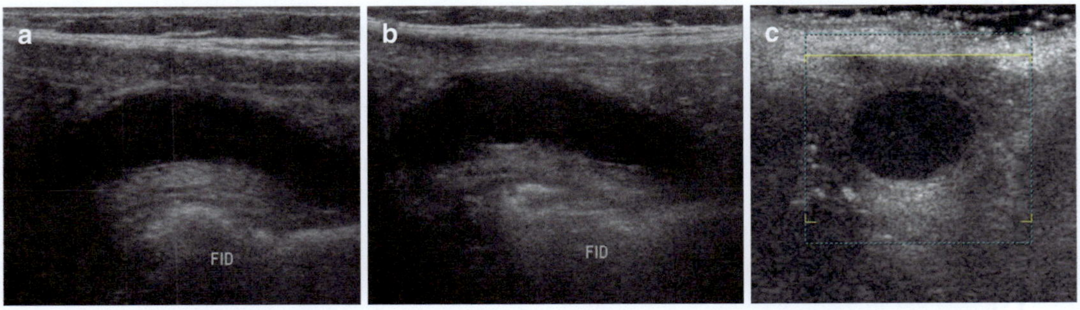

Fig. 10.6 Longitudinal (**a**, **b**) and transverse (**c**) US scan shows inflamed appendix as a fluid-filled, noncompressible, blind-ended tubular structure, with maximal appendiceal diameter greater than 6 mm

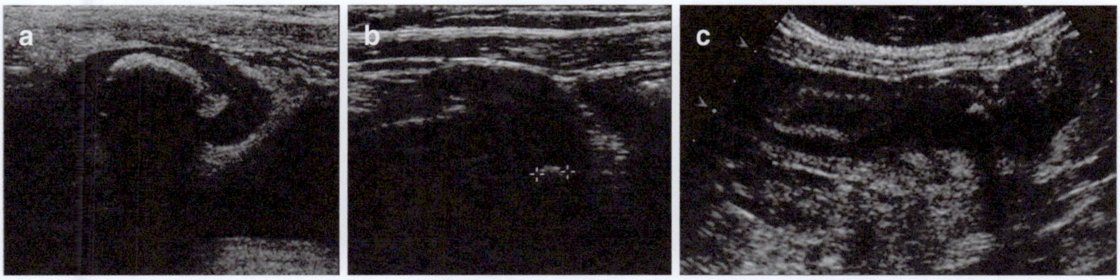

Fig. 10.7 (**a**–**c**) US images show a dilated appendix that contains an appendicolith, which appears as echogenic foci with acoustic shadowing

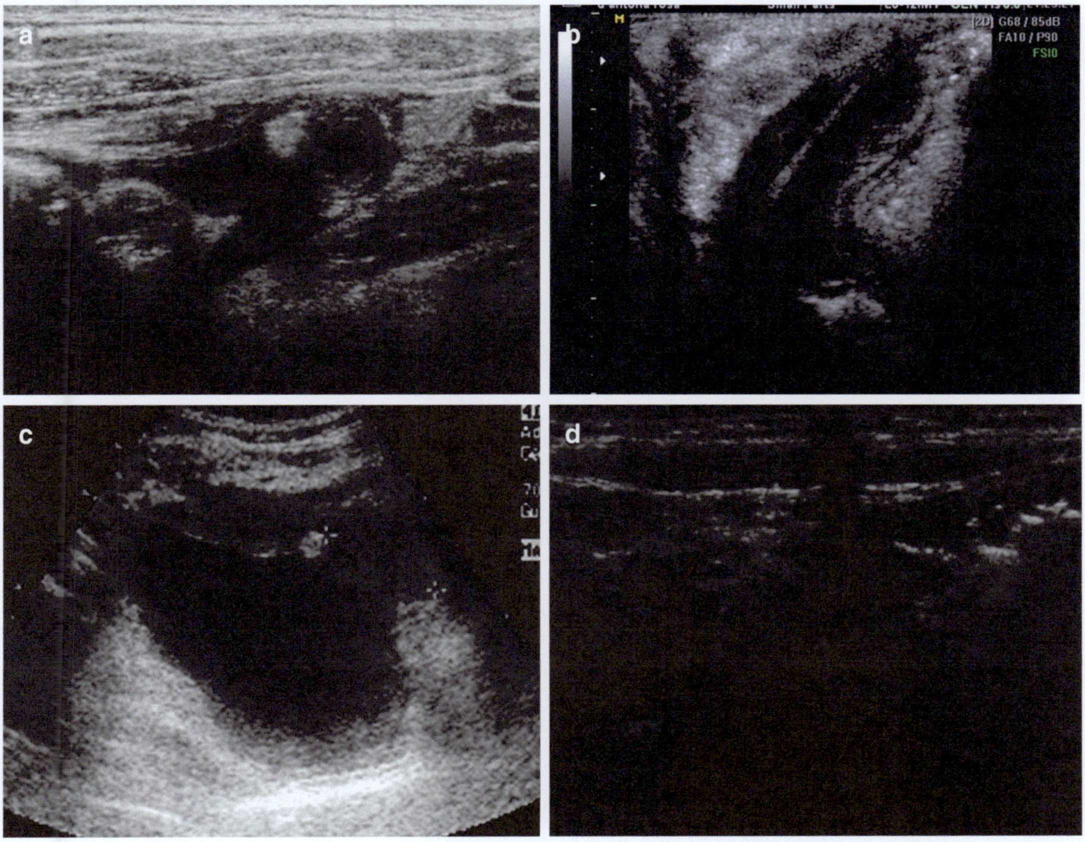

Fig. 10.8 Ultrasonographic findings in appendicitis, such as pericecal or periappendiceal fluid (**a**) and increased periappendiceal echogenicity that represents fat infiltration (**b**)

vein in the pelvis). Appendices were classified as deep pelvic when they extended beyond the iliac vessels toward the pelvis minor or when the cecum was located in a lower position in relation to these vessels.

The course of appendicitis can be variable.

The presence of appendicoliths appears as bright, echogenic foci with distal acoustic shadowing. Their identification within the appendix or in the adjacent perienteric soft tissue after perforation is highly associated with a positive diagnosis (Lovrenski et al. 2016).

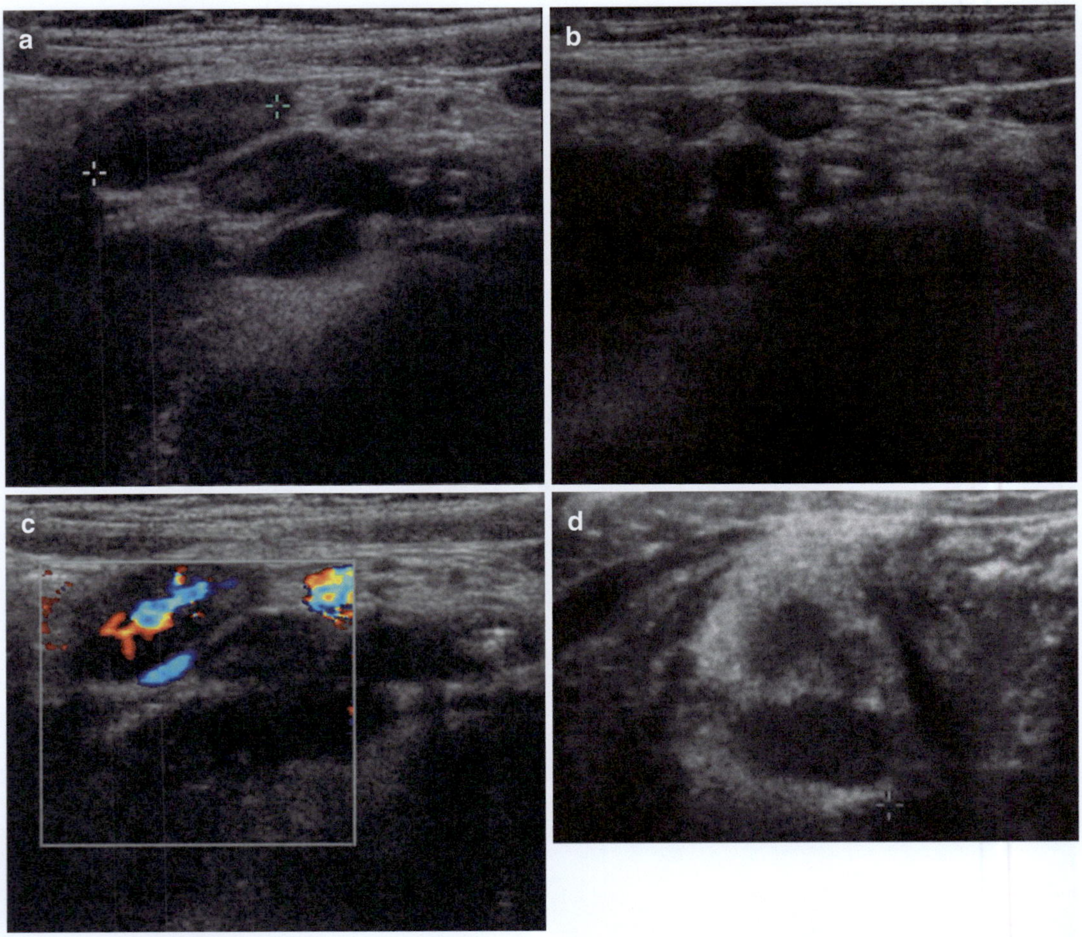

Fig. 10.9 Ultrasonographic findings of appendicitis, such as increased periappendiceal echogenicity that represents fat infiltration (**a**) and enlarged mesenteric lymph nodes (**a**–**d**)

Phlegmonous change manifests as hypoechoic zones with poor margination within the inflamed fat that blend imperceptibly at its margins with the fatty tissue. Liquefaction and abscess formation will manifest as an actual fluid component (Fig. 10.11).

Some authors proposed the use of contrast-enhanced ultrasound (CEUS) to differentiate abdominal phlegmon and abscess. CEUS should be used to confirm these conditions primarily identified at US (Ripollès et al. 2013).

Although this method is still little used in non-traumatic pediatric emergencies (Catalano et al. 2004; Farina et al. 2015), its use however is well established in traumatic pediatric emergencies (Pinto et al. 2014, 2015; Miele et al. 2015, 2016a, b, c; Sessa et al. 2015; Menichini et al. 2015).

Gas bubbles within a collection suggest perforation (Blumfield et al. 2013).

In conclusion the most accurate US finding for acute appendicitis is an outer wall diameter greater than 6 mm under compression, with reported positive and negative predictive values of 98 % (Cohen et al. 2015).

Less sensitive and specific US findings for appendicitis include hyperemia within the appendiceal wall on color Doppler images, echogenic inflamed periappendiceal fat (Trout et al. 2012), and the presence of an appendicolith.

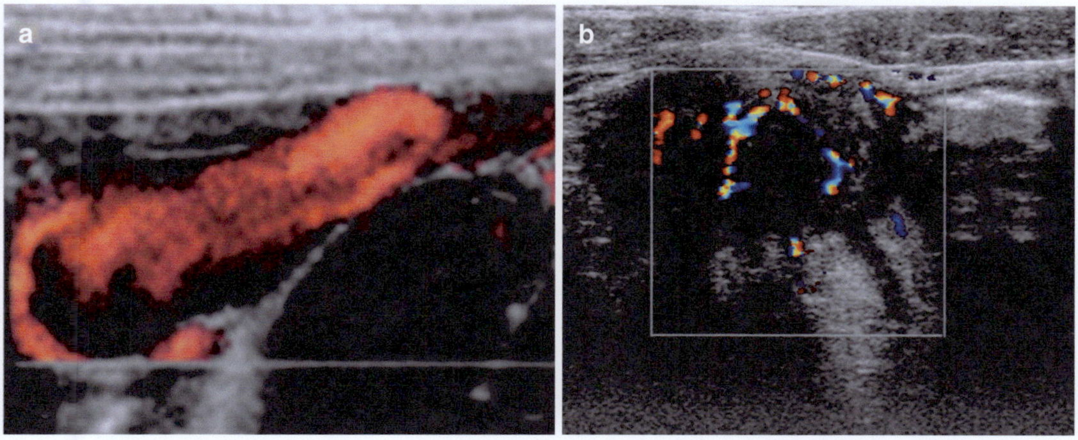

Fig. 10 10 (**a**, **b**) The color Doppler US demonstrates peripheral wall hyperemia, reflecting inflammatory hyperperfusion

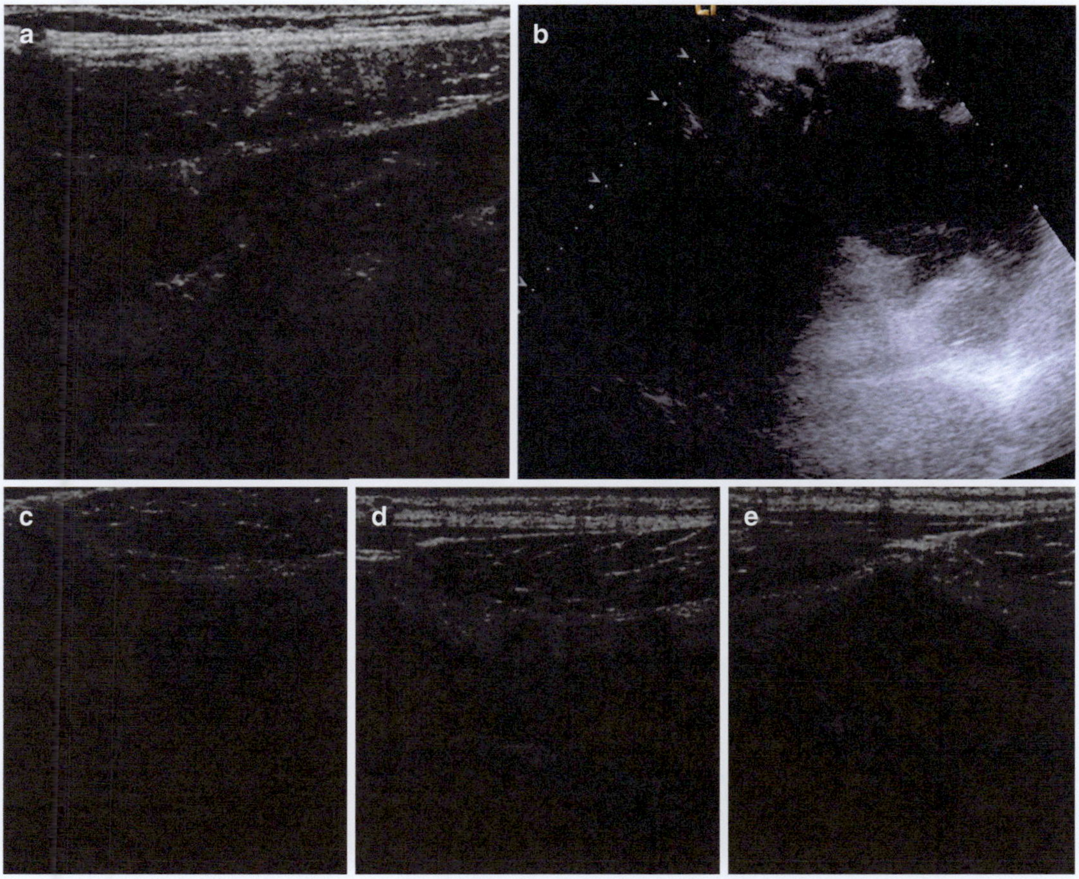

Fig. 10.11 (**a–e**) US scan demonstrates hypoechoic zones with poor margination within the inflamed fat corresponding to phlegmonous appendicitis. Liquefaction and abscess formation will manifest as an actual fluid component

The principal advantages of US are its lower cost and wide availability, its lack of ionizing radiation, and its ability to assess vascularity through color Doppler analysis, provision of dynamic information through graded compression, and delineation of gynecologic disease which is a common mimic of acute appendicitis.

However US is operator dependent, and often technical failures are due to the presence of severe pain or patient obesity.

10.8 US of Perforation

Despite the relatively high incidence of appendicitis, the clinical diagnosis is very commonly delayed or missed, leading to high rates of appendiceal perforation, particularly in young children less than 5 years of age. Because diagnostic delays arise from the interpretation of the history and physical examination results, diagnostic imaging has become an essential tool in the evaluation of children suspected of having appendicitis.

The classic findings of bowel perforation, abscess, and extraluminal air are well known but are not always present in patients with perforated appendicitis (Pinto et al. 2016).

The presence of an appendicolith in a child with appendicitis has been associated with earlier and higher rate of perforation.

If perforation has occurred, the appendix may not be recognizable as a discrete structure.

The US features of perforation include loss of the echogenic submucosal layer and presence of a loculated periappendiceal or pelvic fluid collection or abscess.

These findings occur in 50–70 % of cases of perforated appendicitis.

Color Doppler findings of appendiceal perforation include hyperemia in the periappendiceal soft tissues or within a well-defined abscess.

Specific findings indicative of perforated appendicitis are abscess, phlegmon, extraluminal air, extraluminal appendicolith, and a defect in the enhancing appendiceal wall (Fig. 10.12).

An abscess was characterized by a well-delineated, discrete collection with rim enhancement (Fig. 10.13).

A phlegmon was characterized by diffuse and substantial inflammation of the periappendiceal fat with ill-defined fluid collections (Fig. 10.14).

Preoperative knowledge of whether the appendix is perforated has clinical relevance (Kaiser et al. 2004).

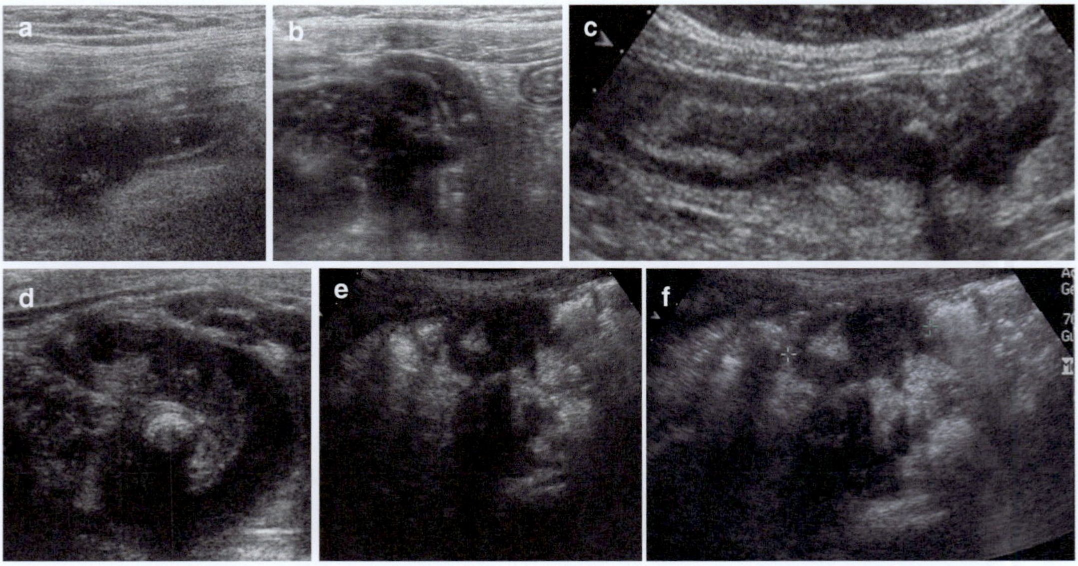

Fig. 10.12 (**a–f**) US of perforation: US findings include loss of the echogenic submucosal layer, hyperemia in the periappendiceal soft tissues, and the presence of a loculated periappendiceal or pelvic fluid collection or abscess. The appendix may not be recognizable as a tubular structure

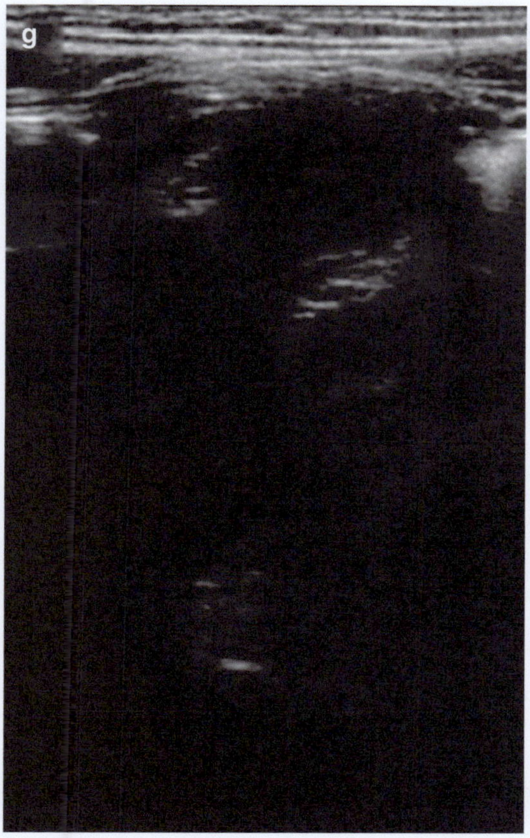

Fig. 10.12 (continued)

Once perforation has occurred, the complications increase.

US criteria for perforation include loculated pericecal fluid, prominent pericecal fat greater than 10 mm, and circumferential loss of the echogenic submucosal layer. For perforation, the reported US sensitivities vary from a low of 29 % (Mazeh et al. 2009) to a high of 84 % (Lim et al. 1996).

But extraluminal air, extraluminal appendicoliths, and interloop abscesses are more easily detected with the use of CT that demonstrates more sensitivity than US for perforated appendicitis (Cogley et al. 2012).

10.9 Pitfalls and Differential Diagnosis

Although common, acute appendicitis can be a difficult diagnosis to make on clinical grounds alone, because a number of other common pathologic abdominal processes share a similar clinical presentation (Levine et al. 2004).

Relatively low sensitivity or specificity has been reported for individual symptoms and signs in patients clinically suspected of having appendicitis, including nausea (sensitivity of 67.5 %, specificity of 38.9 %), anorexia (sensitivity of 61.0 %, specificity of 59.3 %), fever (sensitivity of 17.9 %, specificity of 72.2 %), chills (sensitivity of 6.9 %, specificity of 96.3 %), right lower quadrant pain (sensitivity of 95.9 %, specificity of 3.7 %), and rebound tenderness (sensitivity of 69.5 %, specificity of 38.9 %).

The most common sources of error in the overdiagnosis of appendicitis with US include misinterpretation of the terminal ileum as the appendix and misinterpretation of a normal appendix as an inflamed appendix. The terminal ileum, in contrast to the appendix, does not attach to the base of the cecum, is not blind ended, and shows frequent peristaltic activity.

Also, the terminal ileum usually is oval in cross section as compared with the appendix, which is round.

Another cause of a false-positive examination is periappendiceal inflammation due to Crohn disease; interpretation of US findings may be difficult since the appendix may be involved in the inflammatory process of Crohn disease, or, conversely, appendicitis may be the first manifestation of this disease (Sung et al. 2006).

More causes of a false-positive examination that may mimic acute appendicitis are inflamed Meckel's diverticulum (Marin et al. 2016; Miele et al. 2001) and pelvic inflammatory disease (Miele et al. 2002).

Other problems in diagnosis may be related to a position of the appendix that makes it more difficult to appreciate, in particular when it is in the true pelvis and when it is retrocecal.

The most common alternate diagnoses included mesenteric adenitis, ovarian abnormality, constipation, colitis, intussusception, and pyelonephritis.

Mesenteric adenitis has been reported as the second most common cause of right lower quadrant pain after appendicitis (Xu et al. 2016). The clinical presentation may mimic that of

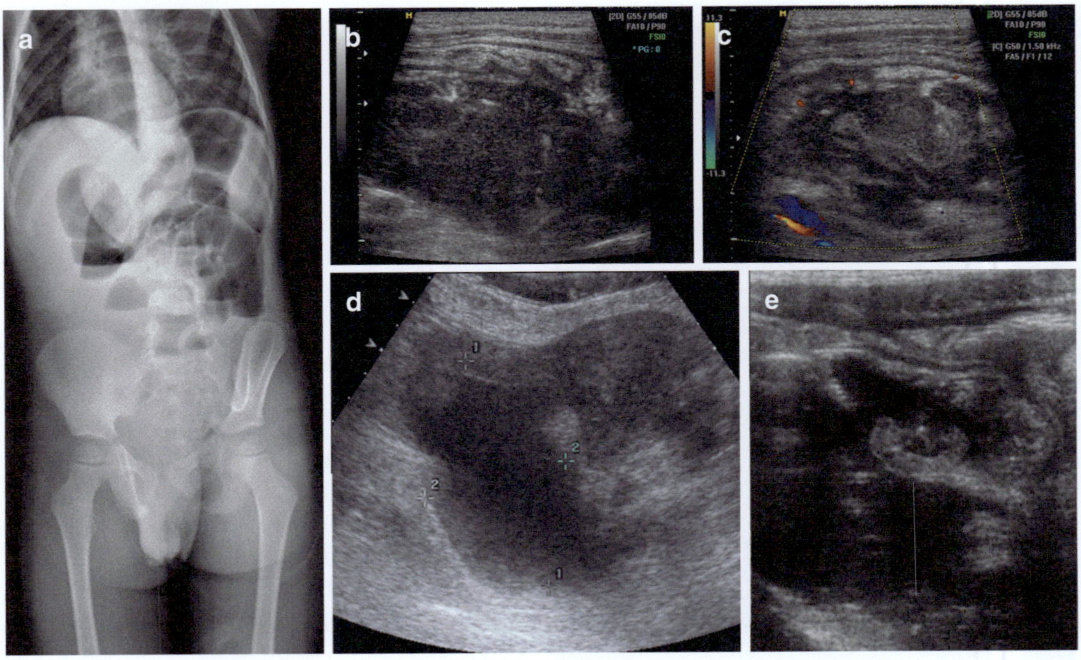

Fig. 10.13 (**a**) X-ray and (**b–e**) US scan of abscess; the RX image shows intestinal obstruction with air-fluid levels; the US demonstrates a well-delineated fluid collection with rim enhancement and peripheral wall hyperemia

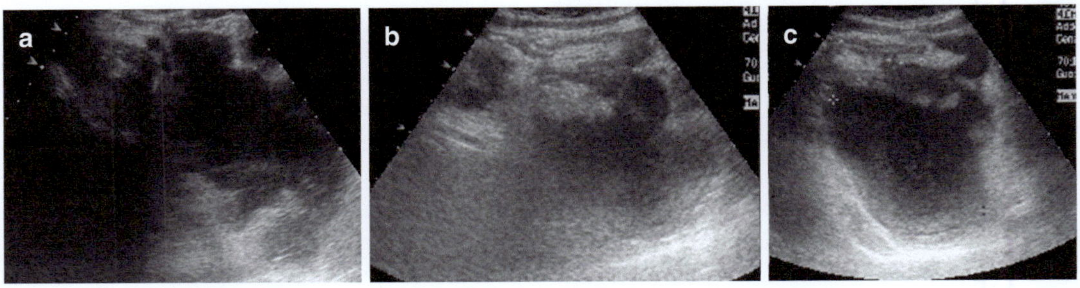

Fig. 10.14 (**a–c**) US of phlegmon: diffuse inflammation of the periappendiceal fat with ill-defined fluid collections

appendicitis; however, it is a benign self-limiting condition that does not require surgery. US findings consist of multiple enlarged RLQ mesenteric lymph nodes in the absence of other diseases.

Another nonsurgical mimic of appendicitis is terminal *ileitis-ileocecitis of infectious* (*Yersinia*, *Salmonella*, or *Campylobacter* species) or inflammatory (e.g., Crohn disease) origin. Acute or subacute RLQ pain is the predominant symptom, and diarrhea may be absent or only mild in cases with an infectious origin.

Up to one-third of patients with Crohn disease initially present with acute onset of symptoms mimicking appendicitis. A thickened terminal ileum may be the only finding at US (Fig. 10.15), and it is imperative not to confuse terminal ileitis with a dilated appendix.

Only when US findings were equivocal and the diagnosis cannot be certain should be considered to use the CT subsequent to US to avoid invasive interventions when they are not needed.

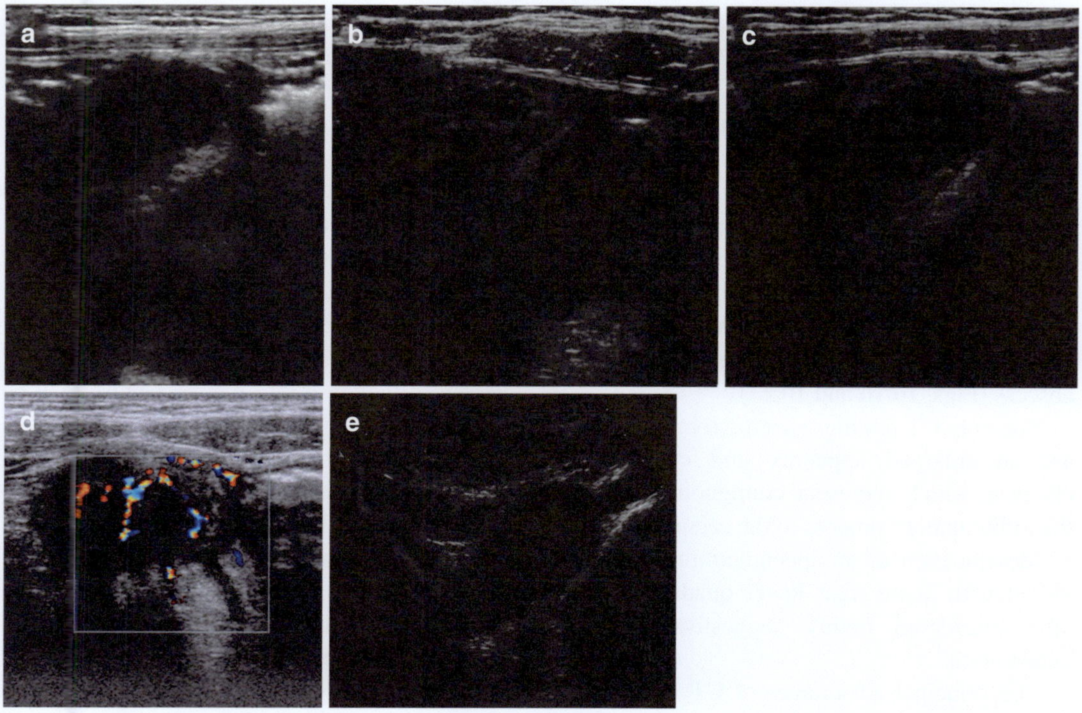

Fig. 10.15 (a–e) US images demonstrates thickened terminal ileum that may be the only finding at US for Crohn disease presentation

10.10 CT

Computed tomography (CT) has become the predominant imaging method used to diagnose appendicitis in children in the United States.

The diagnosis of appendicitis with CT is made by identifying an abnormal appendix and periappendiceal signs of appendicitis, whereas exclusion of appendicitis is predicated on visualization of a normal appendix and the absence of indirect signs of appendicitis.

Pediatric abdominopelvic CT with nonvisualization of the appendix has a high negative predictive value (98.7 %) for appendicitis, which does not differ significantly from that in cases with a partially or even fully visualized normal appendix.

Helical CT has been shown to be a highly sensitive and specific modality for the diagnosis of acute appendicitis in children and adults.

The reported sensitivities of CT are 90–100 %, specificities of 91–99 %, accuracies of 94–98 %, positive predictive values of 92–98 %, and negative predictive values of 95–100 % for the diagnosis of acute appendicitis (Kim et al. 2015).

The advantages of CT over US are reduced operator dependence, superior contrast sensitivity, and the capability for viewing the entire range of air, soft tissue, fat, and bone attenuation values inherent to the abdomen. CT is also more useful than US for evaluating complications of acute appendicitis, such as phlegmon and abscess. It can precisely delineate the location and extent of associated fluid collections including interloop abscesses, which facilitates drainage procedures (Doria et al. 2006).

The normal appendix can be identified at CT in over three-fourths of children. The appendix arises from the posteromedial wall of the cecum, approximately 1–2 cm below the ileocecal junction (Ozturkmen Akay et al. 2007).

The maximal normal appendiceal diameter is variable; although it usually is 7 mm or less, it may occasionally be larger.

CT features of acute appendicitis include a distended appendix greater than 7 mm in maximal diameter, appendiceal wall thickening and enhancement, the presence of appendicolith, circumferential or focal apical cecal thickening, pericecal fat stranding, adjacent bowel wall thickening, free peritoneal fluid, mesenteric lymphadenopathy, intraperitoneal phlegmon, or abscess (Figs. 10.16 and 10.17).

The only CT findings specific for appendicitis are an enlarged appendix and cecal apical changes, which represent contiguous spread of the inflammatory process to the cecum.

Identification of an appendicolith in an individual with acute right lower quadrant pain is also considered highly suggestive of acute appendicitis.

The principal advantages of CT include less operator dependency than US and enhanced delineation of disease extent in perforated appendicitis. Furthermore CT is particularly valuable in obese patients, since they are typically difficult to evaluate with US (Wan et al. 2009).

The most popular and conservative approach is to perform helical CT scanning of the entire abdomen and pelvis with intravenous contrast material, since contrast-enhanced CT is essential in the diagnosis and staging of numerous inflammatory diseases that may cause acute abdominal pain and may simulate appendicitis.

When seen, the normal appendix appears as a tubular or ringlike pericecal structure that is either totally collapsed or partially filled with fluid, contrast material, or air. In our experience, the normal appendiceal wall measures less than 1–2 mm in thickness.

The periappendiceal fat should appear homogeneous, although a thin mesoappendix may be present.

The CT findings are most subtle in patients with mild, nonperforating appendicitis who undergo scanning shortly after the onset of symptoms. In these patients, the appendix may appear as a minimally distended, fluid-filled, tubular structure 5–6 mm in diameter surrounded by the homogeneous fat attenuation of the normal mesentery. This appearance is seen in only the most incipient forms of acute appendicitis (Horrow et al. 2003).

The main CT criteria for the diagnosis of acute appendicitis include identification of a thickened appendix with a wall diameter greater than 6.0–7.0 mm, periappendiceal inflammatory changes, and a calcified appendicolith (Fig. 10.18). Circumferential and symmetric wall thickening is nearly always present and is best demonstrated on

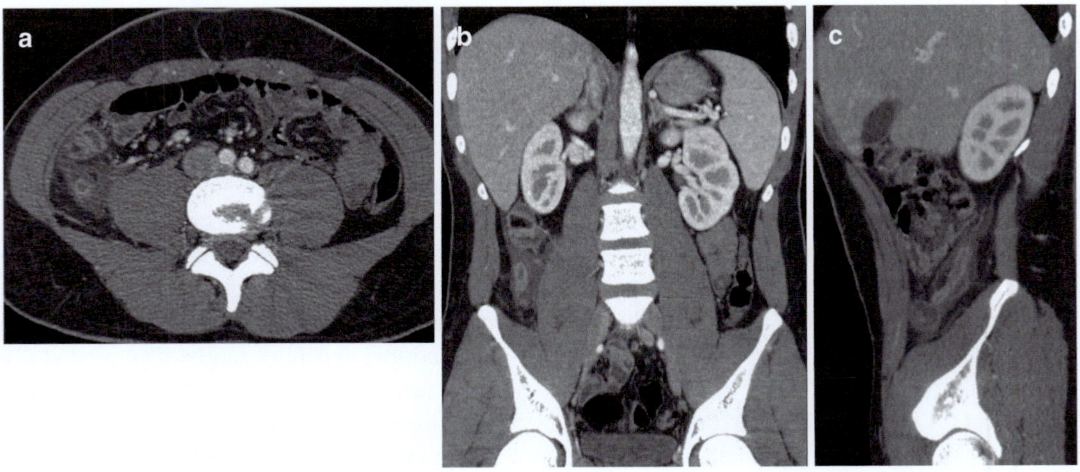

Fig. 10.16 CT axial (**a**) and coronal and sagittal reconstruction (**b–c**) images demonstrate features of acute appendicitis: distended appendix greater than 7 mm in maximal diameter, appendiceal wall thickening and enhancement, pericecal fat stranding, and free peritoneal fluid

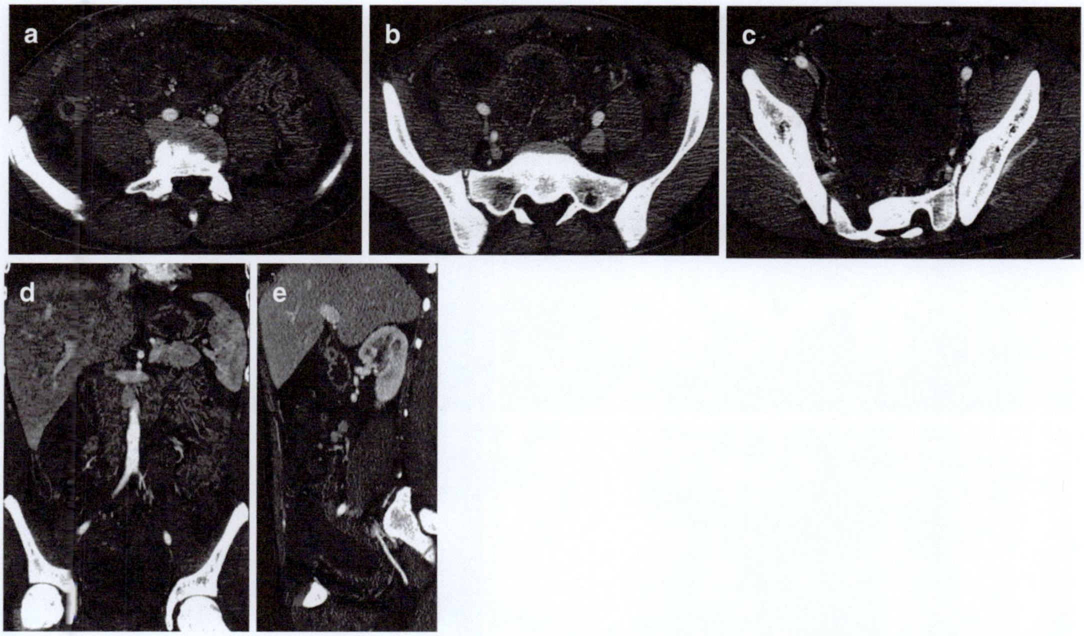

Fig. 10.17 (**a–c**) CT, axial scans and (**d–e**) coronal and sagittal reconstructions show a fluid-filled appendicitis, with thickened wall and periappendiceal inflammatory changes. CT demonstrates the real extent of periappendiceal inflammation and the presence of periappendiceal abscess

images obtained with intravenous contrast material enhancement. The thickened wall usually is homogeneously enhanced, although mural stratification in the form of a target sign may be noted.

Periappendiceal inflammation is present in 98 % of patients with acute appendicitis.

Perforated appendicitis is usually accompanied by pericecal phlegmon or abscess formation. Associated findings include extraluminal air, marked ileocecal thickening, localized lymphadenopathy, peritonitis, and small-bowel obstruction (Fig. 10.19).

CT can be used to accurately stage the extent of periappendiceal inflammation and to reliably differentiate periappendiceal abscess from phlegmon. This distinction is of critical importance to the surgeon.

10.11 US Versus CT

There are several fundamental differences between CT and US that affect the diagnostic accuracy achieved by using each.

The sensitivity of US ranges between 44 % and 98 %, and its specificity ranges between 47 % and 95 %, whereas the sensitivity and specificity of CT range between 87 % and 100 % and 89 % and 99 %, respectively (Shah et al. 2014).

US is rapid, noninvasive, and inexpensive and requires no patient preparation or contrast material administration. Because US involves no ionizing radiation and excels in the depiction of acute gynecologic conditions, it is recommended as the initial imaging study in children.

Operator dependency is the major disadvantage of US in evaluating for appendicitis.

Another important limitation of US is the sensitivity and specificity for perforated appendicitis.

CT is preferred in patients suspected to have appendiceal perforation because diagnostic accuracy remains high and because CT is particularly useful for characterizing periappendiceal inflammatory masses.

CT was shown to be more accurate in staging periappendiceal inflammation, more useful in diagnosing acute abdominal conditions unrelated to appendicitis, and more sensitive in

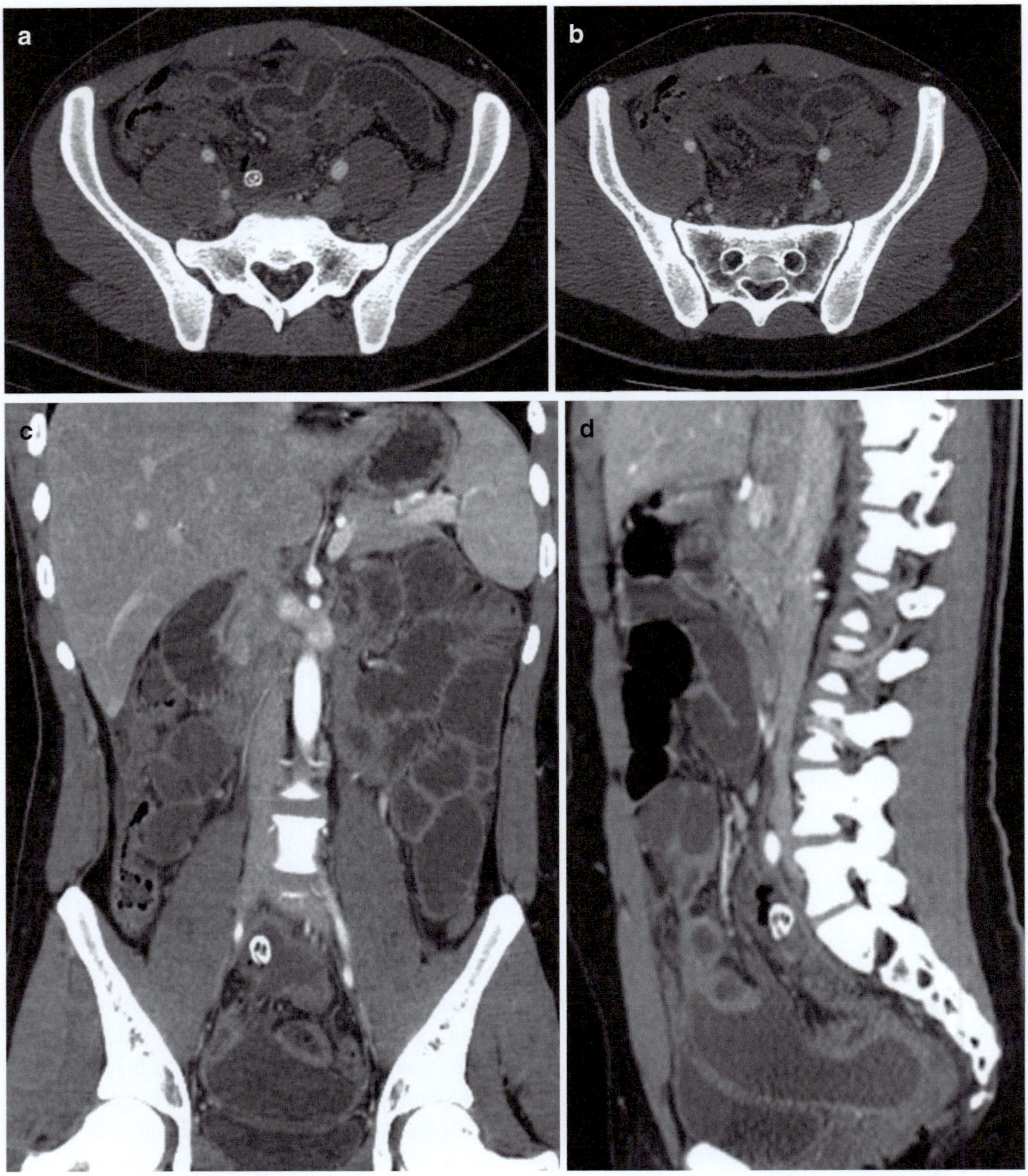

Fig. 10.18 (**a–b**) CT, axial scans and (**c–d**) coronal and sagittan reconstructions: acute appendicitis. The figures show a thickened appendix with a wall diameter greater than 6.0–7.0 mm, periappendiceal inflammatory changes, and a calcified appendicolith in an individual with acute right lower quadrant pain. This condition is considered highly suggestive of acute appendicitis. Perforated appendicitis is usually accompanied by pericecal phlegmon or abscess formation, extraluminal air, marked ileocecal thickening, localized lymphadenopathy, peritonitis, and small-bowel obstruction

demonstrating a normal appendix and in excluding acute appendicitis from the differential diagnosis.

Analysis of the data for CT and US revealed similar specificities (89 % vs 91 %, respectively) and positive predictive values (96 % vs 95 %, respectively); however, CT demonstrated higher sensitivity (96 % vs 76 %), accuracy (94 % vs 83 %), and negative predictive value (95 % vs 76 %).

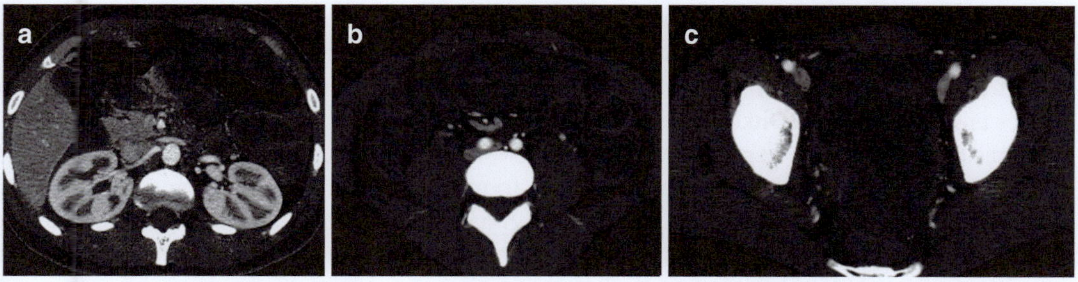

Fig. 10.19 (**a–c**) CT axial, same patient: evidence of small-bowel obstruction and peritonitis

US is able to differentiate many pathologic processes in the female pelvis that may cause pain. Because the symptoms in such patients and the symptoms of girls with appendicitis often overlap and radiation exposure may be avoided with US, US is clearly the imaging modality of choice in the adolescent female with right lower quadrant or pelvic pain.

US has limitations in large or obese patients in the presence of abundant bowel gas and in anomalous appendiceal location. These are not limitations with CT (Yiğiter et al. 2011).

Another limitation of US is the inability to see the appendix in most patients when it is normal and the inability to see the entirety of the normal appendix.

Conversely CT may require sedation or general anesthesia, and the use of intravenous contrast material is not without complications, such as contrast material extravasation, anaphylactoid reactions, and contrast material-induced nephropathy.

The overriding disadvantage of CT, however, is the dependence of CT on ionizing radiation. The approximate dose to a child for single-phase CT of the abdomen and pelvis performed with appropriate, age-adjusted CT parameters is 5 mSv. Although this dose is small, it is not negligible. Younger patients, including young adults, are more radiosensitive (Bachur et al. 2015).

US can help us to use CT more effectively and in the practice the US examination must precede the use of CT.

Whenever the diagnosis can be definitively made at US, CT is avoided, as the patient can undergo surgery directly. Whenever an alternative diagnosis is made at US, CT is avoided.

In conclusion, a staged US and CT imaging protocol in which US is performed first for suspected acute appendicitis in children is highly accurate and offers the opportunity to substantially reduce radiation. A definitive US result, either positive or negative, is sufficiently accurate to guide therapy without performing subsequent CT.

Patients with right lower quadrant pain and an equivocal clinical diagnosis should be triaged to imaging examination, with US as the primary imaging modality in patients who are suspected of having gynecologic abnormalities. US may be used first in patients who are suspected of having appendicitis, but a US examination with negative findings should not lead to a dismissal of the diagnosis.

CT scans should be used judiciously, by using scanning parameters that are appropriate for patient size, and should be optimized for diagnosis with a single pass; additional passes are additional examinations, which are typically unnecessary (Srinivasan et al. 2015; Miele et al. 2006; Miele and Di Giampietro 2014).

10.12 RM

Children are particularly at risk for the adverse effects of ionizing radiation, and even low-dose radiation is associated with a small but significant increase in lifetime risk of fatal cancer.

Magnetic resonance (MR) imaging can be used to evaluate for abdominal disease without the use of ionizing radiation. In most emergency departments, however, the use of MR imaging as a primary modality for the evaluation of a child with abdominal pain is still impractical due to its high cost, its limited availability, and the frequent need for sedation to obtain diagnostic-quality images in young children (Ditkofsky et al. 2014).

Ultrasonography (US) remains the standard imaging technique to investigate acute appendicitis.

MR imaging may be used as a complementary examination when US is inconclusive or when it is important to avoid exposure to CT radiation or contrast material in children with signs and symptoms of appendicitis (Aspelund et al. 2014; Herliczek et al. 2013).

Magnetic resonance (MR) imaging has been proposed as an alternative to CT for imaging suspected acute appendicitis. Like US, MR imaging does not expose patients to ionizing radiation. Unlike US, it is readily available at many adult facilities due to the need for 24-h-a-day stroke imaging and is less operator dependent.

MR imaging without contrast material demonstrates high diagnostic performance for suspected pediatric appendicitis with sensitivity of 93.3 %, specificity of 98 %, positive predictive value of 96.5 %, and negative predictive value of 96.2 % (Orth et al. 2014).

MR imaging must be conducted with an equipment from 1.5-T imager and a surface phased-array coil.

Four sequences were performed: axial T1-weighted fast SE, axial T2-weighted fast SE, axial T2-weighted fat-saturated fast SE, and coronal T2-weighted fast SE.

The sequences were acquired at a 4-mm section thickness without intersection gaps.

All images were obtained with the patient free breathing.

The coronal T2-weighted sequence was performed to identify the position of the cecum. Axial sections were defined according to the position of the cecum in each subject. The cranial section was at least 10 cm above the cecum and extended to the most caudal point of the pubic symphysis.

The axial T2-weighted fast SE sequence was the most useful in the detection of the normal appendix, with the appendix being detected in 48 % of cases, as compared with lower detection rates for axial T1-weighted (15 %), axial T2-weighted fat-saturated (10 %), and coronal T2-weighted (10 %) fast SE sequences.

The internal appendiceal contents were hyperintense on the T2-weighted images (Fig. 10.20). On the T1-weighted images, the internal contents were hypointense.

The appendiceal walls were isointense on T1- and T2-weighted images (Chang et al. 2016).

Each examination lasted 7 min for the four sequences. The total examination time was 20 min and included intervals between sequences, stops during acquisition, subject's entry into the room, positioning, and exit. All examinations were performed without intravenous contrast material (Rosines et al. 2014).

The criterion to define the normal appendix was the visualization of a blind-ended tubular

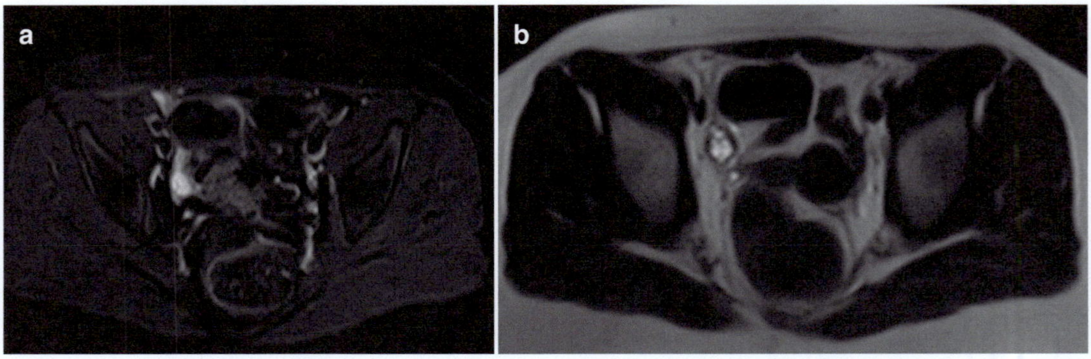

Fig. 10.20 MRI, (**a**) axial T2- weighted fat sarutated fast SE and (**b**) axial T2 weighted fast SE demonstrate the internal appendiceal contents hyperintense on the T2-weighted images

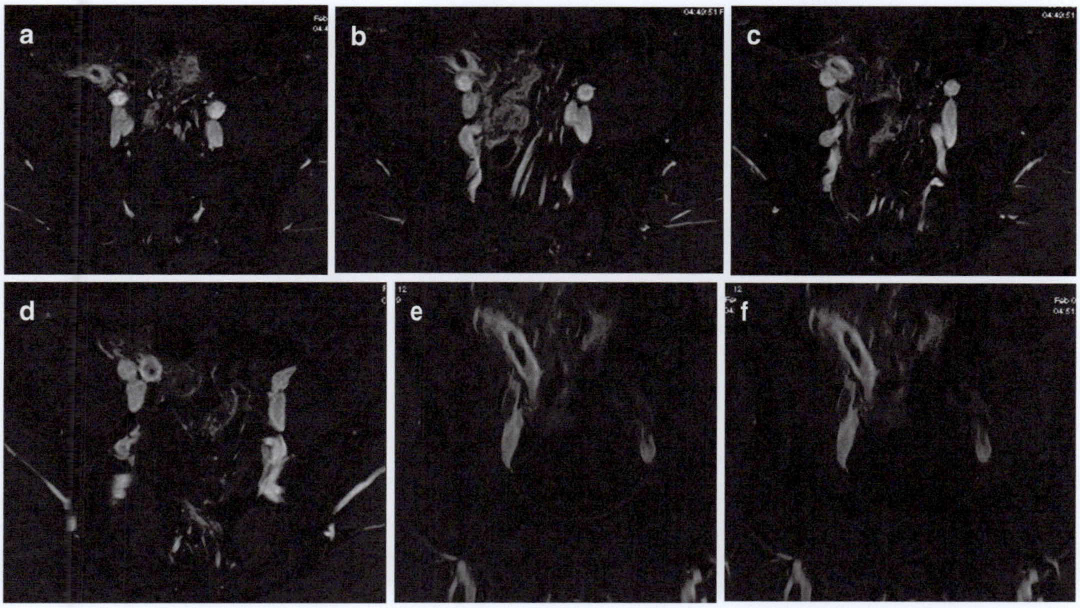

Fig. 10.21 (a–f) MRI with gadolinium: the appendiceal walls were hyperintense on T1-weighted images. The normal appendix was the visualization of a blinded tubular structure that extended from the cecum and had a transverse diameter less than or equal to 6 mm. MRI images show distended appendix greater than 7 mm in maximal diameter, appendiceal wall thickening and enhancement, and free peritoneal fluid

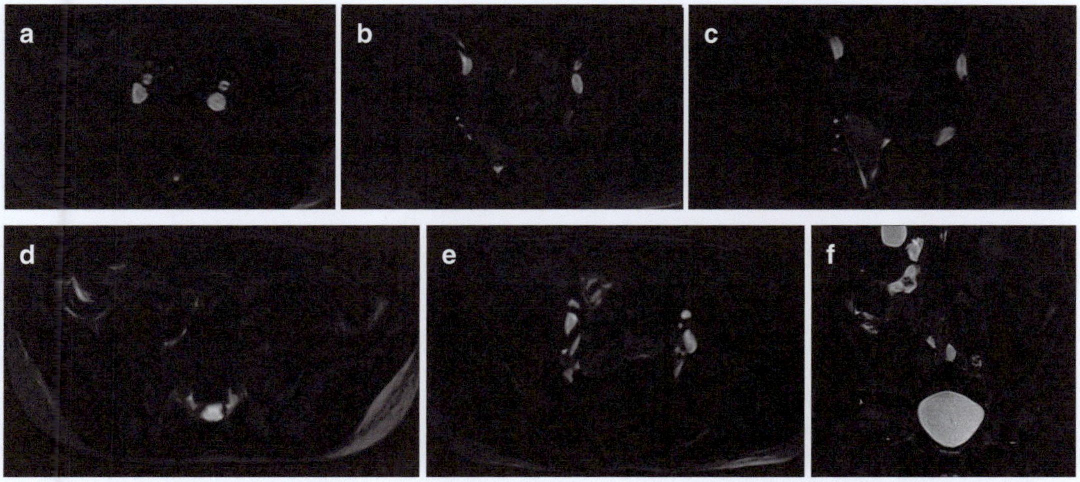

Fig. 10.22 (a–f) MRI with gadolinium: the appendiceal walls were isointense on T2-weighted images. The normal appendix was the visualization of a blinded tubular structure that extended from the cecum and had a transverse diameter less than or equal to 6 mm: MRI images show distended appendix greater than 7 mm in maximal diameter, appendiceal wall thickening and enhancement, and free peritoneal fluid

structure that extended from the cecum and had a transverse diameter less than or equal to 6 mm (Swenson et al. 2016).

This criterion is the same one used for the detection of the normal appendix at CT and US.

The detection of the appendix was positive when it was visualized with at least one MR sequence (Figs. 10.21 and 10.22).

One of the greatest limitations of US is the detection of retrocecal appendices.

With the use of MR imaging, however, appendices in this position were easily detected, particularly because of the fat between the posterior wall of the cecum and the posterior abdominal wall.

MR imaging examinations in children and adolescents were easily performed.

However MR imaging is expensive, and sedation is necessary to examine some pediatric patients. Therefore, MR imaging should be used only in cases in which US studies are not diagnostic: when it is available, MRI is preferable to CT as a second-level investigation, avoiding the use of radiation and contrast media. Nonenhanced MR imaging is highly accurate for the diagnosis of pediatric appendicitis, with test performance characteristics similar to those of US.

Nonenhanced MR imaging demonstrates high diagnostic performance similar to that of US for suspected pediatric appendicitis.

In conclusion, graded-compression ultrasonography (US) of the right lower quadrant is a valuable imaging modality for appendicitis, with sensitivities ranging from 75 % to 90 %, although such complications are often better delineated with CT or MRI (Epifanio et al. 2016).

Then, the second-level investigations can therefore be used in the follow-up of complications (e.g., abscesses) or when the clinical and laboratory tests are discordant.

References

Aspelund G, Fingeret A, Gross E, Kessler D, Keung C, Thirumoorthi A, Oh PS, Behr G, Chen S, Lampl B, Middlesworth W, Kandel J, Ruzal-Shapiro C (2014) Ultrasonography/MRI versus CT for diagnosing appendicitis. Pediatrics 133:586–593. doi:10.1542/peds.2013-2128, Epub 2014 Mar 3

Bachur RG, Levy JA, Callahan MJ, Rangel SJ, Monuteaux MC (2015) Effect of reduction in the use of computed tomography on clinical outcomes of appendicitis. JAMA Pediatr 169:755–760. doi:10.1001/jamapediatrics.2015.0479

Binkovitz LA, Unsdorfer KM, Thapa P, Kolbe AB, Hull NC, Zingula SN, Thomas KB, Homme JL (2015) Pediatric appendiceal ultrasound: accuracy, determinacy and clinical outcomes. Pediatr Radiol 45:1934–1944

Blumfield E, Nayak G, Srinivasan R, Muranaka MT, Blitman NM, Blumfield A, Levin TL (2013) Ultrasound for differentiation between perforated and nonperforated appendicitis in pediatric patients. AJR Am J Roentgenol 200(5):957–962

Brennan GD (2006) Pediatric appendicitis: pathophysiology and appropriate use of diagnostic imaging. CJEM 8:425–432

Butler M, Servaes S, Srinivasan A, Edgar JC, Del Pozo G, Darge K (2011) US depiction of the appendix: role of abdominal wall thickness and appendiceal location. Emerg Radiol 18:525–531

Catalano O, Lobianco R, Sandomenico F, Mattace Raso M, Siani A (2004) Real time contrast enhanced sonographic imaging in emergency radiology. Radiol Med 108:454–469

Chang PT, Yang E, Swenson DW, Lee EY (2016) Pediatric emergency magnetic resonance imaging: current indications, techniques, and clinical applications. Magn Reson Imaging Clin N Am 24:449–480. doi:10.1016/j.mric.2015.11.009, Epub 2016 Feb 22

Cogley JR, O'Connor SC, Houshyar R, Al Dulaimy K (2012) Emergent pediatric US: what every radiologist should know. Radiographics 32:651–665. doi:10.1148/rg.323115111

Cohen B, Bowling J, Midulla P, Shlasko E, Lester N, Rosenberg H, Lipskar A (2015) The non-diagnostic ultrasound in appendicitis: is a non-visualized appendix the same as a negative study? J Pediatr Surg 50:923–927

Di Giacomo V, Trinci M, Van der Byl G, Catania VD, Calisti A, Miele V (2015) Ultrasound in newborns and children suffering from nontraumatic acute abdominal pain: imaging with clinical and surgical correlation. J Ultrasound 18:385393. doi:10.1007/s4047701400874, Epub 2014 Apr 9

Ditkofsky NG, Singh A, Avery L, Novelline RA (2014) The role of emergency MRI in the setting of acute abdominal pain. Emerg Radiol 21:615–624. doi:10.1007/s10140-014-1232-2, Epub 2014 May 15

Doria AS (2011) Optimizing the role of imaging in appendicitis. Pediatr Radiol 41(8):993–999

Doria AS, Moineddin R, Kellenberger CJ et al (2006) US or CT for diagnosis of appendicitis in children and adults? A meta-analysis. Radiology 241:283–294

Epifanio M, Antonio de Medeiros Lima M, Epifanio M, Corrêa P, Baldisserotto M (2016) An imaging diagnostic protocol in children with clinically suspected acute appendicitis. Am Surg 82(5):390–396

Farina R, Catalano O, Stavolo C, Sandomenico F, Petrillo RL (2015) Emergency radiology. Radiol Med 120:73–84. doi:10.1007/s1154701404802121

Fonio P, Coppolino F, Russo A, D'Andrea A, Giannattasio A, Reginelli A, Grassi R, Genovese EA (2013) Ultrasonography (US) in the assessment of pediatric non traumatic gastrointestinal emergencies. Crit Ultrasound J 15(5 Suppl 1):S12

Gaitini D (2011) Imaging acute appendicitis: state of the art. J Clin Imaging Sci 1:49. doi:10.4103/2156-7514.85778, Epub 2011 Oct 7

Gendel I, Gutermacher M, Buklan G, Lazar L, Kidron D, Paran H, Erez I (2011) Relative value of clinical, laboratory and imaging tools in diagnosing pediatric acute appendicitis. Eur J Pediatr Surg 21:229–233
Goldin AB, Khanna P, Thapa M, McBroom JA, Garrison MM, Parisi MT (2009) Revised ultrasound criteria for appendicitis in children improve diagnostic accuracy. Pediatr Radiol 39(Suppl 2):S144–S148
Hagendorf BA, Clarke JR, Burd RS (2004) The optimal initial management of children with suspected appendicitis: a decision analysis. J Pediatr Surg 39:880–885
Herliczek TW, Swenson DW, Mayo-Smith WW (2013) Utility of MRI after inconclusive ultrasound in pediatric patients with suspected appendicitis: retrospective review of 60 consecutive patients. AJR Am J Roentgenol 200:969–973. doi:10.2214/AJR.12.10078
Horrow MM, White DS, Horrow JC (2003) Differentiation of perforated from nonperforated appendicitis at CT. Radiology 227:46–51
Hryhorczuk AL, Mannix RC, Taylor GA (2012) Pediatric abdominal pain: use of imaging in the Emergency Department in the United States from 1999 to 2007. Radiology 263:778–785
Je BK, Kim SB, Lee SH, Lee KY, Cha SH (2009) Diagnostic value of maximal-outer-diameter and maximal-mural-thickness in use of ultrasound for acute appendicitis in children. World J Gastroenterol 15:2900–2903
Kaiser S, Jorulf H, Söderman E, Frenckner B (2004) Impact of radiologic imaging on the surgical decision-making process in suspected appendicitis in children. Acad Radiol 11:971–979
Kearl YL, Claudius I, Behar S, Cooper J, Dollbaum R, Hardasmalani M, Hardiman K, Rose E, Santillanes G, Berdahl C (2016) Accuracy of magnetic resonance imaging and ultrasound for appendicitis in diagnostic and nondiagnostic studies. Acad Emerg Med 23:179–185
Kim ME, Orth RC, Fallon SC, Lopez ME, Brandt ML, Zhang W, Bisset GS (2015) Performance of CT examinations in children with suspected acute appendicitis in the community setting: a need for more education. AJR Am J Roentgenol 204:857–860. doi:10.2214/AJR.14.12750
Klein MD (2007) Clinical approach to a child with abdominal pain who might have appendicitis. Pediatr Radiol 37:11–14, Epub 2006 Oct 17
Koike Y, Uchida K, Matsushita K, Otake K, Nakazawa M, Inoue M, Kusunoki M, Tsukamoto Y (2014) Intraluminal appendiceal fluid is a predictive factor for recurrent appendicitis after initial successful non-operative management of uncomplicated appendicitis in pediatric patients. J Pediatr Surg 49(7):1116–1121
Krishnamoorthi R, Ramarajan N, Wang NE, Newman B, Rubesova E, Mueller CM, Barth RA (2011) Effectiveness of a staged US and CT protocol for the diagnosis of pediatric appendicitis: reducing radiation exposure in the age of ALARA. Radiology 259:231–239
Leeson K, Leeson B (2013) Pediatric ultrasound: applications in the emergency department. Emerg Med Clin North Am 31:809–829
Levine CD, Aizenstein O, Wachsberg RH (2004) Pitfalls in the CT diagnosis of appendicitis. Br J Radiol 77:792–799
Lim HK, Lee WJ, Lee SJ, Namgung S et al (1996) Focal appendicitis confined to the tip: diagnosis at US. Radiology 200:799–801
Lovrenski J, Jokić R, Varga I (2016) Sonographically detected free appendicolith as a sign of retrocecal perforated appendicitis in a 2-year-old child. J Clin Ultrasound 44(6):395–398. doi:10.1002/jcu.22337
Marin JR, Kornblith AE, Doniger SJ (2016) Point-of-care ultrasonography for appendicitis uncovers two alternate diagnoses. Pediatr Emerg Care 32:262–265
Mazeh H, Epelboym I, Reinherz J, Greenstein AJ, Divino CM (2009) Tip appendicitis: clinical implications and management. Am J Surg 197:211–215
Menichini G, Sessa B, Trinci M, Galluzzo M, Miele V (2015) Accuracy of contrast enhanced ultrasound (CEUS) in the identification and characterization of traumatic solid organ lesions in children: a retrospective comparison with baseline US and CEMDCT. Radiol Med 120:9891001. doi:10.1007/s115470150535z, Epub 2015 Mar 31
Miele V, Di Giampietro I (2014) Diagnostic imaging in emergency. Salute Soc, (2EN):127–138. doi:10.3280/SES2014-002010EN
Miele V, De Cicco ML, Andreoli C, Buffa V, Adami L, David V (2001) US and CT findings in complicated Meckel diverticulum. Radiol Med 101:230–234
Miele V, Andreoli C, Cortese A, De Cicco ML, Luzietti M, Stasolla A, David V (2002) Hemoperitoneum following ovarian cyst rupture: CT usefulness in the diagnosis. Radiol Med 104:122–126
Miele V, Andreoli C, Grassi R (2006) The management of emergency radiology: key facts. Eur J Radiol 59:311–314, Epub2006 Jun27
Miele V, Di Giampietro I, Ianniello S, Pinto F, Trinci M (2015) Diagnostic imaging in pediatric polytrauma management. Radiol Med 120:3349. doi:10.1007/s115470140469x.Epub2014Nov7
Miele V, Piccolo CL, Sessa B, Trinci M, Galluzzo M (2016a) Comparison between MRI and CEUS in the follow up of patients with blunt abdominal trauma managed conservatively. Radiol Med 121:27–37. doi:10.1007/s1154701505781Epub2016Jan8
Miele V, Piccolo CL, Galluzzo M, Ianniello S, Sessa B, Trinci M (2016b) Contrast enhanced ultrasound (CEUS) in blunt abdominal trauma. Br J Radiol 89(1061):20150823. doi:10.1259/bjr.20150823Epub2016Jan8
Miele V, Piccolo CL, Trinci M, Galluzzo M, Ianniello S, Brunese L (2016c) Diagnostic imaging of blunt abdominal trauma in pediatric patients. Radiol Med 121:409–430. doi:10.1007/s11547-016-0637-2, Epub 2016 Apr 13

Orth RC, Guillerman RP, Zhang W, Masand P, Bisset GS III (2014) Prospective comparison of MR imaging and US for the diagnosis of pediatric appendicitis. Radiology 272:233–240

Ozturkmen Akay H, Akpinar E, Akgul Ozmen C, Ergun O, Haliloglu M (2007) Visualization of the normal appendix in children by non-contrast MDCT. Acta Chir Belg 107:531–534

Pastore V, Cocomazzi R, Basile A, Pastore M, Bartoli F (2014) Limits and advantages of abdominal ultrasonography in children with acute appendicitis syndrome. Afr J Paediatr Surg 11:293–296

Pinto F, Miele V, Scaglione M, Pinto A (2014) The use of contrast-enhanced ultrasound in blunt abdominal trauma: advantages and limitations. Acta Radiol 55:776784. doi:10.1177/0284185113505517.Epub2013Sep23

Pinto F, Valentino M, Romanini L, Basilico R, Miele V (2015) The role of CEUS in the assessment of haemodinamically stable patients with blunt abdominal trauma. Radiol Med 120:311. doi:10.1007/s1154701404553.Epub2014Aug21

Pinto A, Miele V, Schillirò ML, Nasuto M, Chianese V, Romano L, Guglielmi G (2016) Spectrum of signs of pneumoperitoneum. Semin US CT MRI 37:39. doi:10.1053/j.sult.2015.10.008Epub2015Oct28

Prendergast PM, Poonai N, Lynch T, McKillop S, Lim R (2014) Acute appendicitis: investigating an optimal outer appendiceal diameter cut-point in a pediatric population. J Emerg Med 46:157–164

Ripollès T, Martinez-Perez MJ, PAredes JM, Vizuete J, Garcìa-Martinez E, Jimènez-Restrepo DH (2013) Contrast-enhanced ultrasound in the differentiation between phlegmon and abscess in Crohn's disease and other abdominal conditions. Eur J Radiol 82:e525–e531

Rosines LA, Chow DS, Lampl BS, Chen S, Gordon S, Mui LW, Aspelund G, Ruzal-Shapiro CB (2014) Value of gadolinium-enhanced MRI in detection of acute appendicitis in children and adolescents. AJR Am J Roentgenol 203:W543–W548. doi:10.2214/AJR.13.12093

Sessa B, Trinci M, Ianniello S, Menichini G, Galluzzo M, Miele V (2015) Blunt abdominal trauma: role of contrast enhanced ultrasound in the detection and staging of abdominal traumatic lesions compared with US and CEMDCT. Radiol Med 120:180189. doi:10.1007/s1154701404259, Epub 2014 Jun 25

Shah BR, Stewart J, Jeffrey RB, Olcott EW (2014) Value of short-interval computed tomography when sonography fails to visualize the appendix and shows otherwise normal findings. J Ultrasound Med 33:1589–1595

Simonovsky V (2002) Normal appendix: is there any significant difference in the maximal mural thickness at US between pediatric and adult populations? Radiology 224:333–337

Sivit CJ (2004) Imaging the child with right lower quadrant pain and suspected appendicitis: current concepts. Pediatr Radiol 34:447–453

Srinivasan A, Servaes S, Peña A, Darge K (2015) Utility of CT after sonography for suspected appendicitis in children: integration of a clinical scoring system with a staged imaging protocol. Emerg Radiol 22(1):31–42. doi:10.1007/s10140-014-1241-1, Epub 2014 Jun 12

Strouse PJ (2010) Pediatric appendicitis: an argument for US. Radiology 255:8–13

Sung T, Callahan MJ, Taylor GA (2006) Clinical and imaging mimickers of acute appendicitis in the pediatric population. AJR Am J Roentgenol 186:67–74

Swenson DW, Schooler GR, Stamoulis C, Lee EY (2016) MRI of the normal appendix in children: data toward a new reference standard. Pediatr Radiol 46:1003–1010

Taylor GA (2004) Suspected appendicitis in children: in search of the single best diagnostic test. Radiology 231:293–295

Trout AT, Sanchez R, Ladino-Torres MF (2012) Reevaluating the sonographic criteria for acute appendicitis in children: a review of the literature and a retrospective analysis of 246 cases. Acad Radiol 19:1382–1394

Tseng P, Berdahl C, Kearl YL, Behar S, Cooper J, Dollbaum R, Hardasmalani M, Hardiman K, Rose E, Santillanes G, Lam C, Claudius I (2016) Does right lower quadrant abdominal ultrasound accurately identify perforation in pediatric acute appendicitis? J Emerg Med 50(4):638–642

Wan MJ, Krahn M, Ungar WJ, Caku E, Sung L, Medina LS, Doria AS (2009) Acute appendicitis in young children: cost-effectiveness of US versus CT in diagnosis—a Markov decision analytic model. Radiology 250:378–386

Xu Y, Jeffrey RB, DiMaio MA, Olcott EW (2016) Lymphoid hyperplasia of the appendix: a potential pitfall in the sonographic diagnosis of appendicitis. AJR Am J Roentgenol 206(1):189–194. doi:10.2214/AJR.15.14846

Yiğiter M, Kantarci M, Yalçin O, Yalçin A, Salman AB (2011) Does obesity limit the sonographic diagnosis of appendicitis in children? J Clin Ultrasound 39:187–190. doi:10.1002/jcu.20782, Epub 2010 Dec 28

Meckel's Diverticulum

11

Maria Elena Latini, Sara Riccioni, Maria Napoletano, Nicola Recchia, and Michele Scialpi

11.1 Epidemiology

Meckel's diverticulum is the most common congenital anomaly of the gastrointestinal tract, occurring in 2–3% of the population, with equal frequency in both sexes. Described for the first time by Wilhelm Fabricius Hildanus in 1598, it is named after Johann Friedrich Meckel, the German anatomist who explained its embryological origin in 1809. Its clinical importance depends on the high frequency of related complications, as inflammation, hemorrhage, and bowel obstruction. The risk of complications ranges from 4% to 40% in several studies, three times more common in male patients. Complications may occur at all ages, but they are more frequent in children than adults, with major incidence in the first decade (more than 50% in the first 2 years), decreasing during lifetime.

11.2 Etiopathology

Meckel's diverticulum is the main abnormality among a group of anomalies which derives from an incomplete obliteration of the omphalomesenteric (vitelline) duct.

Before the fifth week of embryogenesis, the omphalomesenteric duct represents the communication between the yolk sac and the developing midgut, through which the vitelline vessels provide fetal nutrition. Subsequently, the omphalomesenteric duct merges with the allantois to produce the umbilical cord. Between the fifth and the seventh week of gestation, the omphalomesenteric duct becomes completely obliterated along its entire course and turns into a thin fibrous band, which is eventually absorbed afterward.

If the duct fails to fully atrophy, different types of anomalies appear, according to the time and the way of failed obliteration (Fig. 11.1): (1) *umbilicoileal fistula*, when the duct remains completely patent (Fig. 11.2); (2) *omphalomesenteric duct sinus*, if the distal (umbilical) end of the duct fails to regress and forms a sinus tract, which extends for a variable length (Fig. 11.3); (3) *omphalomesenteric duct cyst*, when only the central portion of the duct is patent, while the umbilical and intestinal ends close; (4) *fibrous connection of the ileum to the umbilicus*, if the duct becomes atrophic but not obliterated and absorbed; and (5) *Meckel's diverticulum*, the most common of all (98%), when only the proximal (intestinal) end of the duct fails to obliterate and remains patent.

Meckel's diverticulum is a true diverticulum, containing all layers of the ileal wall. In 90% of cases, it is localized in the ileum in a tract

M.E. Latini (✉) • S. Riccioni • M. Napoletano
N. Recchia • M. Scialpi
Division of Radiology, Department of Surgical and Biomedical Sciences, S. Maria della Misericordia Hospital, S. Andrea delle Fratte, Perugia, Italy
e-mail: elenalatini@hotmail.com

V. Miele, M. Trinci (eds.), *Imaging Non-traumatic Abdominal Emergencies in Pediatric Patients*,
DOI 10.1007/978-3-319-41866-7_11

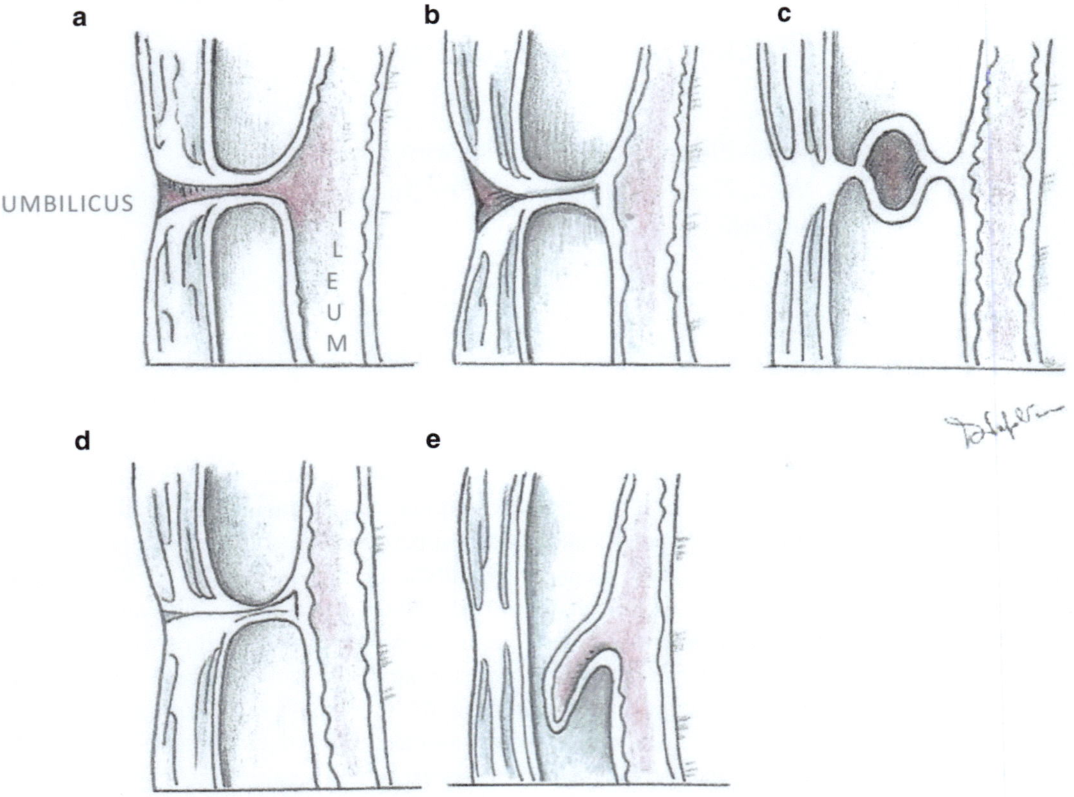

Fig. 11.1 Different types of anomalies from the incomplete obliteration of the omphalomesenteric duct: (**a**) umbilicoileal fistula, (**b**) omphalomesenteric duct sinus, (**c**) omphalomesenteric duct cyst, (**d**) fibrous connection of the ileum to the umbilicus, and (**e**) Meckel's diverticulum

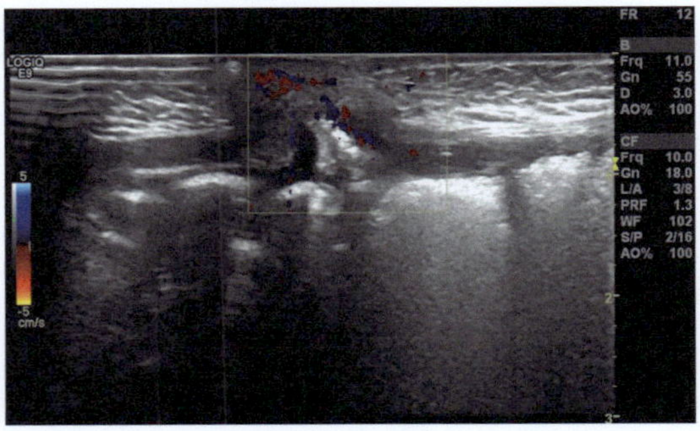

Fig. 11.2 Umbilicoileal fistula in a 1-month-old child presenting with fecal drainage from the umbilicus

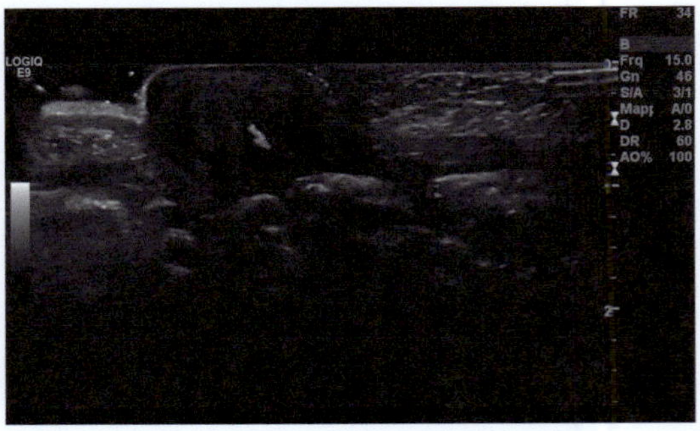

Fig. 11.3 Omphalomesenteric duct sinus in a 2-month-old child came to clinical attention because of mucus discharge from the umbilicus

40–100 cm proximal to the ileocecal valve, arising from its antimesenteric border, although case reports have also described a mesenteric location. Its length ranges from 1 to 10 cm, with a diameter up to 3 cm. Rare cases of diverticula larger than the ileal loops have been reported (giant Meckel's diverticula).

The tip of the diverticulum is free in 75 % of cases, while it is connected to the anterior abdominal wall or to the mesentery through fibrous bands in the remaining cases. The vitelline ligament is a cordlike structure which joins the diverticulum to the umbilical region.

The diverticulum is usually supplied by the omphalomesenteric artery, a remnant of the vitelline artery, which arises from an ileal branch of the superior mesenteric artery, running within a different fold of the small bowel mesentery, thus creating a support for the diverticulum or along the surface of the diverticulum itself.

Meckel's diverticulum is typically lined by ileal mucosa, but heterotopic mucosa is often found: gastric mucosa is the most common (62 % of cases), followed by pancreatic tissue (6 %), both gastric mucosa and pancreatic tissue (5 %), jejunal mucosa (2 %), Brunner's glands (2 %), and combined gastric and duodenal mucosa (2 %). In rare cases colonic, rectal, endometrial, or hepatobiliary tissues have been found.

11.3 Clinical Presentation

Most Meckel's diverticula are asymptomatic and incidentally found during autopsy, surgery, or barium studies. Symptoms are typically related to the onset of complications, which are reported to occur in 4–40 % of patients. In a retrospective study, it has been demonstrated that the lifetime risk of developing complications of a Meckel's diverticulum decreases with age: 4 % up to the age of 20 years, 2 % up to the age of 40 years, and zero in the elderly population.

Hemorrhage is the most common complication in the pediatric population (20–30 %). It is due to peptic ulceration from ectopic gastric mucosa within the diverticulum. Bleeding may be acute and massive, resulting in a shock-producing hemorrhage, or chronic and occult, causing weakness and anemia. Children complain of passing bright red blood in the stools, usually without abdominal pain or tenderness.

Intestinal obstruction is the second most common complication (20–25 %), the most recurrent in adult patients. Various mechanisms are involved in its genesis: intussusception and volvulus are the most frequent. If Meckel's diverticulum gets invaginated into the ileum like an inverted finger glove, it may form the lead point of an ileoileal or ileocolic intussusception. Volvulus occurs because of the torsion of a loop of bowel around fibrous bands connecting the diverticulum to the abdominal wall or mesodiverticular bands. Other causes of intestinal obstruction in Meckel's diverticulum include luminal blockage from foreign bodies (enteroliths, fecaliths); Littré hernia, which represents the entrapment of the diverticulum in a hernia (50 % of cases in the inguinal region); and tumors originating in the diverticulum.

Diverticulitis occurs in 10–20 % of symptomatic patients. It may mimic symptoms of acute appendicitis: intermittent crampy abdominal pain and tenderness in the periumbilical area, sometimes associated with fever and vomiting. A persistent pain around the umbilicus delaying in moving to the right iliac fossa as well as a normal appendix found at laparotomy for presumptive appendicitis should always raise the suspicion of Meckel's diverticulitis. Like appendicitis, Meckel's diverticulitis may lead to perforation and peritonitis (Chohan et al. 2010).

Neoplasms arising in Meckel's diverticulum have been reported in 3–5 % of cases. Leiomyoma is the most common type, followed by leiomyosarcoma, carcinoid tumor, and fibroma. Rare cases of adenocarcinomas originating from ectopic gastric mucosa have been described.

Intestinal obstruction is the most common complication in newborns. A rectal bleeding or an abdominal appendicitis-like pain is usually the first symptomatic manifestations in older children, while adults may incur bowel obstruction or carcinoid syndrome.

11.4 Imaging Diagnosis

Preoperative diagnosis of Meckel's diverticulum may be difficult. A study by Yamaguchi et al. demonstrated that only 6 % of diverticula have a presurgical diagnosis.

The radiological diagnosis of Meckel's diverticulum is greatly significant in those patients presenting with clinical sign and symptoms of its complications (Levy and Hobbs 2004; Rossi et al. 1996; Parigi 2005; Di Giacomo et al. 2015; Elsayes et al. 2007).

Plain Abdominal Radiographs. They may reveal nonspecific signs of intestinal obstruction, as air-fluid levels eventually associated with enteroliths within the diverticulum (Fig. 11.4).

Barium Studies (small bowel follow-through, enteroclysis, enema). They may make virtually certain diagnosis by showing the presence of a saccular, blind-ending pouch on the antimesenteric border of the ileum, with a triradiate fold pattern (when loops are collapsed) or a mucosal triangular plateau (when loops are distended) at the junction of the diverticulum with the ileum, which represents the site of omphalomesenteric duct attachment to the small bowel (Fig. 11.5).

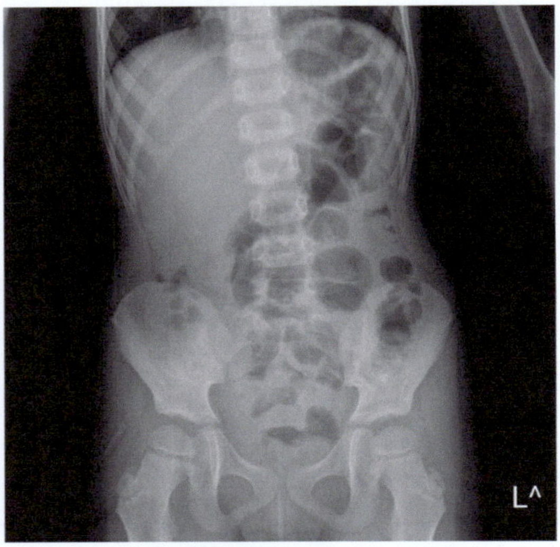

Fig. 11.4 The erect abdominal radiography demonstrates multiple air-fluid levels in the hypogastrium and right iliac fossa

Enteroliths and fecaliths may appear as defects of opacification.

Solitary diverticulum of the ileum, communicating enteric duplications, and cavitating malignant masses of the small bowel should be considered in the differential diagnosis. An inverted Meckel's diverticulum defines a tubular defect of opacification, resembling an intestinal polyp. False-negative studies may be related to small-mouthed diverticula, stenosis of the ostium, blood clots within the pouch, and rapid emptying due to peristaltic activity.

Ultrasonography. It is usually a first-line method in the diagnosis of Meckel's diverticulum nowadays, but of little use in uncomplicated cases. Ultrasonography may show a blind-ending peristaltic tubular structure connected to the small bowel. When obstructed, the diverticulum appears overdistended and fluid filled.

In case of diverticulitis (Fig. 11.6), ultrasonography may find a round or tubular, cyst-like, noncompressible, aperistaltic formation, with a thick irregular hyperechoic internal wall and a hypoechoic external wall ("gut signature"). Internal echoes may be related to the intraluminal presence of enteroliths, fecaliths, or inflammatory debris. Color Doppler sonographic findings of inflammation include bowel wall hyperemia, compared with a normal adjacent intestinal loop, and the presence of a large-caliber artery supplying blood to the diverticulum, while an avascular wall most often characterizes an intestinal ischemia (Baldisserotto 2004). A variable amount of free fluid may be found in the peritoneal cavity.

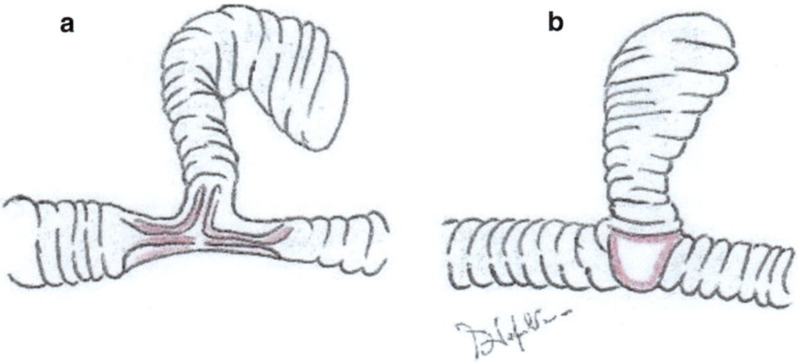

Fig. 11.5 (**a**) Triradiate fold pattern with collapsed loops; (**b**) mucosal triangular plateau with distended loops

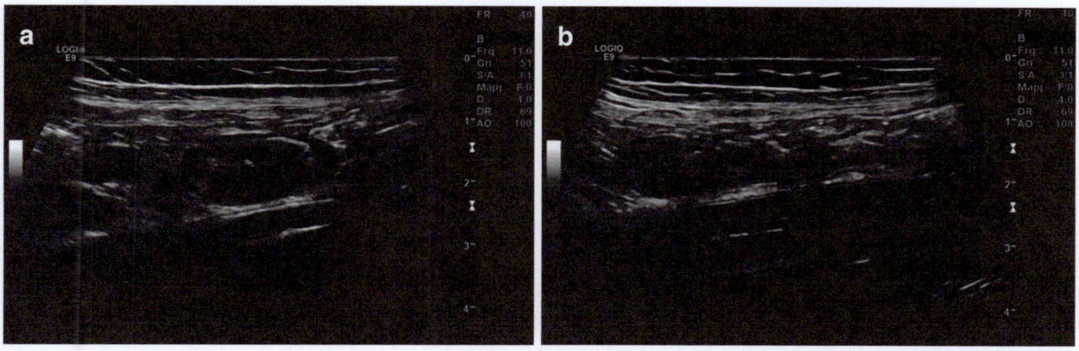

Fig. 11.6 The transverse (**a**) and longitudinal (**b**) ultrasonographic views show a Meckel's diverticulitis with *gut signature* appearance: a thick irregular hyperechoic internal wall (mucosa and submucosa) and a hypoechoic external wall (muscularis propria)

When a hyperechoic layer surrounds the diverticulum, perforation should be suspected.

An intussuscepted Meckel's diverticulum may appear as a "double target sign": a target-like mass with a central area of hyperechogenicity from the core of mesenteric fat, due to a twofold intussusception, i.e., the diverticulum into the ileum and the ileum into the colon (Fig. 11.7).

Computed Tomography. It is of limited diagnostic value in uncomplicated cases, because the diverticulum may resemble a normal bowel loop (Fig. 11.8). Furthermore, because the CT scan exposes children to the risk of contrast and radiation, it should not be used as the first diagnostic test.

If a strong suspicion of volvulus exists, together with the finding of a blind-ending diverticular sac communicating with the small bowel at the level of obstruction, the detection of the vitelline ligament or mesodiverticular bands, however difficult it is, significantly increases the degree of diagnostic confidence. Other findings to consider are abrupt change in caliber between the proximal dilated bowel loops and the collapsed distal ones and stretched whirling vessels converging toward the volvulated loops. The diverticulum may contain fluid, air, enteroliths/fecaliths, or fecal matter.

Intussuscepted Meckel's diverticulum may appear as an abnormal multilayered target-like image, with a diameter larger than the normal bowel, although the direct visualization of the diverticulum as the lead point is often difficult.

Ischemic sufferance of the intestine is indicated by thickened and increased attenuation of the bowel wall, "halo sign", pneumatosis intestinalis, portal venous gas, localized fluid, or hemorrhage in the mesentery.

Thickened and hyperenhanced wall, with inner and outer high-attenuation layers and an intervening low-attenuation one, adjacent mesenteric fat stranding, and fluid collections are indicative of inflammation.

Diverticular bleeding is suggested by leakage of contrast within the diverticulum.

Magnetic Resonance. It is a radiation-free nonroutine method for the diagnosis of Meckel's diverticulum (Fig. 11.9).

Bleeding from Meckel's diverticulum may be detected at magnetic resonance as a cyst-like structure with a teardrop shape and high-intensity signal on non-enhanced T1-weighted images in the right iliac fossa (Epifanio et al. 2015; Zhou et al. 2013).

In case of inverted Meckel's diverticulum as a lead point for intussusception, a hypointense loop-in-loop lesion in the ileum appears on T1- and T2-weighted images, without contrast enhancement (Dujardin et al. 2002).

Nuclear Medicine. Scintigraphy with ^{99m}Tc-pertechnetate (also referred to as "Meckel scan") is historically the modality of choice for evaluating pediatric patients with gastrointestinal bleeding and suspected Meckel's diverticulum. ^{99m}Tc-pertechnetate is preferentially accumulated and secreted by the mucus cells of gastric mucosa

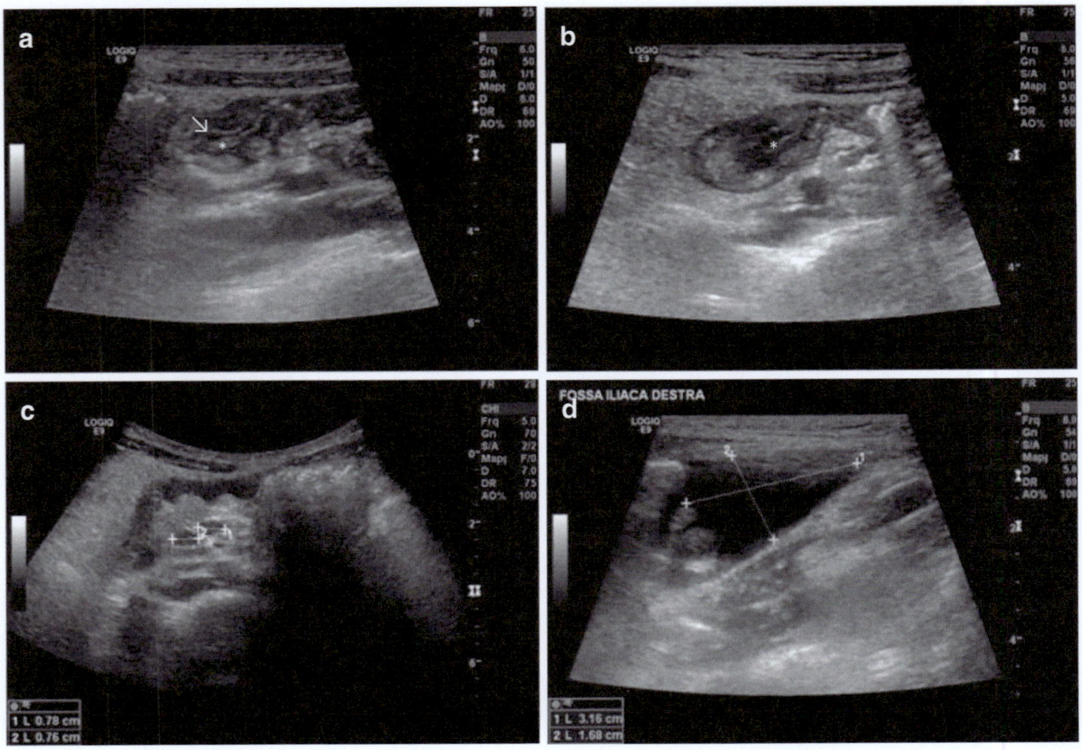

Fig. 11.7 Ultrasonographic features of inverted Meckel's diverticulum with ileocolic intussusception. (**a**) The transverse view shows the *double target sign*: alternating concentric layers of high and low echogenicity with an additional central area of hyperechogenicity, composed of mesenteric fat (*) and small mesenteric lymph nodes (*arrow*). (**b**) The longitudinal view of the same area shows invaginated mesenteric fat (*) within the colon (intussuscipiens). (**c**) The adjacent mesentery appears thickened and edematous, with reactive lymph nodes. (**d**) A moderate amount of pelvic free fluid is found

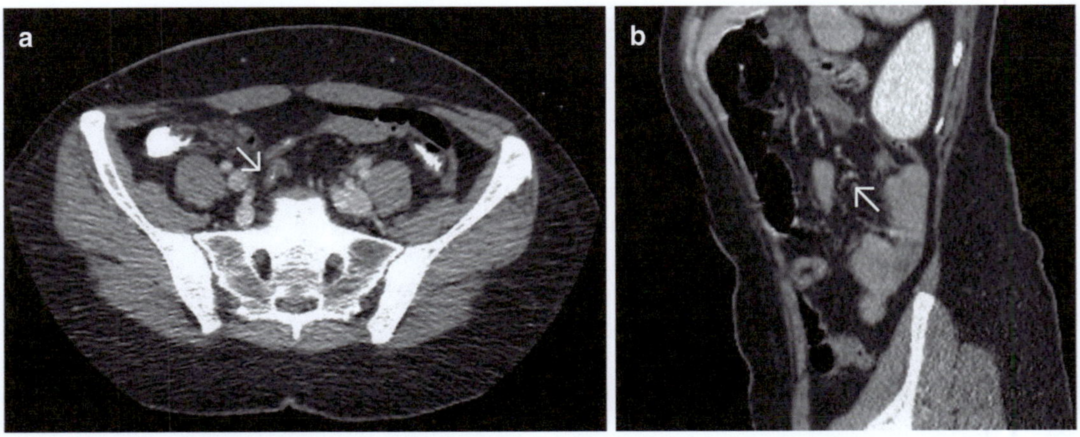

Fig. 11.8 A contrast-filled Meckel's diverticulum (*white arrows*) incidentally found on a CT scan in a 50-year-old woman, who was given positive oral contrast. Axial (**a**) and sagittal (**b**) view

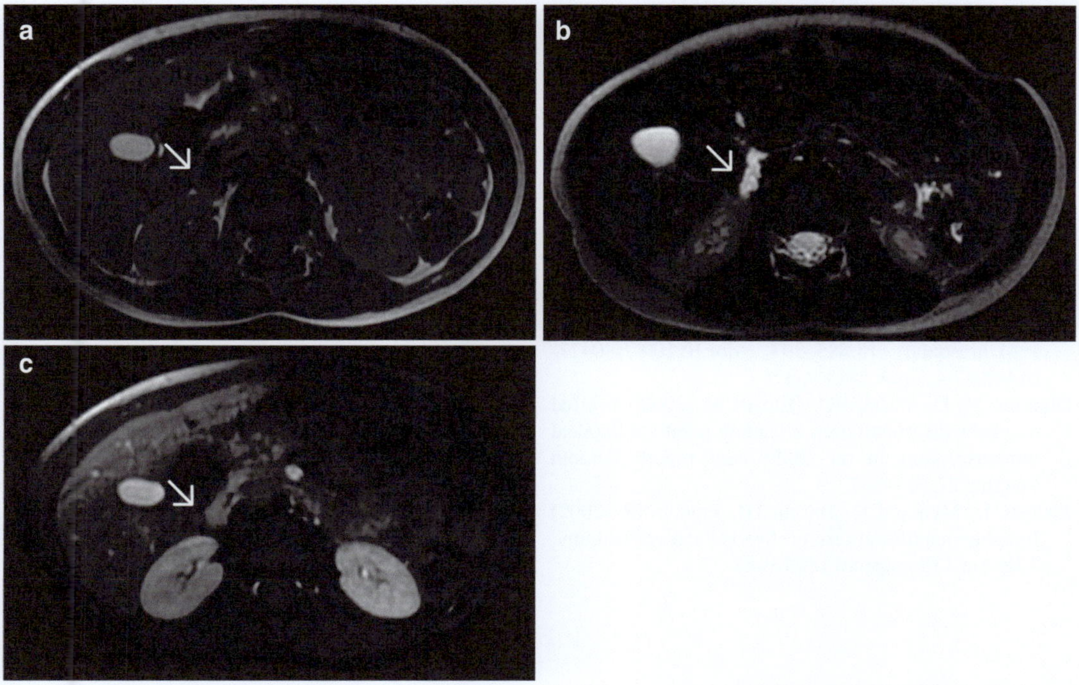

Fig. 11.9 In a 4-year-old child, the magnetic resonance demonstrates a tubular structure (*white arrows*) connected to the small bowel, which appears hypointense on T1-weighted (**a**) and hyperintense on T2-weighted images (**b**), with parietal contrast enhancement (**c**)

and ectopic gastric epithelium in the diverticulum. Within 30 min after intravenous injection of the radioisotope, a Meckel's diverticulum containing at least 1.8 cm^2 of ectopic gastric tissue appears as a focal area of increased uptake in the right lower quadrant.

In the pediatric population, scintigraphy has a sensitivity of 85 % and a specificity of 95 %, which become 63 % and 2 % in adults, respectively, because the prevalence of heterotopic gastric mucosa decreases in patients older than 30 years. The sensitivity may be increased using an H2 antagonist, pentagastrin, or glucagon. False-positive results may be related to gastric duplication, islets of ectopic gastric mucosa in the small bowel outside of the diverticulum, and all conditions of intestinal hyperemia.

Active or recurrent bleeding may be detected by using ^{99m}Tc-sulfur colloid or ^{99m}Tc-labeled red blood cells, but neither technique is specific.

Angiography. Superior mesenteric angiography may be useful to localize the site of acute bleeding to a Meckel's diverticulum, undetected at scintigraphy, but it requires a 0.5–1 ml/min blood loss to be effective. Discovery of the omphalomesenteric artery supplying the diverticulum and extravasation of contrast during the active phase of bleeding make diagnosis. Angiographic procedure may be therapeutic also, stopping bleeding through the selective embolization of the anomalous blood vessel.

In emergency Meckel's diverticulum may mostly appear as inflammatory complication or intussusception. In both cases it represents a diagnostic and therapeutic challenge, because of the lack of pathognomonic imaging signs. Ultrasonography remains, however, the first-level diagnostic method in pediatric patients who complain of an abdominal pain typically localized in the periumbilical region.

References

Baldisserotto M (2004) Color doppler sonographic findings of inflamed and perforated Meckel diverticulum. J Ultrasound Med 23:843–848

Chohan TA, Tabook SA, Elmukashfi E, Skroon SM (2010) Acute appendicitis or… is it Meckel's diverticulitis? Oman Med J 25:2010

Di Giacomo V, Trinci M, Van der Byl G, Catania VD, Calisti A, Miele V (2015) Ultrasound in newborns and children suffering from nontraumatic acute abdominal pain: imaging with clinical and surgical correlation. J Ultrasound 18:385–393. doi:10.1007/s40477-014-0087-4, Epub 2014 Apr 9

Dujardin M, De Beeck BO, Osteaux M (2002) Inverted Meckel's diverticulum as a leading point for ileoileal intussusception in an adult: case report. Abdom Imaging 27:563–565

Elsayes K, Menias CO, Harvin HJ, Francis IR (2007) Imaging manifestations of Meckel's diverticulum». AJR Am J Roentgenol 189:81–88

Epifanio M, Terrazas E, Spolidoro J, Bastos JC, Mattiello R, Baldisserotto M (2015) Magnetic resonance findings of a Meckel's diverticulum at 3 Tesla. J Pediatr Gastroenterol Nutr. [Epub ahead of print]. PMID: 25643017. doi:10.1097/MPG.0000000000000746

Levy AD, Hobbs MC (2004) From the archives of the AFIP – Meckel diverticulum: radiologic features with pathologic correlation. RadioGraphics 24:565–587

Parigi GB (2005) Chirurgia pediatrica. Masson Editore, Milano, pp 327–329

Rossi P, Gourtsoyiannis N, Bezzi M, Raptopoulos V, Massa R, Capanna G, Pedicini V, Coe M (1996) Meckel's diverticulum: imaging diagnosis. AJR Am J Roentgenol 166:567–573

Zhou FR, Huang LY, Xie HZ (2013) Meckel's diverticulum bleeding diagnosed with magnetic resonance enterography: a case report. World J Gastroenterol 19:2727–2730

Part III

Neonatal and Pediatric GU Emergencies

Neonatal Adrenal Hemorrhage

12

Margherita Trinci, Caterina Maria Trinci,
Michele Galluzzo, Eugenio Rossi,
Massimo Zeccolini, and Vittorio Miele

12.1 Anatomy

The adrenal (suprarenal) glands are paired organs and belong to the endocrine system; they are enclosed in the perirenal fascia in the retroperitoneal space and lie superior and anteromedial to the upper pole of the kidneys, at the side of the spine (Fig. 12.1). The right adrenal gland posteriorly lies on the right crus of the diaphragm, which separates it from the 12th thoracic vertebra and the initial part of the corresponding cost; medially and anteriorly it is related to the inferior vena cava and on the anterolateral side to the right lobe of the liver (bare area).

The left adrenal gland posteriorly lies on the left crus of the diaphragm which separates it from the 12th thoracic vertebra and the first lumbar vertebra. Its anterior surface is covered by the peritoneum, and anteriorly it is related to the posterior surface of the stomach to the pancreas and the spleen. The medial border of the left adrenal gland is related to the aorta (Westra et al. 1994; Miele et al. 1994).

Both glands are roughly pyramidal in shape and have a body and two limbs, medial and lateral. In particular, the right adrenal gland appears as a V shape or comma shape, and the left adrenal gland appears as a triangular or Y shape (Rahman et al. 1997) (Fig. 12.2). The size and weight are variable according to age, sex, and physiological conditions. Proportionately, the adrenal size is larger in newborn and infants than in adult, being almost one-third of the size of the kidney in the fourth month of pregnancy and during the following months of fetal life, and then until the first year of life, this gland tends to shrink in size, mainly at the expense of the medulla. The adrenal glands in the newborn have a very large size and are about one-third the size of the kidney. After birth the dimensions decrease in time; the right adrenal body should measure ≤8 mm and limbs 5–9; the left adrenal gland body should measure ≤10 mm and limbs 5–9 mm.

Some anatomical variants have to be kept into consideration: horseshoe adrenal gland, pancake adrenal gland, and adrenal gland hyperplasia, hypoplasia, or agenesis, and accessory adrenal nest soften near adrenal glands but may be found anywhere in the abdomen, pelvis, or scrotum.

The adrenal gland is surrounded by a fibrous capsule and has a thick outer cortex and a thin inner medulla. These glands are responsible for the release of hormones that regulate the immune system function, the metabolism, and the salt-water balance in the bloodstream; they also

M. Trinci (✉) • C.M. Trinci • M. Galluzzo • V. Miele
Department of Emergency Radiology,
S. Camillo Hospital, Rome, Italy
e-mail: margherita.trinci@libero.it

E. Rossi • M. Zeccolini
Department of Pediatric Radiology, Pausilipon
Oncologic Pediatric Hospital, Naples, Italy

V. Miele, M. Trinci (eds.), *Imaging Non-traumatic Abdominal Emergencies in Pediatric Patients*,
DOI 10.1007/978-3-319-41866-7_12

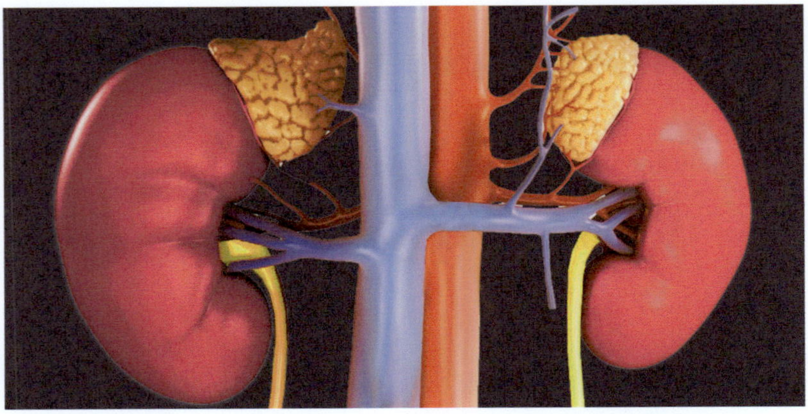

Fig. 12.1 Adrenal gland anatomy. (Thanks to Edoardo Saperi for the drawing)

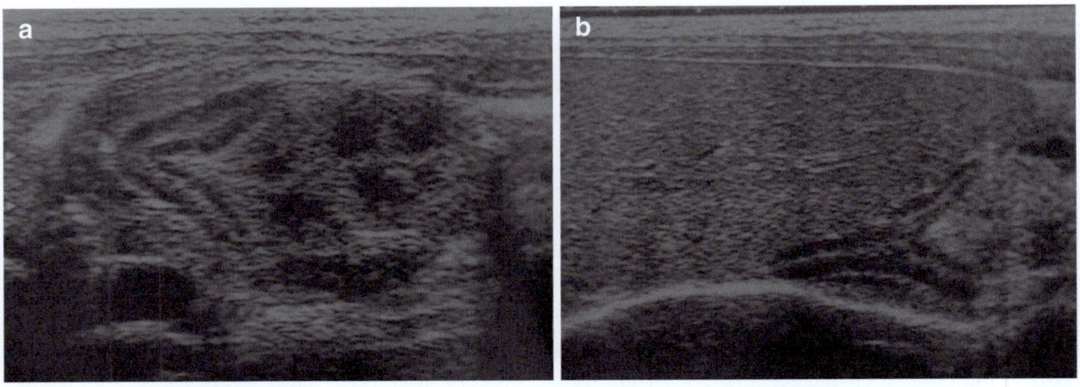

Fig. 12.2 Sonographic aspects of normal adrenal glands in newborn. (**a**) Right adrenal gland, V shape. (**b**) Left adrenal gland, Y shape

contribute in the body's response to stress. The medullar zone is responsible for the production of catecholamines (adrenaline, noradrenaline) as well as dopamine.

12.2 Ultrasound (US)

Unlike what happens in adult patients where the adrenal gland is difficult to see by ultrasound, this technique is the best approach in pediatric patients (Westra et al. 1994). Ultrasound study, in fact, is able to easily assess the organs of the abdominal cavity in a short time, it can be easily repeatable, and it is not painful and does not expose the patient to radiation (Kawashima et al. 1999). The study in newborn is performed with a high-frequency linear probe adapted to the size of the baby (from 10 to 7.5 MHz); in pediatric patients convex probe (3.5 MHz) could be used to complete the exam. The gland is evaluated with anterior transverse scanning. While neonatal adrenal glands are always visible, in older children the adrenal glands are not always visible to the physical constitution.

Left adrenal gland is more difficult to visualize than the right because it is often posterior to the stomach and is obscured by gas; this can be overcome by intercostal scanning with the left side of the patient up.

At ultrasound exam the corticomedullary differentiation is easy to see: in fact the cortex has lower echogenicity than medulla, and this differentiation varies over the time. In healthy newborn

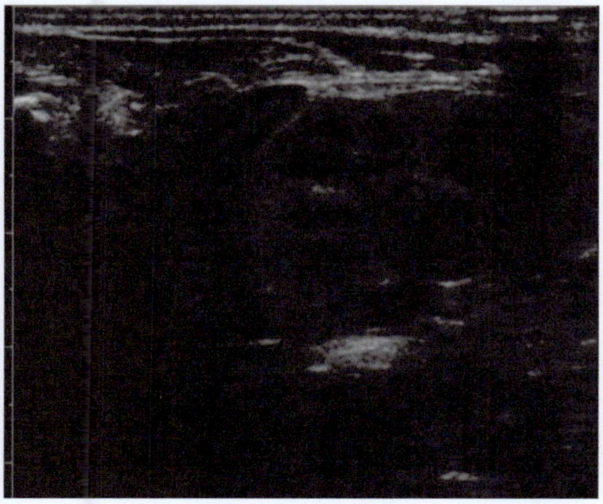

Fig. 12.3 In a 10-day-old female, ultrasound shows the normal aspect of the adrenal gland with the typical corticomedullary differentiation due to the cortex that is lower echogenicity than medulla

the cortex is also prominent; it is due to the presence of a transient fetal cortical zone that is possible to visualize at the perimeter of the gland as a thin echogenic line performing the exam with high-resolution probe (Fig. 12.3) (Westra et al. 1994).

12.3 Computed Tomography (CT)/ Magnetic Resonance Imaging (MRI)

In cases in which a second level evaluation is required, especially in pediatric patients, MRI is preferred to CT that uses ionizing radiation (Miele and Di Giampietro 2014); the lack of retroperitoneal fat in new born may make difficult the assessment of the adrenal gland. Sedation often can be necessary in younger patient for both procedures.

Both the exams detect the gland, the shape, the presence, and the kind of a mass and are more accurate than ultrasonography in the evaluation of the extension of the tumor (Westra et al. 1994).

On CT exam the adrenal glands enhance after contrast administration to approximately 50–60 HU. Hyperenhancement of the adrenal gland is concerning for hypovolemic shock.

12.4 Related Pathology and Clinical Presentation

12.4.1 Adrenal Hemorrhage

Neonatal adrenal gland hemorrhage is not uncommon (1.7 per 1,000 births); it has been described for the first time by Spencer in 1892 in alive infants [2 Rahman, 12 Gyurkovitz]. The etiology remains unclear; hypoxia antenatal, labor-induced or a difficult delivery, prematurity, macrosomic neonates, and coagulation disorders are often reported in obstetrical history (Westra et al. 1994; Miele et al. 1994; Rahman et al. 1997). The same causes are also frequently associated with neonatal renal vein thrombosis; for this reason we can find the adrenal hemorrhage and renal vein thrombosis in the same patient (Westra et al. 1994; Miele et al. 1994; Lau et al. 2007). Adrenal hemorrhage has been observed during the prenatal life in utero generally occurring around birth (Schrauder et al. 2008; Gyurkovitz et al. 2015).

Its significant vascularization provides from the inferior phrenic artery, abdominal aorta, and renal artery, and the large size of adrenal gland, about 20 times the relative size in the adult, leads to hemorrhage (Miele et al. 1994).

The hemorrhage can be bilateral in 5–10 % of cases (Gyurkovitz et al. 2015) but is more frequent in the involvement of the right adrenal gland; this is due to its anatomical position between the liver and the spine that cause its susceptibility to the compression. Even the direct drainage of the right adrenal vein into the inferior vena cava makes the right adrenal gland more susceptible to rapidly increasing venous pressure compared to the left adrenal gland where the adrenal veins are directly connected to the renal vein (Kuhn et al. 1971).

Clinical assessment could show an abdominal mass in the upper left or right abdominal side. Symptoms depend on the severity of the hemorrhage and include jaundice, anemia, and if the capsule breaks up to the shock associated with severe blood loss especially when the blood pass from the retroperitoneal space to the peritoneal space (Singh et al. 2016; Alabsi and Layland 2015; Fadil et al. 2014; Mutlu et al. 2011; Demirel et al. 2011; Abdu et al. 2009).

In some cases the hematoma drains along the retroperitoneal space and emerges in the groin, manifesting itself as scrotal hematoma (Fig. 12.4) (Adorisio et al. 2007; Avolio et al. 2002; Miele et al. 1997, 2000). Instead if the hemorrhage is contained in retroperitoneal space, the inferior vena cava and/or the kidney may be obstructed from the mass. Clinically whereas a minor bleeding into the adrenal cortex may remain asymptomatic, a severe blood loss can be life-threatening, with hypovolemic shock (Gyurkovitz et al. 2015).

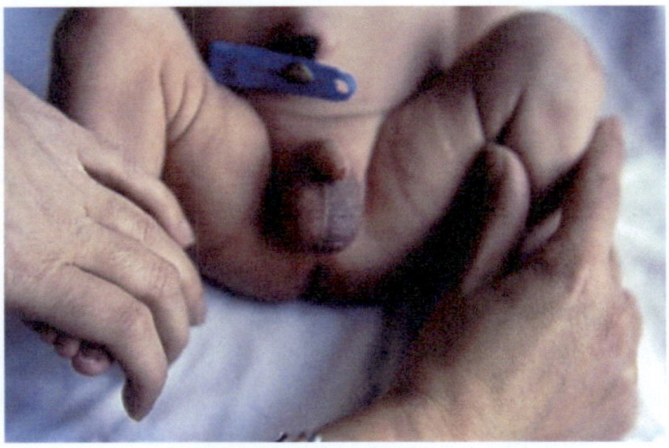

Fig. 12.4 Clinical presentation of scrotal hematoma due to adrenal hemorrhage

In the rare case of both glands are involved, there will be an acute adrenal failure. Residual functioning adrenal tissue in the subcapsular region is left in most cases, when more than 90 % of each gland is destroyed and the adrenal insufficiency is clinically manifested.

12.4.2 US Findings

Normal adrenal gland is easily visualized in the newborn by ultrasound and consists of a hypoechoic cortex and a thin echogenic medulla. The gland is located above the upper pole of the kidney and has a triangular shape.

Adrenal hemorrhage shows a typical sonographic aspect: the gland will be enlarged depending on the amount of bleeding, and its echogenicity will change depending on the timing at which it is observed (Fig. 12.5) (Velaphi and Perlman 2001). We must emphasize, however, that the appearance of the hematoma is very variable depending on the hemorrhagic component; therefore, we can have aspects cystic-like or solid-like (Miele et al. 1994). In some cases the differentiation between a suprarenal hemorrhagic mass and a solid mass can be difficult (Calisti et al. 2012). In every case, it is necessary to differentiate an adrenal mass from a renal mass; in case of any

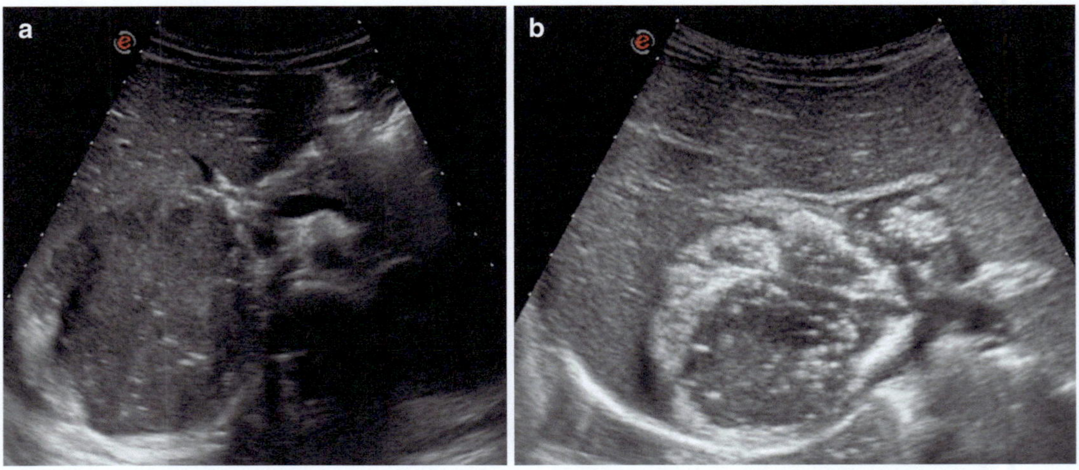

Fig. 12.5 Adrenal hemorrhage. The hemorrhagic mass shows a complex aspect, fluid-corpusculated homogeneous at onset examination (**a**), very inhomogeneous in the control exam after 14 days (**b**)

suprarenal mass, the kidney is displaced inferiorly, laterally, and anteriorly. Any right adrenal mass displaced anteriorly and medially the inferior vena cava.

At ultrasound exam, the mass will keep the original triangular shape of normal gland, remains included in the adrenal capsule, and depending on the size of the hematoma, it may be observed a concave pressure defect on the superior renal pole.

As we previously discussed, because of its hemorrhagic component, the pattern of echogenicity of the mass changes over time:

- Early stage: fresh clot following active bleeding appears as echogenic homogeneous or inhomogeneous solid mass with dense echoes (Figs. 12.6a and 12.7a) (Miele et al. 1994; Rahman et al. 1997).
- Later stage: the liquefaction occurs, and the ultrasound exam shows progressive loss of echogenicity; the mass decrease in size and becomes hypoechoic and can become completely anechoic "cyst-like" (Figs. 12.6b and 12.7b). Over time as the size decreases, the inner hypoechoic component is reabsorbed and the edges of the mass become more echogenic; sometimes there could remain few dystrophic calcifications (Westra et al. 1994; Miele et al. 1994; Rahman et al. 1997).
- Power or color Doppler examination shows the absence of flow within the mass, and it is possible to see few vessels within the capsule "rim-like Doppler pattern."

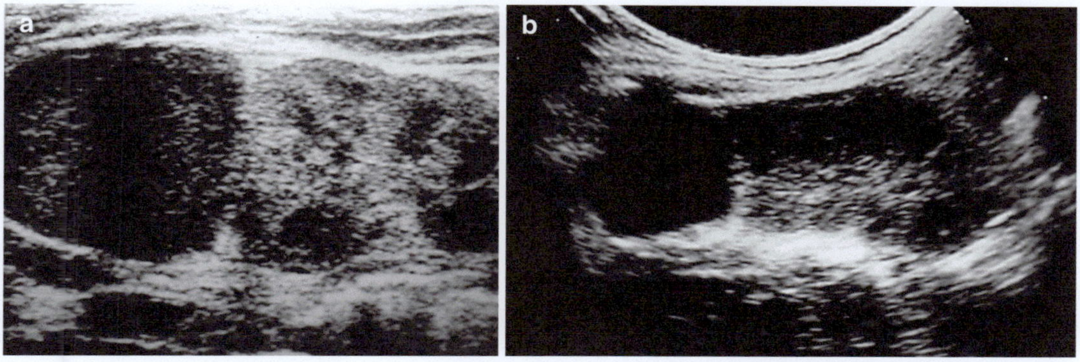

Fig. 12.6 (**a**) US, early stage: in this large adrenal gland hematoma, fresh clot appears as echogenic homogeneous solid mass with dense echoes. (**b**) US, later stage: the liquefaction occurs, and the ultrasound exam shows decreasing in size and progressive loss of echogenicity "cyst-like"

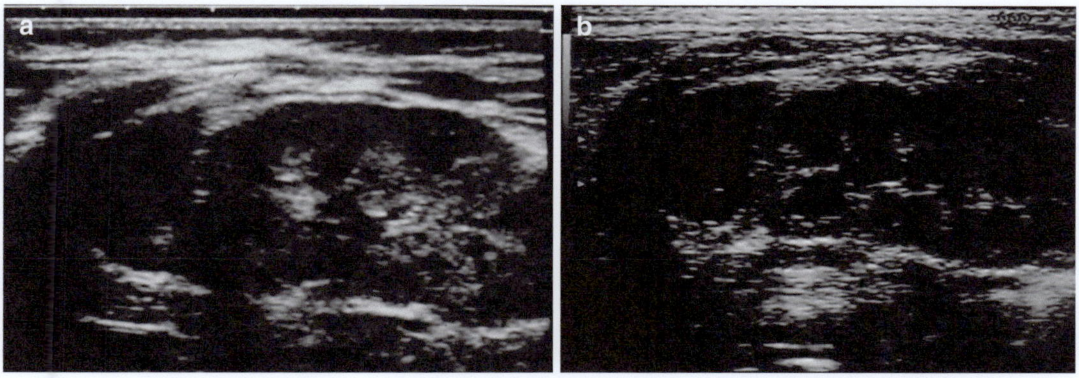

Fig. 12.7 In this case also, a smaller hematoma presents similar aspects. (**a**) In early stage, echogenic homogeneous "solid" mass with dense echoes. (**b**) In later stage, progressive loss of echogenicity, with "cyst-like" aspect

The progressive decrease in size of the lesion and the changing of the sonographic appearance allow the diagnosis of adrenal hemorrhage. In newborn, the use of high-frequency linear probe allows to determinate accurately the size, shape, and echographic structure of the hemorrhagic mass (Fig. 12.8). A follow-up examination may reveal a suprarenal calcification as early as 1–2 weeks.

In case of breakage of the adrenal capsule, blood flows mostly in the retroperitoneal space and dissects retroperitoneal fat tissue to reach the inguinal canal and to emerge at the scrotal sac, causing the hemorrhage of the superficial structures, resulting in a ipsilateral scrotal hematoma, which can mimic testicular torsion (see Fig. 12.3) (Schrauder et al. 2008; Adorisio et al. 2007; Avolio et al. 2002; Miele et al. 1997). In very rare cases, the occurrence of a scrotal hematoma contralateral to the adrenal lesion has also been reported (Miele et al. 2000).

Infrequently the blood can even achieve to peritoneal space, and if the peritoneal-vaginal duct is open, it can arrive into scrotal sac causing hematocele (Fig. 12.9) (Miele et al. 1997, 2000).

In case of association with renal vein thrombosis, the typical aspects of the disease can be found: enlargement of the kidney, enlarged renal vein with the presence of intraluminal echogenic material, and loss of the flow signal in the renal vein at color Doppler study (Fig. 12.10).

Usually within 3 months of life, the mass has completely regressed, and by the 10–12 weeks of life, it can be found glandular calcifications as the result of previous hemorrhage.

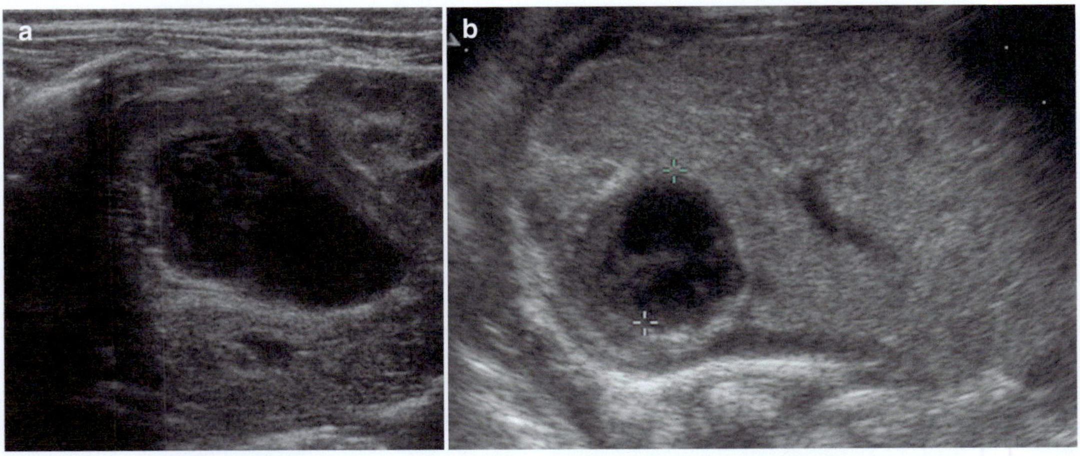

Fig. 12.8 (**a**) Ultrasound scan with linear probe and with (**b**) convex probe on an infant with an adrenal hemorrhage shows the best definition of the linear probe compared to the wider panoramic of the convex probe

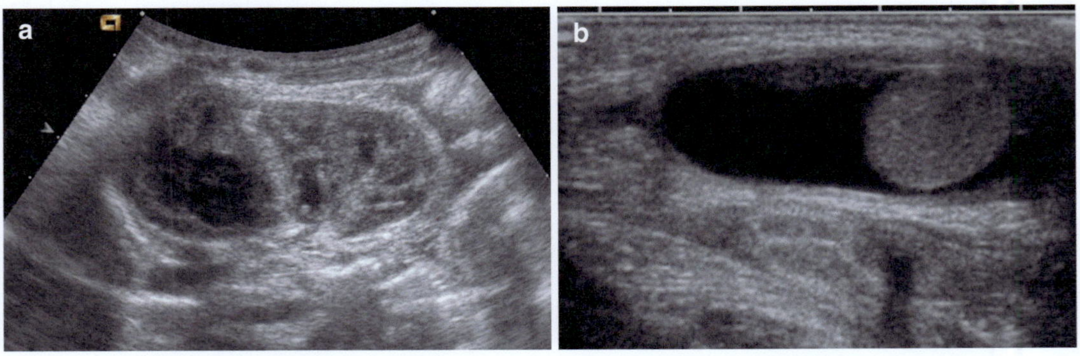

Fig. 12.9 (**a**) Adrenal hemorrhage. The hemorrhagic mass displaces inferiorly the kidney. (**b**) Ipsilateral scrotal hematoma, with hematocele

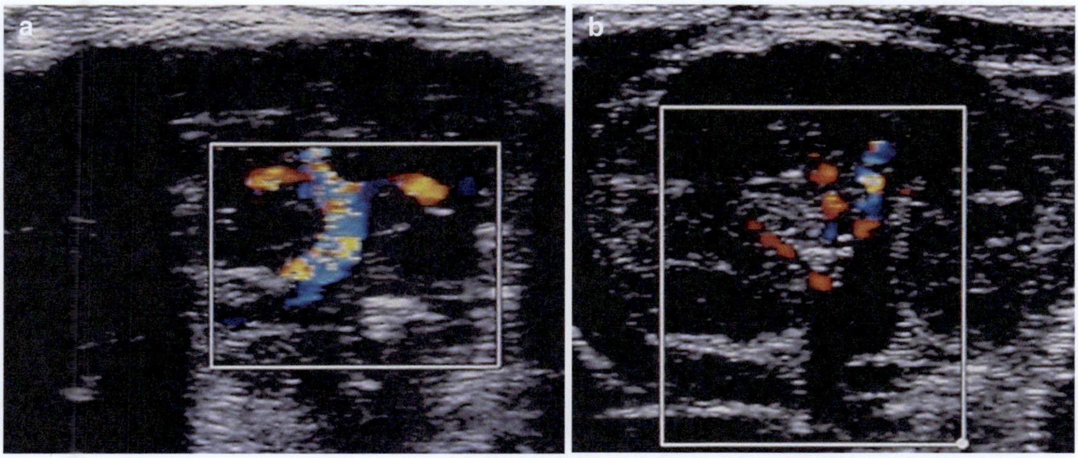

Fig. 12.10 Color Doppler ultrasound. (**a**) Normal right renal vein. (**b**) Left renal vein thrombosis: the absence of color signal and the presence of echoes in the vessel

The use of contrast-enhanced ultrasound (CEUS), in pediatric patients and especially in the newborn, is not routinely performed, but this technique could be useful in the differential diagnosis with vascularized adrenal mass. Actually CEUS is used in nontraumatic emergencies, most often in adult patients (Catalano et al. 2004; Farina et al. 2015); its use, even in pediatric patients, is much established in the study of focal lesions and traumatic emergencies (Pinto et al. 2014, 2015; Sessa et al. 2015; Menichini et al. 2015 Miele et al. 2015, 2016a, b, c).

12.4.3 CT Findings

Even in the CT examination, we have the same morphological aspects as reported in the ultrasound findings. In the CT exam, it is easy to see the fat tissue surrounding adrenal gland and to determine clearly if the mass is renal or adrenal in origin. During the CT scan, it is also easier to evaluate possible complications such as retroperitoneal hemorrhage and thrombosis of renal vein.

According to the stage of the hemolysis, the attenuation value of an adrenal hematoma depends on its age.

In the early stage, in non-contrast-enhanced CT acute and subacute, hematoma contains areas of high attenuation, ranging from 50 to 90 HU. After the administration of contrast medium, the hematoma doesn't enhance because no vessels are in the mass and will be only a thin capsular enhance (Kawashima et al. 1999) (Fig. 12.11). The use of CT can be very useful in case of adrenal hemorrhage with complex mass aspect, in which differential diagnosis with neuroblastoma can be difficult (Fig. 12.12).

Adrenal hematoma decreases in size and attenuation over time. In the later stage, if it is not completely resolved, organized chronic hematoma can appear as a calcified cystic mass.

12.4.4 MRI Findings

The same concepts previously discussed for CT are valid for MRI exam. Even in the MRI exam, the hematoma has different stages depending on the time:

Early stage <7 days: the hematoma typically appears isointense or slightly hypointense on T1-weighted images and highly hypointense on T2-weighted images.

Subacute stage, from 7 days to 7 weeks: the hematoma appears hyperintense on T1- and T2-weighted images (Kawashima et al. 1999).

Later chronic stage >7 weeks: a hypointense rim is present on T1- and T2-weighted images, which is due to the presence of a fibrous capsule and to hemosiderin deposition (Jordan et al. 2012).

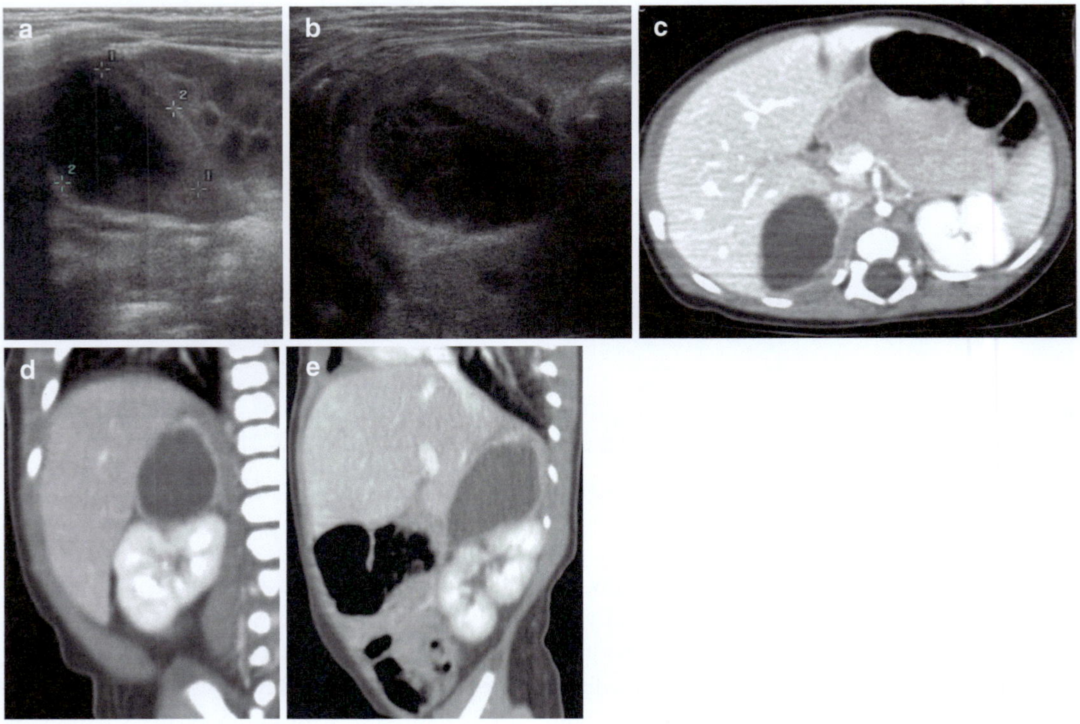

Fig. 12.11 (**a**) Ultrasound performed with linear high-frequency probe shows an inhomogeneous and enlarged right adrenal gland within internal echoes and fluid. (**b**) Two weeks later US still shows a fluid-corpusculated mass with thickened walls. (**c**) Axial contrast-enhanced CT scan shows a homogenous nonenhanced adrenal mass. (**d**) Coronal and (**e**) sagittal reconstruction clearly show the anatomical relationships between the adrenal hemorrhagic mass and the right kidney

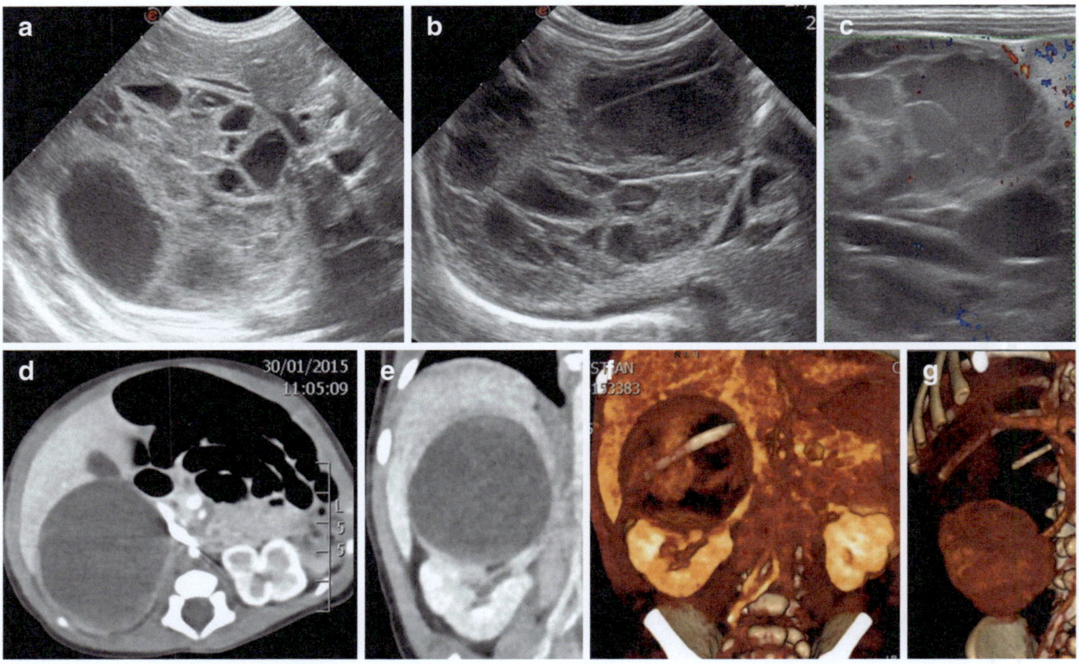

Fig. 12.12 Male, 3 days of life. (**a–c**) US shows a rounded left flank lobulated mass. (**d–g**) Contrast-enhanced CT exam, in axial view (**d**), and the 2d (**e**) and 3d (**f–g**) reconstructions allow to exclude the diagnostic hypothesis of neuroblastoma and to confirm the diagnosis of adrenal hemorrhage

In the MRI exam, using balanced fast-field echo (FFE) sequences, the evaluation of the renal vein and of the inferior cava vein is more easy than in CT or ultrasound exam; this is important for the visualization of an eventual thrombosis that can be the cause of the hemorrhage.

12.4.5 X-Ray Findings

A suprarenal mass is rarely viewable on plain film. Radiographic evidence on the first day of life, of a thin curvilinear shape calcification, displaying typically suprarenal, is suggestive for an adrenal gland calcification and confirms the theory that a substantial number of cases of adrenal hemorrhage occur during fetal life, well before delivery.

A small pleural effusion or lung atelectasis can be visualized ipsilateral to the adrenal hemorrhage.

Even in adult patient, the presence of a calcification in the adrenal site has to also think about a hemorrhagic event.

Many years ago, the way to study adrenal hematoma was the excretory urography in which the hematoma appears as a relatively lucent suprarenal mass and the angiography that rarely shows the contour of the hematoma; nowadays actually these techniques have been abandoned.

12.5 Differential Diagnoses and Complications

The differential diagnosis that we have to consider in case of suprarenal masses should include above all neuroblastoma because it is the predominant neonatal malignancy, teratoma, subdiaphragmatic extralobar pulmonary sequestration, vascular thrombosis, congenital adrenal cystic lesions, and other causes of abdominal emergencies in newborns (Gyurkovitz et al. 2015; Di Giacomo et al. 2015).

Neuroblastoma is the most common solid extracranial tumor in infants with an incidence of approximately 6 out of 1,000 liveborns (Schrauder et al. 2008) and is the most important diagnosis to exclude because the adrenal gland is the primary site (Calisti et al. 2012; Eo et al. 2011). It is related with the increase of catecholamines and there is no association with jaundice. Frequently these infants have hepatic or subcutaneous metastases at the time of the diagnosis. Clinical evaluation shows in the flank a hard nodular mass. At the sonographic exam, it can be solid, cystic, or mixed pattern (Miele et al. 1994) (Fig. 12.13).

A significant data is that the neuroblastoma distorts adrenal shape, does not reduce its size, and does not change progressively its echogenicity over time.

The power/color Doppler evaluation often shows a network of microscopic vessels with characteristic high-velocity Doppler shifts inside the tumor and stippled calcifications (Eo et al. 2011).

However sometimes, the differential diagnosis can be difficult especially because the neuroblastoma can be complicated by hemorrhage or can have a cystic aspect (Yao et al. 2013; Deeg et al. 1998; Yamamoto et al. 1998; Meersman et al. 2008).

If there are doubts about the nature of the mass, it may be useful to complete the evaluation with an MRI or CT exam (Fig. 12.14).

Even if in recent years it has been suggested that many of the neonatal cases of neuroblastoma can regress spontaneously, in case of suspect masses that progress or remain unchanged during the first few months, the surgical exploration is requested (Deeg et al. 1998; Yamamoto et al. 1998).

A precise description of radiological findings is carried out in Chap. 21.

Congenital adrenal hyperplasia is as an autosomal recessive disease (*1/5.000–1/15.000* liveborn), characterized by disorders in the biosynthesis of steroid hormones due to a mutation of one of the five enzymes, produced by adrenal cortex, involved in the synthesis process. Most frequently, in around 90 % of cases, the disease is due to the deficiency of the 21-hydroxylase. Consequently the result will be a reduction of glucocorticoid and mineral corticoid hormones and an increase of androgens.

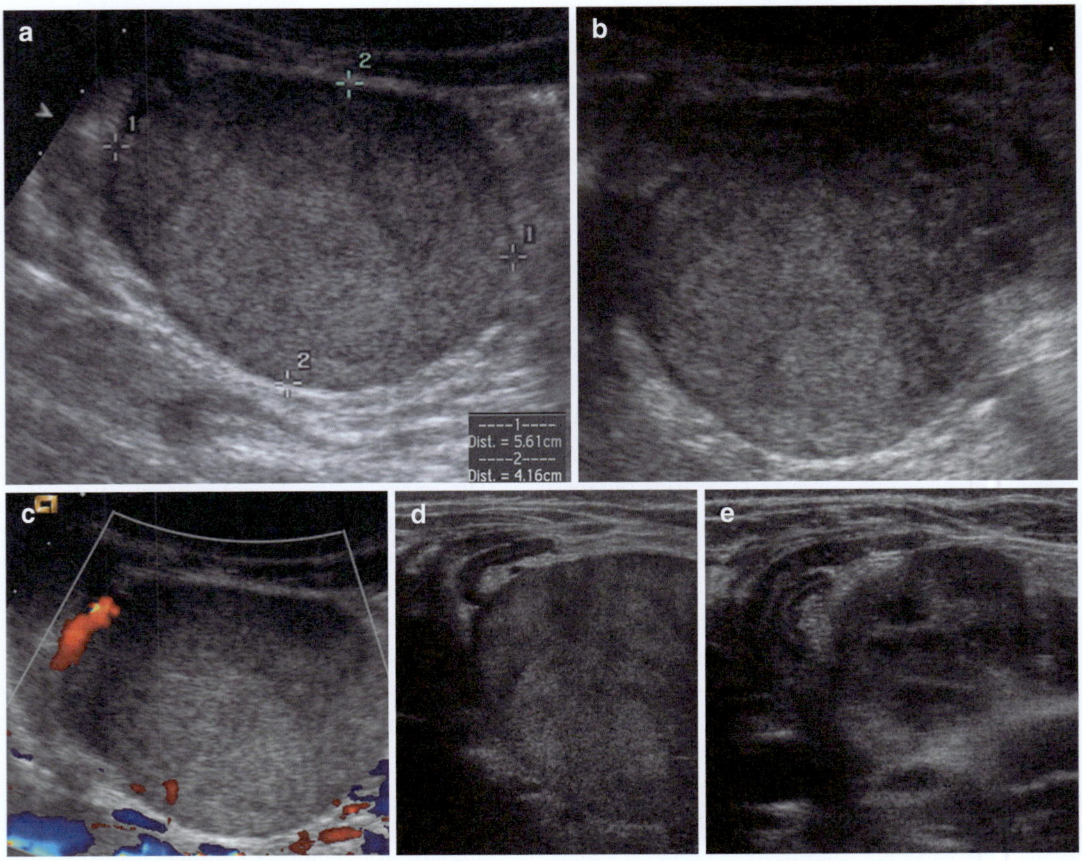

Fig. 12.13 Female, 7 days old, mass in left flank. Neuroblastoma. (**a–e**) US shows a huge mass arising from the limb of left adrenal gland, with solid pattern. Color Doppler study (**c**) shows a little vascular signal within the mass. (**e**) Note the normal aspect of the right adrenal gland

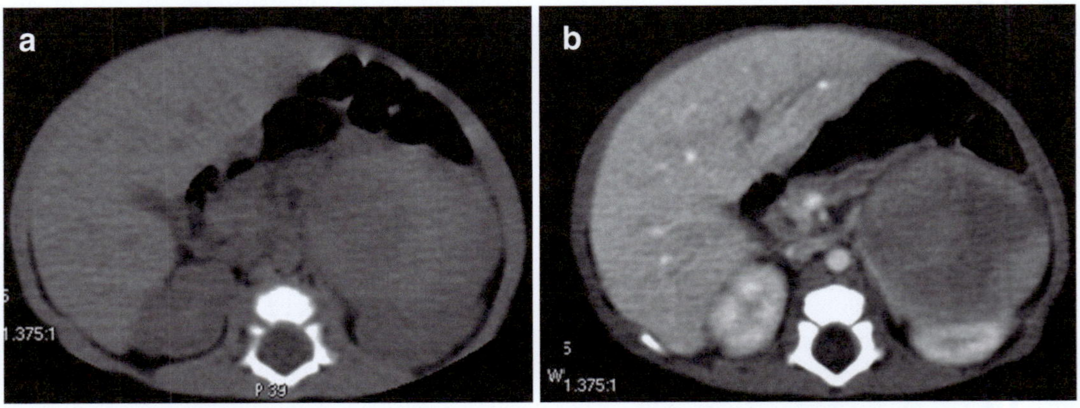

Fig. 12.14 The same patient of Fig. 12.13. Left adrenal gland neuroblastoma. (**a**) Unenhanced and (**b**) contrast-enhanced CT scans show a left inhomogeneous adrenal mass displacing the kidney. The mass is slightly hyperdense in unenhanced CT and has an irregular poor enhancement after contrast medium administration. (**c**) Coronal and (**d**) sagittal reconstructions clearly depict the relationship between the adrenal mass and the left kidney

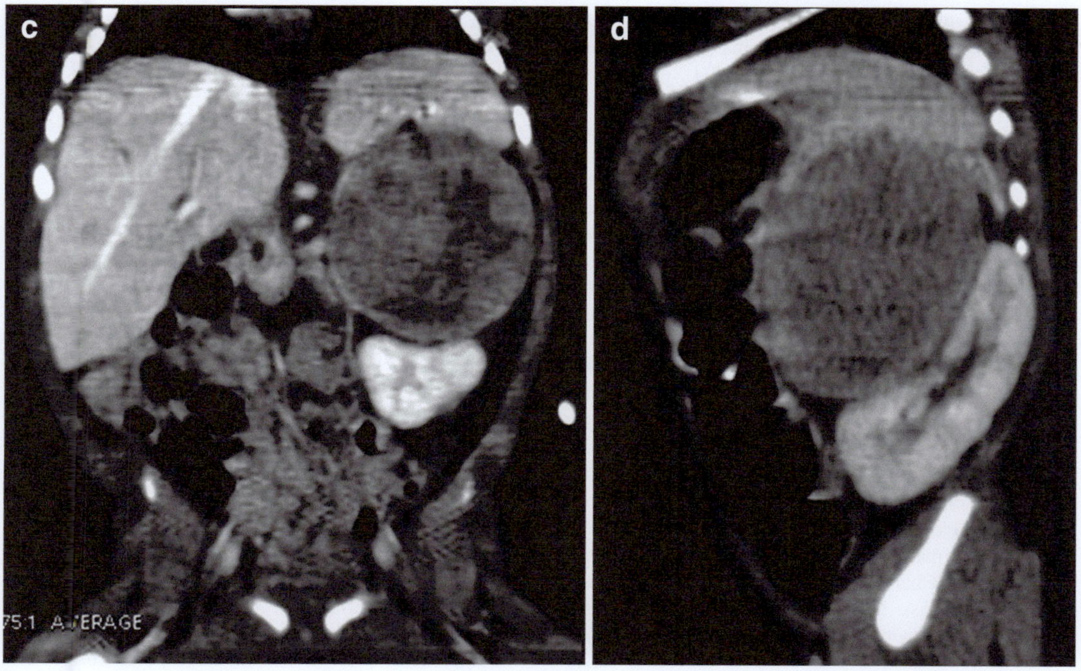

Fig. 12.14 (continued)

The diagnosis is clinical; at the ultrasound exam the hyperplasia involved both the adrenal glands.

The complications are rare: adrenal dysfunction with Addison syndrome especially if both glands are involved, the infection of the hematoma with an abscess mass.

If after 4 weeks from the presentation of the adrenal mass, there is no reduction in size or changes in echogenicity, a malignant mass must be suspected and valuable supplemental information must be obtained by computed tomography and magnetic resonance.

References

Abdu AT, Kriss VM, Bada HS, Reynolds EW (2009) Adrenal hemorrhage in a newborn. Am J Perinatol 26:553–557

Adorisio O, Mattei R, Ciardini E, Centonze N, Noccioli B (2007) Neonatal adrenal hemorrhage mimicking an acute scrotum. J Perinatol 27:130–132

Alabsi SY, Layland T (2015) Adrenal hemorrhage in neonates: unusual presentation. Neonatal Netw 34:220–226

Avolio L, Fusillo M, Ferrari G, Chiara A, Bragheri R (2002) Neonatal adrenal hemorrhage manifesting as acute scrotum: timely diagnosis prevents unnecessary surgery. Urology 59:601

Calisti A, Oriolo L, Molle P, Miele V, Spagnol L (2012) Neonatal adrenal masses: do we have reliable criteria for differential diagnosis and expectant management? Minerva Pediatr 64:313–318

Catalano O, Lobianco R, Sandomenico S, Mattace Raso M, Siani A (2004) Real time, contrast-enhanced sonographic imaging in emergency radiology. Radiol Med 108:454–469

Deeg KH, Bettendorf U, Hofmann V (1998) Differential diagnosis of neonatal adrenal hemorrhage and congenital neuroblastoma by colour coded Doppler sonography and power Doppler sonography. Eur J Pediatr 157:294–297

Demirel N, Baş AY, Zenciroğlu A, Taşci-Yildiz Y (2011) Adrenal bleeding in neonates: report of 37 cases. Turk J Pediatr 53:43–47

Di Giacomo V, Trinci M, Van der Byl G, Catania VD, Calisti A, Miele V (2015) Ultrasound in newborns and children suffering from nontraumatic acute abdominal pain: imaging with clinical and surgical correlation. J Ultrasound 18:385–393. doi:10.1007/s40477-014-0087-4, Epub 2014 Apr 9

Eo H, Kim JH, Jang KM, Yoo SY, Lim JH, Kim MJ, Kim OH (2011) Comparison of clinico-radiological features of congenital cystic neuroblastoma and neonatal adrenal hemorrhagic pseudocyst. Korean J Radiol 12:52–58

Fadil FZ, Lehlimi M, Chemsi M, Habzi A, Benomar S (2014) Neonatal adrenal hematoma: various modes of presentation. Arch Pediatr 21:990–994
Farina R, Catalano O, Stavolo C, Sandomenico F, Petrillo A, Romano L (2015) Emergency radiology. Radiol Med 120:73–84
Gyurkovitz Z, Maroti A, Renes L, Nemeth G, Pal A, Orvos H (2015) Adrenal haemorrhage in term neonates: a retrospective study from the period 2001–2013. J Matern Fetal Neonatal Med 28:2062–2065
Jordan E, Poder L, Courtier J, Sai V, Jung A, Coakley FV (2012) Imaging of nontraumatic adrenal hemorrhage. AJR Am J Roentgenol 199:W91–W98
Kawashima H, Sandler CM, Ernst RD, Takahashi N, Robidoux NA, Goldman SM, Fishman EK, Dunnick NR (1999) Imaging of non traumatic hemorrhage of the adrenal gland. Radiographics 19:949–863
Kuhn J, Jewett T, Munshauer R (1971) The clinical and radiographic features of massive neonatal adrenal hemorrhage. Radiology 99:647–652
Lau KK, Stoffman JM, Williams S, McCusker P, Brandao L, Patel S, Chan AK, Canadian Pediatric Thrombosis and Hemostasis Network (2007) Neonatal renal vein thrombosis: review of the English-language literature between 1992 and 2006. Pediatrics 120:e1278–e1284
Meersman A, Wojciechowski M, Vaneerdeweg W, Jorens P, Michiels E, Ramet J (2008) Acute retroperitoneal hemorrhage and shock as presenting signs of neuroblastoma in an infant. Pediatr Emerg Care 24:37–38
Menichini G, Sessa B, Trinci M, Galluzzo M, Miele V (2015) Accuracy of contrast-enhanced ultrasound in the identification and characterization of traumatic solid organ lesions in children: a retrospective comparison with baseline-US and CE-MDCT. Radiol Med 120:989–1001
Miele V, Di Giampietro I (2014) Diagnostic imaging in emergency. Salute e Società (2EN):127–138. doi:10.3280/SES2014-002010EN
Miele V, Patti G, Cappelli L, Calisti A, Valenti M (1994) Ultrasonography in the diagnosis of neonatal adrenal hemorrhage. Radiol Med 87:111–117
Miele V, Galluzzo M, Patti G, Mazzoni G, Calisti A, Valenti M (1997) Scrotal hematoma due to neonatal adrenal hemorrhage: the value of ultrasonography in avoiding unnecessary surgery. Pediatr Radiol 27:672–674
Miele V, Galluzzo M, Pedicelli C, Adami L, Calisti A (2000) Neonatal adrenal hemorrhage associated with a scrotal hematoma. Radiol Med 99:299–301
Miele V, Di Giampietro I, Ianniello S, Pinto F, Trinci M (2015) Diagnostic imaging in pediatric polytrauma management. Radiol Med 120:33–49
Miele V, Piccolo CL, Sessa B, Trinci M, Galluzzo M (2016a) Comparison between MRI and CEUS in the follow-up of patients with blunt abdominal trauma managed conservatively. Radiol Med 121:27–37
Miele V, Piccolo CL, Galluzzo M, Ianniello S, Sessa B, Trinci M (2016b) Contrast enhanced ultrasound (CEUS) in blunt abdominal trauma. Br J Radiol 89(1061):20150823. doi:10.1259/bjr.20150823, Epub 2016 Jan 8
Miele V, Piccolo CL, Trinci M, Galluzzo M, Ianniello S, Brunese L (2016c) Diagnostic imaging of blunt abdominal trauma in pediatric patients. Radiol Med 121:409–430. doi:10.1007/s11547-016-0637-2, Epub 2016 Apr 13
Mutlu M, Karagüzel G, Aslan Y, Cansu A, Okten A (2011) Adrenal hemorrhage in newborns: a retrospective study. World J Pediatr 7:355–357
Pinto F, Miele V, Scaglione M, Pinto A (2014) The use of contrast-enhanced ultrasound in blunt abdominal trauma: advantages and limitations. Acta Radiol 55:776–784
Pinto F, Valentino M, Romanini L, Basilico R, Miele V (2015) The role of CEUS in the assessment haemodinamically stable patients with blunt abdominal trauma. Radiol Med 120:3–11
Rahman S, Ohlsson A, Fong KW, Glanc P (1997) Fetal adrenal hemorrhage in a diamniotic, dichorionic twin: case report and review of controversies in diagnosis and management. J Ultrasound Med 16:297–300
Schrauder MG, Hammersen G, Siemer J, Goecke TW, Meurer B, Hart N, Beckmann MW, Schild RL (2008) Fetal adrenal haemorrhage – two-dimensional and three-dimensional imaging. Fetal Diagn Ther 23:72–75
Sessa B, Trinci M, Ianniello S, Menichini G, Galluzzo M, Miele V (2015) Blunt abdominal trauma: role of contrast-enhanced ultrasound in the detection and staging of abdominal traumatic lesions compared with US and CE-MDCT. Radiol Med 120:180–189
Singh J, Dalal P, Bhalla K, Rattan KN (2016) Neonatal adrenal hemorrhage presenting as prolonged hyperbilirubinemia. J Neonatal Surg 10:5–22
Velaphi SC, Perlman JM (2001) Neonatal adrenal hemorrhage: clinical and abdominal sonographic findings. Clin Pediatr (Phila) 40:545–548
Westra SJ, Zaninovic AC, Hall TR, Kangarloo H, Boechat MI (1994) Imaging of adrenal gland in children. Radiographics 14:1323–1340
Yamamoto K, Hanada R, Kikuchi A, Ichikawa M, Aihara T, Oguma E, Moritani T, Shimanuki Y, Tanimura M, Hayashi Y (1998) Spontaneous regression of localized neuroblastoma detected by mass screening. J Clin Oncol 16:1265–1269
Yao W, Li K, Xiao X, Zheng S, Chen L (2013) Neonatal suprarenal mass: differential diagnosis and treatment. J Cancer Res Clin Oncol 139:281–286

13 Hydrometrocolpos: Hematocolpos/Colpo-hematometra

Stefania Ianniello, Maria Gabriella Merola, Marinella Nanni, Cinzia Orazi, Paolo Schingo, and Margherita Trinci

13.1 Genesis

Congenital genital malformations occurring in the female population have an incidence of 5 per 1,000 live births, or 0.5 % (Brucker et al. 2011), and underlie congenital developmental defects of Müllerian derivates.

The anomalous embryological development of Wolffian and Müllerian ducts may prejudice their canalization (= gynatresias) or their fusing, sometimes combined with each other, or more rarely, may cause uterovaginal agenesis (<5 %) (Hořejší 2012).

These anomalies are typically associated with infertility, abortion, stillbirth, preterm delivery, and other organ abnormalities.

S. Ianniello (✉) • M. Nanni • M. Trinci
Department of Emergency Radiology, S. Camillo Hospital, Rome, Italy
e-mail: stefianni66@gmail.com

M.G. Merola
Department of Emergency Radiology, S. Camillo Hospital, Rome, Italy

Department of Advanced Biomedical Sciences - Diagnostic Imaging, University of Naples Federico II, Naples, Italy
e-mail: stefianni66@gmail.com

C. Orazi • P. Schingo
Department of Emergency Radiology, S. Camillo Hospital, Rome, Italy

Department of Diagnostic Imaging, Children's Hospital Bambino Gesù, Rome, Italy

Moreover, these malformations involving the internal genitalia (uterus and vagina) and/or the external genitalia are often in combination with each other, sometimes as component of a syndrome; Mayer-Rokitansky-Kuster, Kaufman-McKusick, Fraser, Winter, and congenital adrenal hyperplasia syndromes are the known examples of such associations (Blask et al. 1991).

According to Maneschi (Maneschi 1994), the female genital tract malformation obstruction can be classified in three categories:

- Uterine obstructions: Due to horns often equipped with rudimentary cavity with functional endometrium that, therefore periodically bleeds, but which do not communicate with the vagina or the normal hemi-uterus, causing hematometra; for example, unicornuate uterus by nonunion of Mullerian ducts with a rudimentary horn or didelphys uterus with two separate uterine cavities connected to the respective fallopian tube and ovary. Other types of uterine obstructions, although rather rare, are those that involve the cervix, such as atresia and aplasia of the uterine cervix, causing hematometra in approximately 20 % of the cases. More often, in fact, the cervix is associated with uterine abnormalities, such as bicornuate or septate uterus with cervical duplication.
- Vaginal obstructions: due to complete agenesis of the vagina from the non-fusion or channeling of Mullerian ducts, or to a partial

V. Miele, M. Trinci (eds.), *Imaging Non-traumatic Abdominal Emergencies in Pediatric Patients*,
DOI 10.1007/978-3-319-41866-7_13

aplasia when the vagina is less than 1 cm, or to vaginal transverse imperforate septa.
- Mixed obstructions: due to the combination of vaginal and uterine obstructive anomalies (Martínez-Escoriza et al. 2013; Ludwin et al. 2013).

These malformations may result in the obstruction of the normal menstrual blood flow, causing a condition known as "cryptomenorrhea."

In fact, a functional endometrium makes menstrual flow regularly, but at the same time, the blood collects in the vaginal cavity and then into the uterine cavity with the formation first of a hematocolpos and then a colpo-hematometra, with a tendency to flow back through the tube and into the peritoneal cavity, sometimes with the clinical presentation of the acute abdomen.

Another important cause of hematocolpos and colpo-hematometra, until hematosalpinx, are external genitalia malformations and, specifically, the imperforate or atretic hymen, with an incidence of 0.0014–0.1 % in full-term newborns (Messina et al. 2004; Winderl and Silverman 1995), occurring sporadically, rarely associated with other female genital tract malformations.

Hydrometrocolpos can present during two different stages in life, understandable with the knowledge of the functional features of endometrium:

1. Newborn-infanthood-childhood: although an unusual finding in newborn infants, the endogenous maternal estrogenic stimulation leads to the accumulation of cervical and endometrial gland secretions within the blind vagina and presenting as hydrocolpos; rarely it occurs in fetus where obstetric ultrasound suspects the diagnosis (Messina et al. 2004; Winderl and Silverman 1995) to be confirmed postnatally.
2. At puberty: it is the typical onset around the age of 9–13 years (Glavan et al. 2015) because it is usually asymptomatic until menstruation starts. After menarche, in fact, the cyclic menstrual blood collects in the distal closed vagina producing hematocolpos and colpo-hematometra.

13.2 Clinical Findings

In young girls, the typical clinical finding of these conditions is the primary normogonadotropic amenorrhea (Posner and Spandorfer 2005) in the presence of well-developed secondary sexual characteristics, with painful hypogastric crises and pelvic colic pain, typically repeated cyclically and progressively more intense as it happens in the acute abdomen (Le Hors-Albouze et al. 2011; Fischer and Kwan 2014; Di Giacomo et al. 2015). The age of the patient and the cyclical nature of painful crises, similar to menstrual cycles, point us toward the right diagnosis (Daboiko et al. 2011).

In newborn infants, instead, the clinical findings are often doubtful, sometimes hypogastric and pelvic colic pain, or abdominal distension, due to a palpable abdominal/pelvic mass and possibly lower-limb swelling (Nagaraj et al. 2016).

Moreover, hematocolpos or colpo-hematometra can cause a mechanical obstruction on the urethra and bladder, resulting in acute urinary retention and/or recurrent urinary tract infections, albeit rather infrequently (Nagaraj et al. 2016; Gyimadu et al. 2009; Salhan et al. 2013; Bursać et al. 2012).

The failure outflow and the resulting accumulation of menstrual blood in the vaginal cavity, and then in the uterine cavity, causes a progressive increase in volumetric endopelvic organs like the uterus; in fact, the abdominal palpation may appreciate a suprapubic, well-demarcated, roundish mass, with tense-elastic consistency.

In case of imperforate hymen, diagnosis is easier by clinical gynecological examination that shows bulging integrated membrane typically with blue appearance due to the blood collected behind it in the vaginal cavity. This typical feature is not detectable in a newborn child, where cervical and endometrial gland secretions collect within the blind vagina showing a whitish appearance.

13.3 Instrumental and Imaging Evaluation

Correct diagnosis of hydrometrocolpos, or hematocolpos, and hematometra is often very difficult based on clinical examination and imaging evaluation. Imaging techniques in the emergency setting include ultrasonography and, although rarely used, CT or MRI (Miele et al. 2006; Miele and Di Giampietro 2014).

13.3.1 US

Ultrasound evaluation is the first step in patients with primary amenorrhea and cyclical chronic pelvic pain because of the easy accessibility, the lack of ionizing radiation, and the good visualization of the pelvic organs.

Because the typical onset of these symptoms is around the age of 9–13 years, usually, the US examination is performed using a transabdominal approach with a conventional convex probe (3.5–5 MHz) or a pediatric sector probe (5–8 MHz) and requiring proper filled bladder.

Ultrasonography, in fact, is able to visualize the anatomy and/or the pathology of the internal genitalia and to discriminate between the many causes of pelvic pain (FischerKwan 2014; Valentin 2009; Doganay et al. 2010; Drakonaki et al. 2010).

In the presence of hematocolpos and hematometra, it is possible, by ultrasound examination, to appreciate a significant expansion of the uterus and vagina cavities because of a massive collection of menstrual blood, appearing as a large, inhomogeneous hyperechoic and fluid-corpusculated cystic mass in the lower abdomen and pelvis (Figs. 13.1, 13.2, 13.3. 13.4, 13.5, 13.6, and 13.7). Ultrasonography, furthermore, is able to distinguish

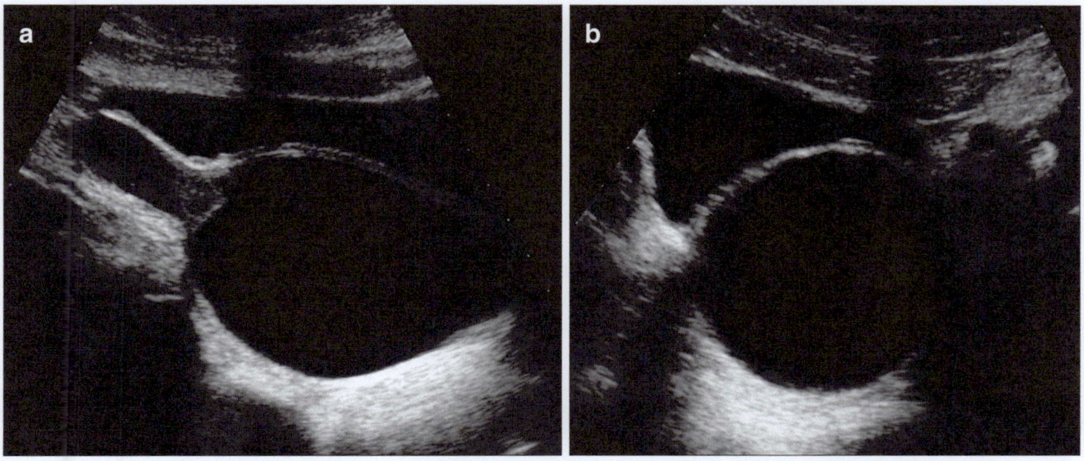

Fig. 13.1 (**a**, **b**) Imperforate hymen. The US imaging shows a significant expansion of the vagina cavity because of a massive collection of blood material, appearing as a large, fluid anechoic mass

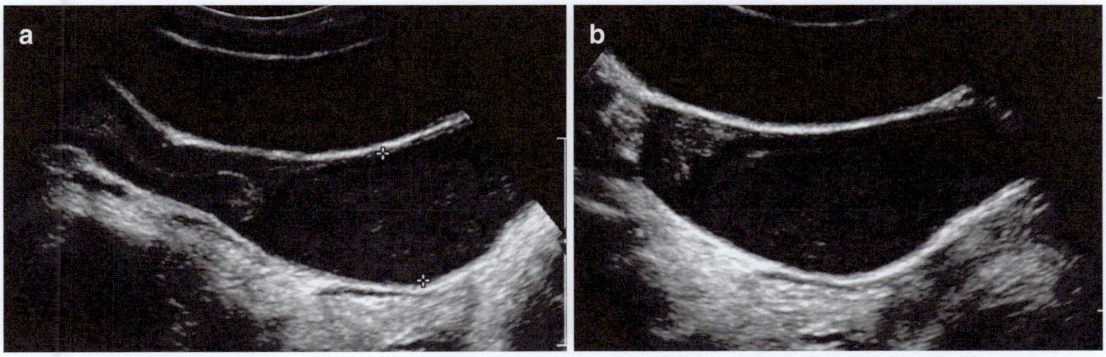

Fig. 13.2 (**a**, **b**) Imperforate hymen. In this case, the vaginal cavity is filled by a fluid-corpusculated cystic mass

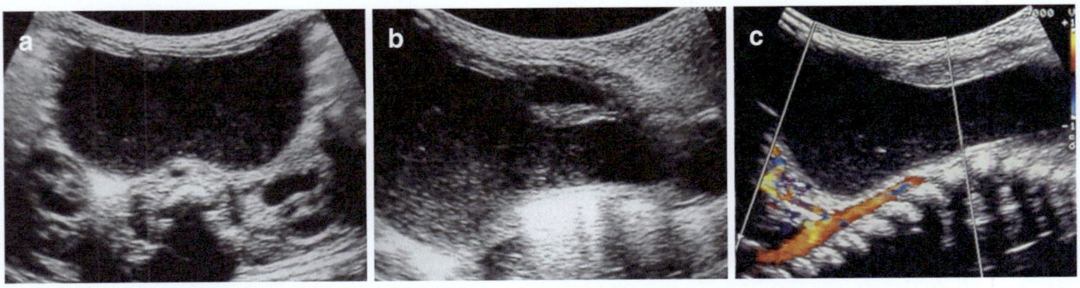

Fig. 13.3 (**a**–**c**) The US imaging shows the expansion of the uterine cavity by inhomogeneous hyperechoic and fluid-corpusculated material in a newborn child with imperforate hymen. Note the relationship of the mass with abdominal vessels and the superior mesenteric artery displacement

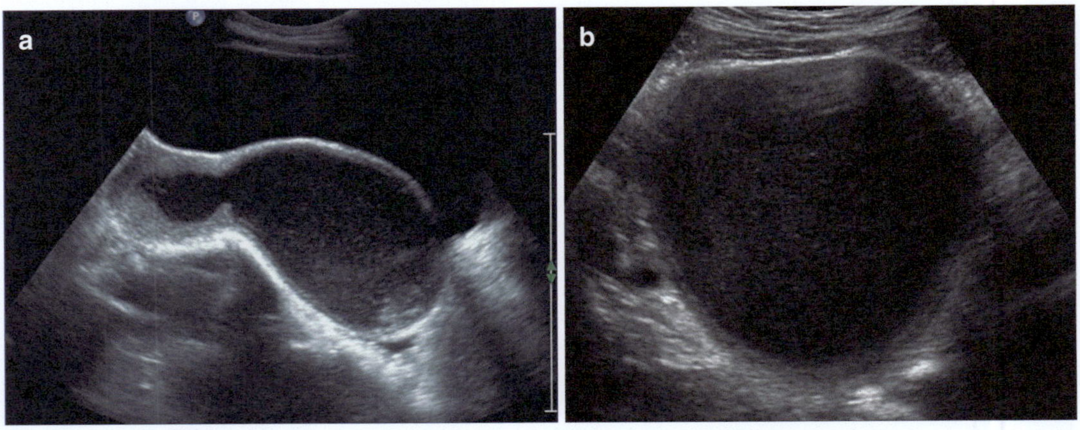

Fig. 13.4 (**a**, **b**) The US imaging shows the expansion of the uterine cavity by inhomogeneous hyperechoic and fluid-corpusculated material due to complete vaginal agenesis because of the complete absence of echoes in the distal genital tract

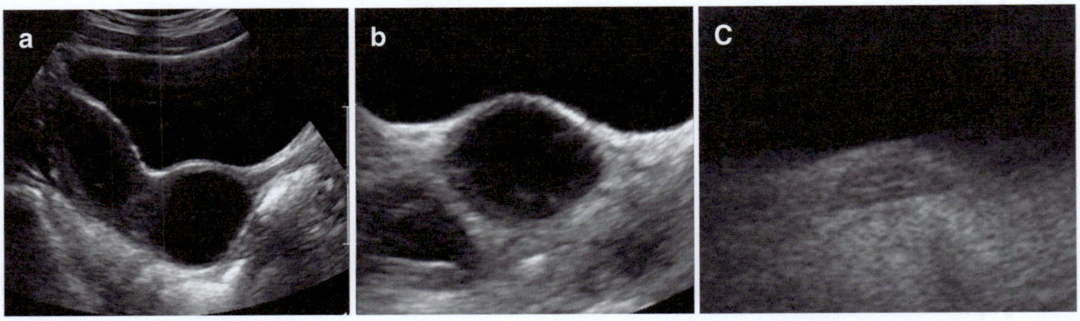

Fig. 13.5 (**a**–**c**) The US imaging shows the expansion of the uterus and of the proximal tract of vaginal cavity in a patient with partial vaginal aplasia as when the vagina is less than 1 cm or there are vaginal transverse imperforate septa because of the presence of echoes in the distal genital tract

the different pathologies of the internal genitalia, such as uterine or cervical obstruction, or a vaginal obstruction, or even a mixed obstruction, due to the combination of vaginal and uterine obstructive anomalies; for example, US imaging could detect a didelphys uterus with unilateral obstruction and subsequent expansion of the corresponding hemi-vagina, hemi-uterus, and fallopian tube (Fig. 13.8).

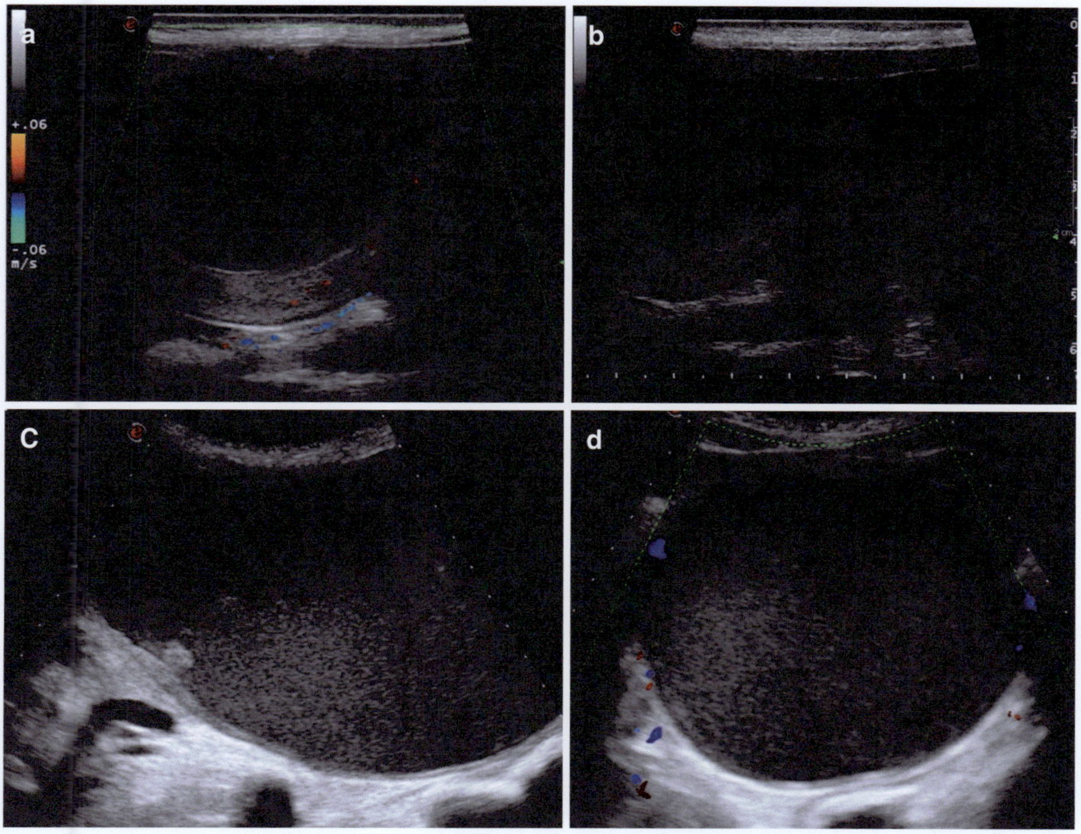

Fig. 13.6 (**a–d**) The US imaging shows the massive expansion of both the uterine and vaginal cavity in a patient with partial vaginal aplasia due to a transverse imperforate septum in the distal tract

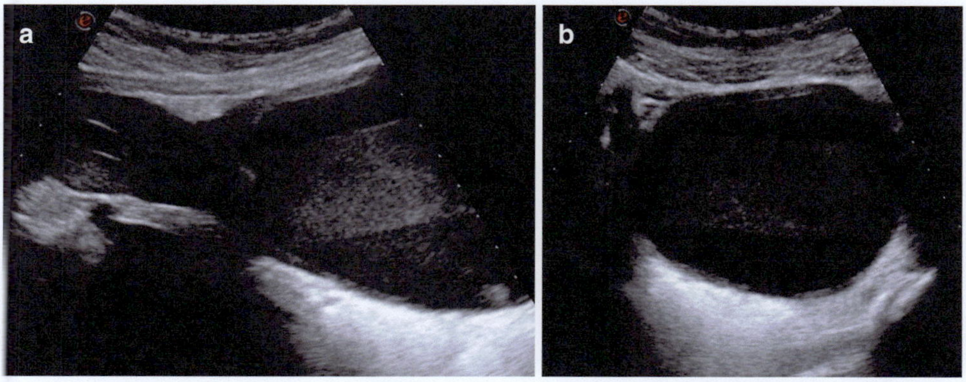

Fig. 13.7 (**a**, **b**) The US imaging shows the expansion of the vaginal cavity with fluid-fluid level of corpusculated contents in a patient with partial vaginal aplasia due to a vaginal transverse imperforate septum

Sometimes the uterus could overly expand in the abdomen, compressing or displacing other intra-abdominal organs, such as the bladder, or the urinary tract with dilation of renal pelvicaly-ceal systems (Fig. 13.9), or the bowel loops, or even big abdominal vessels.

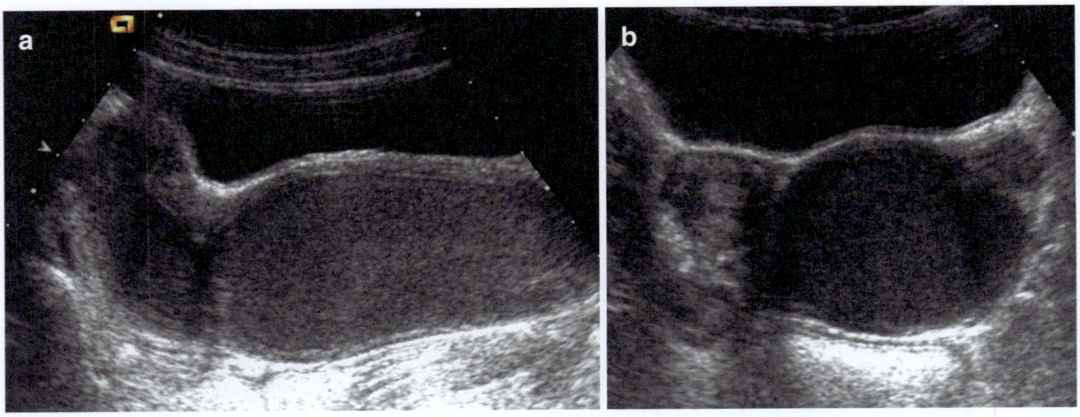

Fig. 13.8 (**a**, **b**) The US imaging shows a rare condition of didelphys uterus with left obstruction and subsequent expansion of the corresponding hemi-vagina, hemi-uterus, and left fallopian tube

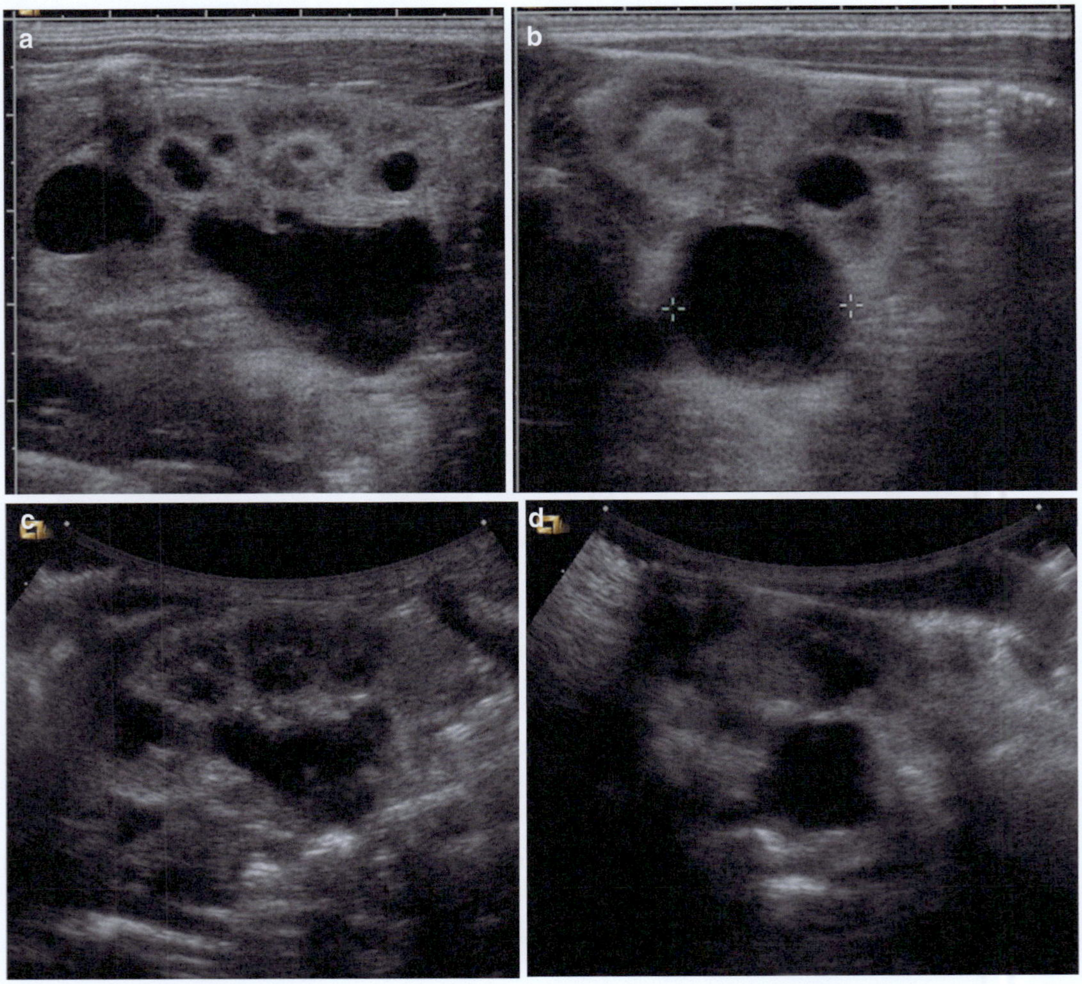

Fig. 13.9 The US imaging shows a significant ectasia of renal pelvicalyceal systems due to the compression by the pelvic cystic mass, respectively, in a newborn (**a**, **b**) and in an infant child (**c, d**)

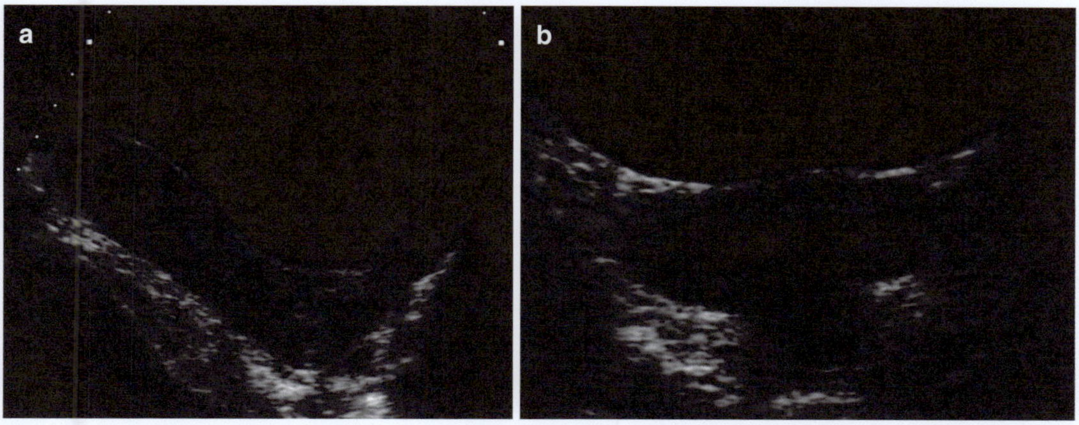

Fig. 13.10 (**a**, **b**) The US imaging shows the complete resolution of the hematocolpos after the incision of the hymenal membrane and the drainage of blood intravaginal collection, with a residual transient and mild thickening of the vaginal walls

Rarely, the uterus could not be identified by ultrasound, because the pelvis is fully occupied by the complex mass due to hematometra.

Sometimes blood can flow back and even expand the tube resulting in hematosalpinx or also flow back into the peritoneal cavity.

Moreover, US imaging is able to show the resolution of the hydrometrocolpos or hematocolpos/hematometra after incision of the hymenal membrane and the drainage of blood intravaginal collection, with a normal appearance of the uterus and vagina (Fig. 13.10) and no signs of hydroureter and/or hydronephrosis.

The use of the contrast-enhanced ultrasound (CEUS) is not yet described in this clinical setting; however, it could be useful to detect the blood supply of the pelvic mass and, maximizing the performance of ultrasonography, to make differential diagnosis with other abdominal or pelvic masses. Currently, the use of the contrast-enhanced ultrasound (CEUS) in childhood is limited to the identification and characterization of traumatic solid organ lesions (Pinto et al. 2014, 2015; Sessa et al. 2015; Menichini et al. 2015; Miele et al. 2015, 2016a, b, c), but its use, even in nontraumatic emergencies, is increasing considerably (Catalano et al. 2004; Farina et al. 2015).

13.3.2 CT

CT is not usually employed in young patients with cyclical chronic pelvic pain, especially in girls with suspicion of hydrometrocolpos or hematocolpos/hematometra, because of the radiation exposure and poor cost efficiency compared to US. Nevertheless, sometimes contrast-enhanced CT is useful to make the right diagnosis in patients with equivocal sonographic findings.

The most common CT finding in hydrometrocolpos and hematocolpos/hematometra is a hyperdense, nonenhancing, fluid-filled pelvic mass with typical compression of the bladder and other intra-abdominal organs, possibly associated with complications, such as hydroureter and/or hydronephrosis.

13.3.3 MRI

MRI is the best choice for a more detailed diagnosis, often performed to better delineate the anatomy and assist in surgical planning (Krafft et al. 2012) because of its excellent soft tissue contrast and a safer distinction among all possible causes of hematocolpos, such as vaginal septum or partial agenesis; nevertheless, we

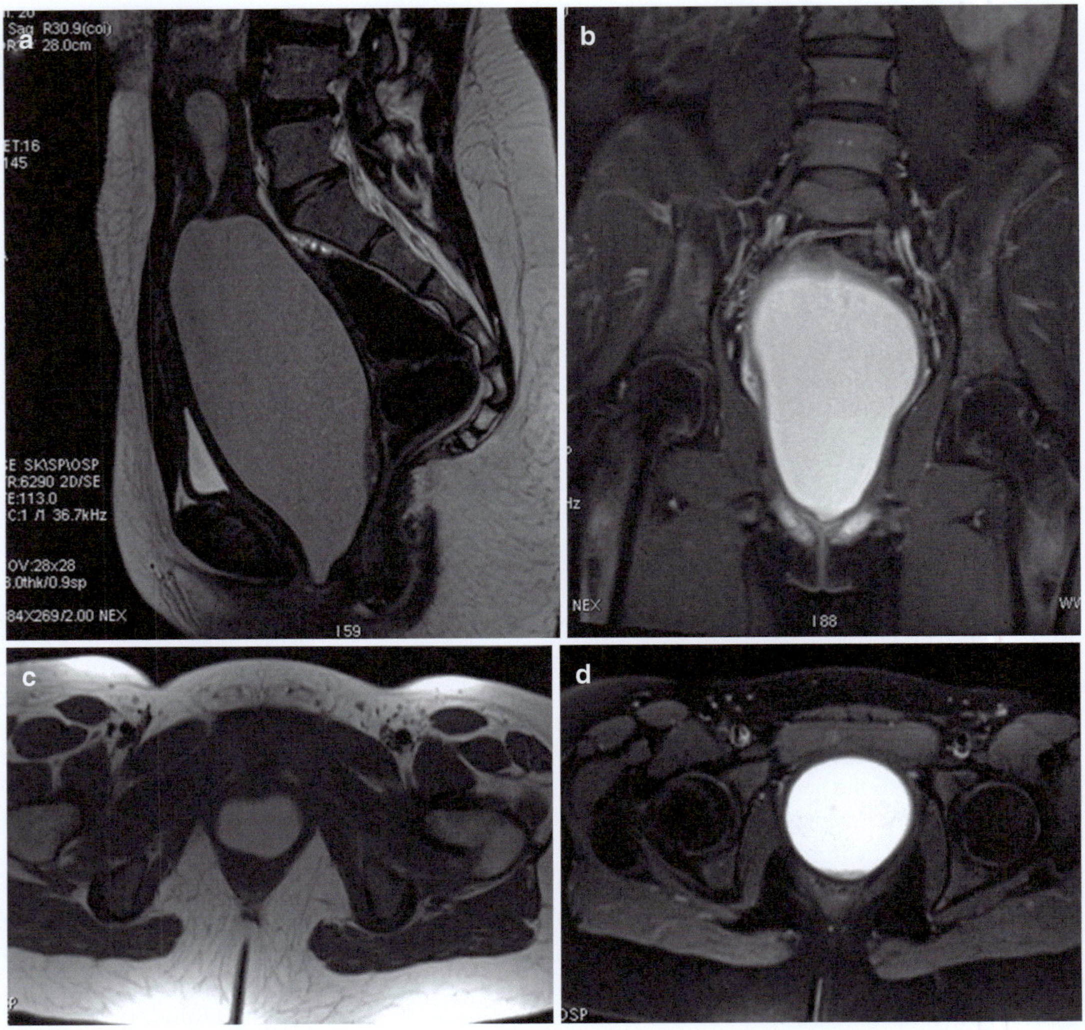

Fig. 13.11 (**a–d**) The MRI shows a large pelvic mass due to the significant expansion of the vagina cavity because of a massive collection of blood material mass appearing as hypointense in T1-weighted fat-suppressed sequences (**a**, **c**) and hyperintense in T2 sequences (**b**, **d**) in a young girl with imperforate hymen

must consider the difficulty to perform this exam in a young patient and the high costs (Fischer and Kwan 2014; Doganay et al. 2010). The hysterosalpingography and/or hysteroscopy are indicated in case of uterine obstruction; sometimes diagnostic laparoscopy is also used.

Magnetic resonance imaging (MRI) of the abdomen and pelvis needs a 1.5 Tesla MRI machine and requires a standard MRI protocol including T1-weighted fat-suppressed sequences and T2 sequences, to identify the hemorrhagic fluid-corpusculated contents within the vagina and endometrial cavity, appearing as a pelvic mass which had several fluid layers indicative of blood products (Fig. 13.11).

The accurate diagnosis of the female genital tract malformation obstruction and careful preoperative set-up (Fig. 13.12), including evaluation of associated anomalies, bowel preparation, available vaginal stents, and a multidisciplinary approach for the potential need for grafts, may be a key to success (Ugur et al. 2012).

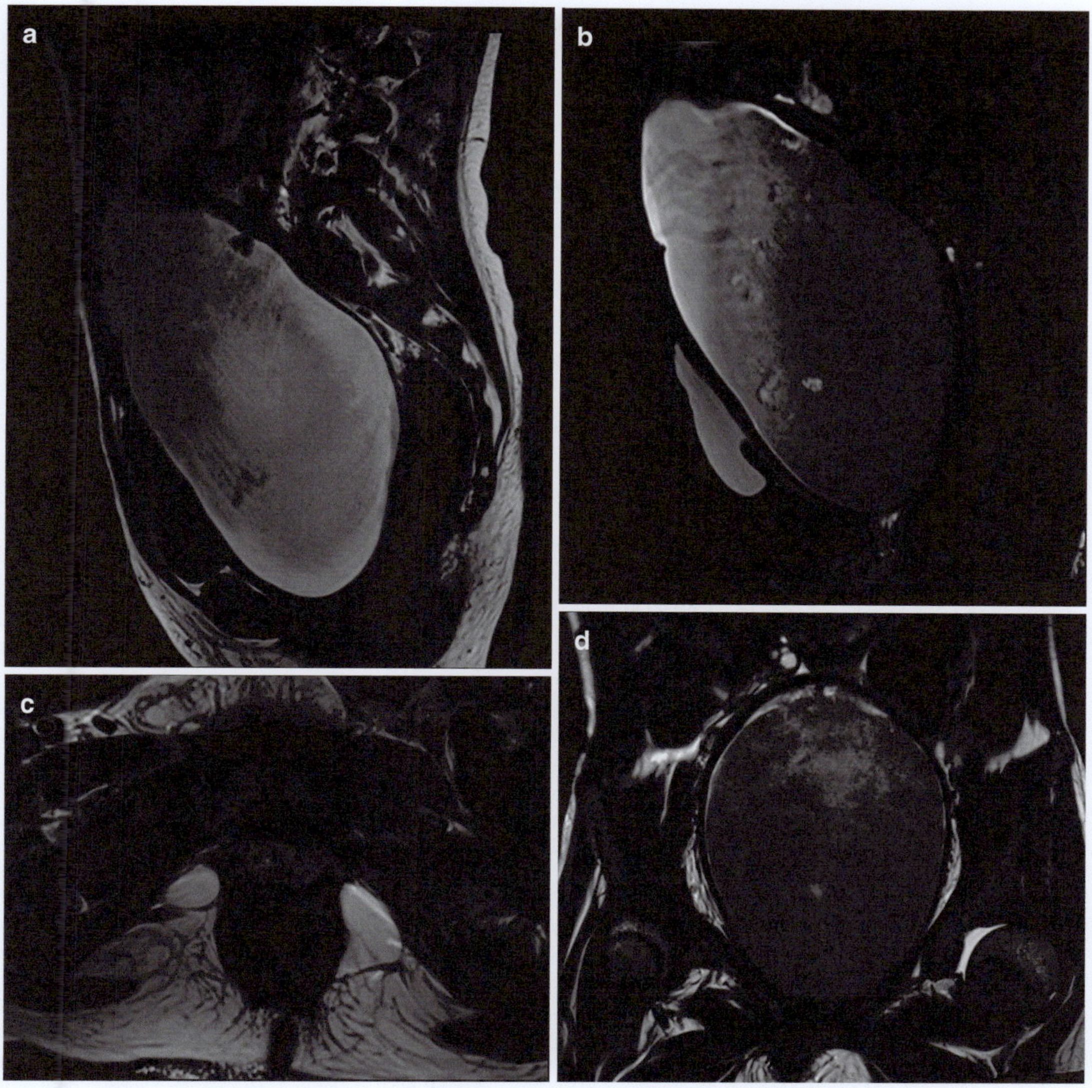

Fig. 13.12 (**a–d**) The MRI T1-weighted sequences and T2-weighted imaging show hematocolpos/hematometra as enlarged uterine and vaginal cavities in the same patient previously described in Fig. 13.7, with partial vaginal aplasia, due to a transverse imperforate septum in the distal tract

13.4 Differential Diagnosis

As already known, hydrometrocolpos can occur during two main stages in life: newborn-infanthood-childhood or during puberty; several diseases can mimic this condition, so it is suitable to exploit all instrumental diagnostic possibilities to make the right diagnosis and proper therapy.

The most common differential diagnosis of a perinatally identified abdominal mass should consider primarily ovarian cysts, especially those complicated, such as prenatal adnexal torsion, where the pelvic mass has a round shape and the involved adnexa shows a volumetric increase and a heterogeneous appearance due to internal echoes.

Other pathologies in differential diagnosis are neonatal cystic abdominal masses, such as mesenteric cyst, lymphangioma, bowel duplication cyst, intra-abdominal sacrococcygeal teratoma (type IV), neuroblastoma (Calisti et al. 2012), mesoblastic nephroma, genital/urinary anomalies

(Calisti et al. 2008), and anterior sacral meningocele.

After menarche, instead, differential diagnosis of an abdominal mass should exclude complicated ovarian cysts, such as adnexal torsion or hemorrhagic cysts, where, however, the imaging findings, US, CT, and MRI, are typically characterized by an ovarian enlargement with heterogeneous appearance and hemoperitoneum (Miele et al. 2002), or free pelvic fluid, especially if centered around the ovary, ever detected in the case of hydrometrocolpos.

Sometime, however, the definitive diagnosis is possible only after surgery.

References

Blask ANR, Sanders RC, Rock JA (1991) Obstructed uterovaginal anomalies: demonstration with sonography. Radiology 179:84–88

Brucker SY, Rall K, Campo R, Oppelt P, Isaacson K (2011) Treatment of congenital malformations. Semin Reprod Med 29:101–112

Bursać D, Duic Z, Partl JZ, Valetic J, Stasenko S (2012) Hematocolpos resulting from an imperforated hymen diagnosed by ultrasound in a patient with recurrent urinary tract infections. J Pediatr Adolesc Gynecol 25:340–341

Calisti A, Perrotta ML, Oriolo L, Ingianna D, Miele V (2008) The risk of associated urological abnormalities in children with pre- and postnatal occasional diagnosis of solitary, small or ectopic kidney: is a complete urological screening always necessary? World J Urol 26:281–284. doi:10.1007/s00345-008-0249-0, Epub 2008 Mar 29

Calisti A, Oriolo L, Molle P, Miele V, Spagnol L (2012) Neonatal adrenal masses: do we have reliable criteria for differential diagnosis and expectant management? Minerva Pediatr 64:313–318

Catalano O, Lobianco R, Sandomenico S, Mattace Raso M, Siani A (2004) Real time, contrast-enhanced sonographic imaging in emergency radiology. Radiol Med 108:454–469

Daboiko JC, Gbané-Koné M, Ouattara B (2011) Low-back pain in adolescents: consider haematocolpometra by imperforate hymen in the case of a premenarchal girl. Clin Exp Rheumatol 29:146

Di Giacomo V, Trinci M, Van der Byl G, Catania VD, Calisti A, Miele V (2015) Ultrasound in newborns and children suffering from nontraumatic acute abdominal pain: imaging with clinical and surgical correlation. J Ultrasound 18:385–393. doi:10.1007/s40477-014-0087-4, Epub 2014 Apr 9

Doganay S, Yikilmaz A, Kahriman G, Tuna IS, Coskun A (2010) Medical image. Haematometrocolpos secondary to vaginal atresia: US and MRI findings. N Z Med J 123:114–116

Drakonaki EE, Tritou I, Pitsoulis G, Psaras K, Sfakianaki E (2010) Hematocolpometra due to an imperforate hymen presenting with back pain: sonographic diagnosis. J Ultrasound Med 29:321–322

Farina R, Catalano O, Stavolo C, Sandomenico F, Petrillo A, Romano L (2015) Emergency radiology. Radiol Med 120:73–84

Fischer JW, Kwan CW (2014) Emergency point-of-care ultrasound diagnosis of hematocolpometra and imperforate hymen in the pediatric emergency department. Pediatr Emerg Care 30:128–130

Glavan N, Haller H, Brnčić-Fischer A, Glavan-Gačanin L, Miletić D, Jonjić N (2015) Imperforate hymen presenting as vaginal cyst in a 16-month-old child – considerations for an early diagnosis. Scott Med J. pii: 0036933015615263. [Epub ahead of print]

Gyimadu A, Sayal B, Guven S, Gunalp GS (2009) Hematocolpos causing severe urinary retention in an adolescent girl with imperforate hymen: an uncommon presentation. Arch Gynecol Obstet 280:461–463

Hořejší J (2012) Congenital developmental defects of derivates of müllerian ducts. Endocr Dev 22:251–270

Krafft C, Hartin CW Jr, Ozgediz DE (2012) Magnetic resonance as an aid in the diagnosis of a transverse vaginal septum. J Pediatr Surg 47:422–425

Le Hors-Albouze H, Boutin A, Louis-Borrione C, Jouve JL (2011) Girls' abdominal pains and gynaecological emergencies. Rev Prat 61:635–638

Ludwin A, Ludwin I, Pityński K, Banas T, Jach R (2013) Differentiating between a double cervix or cervical duplication and a complete septate uterus with longitudinal vaginal septum. Taiwan J Obstet Gynecol 52:308–310

Maneschi F (1994) Le malformazioni uterine. CIC Edizioni Internazionali, Roma

Martínez-Escoriza JC, Palacios-Marqués A, Oliva-García AB, Ballester-Galiana H (2013) Uterine duplicity without communication between both hemiuteri and cervicovaginal atresia: importance of a thorough diagnosis before treatment. BMJ Case Rep. doi:10.1136/bcr-2013-200923.2013Sep30

Menichini G, Sessa B, Trinci M, Galluzzo M, Miele V (2015) Accuracy of contrast-enhanced ultrasound in the identification and characterization of traumatic solid organ lesions in children: a retrospective comparison with baseline-US and CE-MDCT. Radiol Med 120:989–1001

Messina M, Severi FM, Bocchi C, Ferrucci E, Di Maggio G, Petraglia F (2004) Voluminous perinatal pelvic mass: a case of congenital hydrometrocolpos. J Matern Fetal Neonatal Med 15:135–137

Miele V, Di Giampietro I (2014) Diagnostic imaging in emergency. Salute Soc, (2EN):127–138. doi:10.3280/SES2014-002010EN

Miele V, Andreoli C, Cortese A, De Cicco ML, Luzietti M, Stasolla A, David V (2002) Hemoperitoneum following ovarian cyst rupture: CT usefulness in the diagnosis. Radiol Med 104:316–321

Miele V, Andreoli C, Grassi R (2006) The management of emergency radiology: key facts. Eur J Radiol 59:311–314

Miele V, Di Giampietro I, Ianniello S, Pinto F, Trinci M (2015) Diagnostic imaging in pediatric polytrauma management. Radiol Med 120:33–49

Miele V, Piccolo CL, Sessa B, Trinci M, Galluzzo M (2016a) Comparison between MRI and CEUS in the follow-up of patients with blunt abdominal trauma managed conservatively. Radiol Med 121:27–37

Miele V, Piccolo CL, Galluzzo M, Ianniello S, Sessa B, Trinci M (2016b) Contrast enhanced ultrasound (CEUS) in blunt abdominal trauma. Br J Radiol 89(1061):20150823. doi:10.1259/bjr.20150823 Epub2016Jan8

Miele V, Piccolo CL, Trinci M, Galluzzo M, Ianniello S, Brunese L (2016c) Diagnostic imaging of blunt abdominal trauma in pediatric patients. Radiol Med 121:409–430. doi:10.1007/s11547-016-0637-2, Epub 2016 Apr 13

Nagaraj BR, Basavalingu D, Paramesh VM, Nagendra PD (2016) Radiological diagnosis of neonatal hydrometrocolpos- a case report. J Clin Diagn Res 10:TD18–TD19

Pinto F, Miele V, Scaglione M, Pinto A (2014) The use of contrast-enhanced ultrasound in blunt abdominal trauma: advantages and limitations. Acta Radiol 55:776–784

Pinto F, Valentino M, Romanini L, Basilico R, Miele V (2015) The role of CEUS in the assessment haemodynamically stable patients with blunt abdominal trauma. Radiol Med 120:3–11

Posner JC, Spandorfer PR (2005) Early detection of imperforate hymen prevents morbidity from delays in diagnosis. Pediatrics 115:1008–1012

Salhan B, Omisore OT, Kumar P, Potter J (2013) A rare presentation of imperforate hymen: a case report. Case Rep Urol 2013:731019

Sessa B, Trinci M, Ianniello S, Menichini G, Galluzzo M, Miele V (2015) Blunt abdominal trauma: role of contrast-enhanced ultrasound in the detection and staging of abdominal traumatic lesions compared with US and CE-MDCT. Radiol Med 120:180–189

Ugur MG, Balat O, Ozturk E, Bekerecioglu M, Dikensoy E (2012) Pitfalls in diagnosis and management of distal vaginal agenesis: 10-year experience at a single centre. Eur J Obstet Gynecol Reprod Biol 163:85–90

Valentin L (2009) Characterizing acute gynaecological pathology with ultrasound: an overview and case examples. Best Pract Res Clin Obstet Gynaecol 23:577–593

Winderl LM, Silverman RK (1995) Prenatal diagnosis of congenital imperforate hymen. Obstet Gynecol 85:857–860

14 Ovarian Torsion

Marinella Nanni, Maria Gabriella Merola,
Stefania Ianniello, Cinzia Orazi,
Paolo Maria Schingo, and Margherita Trinci

14.1 Introduction

Pediatric ovarian torsion is an uncommon cause of acute abdominal pain. It represents approximately 15 % of all cases of ovarian torsion and accounts for 2–3 % of all consultations for abdominal pain in pediatric emergency departments (Ngo et al. 2015; Schmitt et al. 2013).

The course of the disease results to a partial or total rotation of the ovary, the fallopian tube, or both around its vascular axis. This twisting initially leads to the obstruction of venous outflow and lymphatic drainage with edema and adnexal enlargement. If the torsion becomes complete and untreated, necrosis, infection, peritonitis, or loss of adnexa may occur (Ngo et al. 2015).

Ovarian torsion should be considered in any pediatric age (from 1 day to 18 years), but most cases occur between 9 and 14 years of age, with a mean age of presentation of 12 years (Schmitt et al. 2013). The disease is most frequently unilateral, although cases of bilateral synchronous or asynchronous ovarian torsion in childhood have been reported in English literature since 1934 (Celik et al. 2005). The right side is more commonly involved, probably because of the decreased space on the left side of the lower abdomen, occupied by the sigmoid colon which is relatively fixed compared to hypermobility of the cecum and ileum. Furthermore the mesosalpinx and the utero-ovarian ligament are slightly longer on the right side, resulting to excess mobility of the adnexa (Varras et al. 2004; Spinelli et al. 2015).

The diagnosis in children is often difficult because they cannot explain related symptoms accurately and the clinical presentation can mimic other acute abdominal conditions (genital, urinary, and gastrointestinal diseases), which make its differential diagnosis challenging. However, prompt diagnosis and treatment are critical to prevent irreversible ovarian damage, and the radiologist plays a crucial role in this regard. Ultrasound is the diagnostic modality of choice to assess torsion. But sometimes a misleading presentation or equivocal sonographic findings involve the use of CT scan or MRI. For these reasons, it is imperative to know the findings of ovarian torsion across multiple imaging modalities to timely diagnosis and to improve clinical outcome.

14.2 Clinical Findings

The clinical presentation is variable and depends on whether the torsion is complete, incomplete, or intermittent with spontaneous detorsion

M. Nanni (✉) • M.G. Merola • S. Ianniello • M. Trinci
Department of Emergency Radiology,
S. Camillo Hospital, Rome, Italy
e-mail: marinellananni@inwind.it

C. Orazi • P.M. Schingo
Department of Diagnostic Imaging, Children's
Hospital Bambino Gesù, Rome, Italy

V. Miele, M. Trinci (eds.), *Imaging Non-traumatic Abdominal Emergencies in Pediatric Patients*,
DOI 10.1007/978-3-319-41866-7_14

(Varras et al. 2004). The most common symptom is the sudden onset of lower abdominal pain, usually isolated to one side (Sasaki and Miller 2014). The characteristic of the pain is non-radiating, mild, or intense. Its duration can be variable (hours, days, or even weeks) and sometimes the clinical history consists of transient episodes of pain alternated with asymptomatic intervals thought to represent intermittent torsion. It can be associated with nausea, vomiting, and anorexia. Low-grade fever with moderate leukocytosis can occur (Oltmann et al. 2009; Kokoska et al. 2000; Meyer et al. 1995). Occasionally high serum levels of tumor markers (CA125, alpha-fetoprotein) are described in the torsion of normal ovary that returns to normal after surgery (McCarthy et al. 2010; Takeda et al. 2009). On physical examination, abdominal tenderness is the most relevant sign with or without peritoneal signs. Rarely a palpable pelvic mass is present, because of the high position of the ovaries at pediatric age (Rey-Bellet Gasser et al. 2016; Buss and Lee 1987). Anamnesis of prior ovarian cyst or mass and prior ovarian torsion or current pregnancy should increase the suspicion of torsion (Poonai et al. 2013). Definitive diagnosis requires laparoscopy.

14.3 Anatomical Review, Physiopathology of Torsion and Management

The normal tube and the ovary are extremely mobile. They are capable of rotation of 90° without giving rise to symptoms (Celik et al. 2005). Adnexal structures are contained within the multiple folds of the peritoneum and the broad ligament, which is composed of the mesometrium, mesovarium, and mesosalpinx. The ovary is supported by the suspensory ligament, which contains the ovarian artery and attaches to the ovary laterally, while the ovarian ligament attaches the ovary to the uterus medially.

There is a dual blood supply to the ovary from both the ovarian artery and ovarian branch of uterine artery. The ovarian artery arises from the abdominal aorta, runs along the suspensory ligament, and reaches the mesovarium; here, ovarian artery anastomoses with the ovarian branch of the uterine artery resulting in an arterial arch from which arises the branches distributed to the ovarian parenchyma.

If the ovary twists on the mesovarium or fallopian tube on the mesosalpinx, a true isolated ovarian or fallopian torsion occurs; but they are rare because of the wide attachment of the mesovarium or the mesosalpinx to the rest of the broad ligament, which acts as a fulcrum (Fig. 14.1) The twisting of all the adnexal structures, such as the ovary, fallopian tube, suspensory ligaments, and broad ligament, is more common and represents up to 67 % of cases (Chang et al. 2008). The term ovarian torsion is applied generally to include all.

The adnexa may twist around the suspensory ligament and utero-ovarian ligament, resulting in the compression of ovarian vessels. The degree of ovarian torsion on its vascular axis is variable from 180° up to the rotation of 2,160° (six complete twists), with more severe vascular damage; in fact ovaries with torsion less than 360° rarely develop necrosis (Villalba et al. 2005; Ito et al. 2015).

The venous outflow and the lymphatic drainage are affected first because of the thicker muscular walls of the arterial vessels. The venous and lymphatic engorgement, with stasis and thrombosis, leads to ovarian edema and enlargement, resulting to clinical symptoms. If the torsion persists, arterial blood flow is affected; the ovary becomes ischemic and it takes on a macroscopic aspect called black-bluish. If left untreated, hemorrhagic infarction and necrosis occur within 36 h of vascular occlusion (Ngo et al. 2015; Lourenco et al. 2014). Infection, pelvic thrombophlebitis, hemorrhage, and peritonitis may complicate the clinical presentation (Huchon and Fauconnier 2010).

The surgical management of ovarian torsion is a controversial topic; in the past, salpingo-oophorectomy was a common clinical practice, without detorsion, but to date, a conservative treatment with detorsion, with or without cystectomy, and ovarian saving are the most recommended. The decision to perform a radical

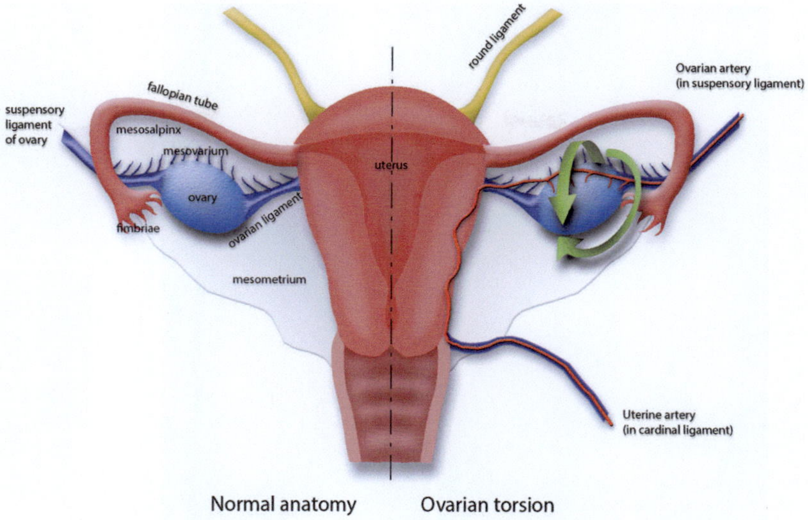

Fig. 14.1 Schematic diagram featuring the normal anatomy of adnexal ligaments (*left* side) and the mechanisms involved in the true isolated ovarian torsion (*small arrow*) and in the adnexal torsion (*large arrow*). (Thanks to Edoardo Saperi for the drawing)

option was motivated by the risk of missing an underlying malignancy by the thromboembolism after detorsion and by a belief that the hemorrhagic ovary (black-bluish) represented nonviable tissue (Celik et al. 2005; Geimanaite and Trainavicius 2013). But there are no reports of malignancy in pediatric patients treated with detorsion alone, and the risk of pulmonary embolism has never been reported in pediatric age. Furthermore it has been demonstrated that a black-bluish ovary, which does not change macroscopic appearance after detorsion, is not a reliable indicator of necrosis, and recovery is still possible (Celik et al. 2005). In fact in the majority of cases, the detorted ovaries have been shown a normal anatomy and follicular development on US follow-up (Spinelli et al. 2015; Geimanaite and Trainavicius 2013).

14.4 Risk Factors

The ovarian torsion can occur at any age but is most common in adolescents and in women of reproductive age.

Approximately 16% of pediatric ovarian torsions are manifested in the first year of age (Oltmann et al. 2009), but the frequency could be underestimated because of unspecific symptoms and limitations in assessing pain in infants. The torsion may occur antenatally, but an antenatal detection of ovarian abnormalities suggestive of torsion in a routine sonographic scan may not be always symptomatic after birth. Embryologically the human ovary originates in the abdomen and later descends into the pelvis; hence, an initial increase in gonadal mobility may have developed propensity to undergo torsion. Moreover, ovarian cysts are common in fetal and neonatal ovaries, resulting from excessive stimulation from placental chorionic gonadotropin and maternal hormones, and serve as a fulcrum for torsion (Nussbaum et al. 1988; Chinchure et al. 2011).

In symptomatic patients, clinical findings are similar to torsion in adult age, with pain, vomiting, fever, abdominal distension, leukocytosis, and peritonitis, while specific sonographic features suggestive of neonatal torsion are described in literature (Fig. 14.2) (Chinchure et al. 2011).

In a female child and an adolescent girl, the twist may involve ovaries anatomically normal or within preexisting physiological or pathological masses that serve as the lead point for torsion. Torsion of normal ovaries is more common in children and adolescent than in adults; in fact up to 25% of pediatric ovarian torsions occur on ovaries without malformations (Geimanaite and Trainavicius 2013).

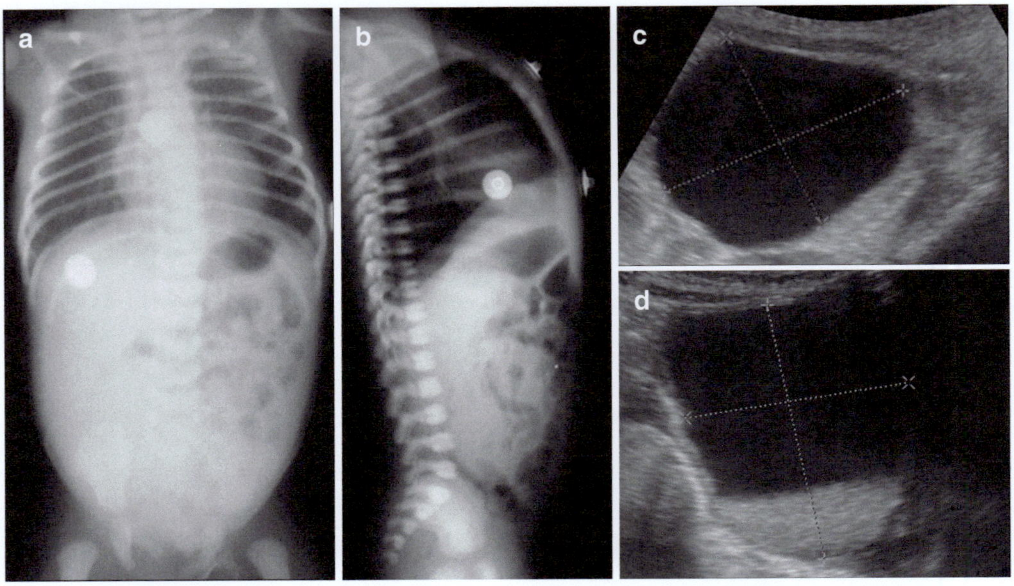

Fig. 14.2 (**a**, **b**) Abdominal radiograph of a 1-month-old girl with vomiting, fever, abdominal distension; the X-ray raises the suspicion of a right abdominal mass displacing the bowel loops; (**c**, **d**) the transabdominal US shows a cystic mass with a fluid-debris level and thin echogenic wall

Various theories have been suggested in this regard: an abnormal congenital length and laxity of adnexal ligaments that increase the mobility of the adnexa structures and the adnexal venous congestion, as in premenarchal activity, due to hyperstimulation that increases ovary size (Poonai et al. 2013; Davis and Feins 1990). Furthermore a possible mechanism involved is the sudden change of the body position or abrupt increase in the intra-abdominal pressure from vomiting and coughing (Schmitt et al. 2013; Spinelli et al. 2015).

On the other hand, most cases of pediatric ovarian torsion are associated with ovarian pathologies, mainly benign cystic or benign neoplasms. In fact torsion is a known complication of physiological follicular or luteal cyst (17 % of twisted ovaries), because they are the most recurring lesions in girls older than 12 years old. Furthermore, pediatric torsion is the most frequent complication of ovarian tumors (from 3 % to 16 %), of which benign dermoid cysts are the most common. Less frequently, other benign lesions are involved, like serous cystadenoma (13 % of twisted ovaries), paratubal cysts, or hydrosalpinx (Duigenan et al. 2012). The risk of torsion of benign masses is likely related to the increased size (5 cm or greater) and weight of the involved ovary, which lead to excessive rotation resulting in torsion. Malignant ovarian neoplasms associated with torsion are extremely rare (only 2 %). This can be explained by the low incidence of malignancy in pediatric age (ovarian dysgerminoma is the most common) and by their ability to invade adjacent structures, caused by adhesions and limited mobility of adnexal structures (Oltmann et al. 2009).

Although most ovarian torsions occur in ovaries with an underlying mass, it is important to remember that most ovarian masses are not twisted and other radiological features are required to suggest diagnosis (Duigenan et al. 2012).

14.5 Imaging Evaluation

Diagnostic imaging plays a main role in diagnosis and management of ovarian torsion. All imaging techniques and all diagnostic techniques used in emergency can give their contribution (Miele et al. 2006; Miele and Di Giampietro 2014). The most useful techniques are US, CT, and MRI.

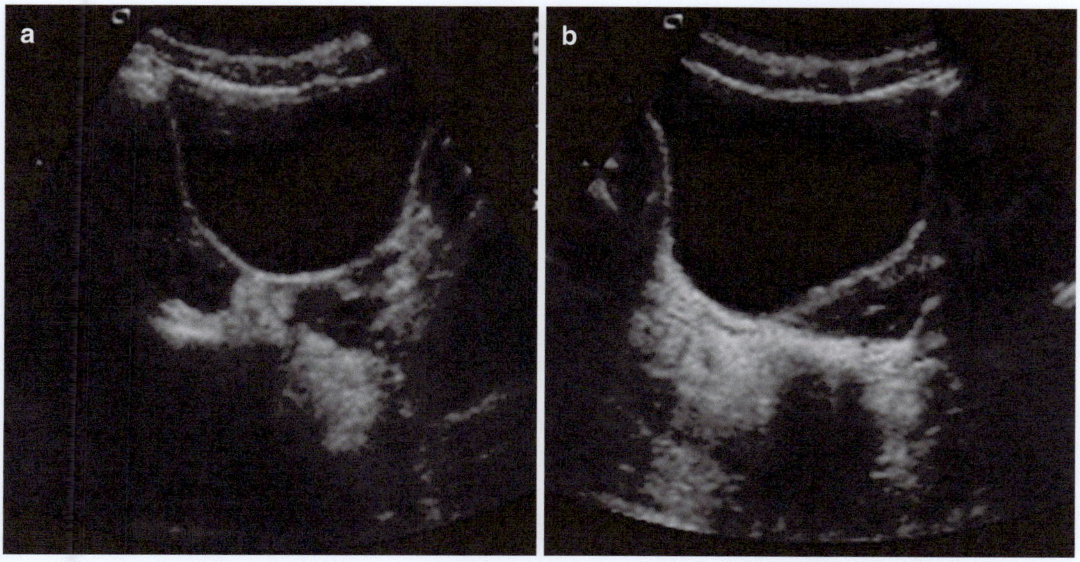

Fig. 14.3 Normal feature of right (**a**) and left (**b**) neonatal ovaries with subcentimeter follicular cysts

14.5.1 Ultrasound Findings in Neonatal Torsion

The ovarian torsion is the most common complication of the neonatal ovarian cyst. The presence of subcentimeter follicular cysts is a frequent and normal feature in neonatal ovaries (Fig. 14.3). They are detected sonographically from the third trimester of pregnancy and in the early infancy, as a result from excessive stimulation from maternal hormones, and regress spontaneously. The cysts that are not retreated may develop complications in utero or in the first year of age, and the most common are torsion and hemorrhage, less frequently autoamputation (Nussbaum et al. 1988); bowel obstruction, pulmonary hypoplasia from thoracic compression, or obstructive uropathy is present if the cyst is huge, filling the entire abdomen (Chinchure et al. 2011).

The ultrasound findings depend on whether the cyst is complicated or not. An uncomplicated cyst appears as an anechoic structure and its wall is imperceptible, while the twisted cyst has a complex sonographic appearance, suggestive of torsion and hemorrhage. If during a routine antenatal sonographic scan the cyst changes from anechoic to cyst with internal echoes, a torsion may occur (Fig. 14.4); even an antenatal uncomplicated cyst may develop internal echoes due to mechanical stress of delivery, causing hemorrhage.

Commonly, torsion occurs in ovaries with a cyst larger than 2.5 cm and the mean volume of twisted cyst measuring 65.5 cm^3 (Chinchure et al. 2011). The twisted cyst contains a fluid-debris level and a retracting clot, indicating hemorrhage within the cyst, and often septa and an echogenic wall (Fig. 14.5), resulting from dystrophic calcification associated with infarction, are seen (Nussbaum et al. 1988). Occasionally a "fishnet" appearance (reticular pattern representing residual fibrin stands) or a solid mass feature (complicated cyst filled with homogeneous internal echoes) has been described (Fig. 14.6) (Chinchure et al. 2011).

Another less frequent complication of twisted neonatal cyst is the autoamputation: when an extreme mobility of the twisted cyst occurs, the cyst pedicle or distal fallopian tube became necrotic, allowing the cyst to break loose and float free in the peritoneal cavity. If not diagnosed in the neonatal period, a calcified pelvic mass can be seen many years later referable to a remotely twisted and calcified free peritoneal ovary (Ngo et al. 2015; Nussbaum et al. 1988).

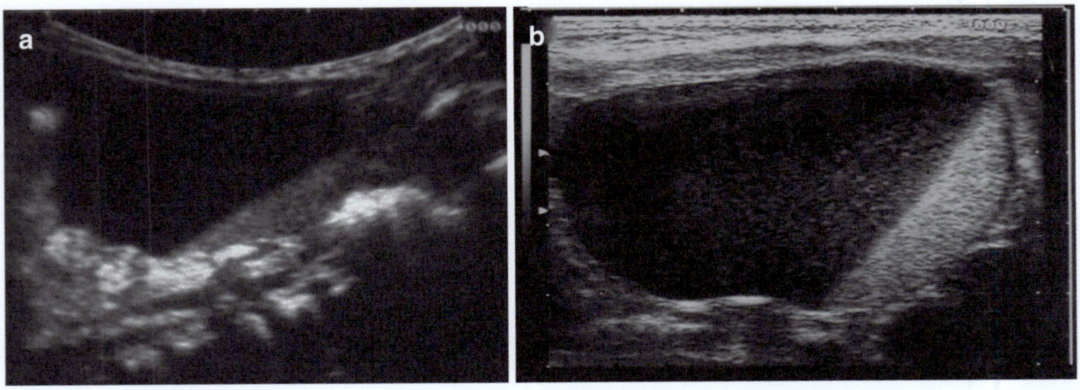

Fig. 14.4 Intrauterine ovarian torsion: a transabdominal US at 36 weeks of pregnancy shows a large cyst (**a**) with a fluid-debris level and internal echoes (**b**), suggestive of torsion

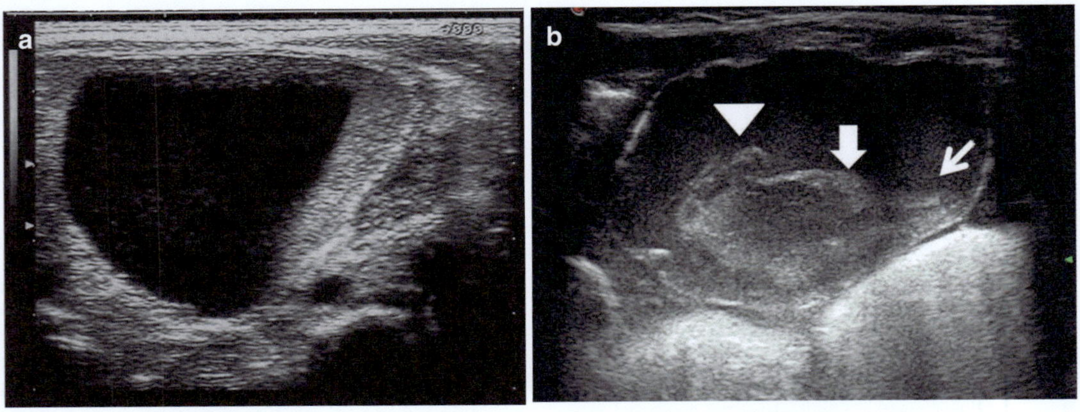

Fig. 14.5 (**a**) Transverse US in a 1-month-old girl with fever and vomiting shows a cyst with markedly thickened and hyperechoic wall, resulting from dystrophic calcification associated with infarction. (**b**) Transverse US in a 2-week-old girl with abdominal distention: a large cyst with fluid-debris level (*arrow*), retracting clot (*large arrow*), and thick septation (*arrowhead*) is seen

The use of Doppler is not helpful in assessing whether the cyst is twisted or not because most of them do not show flow (Chinchure et al. 2011).

14.5.2 Ultrasound Findings in Pediatric Torsion

Ultrasound is the diagnostic modality of choice in girls with pelvic acute pain and clinically suspected ovarian torsion (Ngo et al. 2015), because of easy accessibility, the lack of ionizing radiation, and a good visualization of the pelvic organs. In the premenarchal children, non-sexually active, it is limited to a transabdominal approach using low-frequency convex probe and requiring proper filled bladder to function as an acoustic window. In sexually active female, a transvaginal approach (using high-frequency endovaginal probe with partially void bladder) is preferable, because it is more useful to make the right diagnosis and to exclude others acute abdominal conditions, like ectopic pregnancy.

The most commonly reported sonographic finding associated with pediatric ovarian torsion is unilateral ovarian enlargement, defined as a dimension greater than 5 cm or a volume greater than 20 cm^3, compared with the contralateral side (Oltmann et al. 2009; Lourenco et al. 2014; Huchon and Fauconnier 2010; Houry and Abbott

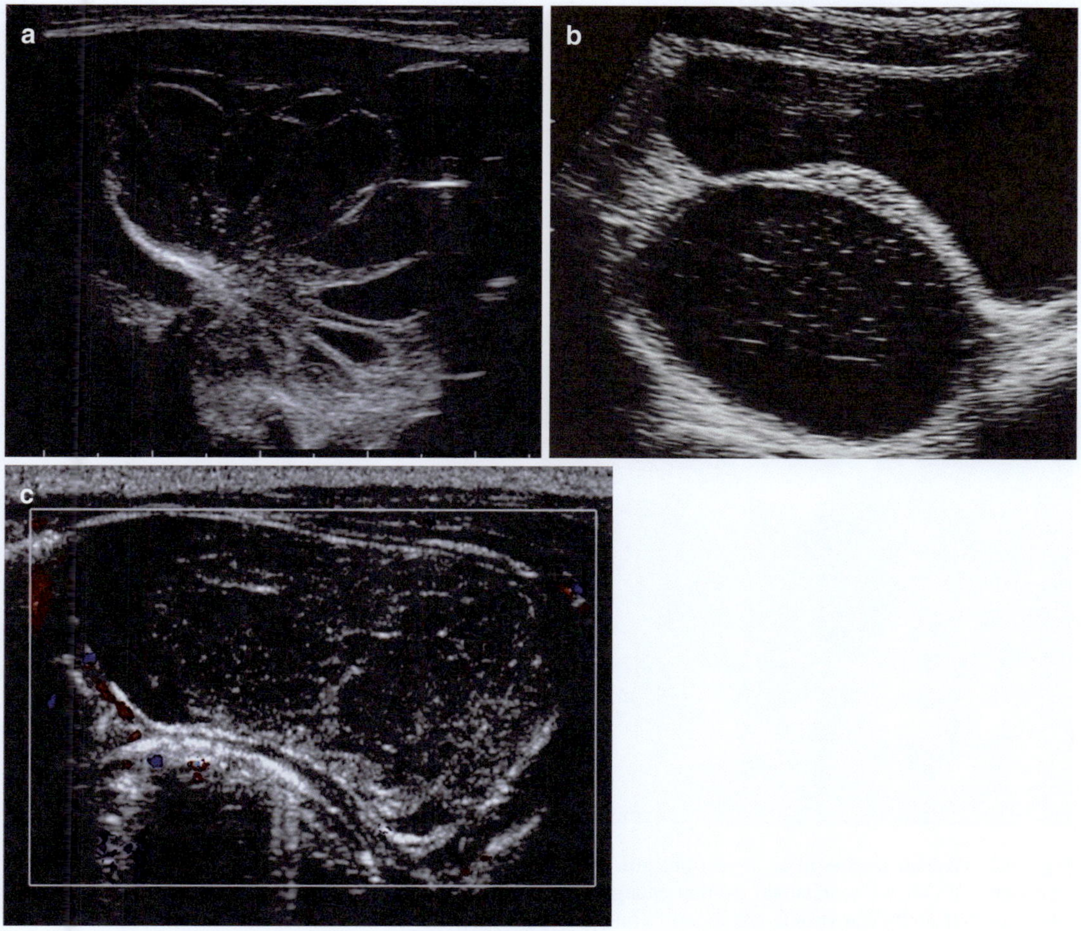

Fig. 14.6 (**a**) Twisted cyst in a 1-month-old girl with multiple thick septations and internal echoes. (**b**) Transverse US in a 1-year-old girl with fever and vomiting shows a cyst with "fish-net" appearance (**c**) Another case: Color Doppler US shows isoechoic or mildly echogenic solid mass without internal vascularity

2001; Chiou et al. 2007; Hiller et al. 2007; Rha et al. 2002; Swenson et al. 2014). The adnexal enlargement may be often the enlarged ovary itself or a cystic, complex, or solid mass is present (Lam et al. 2015). In ovarian torsion, a median volume ratio of the abnormal adnexa has been reported to be 12, compared to the normal adnexa; moreover if the volume ratio is 20 or more, patients are 18 times more likely to have an associated underlying ovarian mass (Servaes et al. 2007). However it is important to remember that in up to 5 % of twisted ovaries the size was reported normal (Rha et al. 2002).

The enlarged ovary is likely secondary to massive ovarian edema, and it is characterized by a central afollicular stroma and a peripheral placement of multiple cortical follicles (8–12 mm), dilated with transudative fluid from the congested ovary (Fig. 14.7); these common ultrasound findings can be visualized in up to 74 % of ovarian torsion cases (Albayram and Hamper 2001; Lee et al. 1998). Another US mark of torsion, seen in 34 % of cases, is the medialization of the twisted ovary: as torsion occurs, the congested adnexal structures, twisted around the broad ligament, which are attached to the uterus and sometimes both ovaries are present on the same side of the pelvis (Servaes et al. 2007; Otjen et al. 2015).

When the adnexal torsion is associated with ovarian pathologies, sonography is able to determine its sonographic features and it is helpful in

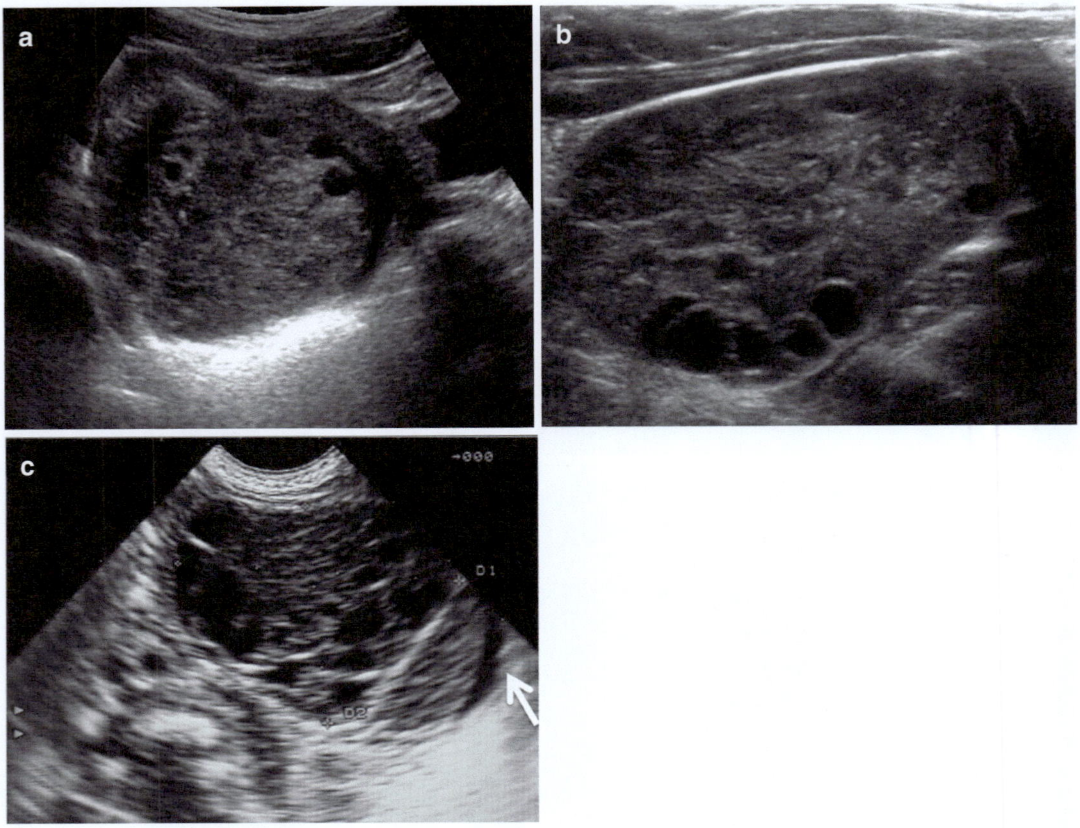

Fig. 14.7 Ovarian torsion in an 8-year-old girl. (**a**, **b**) Transverse US shows a unilateral ovarian enlargement, with a central afollicular stroma and a peripheral placement of multiple cortical follicles. (**c**) The enlarged ovary is surrounded by hyperechoic fat and by a thin fluid flap (*white arrow*)

distinguishing a cystic from a complex mass (Fig. 14.8) (Duigenan et al. 2012).

In cases of suspected ovarian torsion, the utility of Doppler in evaluating the vascular impairment is controversial. In fact in a symptomatic patient, although the absence of blood flow within an abnormal ovary is a useful finding in suggesting the diagnosis, the presence of Doppler blood flow does not exclude the diagnosis of adnexal torsion (Chang et al. 2008). The most common alteration of flow pattern is the decrease or absence of venous flow (93 %), resulting from the collapse of venous walls. While the arterial flow is normal in as many as two-thirds of the patients with surgically proven torsion, as mentioned before, this is because of a late arterial occlusion and a dual arterial vascularization of the ovary (Schmitt et al. 2013). Sometimes, the absence of the end diastolic flow of arterial waveform may be observed (Fig. 14.9) (Chang et al. 2008).

However the utility of Color Doppler might be useful in assessing the viability of the ovary before surgery: the presence of central venous flow in a twisted ovary has been associated with the possibility of viable tissue after the detorsion (Fleischer et al. 1995).

Furthermore Color Doppler is helpful in evaluating the configuration of the adnexal vessels. At ultrasound, the twisted pedicle appears as a hyperechoic round or beaked mass with central multiple concentric hypoechoic rings, result of the twisting of the entire vascular pedicle, tubal structures, and supporting ligaments (Ngo et al. 2015; Lourenco et al. 2014). The use of Color Doppler allows to identify within the echogenic mass the “whirlpool” sign (Fig. 14.10), which is the swirling target appearance of the vessels in

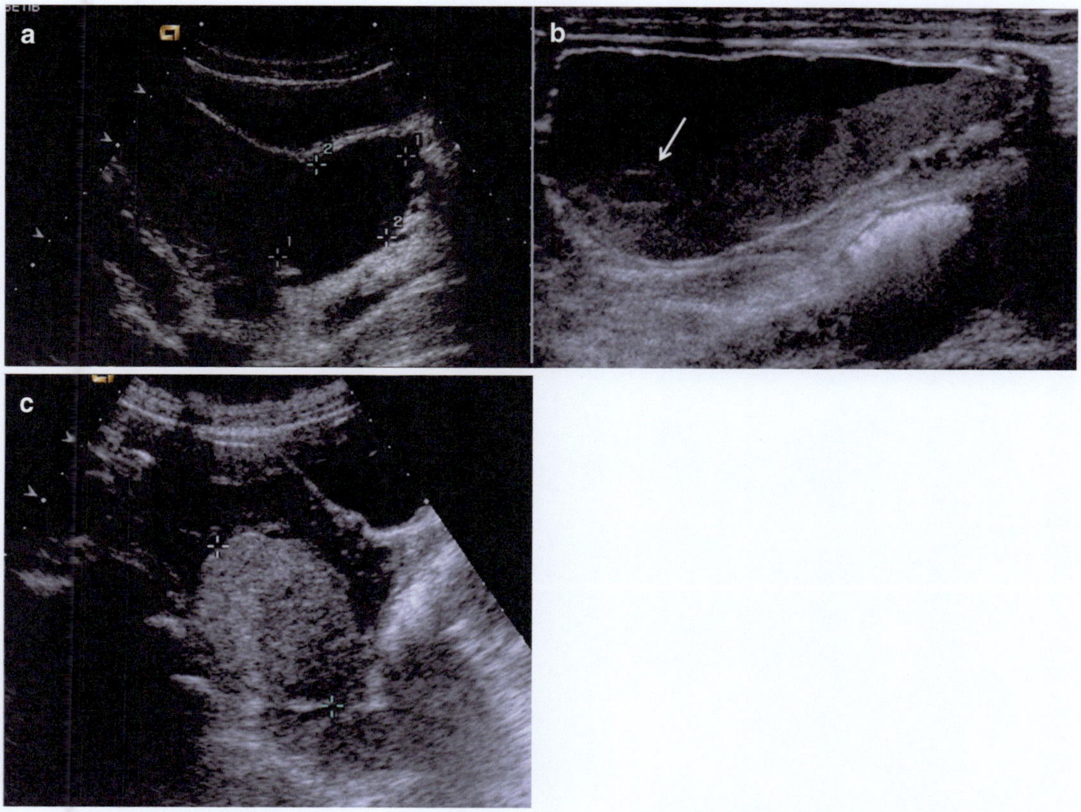

Fig. 14.8 Young girls with sudden onset of lower abdominal pain and surgically proved torsion. The US images show a large paraovarian cyst (**a**), a hemorrhagic luteal cyst with fluid-debris level, retracting clot (*arrow*) and thickened wall (**b**), and a benign teratoma (**c**), which serve as lead point for torsion

the twisted vascular pedicle; when present, it is a highly sensitive and specific finding for ovarian torsion (sensitivity 88 %, specificity 87 %) (Lee et al. 1998).

Another common but nonspecific sonographic finding in adnexal torsion is the free pelvic fluid in the pouch of Douglas. Although this was found in many patients with adnexal torsion, it is also commonly found in asymptomatic women as a result of normal ovulation (Lourenco et al. 2014).

The use of contrast-enhanced ultrasound (CEUS) is not described in this pathology, although it might have a role in assessing the vascularization of the ovarian lesion or in differential diagnosis with other abdominal or pelvic masses. Currently in childhood, the CEUS is mainly used in traumatic emergencies (Pinto et al. 2014, 2015 Sessa et al. 2015; Menichini et al. 2015; Miele et al. 2015, 2016a, b, c); however, the indication for using even in nontraumatic emergencies is increasing (Catalano et al. 2004; Farina et al. 2015).

14.5.3 CT Findings

When ovarian torsion is suspected as the primary diagnosis, CT is not recommended, mainly because of its high doses of radiation and poor cost efficiency compared to US. However in patients with abdominal acute pain, when gastrointestinal or urinary pathologies remain in the clinical differential diagnosis, CT is performed in emergency. In fact CT allows to evaluate the adnexa in the setting of acute pelvic pain (Swenson et al. 2014), and it is helpful in ruling in or ruling out suspected ovarian torsion with a negative predictive value around 100 %.

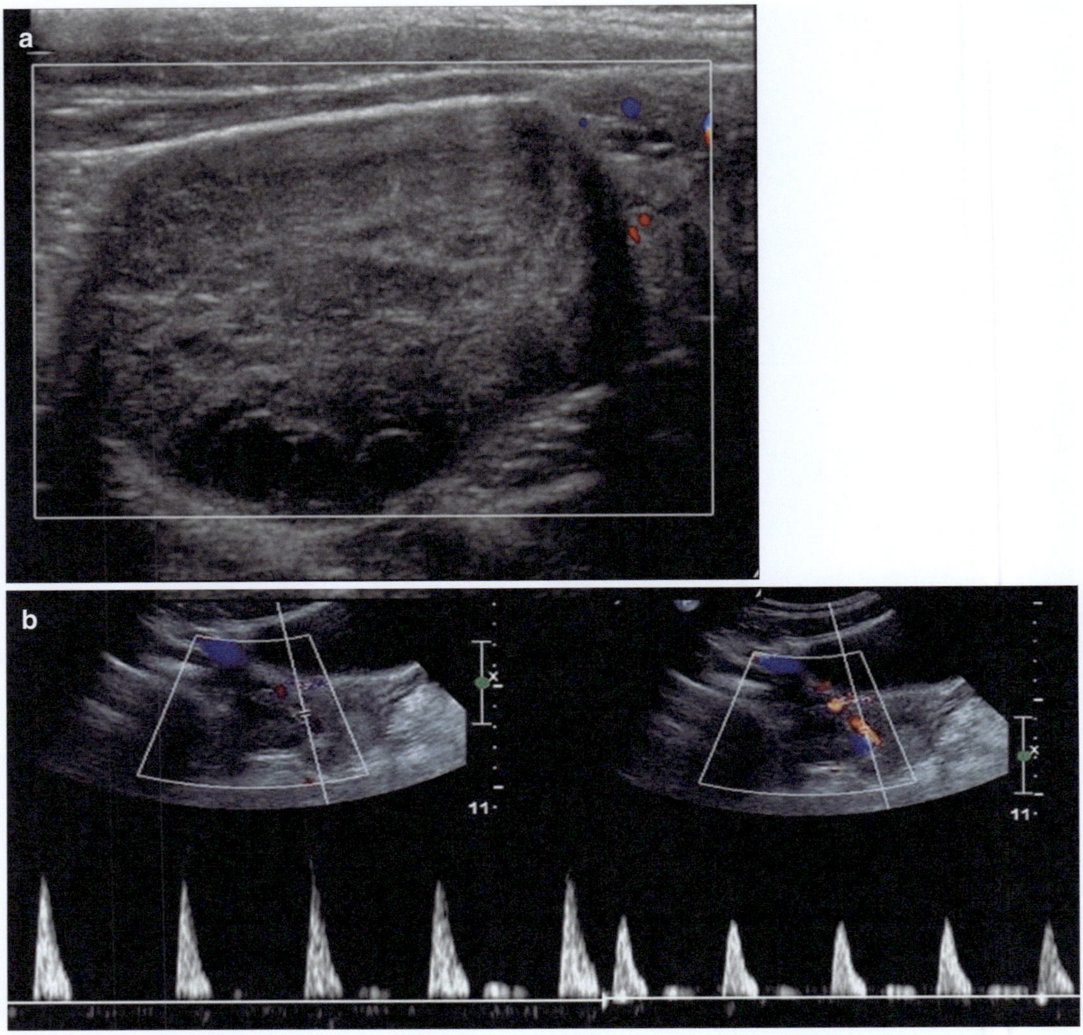

Fig. 14.9 (**a**) The absence of color or spectral flow within an abnormal ovary is suggestive of torsion. (**b**) The use of Color Doppler in an enlarged ovary shows the absence of the end diastolic flow of arterial waveform

The most common CT finding in adnexal torsion is an asymmetric ovarian enlargement or an enlarged adnexal mass (Lourenco et al. 2014; Chinchure et al. 2011), greater than 5 cm (Oltmann et al. 2009). The enlarged ovary with central afollicular stroma and peripheral displacement of the follicles can be identified on contrast-enhanced CT (Fig. 14.11), and it is a specific feature; if the torsion occurs in pathological ovaries, a lead-point mass can be identified on imaging (Fig. 14.12). CT also, comparing to US or MRI, has an increased sensitivity in recognizing calcifications, and this is useful in the diagnosis of teratoma (Fig. 14.13) or in the setting of chronic undetected ovarian torsion because dystrophic calcification may be associated with necrosis.

The "whirlpool sign," a characteristic sonographic finding, can be identified with cross-sectional imaging too. It is detected in less than one-third of the patients, but when present, it is pathognomonic for ovarian torsion (Chinchure et al. 2011). Multiplanar CT reformations demonstrate a twisted vascular pedicle in the broad ligament (Fig. 14.14) with the deviation of the uterus toward the side of torsion (Chinchure et al.

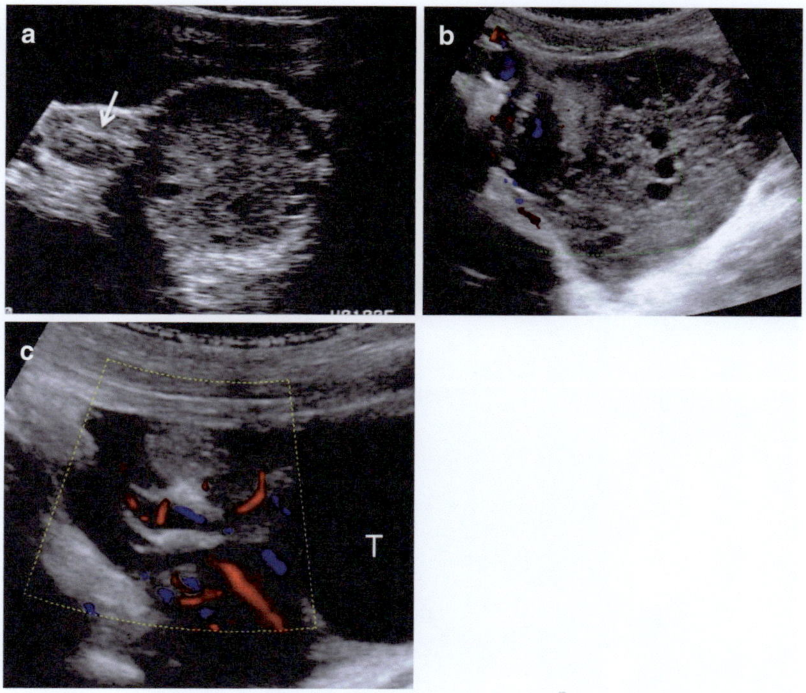

Fig. 14.10 (**a**) The transverse US image shows the twisted pedicle that appears as a hyperechoic round mass (*arrow*). (**b**) The use of Color Doppler identifies the swirling target appearance of the vessels within the echogenic mass ("whirlpool" sign). (**c**) Color Doppler US demonstrates the twisted pedicle in a 13-year-old girl with mature cystic teratoma (T)

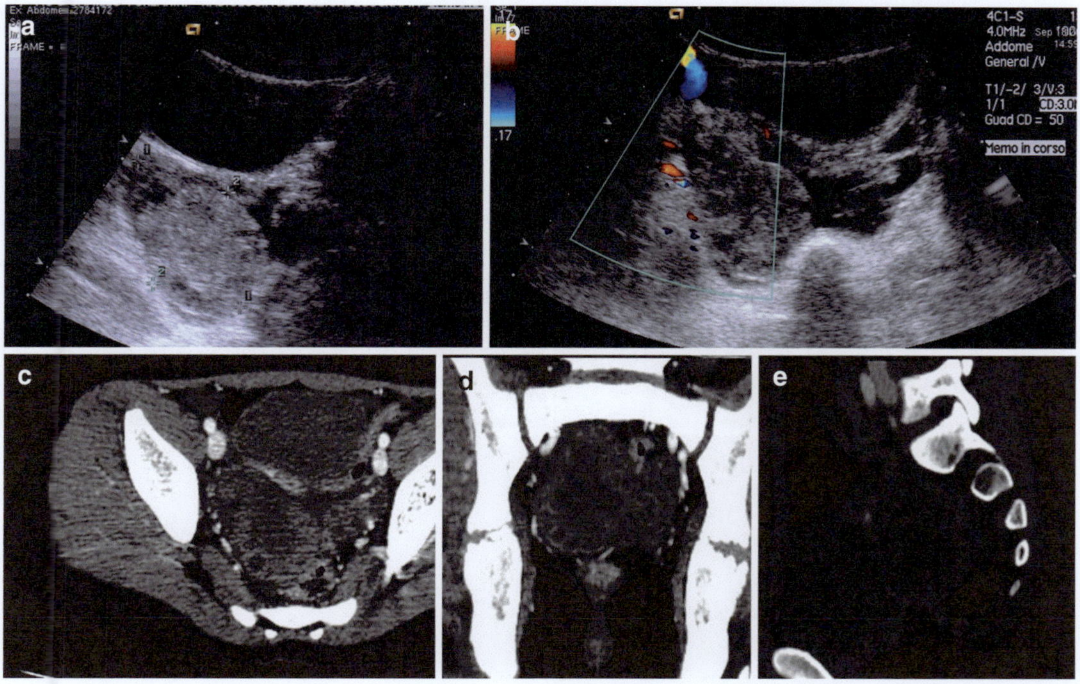

Fig. 14.11 (**a**, **b**) The transverse US and the Color Doppler image show avascular adnexal mass in the pelvis. (**c–e**) Axial, coronal, and sagittal contrast-enhanced CT images show an enlarged right ovary, medialized with central afollicular stroma and peripheral displacement of the follicles. There is no ovarian enhancement compared with the uterine myometrium

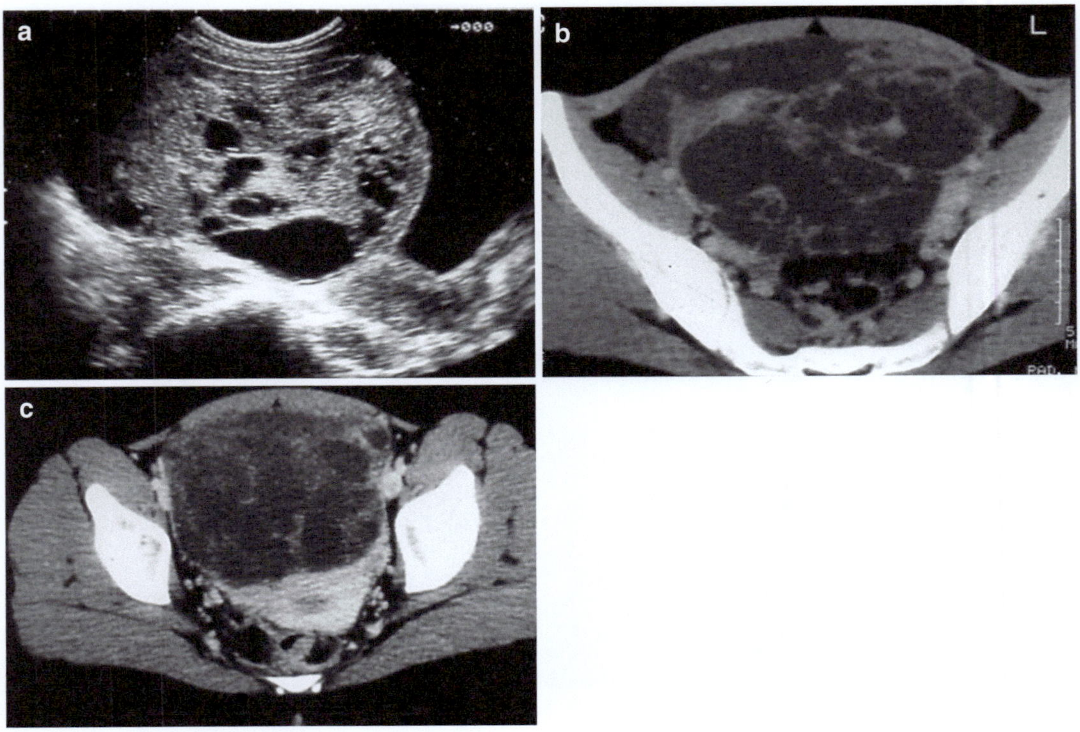

Fig. 14.12 (**a**) Transverse US in a 13-year-old girl with pain and palpable mass shows a large complex mass into the pelvis. (**b**, **c**) Axial contrast-enhanced CT images show a midline pelvic mass with multiple hypodense areas. Surgical evaluation confirmed a twisted right ovary with benign teratoma

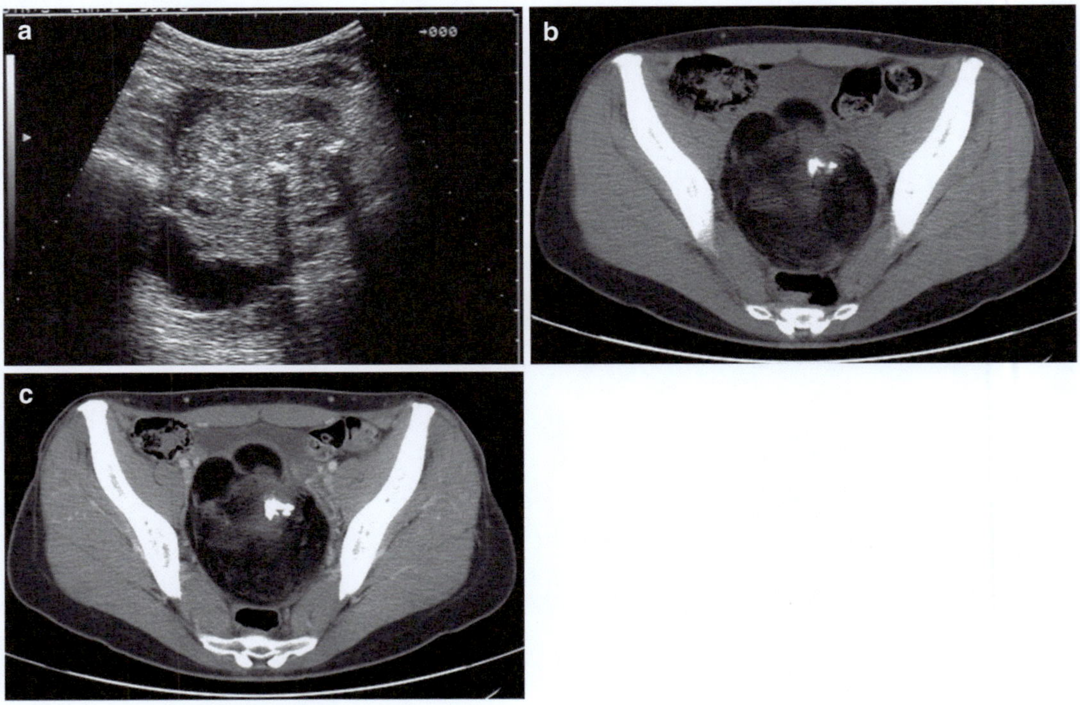

Fig. 14.13 (**a**) The transabdominal US in a 15-year-old girl with acute abdominal pain shows a large midline pelvic complex mass with some hyperechoic spots inside. (**b**) Unenhanced CT confirms the presence of heterogenic, predominantly solid mass with calcifications and posterior fat. (**c**) The contrast-enhanced CT axial image does not show significant enhancement, suggesting torsion

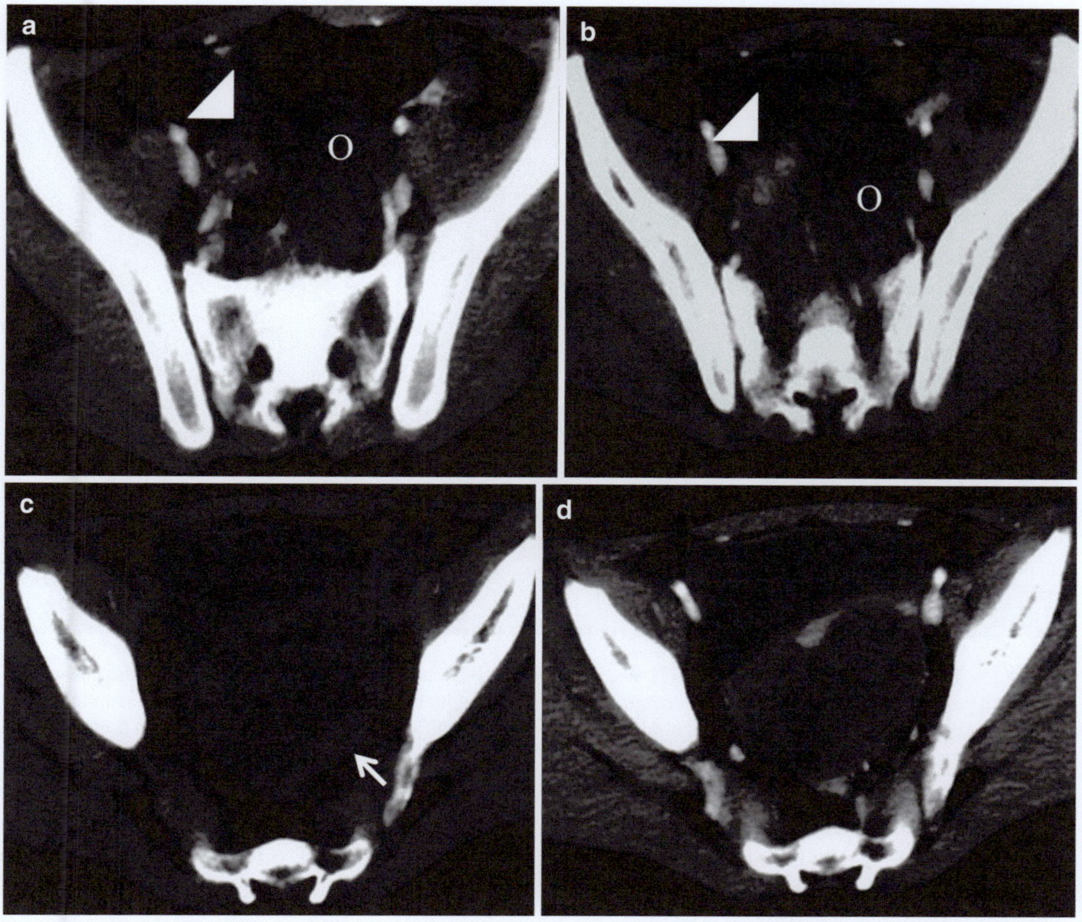

Fig. 14.14 CT in a 16-year-old girl with an acute onset of abdominal pain. (**a**, **b**) Contrast-enhanced CT demonstrates a twisted, enlarged, medialized right ovary (O) with a twisted vascular pedicle in the broad ligament (*arrowhead*). (**c**) Axial unenhanced CT image shows hyperdense areas of subacute hemorrhage in the mass with peripheral displacement of some follicles (*arrow*). (**d**) Axial contrast-enhanced CT image shows a diminished enhancement of the ovary. The surgical evaluation confirmed right ovarian torsion

2011; Hiller et al. 2007). Also the involved ovary changes position and it appears more midline. If the torsion persists, a hemorrhagic infarction of the involved adnexal structures occurs; subacute hemorrhage is best seen on unenhanced CT as an intraovarian hematoma, hematosalpinx, or hemoperitoneum (Fig. 14.15) (Chinchure et al. 2011).

Typical CT findings include smooth wall thickening of an adnexal cystic mass and thickening or enlargement of the fallopian tube (Hiller et al. 2007); the latter appears as an amorphous or tubular mass-like structure with a diameter of 10 mm or more, localized between the twisted adnexa and the uterus (Rha et al. 2002).

Contrast-enhanced CT is useful in identifying an abnormal ovarian enhancement, often described as heterogeneously minimal or absent in comparing with the uterine myometrium (Lourenco et al. 2014; Chinchure et al. 2011; Kimura et al. 1994; Roche et al. 2012). The complete absence of enhancement reflects the evolution of ovarian torsion from ischemia to infarction (Chiou et al. 2007). On the other hand, the presence of enhancement cannot exclude adnexal torsion because of its dual blood supply (Sasaki and Miller 2014; Lourenco et al. 2014), or because of intermittent torsion, or the recent onset.

Other CT findings are the fat stranding adjacent to the ovary and the free pelvic fluid, but they are not specific for ovarian torsion because they are frequent in other gynecologic diseases, including pyosalpinx, tubo-ovarian abscesses,

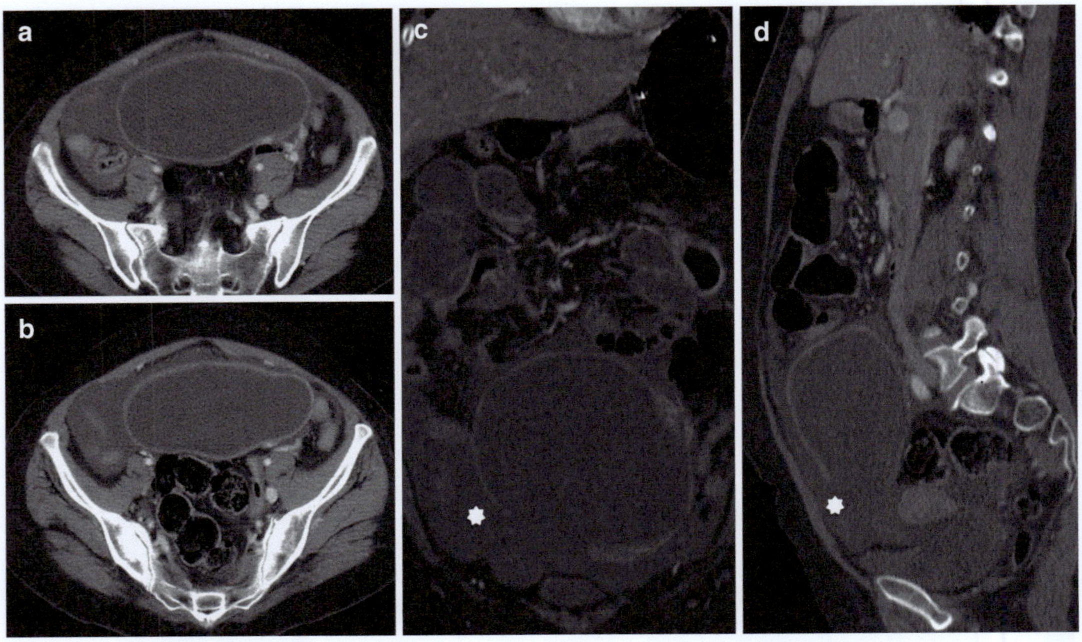

Fig. 14.15 Multiplanar contrast-enhanced CT images in a surgically confirmed twisted serous cystadenoma. (**a**, **b**) The axial images show a large cyst with high-density fluid (60 HU) such as a subacute hemorrhage; the coronal (**c**) and sagittal (**d**) images demonstrate an interruption of the cystic wall with resulting hemoperitoneum (*asterisk*)

and hemorrhagic and endometriotic ovarian cysts (Lourenco et al. 2014; Chinchure et al. 2011; Chiou et al. 2007; Hiller et al. 2007; Swenson et al. 2014; Kimura et al. 1994; Roche et al. 2012; Miele et al. 2000, 2002).

Lastly a CT scan offers better spatial resolution for presurgical planning.

14.5.4 MRI Findings

Magnetic resonance imaging (MRI) is not commonly used in a clinical practice when an adnexal torsion is suspected because of its limited availability in emergency departments and the challenges associated with obtaining a diagnostic image in small patients. However it can be helpful in cases of subacute or intermittent ovarian torsion with equivocal sonographic findings, as well as in pregnant patients where the sonography may be quite difficult because ovaries are displaced out of the pelvis.

MRI features are similar to those seen with the US and CT, but MRI, offering a better soft tissue contrast, allows an optimal representation of the pelvis anatomy and an appropriate preoperative setting.

A standard MRI protocol should include T2 sequences and T1-weighted fat-suppressed sequences, as well as T1-weighted fat-suppressed post-contrast images, to identify, respectively, hemorrhage and a compromised vascular supply, suggesting infarction or necrosis. Diffusion-weighted imaging can show a restricted diffusion expression of adnexal torsion (Wilkinson and Sanderson 2012; Kilickesmez et al. 2009).

As with US and CT, the most common MRI finding of torsion is an enlarged ovary, compared to the contralateral adnexa, with or without an associated ovarian mass. T2-weighted images and post-contrast T1-weighted MRI sequences show an enlarged ovary with central stromal edema and peripherally displaced follicles (Chinchure et al. 2011). A twisted vascular pedi-

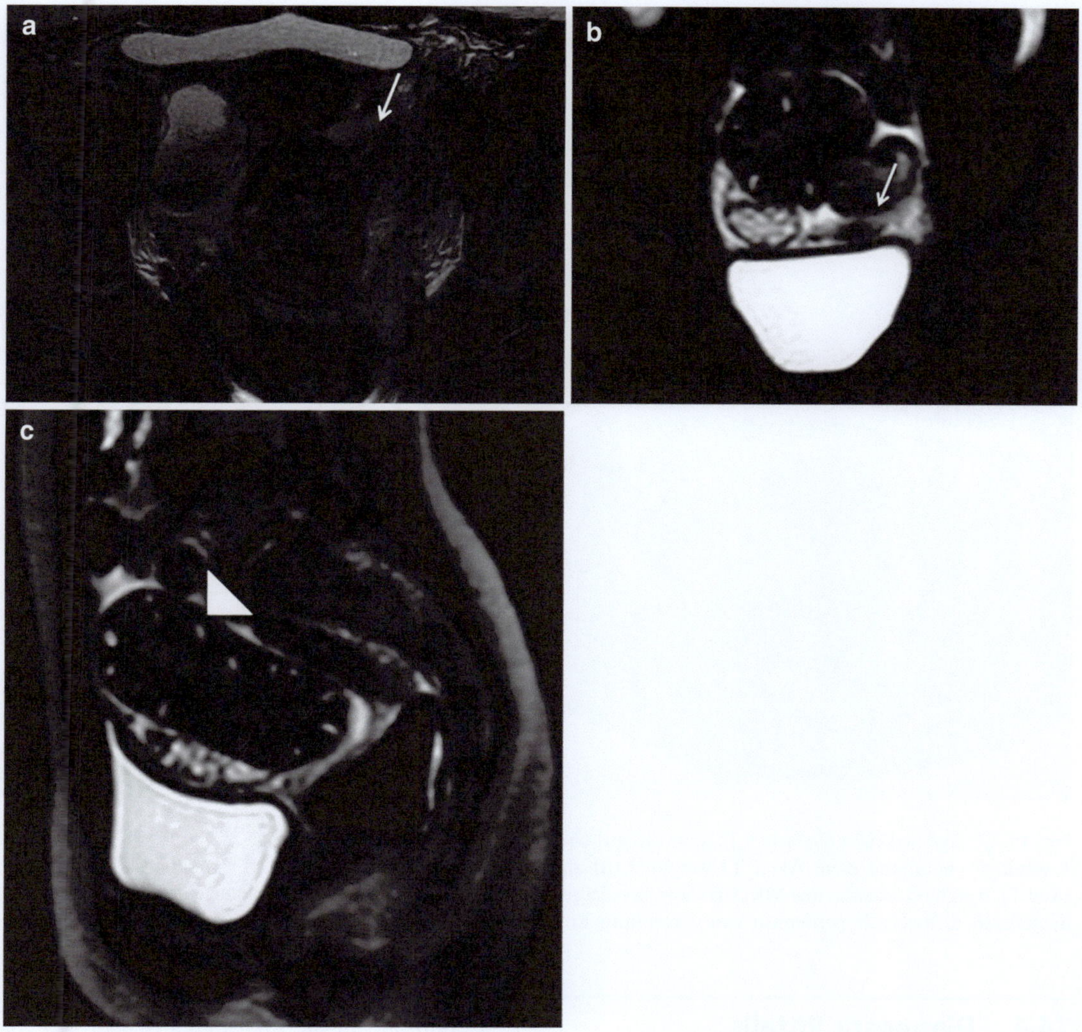

Fig. 14.16 MRI findings of ovarian torsion in a 12-year-old girl: all the images of T2-weighted show an enlarged left ovary with central hyperintense signal for stromal edema and peripherally displaced follicles (*arrowhead*). The axial (**a**) and the coronal (**b**) images show a medialized left ovary with twisted vascular pedicle (*arrow*)

cle can also be seen on multiplanar acquisitions (Fig. 14.16). As the CT scan, an abnormal or absent enhancement within an enlarged ovary and a subacute ovarian hematoma are best seen (Fig. 14.17). Subacute hemorrhage is identified on T1-weighted images with fat saturation as a T1-hyperintense rim in an enlarged ovary.

In cases of adnexal masses greater than 5 cm, MRI is helpful to identify the origin and to determine its specific MRI signal characteristics (Figs. 14.18 and 14.19), allowing definitive diagnosis. The employment of gadolinium-enhanced MRI studies, diffusion-weighted imaging (DWI), and apparent diffusion coefficient (ADC) values leads to distinguish between benign and malignant lesions (Jain 2002).

Lastly on T2-weighted images, free pelvic fluid and fluid placed around the ovary are easily detected and may support the diagnosis of ovarian torsion (Chinchure et al. 2011; Chiou et al. 2007).

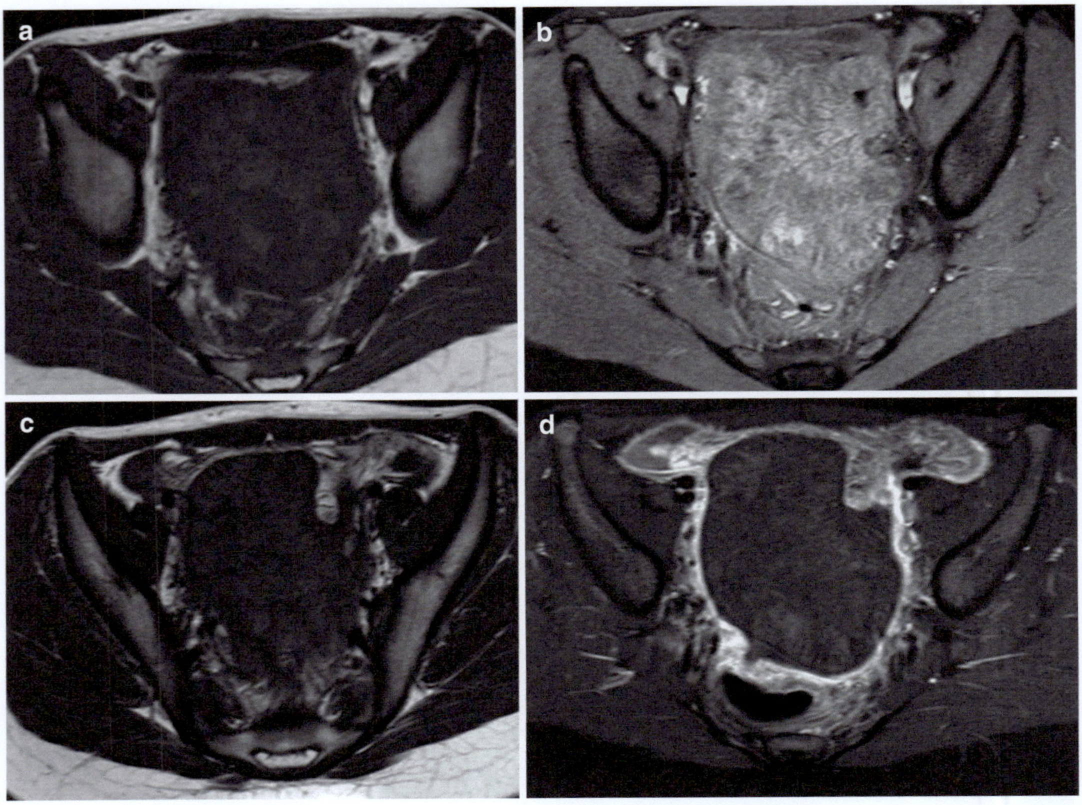

Fig. 14.17 Twisted right ovary in a 14-year-old girl with 1 week of abdominal pain. Axial T1-weighted (**a**) and axial T1-weighted fat-saturated MRI (**b**) show an enlarged medialized diffusely hyperintense ovary resulting to a subacute ovarian hematoma; in the axial T1-weighted post-contrast (**c**) and the axial T1-weighted fat-saturated post-contrast (**d**), an absent enhancement is best seen

14.6 Diagnostic Pitfalls

All the adnexal masses in pediatric patients with acute pelvic pain can mimic the ovarian torsion.

First of all, the hemorrhagic cyst (Fig. 14.20) that occurs in postpubertal girls because the hemorrhage physiologically manifests only after the Graafian follicle ruptures expels the oocyte and rapidly becomes a corpus luteum. Sometimes in these cases, the arterial flow is diminished or absent because of the mass effect, with compression of the adjacent ovarian tissue. The luteal phase of the menstrual cycle and the size of the cyst could aid in the final diagnosis; in fact the hemorrhagic cyst has an average diameter of 3–3.5 cm, while in the torsion, the ovary measures more than 5 cm and have a volume ratio of 15 or more, compared to the normal ovary (Jain 2002). Moreover if US suggests a hemorrhagic cyst, a follow-up in 6–8 weeks is performed to control resolution (Chang et al. 2008).

In sexually active girls, a hemorrhagic adnexal mass can represent an ectopic pregnancy, which is easily excluded with a negative serum β-HCG test.

A massive ovarian edema (Fig. 14.21) from recurrent torsion and detorsion without progres-

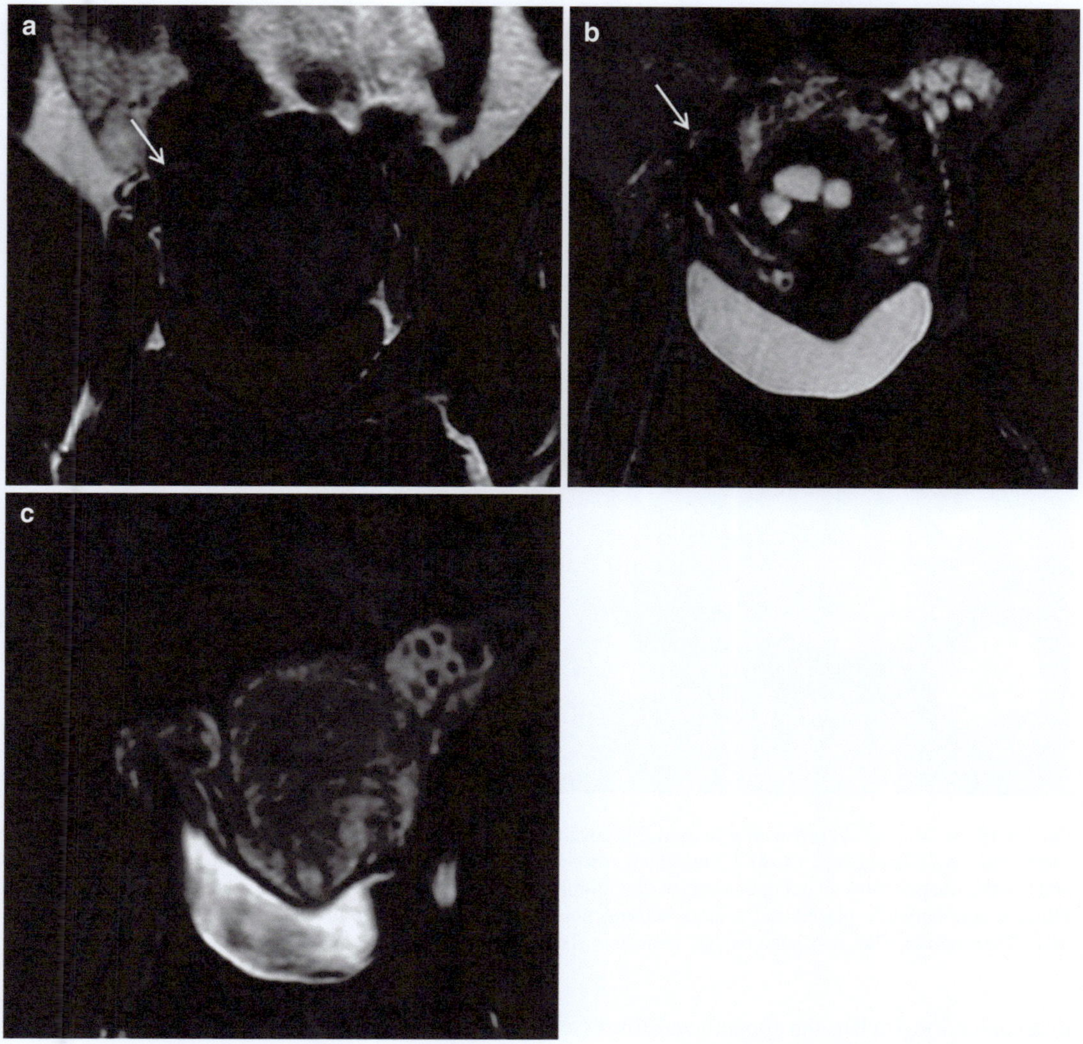

Fig. 14.18 MRI in a 7-year-old girl with surgically confirmed twisted ovarian teratoma. (**a**, **b**) Coronal T1- and T2-weighted images show a heterogenous solid mass with cystic areas inside and associated twisted pedicle. (**c**) Coronal gadolinium-enhanced T1-weighted image confirms torsion with twisted pedicle and shows an abnormal patchy enhancement of the mass because the torsion was not complete at surgical evaluation

sion to infarction simulates an ovarian torsion; on the CT or the MRI with contrast agent, the edema is characterized by the presence of enhancement of the ovarian stroma (Kramer et al. 1997).

Another potential pitfall occurs when the identification of the ovary is difficult because of the loss of its normal architecture due to edema and necrosis of the twisted ovary; in these cases, it is difficult to distinguish ovarian torsion from any other adnexal mass.

Furthermore an inflammatory pelvic mass from adjacent pelvic structures can mimic the

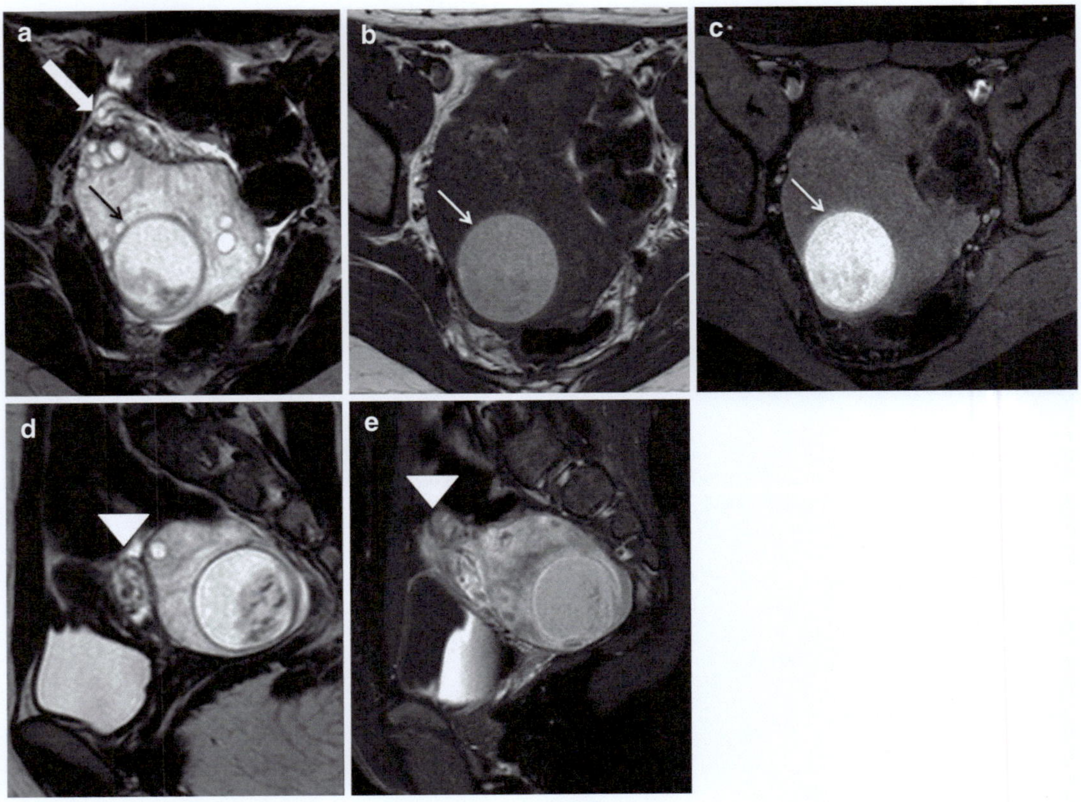

Fig. 14.19 A 14-year-old girl with a twisted right ovary and hemorrhagic luteal cyst. (**a, d**) T2-weighted coronal and sagittal images show an enlarged ovary with multiple follicles peripherically placed and a large heterogenous cyst (*black arrow*). The associated twisted pedicle is also best seen (*arrowhead*). (**b, c**) The T1 and T1 fat-sat weighted images show a hemorrhagic cyst (*arrow*); after gadolinium (**e**) the twisted pedicle (*arrowhead*) is best seen; there is ovarian enhancement because of an incomplete torsion

ovarian torsion, such as the appendiceal abscesses (Fig. 14.22). In these cases, the ultrasound shows a heterogeneous mass on the right side of the lower abdomen very similar to an adnexal mass, and the definitive diagnosis is surgical.

Isolated tubal torsion without ovarian torsion is extremely rare but should also be considered (incidence of 1 case per 1.5 million of females). The clinical presentation is usually indistinguishable from ovarian torsion, but both entities require a timely diagnosis and a prompt surgical intervention. The tube torsion can occur in a normal tube or almost always is associated with tubal pathology such as hydrosalpinx or tubal mass. In the pediatric age, adnexal cysts (either paratubal or paraovarian) are the most common

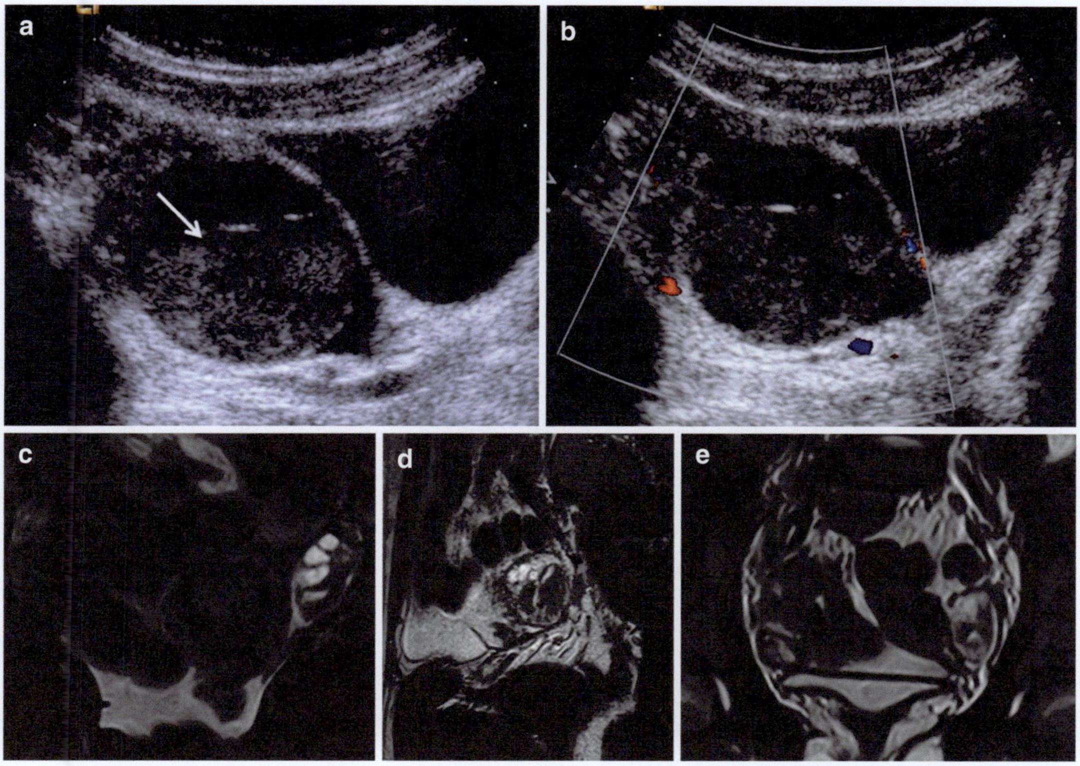

Fig. 14.20 A 13-year-old girl with abdominal pain and hemorrhagic cyst. (**a**) The transverse US shows an enlarged left ovary with a cyst with fluid-debris level (*arrow*); (**b**) no flow at Color Doppler US is seen. (**c**–**e**) At MRI, performed 3 days later, the left ovary is still enlarged with multiple follicles but the cyst disappears

cause. Imaging features include a midline cystic mass, a fusiform dilated tube with thickened echogenic walls and internal debris, or subacute hemorrhage, in the presence of the normal ipsilateral ovary (Fig. 14.23). A pathognomonic sign is the "beak sign," which refers to the tapered end of the dilated fallopian tube (Narayanan et al. 2014; Gross et al. 2005; Richard et al. 1998).

In neonatal ovarian torsion, the common differential diagnosis of ovarian cysts comprises neonatal cystic abdominal masses such as mesenteric cyst, lymphangioma, or enteric duplication cyst (Di Giacomo et al. 2014). Sometimes these pathologies are indistinguishable from complicated ovarian cyst, and the definitive diagnosis is possible only after surgery (Duigenan et al. 2012).

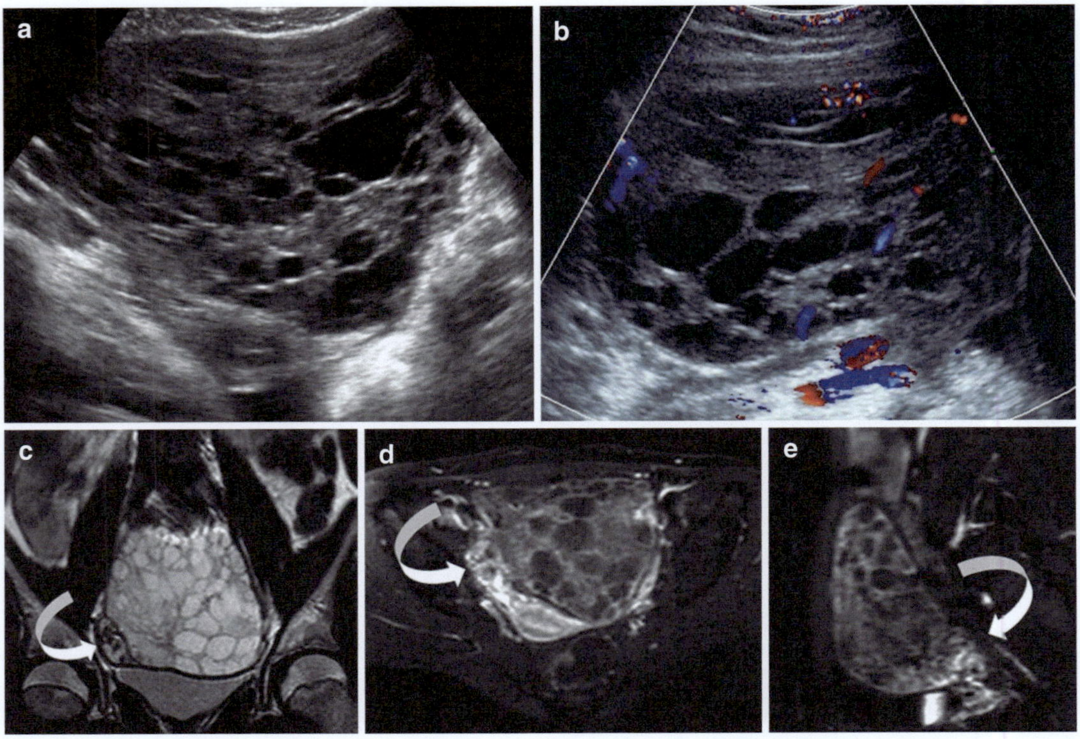

Fig. 14.21 Massive ovarian edema in a 12-year-old girl with recurrent abdominal pain. (**a**) Transverse US shows a complex pelvic mass with multiple cystic areas. (**b**) At Color Doppler, the vascularization is preserved. (**c**) Coronal T2-weighted image shows an enlarged right ovary with multiple follicles and the twisted vascular pedicle that is best seen in the axial and sagittal T1-weighted images post-contrast. (**d**, **e**) The enhancement of the ovarian stroma is preserved

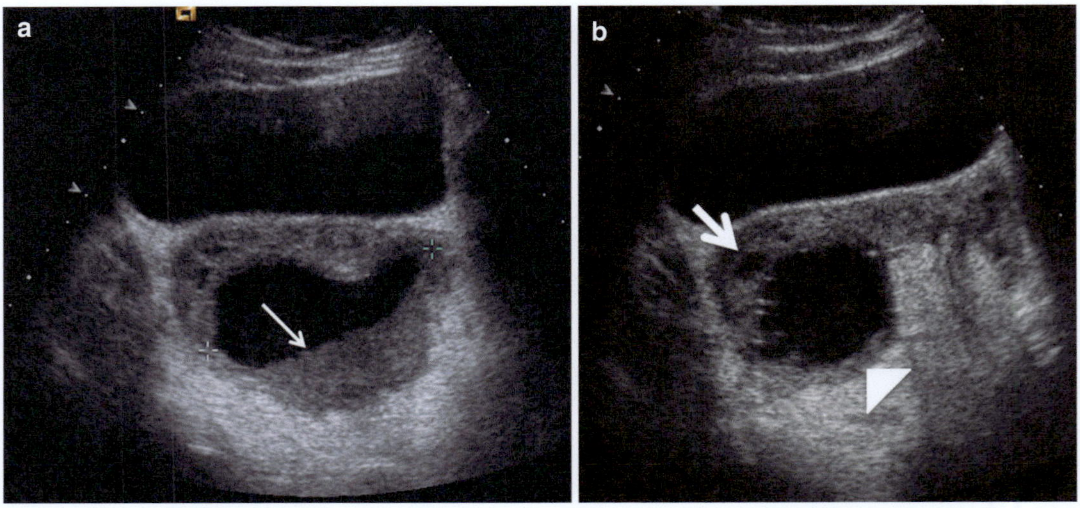

Fig. 14.22 Appendiceal abscess in an 8-year-old girl with abdominal pain, fever, and leukocytosis. (**a**) The transverse US images show a complex mass with a fluid-debris level (*arrow*); (**b**) small peripheric cystic areas (*large arrow*) and a thickened hyperechoic wall (*arrowhead*) are also noted

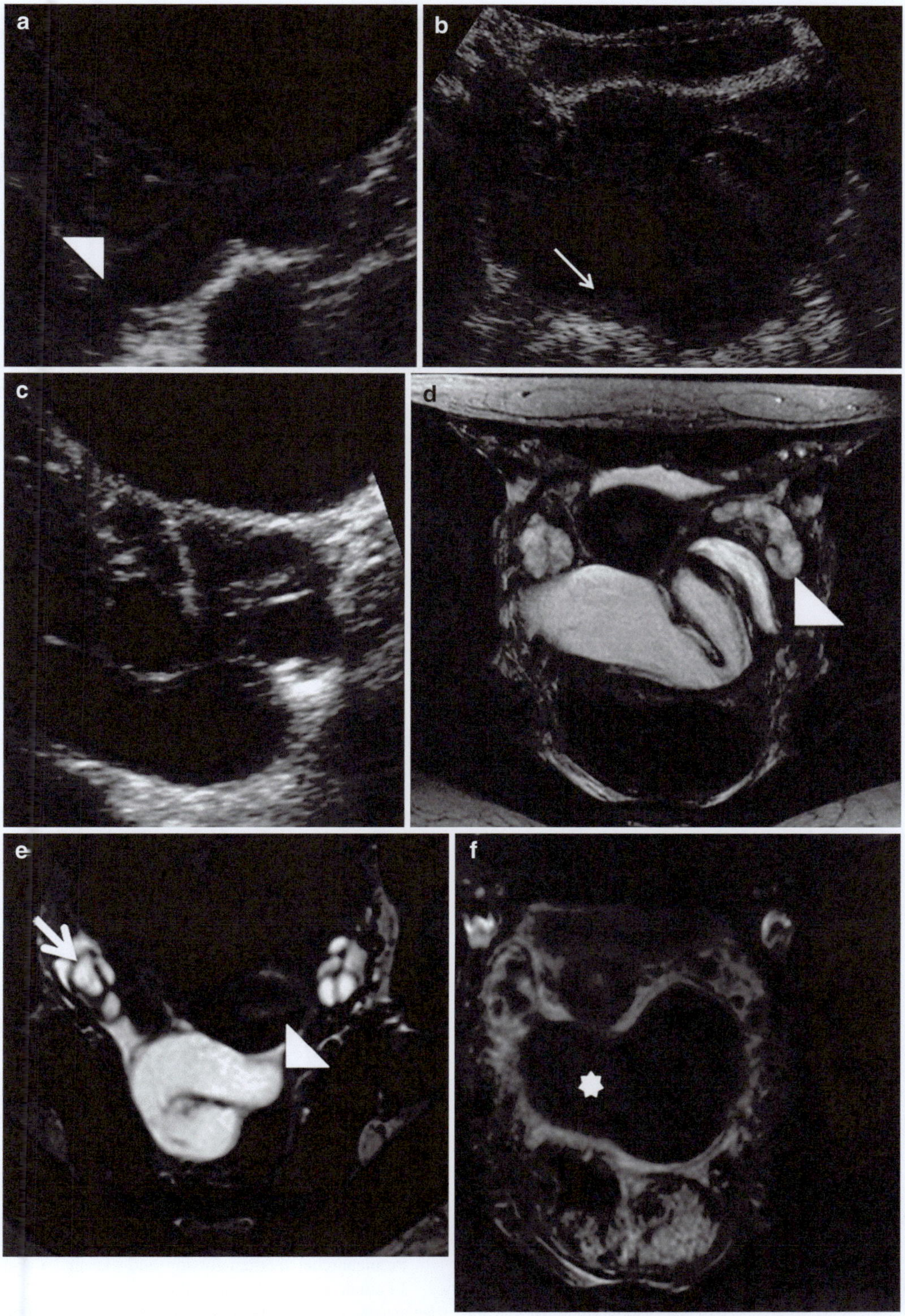

Fig. 14.23 Isolated tubal torsion in a 12-year-old girl, 4 days after menarche. (**a–c**) US images show a dilated tubular structure with internal debris (*arrow*) and the beak sign (*arrowhead*). (**d**, **e**) Axial T2-weighted images show a right enlarged thickened fallopian tube with a tapering end (*arrowhead*); the right ovary is normal (*large arrow*). (**f**) Axial T1-weighted shows hyperintense signal within the dilated tube suggestive of hematosalpinx (*asterisk*)

Conclusion

The pediatric ovarian torsion is an emergency condition. Because the clinical presentation is not specific, radiologists play a crucial role in suggesting diagnosis on cross-sectional imaging.

An asymmetric enlarged ovary with or without adnexal mass, a twisted pedicle, the subacute ovarian hemorrhage, and an abnormal contrast enhancement are not pathognomonic findings of adnexal torsion, but they are suggestive features that combined with the appropriate risk factor or clinical presentation should increase the consideration of torsion. Although the gold standard for the diagnosis of ovarian torsion is the surgery, the radiologic examination with US, CT, or MRI in small patients with acute pelvic pain is useful to recognize torsion and improve patient outcomes.

References

Albayram F, Hamper UM (2001) Ovarian and adnexal torsion: spectrum of sonographic findings with pathologic correlation. J Ultrasound Med 20:1083–1089

Buss JB, Lee RA (1987) Sequential torsion of the uterine adnexa. Mayo Clin Proc 62:623–625

Catalano O, Lobianco R, Sandomenico F et al (2004) Real-time, contrast-enhanced sonographic imaging in emergency radiology. Radiol Med 108:454–469

Celik A, Ergün O et al (2005) Long-term results of conservative management of adnexal torsion in children. J Pediatr Surg 40:704–708

Chang HC, Bhatt S, Dogra V (2008) Pearls and pitfalls in diagnosis of ovarian torsion. Radiographics 28:1355–1368

Chinchure D, Ong CL, Loh AH et al (2011) Neonatal ovarian cysts: role of sonography in diagnosing torsion. Ann Acad Med Singapore 40:291–295

Chiou SY, Lev-Toaff AS, Masuda E et al (2007) Adnexal torsion: new clinical and imaging observations by sonography, computed tomography, and magnetic resonance imaging. J Ultrasound Med 26:1289–1301

Davis AJ, Feins NR (1990) Subsequent asynchronous torsion of normal adnexa in children. J Pediatr Surg 25:687–689

Di Giacomo V, Trinci M, van der Byl G, Catania VD, Calisti A, Miele V (2014) Ultrasound in newborns and children suffering from non-traumatic acute abdominal pain: imaging with clinical and surgical correlation. J Ultrasound 18:385–393

Duigenan S, Oliva E, Lee SI (2012) Ovarian torsion: diagnostic features on CT and MRI with pathologic correlation. Am J Roentgenol 198:W122–W131

Farina R, Catalano O, Stavolo C, Sandomenico F, Petrillo A, Romano L (2015) Emergency radiology. Radiol Med 120:73–84

Fleischer AC, Stein SM, Cullinan JA et al (1995) Color Doppler sonography of adnexal torsion. J Ultrasound Med 14:523–528

Geimanaite L, Trainavicius K (2013) Ovarian torsion in children: management and outcomes. J Pediatr Surg 48:1946–1953

Gross M, Blumstein SL, Chow LC (2005) Isolated fallopian tube torsion: a rare twist on a common theme. AJR Am J Roentgenol 185:1590–1592

Hiller N, Appelbaum L, Simanovsky N et al (2007) CT features of adnexal torsion. Am J Roentgenol 189:124–129

Houry D, Abbott JT (2001) Ovarian torsion: a fifteen-year review. Ann Emerg Med 38:156–159

Huchon C, Fauconnier A (2010) Adnexal torsion: a literature review. Eur J Obstet Gynecol Reprod Biol 150:8–12

Ito K, Utano K, Kanazawa H et al (2015) CT prediction of the degree of ovarian torsion. Jpn J Radiol 33:487–493

Jain KA (2002) Sonographic spectrum of hemorrhagic ovarian cysts. J Ultrasound Med 21:879–886

Kilickesmez O, Tasdelen N, Yetimoglu B et al (2009) Diffusion-weighted imaging of adnexal torsion. Emerg Radiol 16:399–401

Kimura I, Togashi K, Kawakami S et al (1994) Ovarian torsion: CT and MR imaging appearances. Radiology 190:337–341

Kokoska ER, Keller MS, Weber TR (2000) Acute ovarian torsion in children. Am J Surg 180:462–465

Kramer LA, Lalani T, Kawashima A (1997) Massive edema of the ovary: high resolution MR findings using a phased array pelvic coil. J Magn Reson Imaging 7:758–760

Lam A, Nayyar M, Helmy M et al (2015) Assessing the clinical utility of color Doppler ultrasound for ovarian torsion in the setting of a negative contrast-enhanced CT scan of the abdomen and pelvis. Abdom Imaging 40:3206–3213

Lee EJ, Kwon HC, Joo HJ et al (1998) Diagnosis of ovarian torsion with color Doppler sonography: depiction of twisted vascular pedicle. J Ultrasound Med 17:83–89

Lourenco AP, Swenson D, Tubbs RJ et al (2014) Ovarian and tubal torsion: imaging findings on US, CT, and MRI. Emerg Radiol 21:179–187

McCarthy JD, Erickson KM, Smith YR et al (2010) Premenarchal ovarian torsion and elevated CA-125. J Pediatr Adolesc Gynecol 23:47–50

Menichini G, Sessa B, Trinci M, Galluzzo M, Miele V (2015) Accuracy of contrast-enhanced ultrasound in the identification and characterization of traumatic solid organ lesions in children: a retrospective comparison with baseline-US and CE-MDCT. Radiol Med 120:989–1001

Meyer JS, Harmon CM, Harty PM et al (1995) Ovarian torsion: clinical and imaging presentations in children. J Pediatr Surg 30:1433–1436

Miele V, Di Giampietro I (2014) Diagnostic imaging in emergency. Salute e Società, (2EN):127–138. doi:10.3280/SES2014-002010EN

Miele V, Buffa V, Galluzzo M, Stasolla A, Valentini C (2000) Idiopathic retroperitoneal fibrosis. Report of a case studied with spiral computerized tomography. Radiol Med 99:497–499

Miele V, Andreoli C, Cortese A, De Cicco ML, Luzietti M, Stasolla A, David V (2002) Hemoperitoneum following ovarian cyst rupture: CT usefulness in the diagnosis. Radiol Med 104:122–126

Miele V, Andreoli C, Grassi R (2006) The management of emergency radiology: key facts. Eur J Radiol 59:311–314

Miele V, Di Giampietro I, Ianniello S, Pinto F, Trinci M (2015) Diagnostic imaging in pediatric polytrauma management. Radiol Med 120:33–49

Miele V, Piccolo CL, Sessa B, Trinci M, Galluzzo M (2016a) Comparison between MRI and CEUS in the follow-up of patients with blunt abdominal trauma managed conservatively. Radiol Med 121:27–37

Miele V, Piccolo CL, Galluzzo M, Ianniello S, Sessa B, Trinci M (2016b) Contrast enhanced ultrasound (CEUS) in blunt abdominal trauma. Br J Radiol 89(1061):20150823. doi:10.1259/bjr.20150823Epub2016Jan8

Miele V, Piccolo CL, Trinci M, Galluzzo M, Ianniello S, Brunese L (2016c) Diagnostic imaging of blunt abdominal trauma in pediatric patients. Radiol Med 121:409–430. doi:10.1007/s11547-016-0637-2, Epub 2016 Apr 13

Narayanan S, Bandarkar A, Bulas DI (2014) Fallopian tube torsion in the pediatric age group: radiologic evaluation. J Ultrasound Med 33:1697–1704

Ngo AV, Otjen JP, Parisi MT et al (2015) Pediatric ovarian torsion: a pictorial review. Pediatr Radiol 45:1845–1855

Nussbaum AR, Sanders RC, Hartman DS et al (1988) Neonatal ovarian cysts: sonographic-pathologic correlation. Radiology 168:817–821

Oltmann SC, Fischer A, Barber R et al (2009) Cannot exclude torsion – a 15-year review. J Pediatr Surg 44:1212–1216

Otjen JP, Stanescu L, Goldin A et al (2015) A normal ovary in an abnormal location: a case of torsion. J Clin Ultrasound 43:578–580

Pinto F, Miele V, Scaglione M, Pinto A (2014) The use of contrast-enhanced ultrasound in blunt abdominal trauma: advantages and limitations. Acta Radiol 55:776–784

Pinto F, Valentino M, Romanini L, Basilico R, Miele V (2015) The role of CEUS in the assessment haemodynamically stable patients with blunt abdominal trauma. Radiol Med 120:3–11

Poonai N, Poonai C et al (2013) Pediatric ovarian torsion: case series and review of the literature. Can J Surg 56:103–108

Rey-Bellet Gasser C, Gehri M, Joseph JM et al (2016) Is it ovarian torsion? A systematic literature review and evaluation of prediction signs. Pediatr Emerg Care 32:256–261

Rha SE, Byun JY, Jung SE et al (2002) CT and MR imaging features of adnexal torsion. Radiographics 22:283–294

Richard HM 3rd, Parsons RB, Broadman KF et al (1998) Torsion of the fallopian tube: progression of sonographic features. J Clin Ultrasound 26:374–376

Roche O, Chavan N, Aquilina J et al (2012) Radiological appearances of gynaecological emergencies. Insights Imaging 3:265–275

Sasaki KJ, Miller CE (2014) Adnexal torsion: review of the literature. J Minim Invasive Gynecol 21:196–202

Schmitt ER, Ngai SS, Gausche-Hill M et al (2013) Twist and shout! Pediatric ovarian torsion clinical update and case discussion. Pediatr Emerg Care 29:518–523

Servaes S, Zurakowski D, Laufer MR et al (2007) Sonographic findings of ovarian torsion in children. Pediatr Radiol 37:446–451

Sessa B, Trinci M, Ianniello S, Menichini G, Galluzzo M, Miele V (2015) Blunt abdominal trauma: role of Contrast-Enhanced Ultrasound in the detection and staging of abdominal traumatic lesions compared with US and CE-MDCT. Radiol Med 120:180–189

Spinelli C, Piscioneri J, Strambi S (2015) Adnexal torsion in adolescents: update and review of the literature. Curr Opin Obstet Gynecol 27:320–325

Swenson DW, Lourenco AP, Beaudoin FL et al (2014) Ovarian torsion: case-control study comparing the sensitivity and specificity of ultrasonography and computed tomography for diagnosis in the emergency department. Eur J Radiol 83:733–738

Takeda A, Mori M, Sakai K et al (2009) Laparoscopic management of ovarian dysgerminoma presenting with acute abdomen caused by adnexal torsion in a 17-year-old girl. J Pediatr Adolesc Gynecol 22:9–13

Varras M, Tsikini A, Polyzos D et al (2004) Uterine adnexal torsion: pathologic and gray scale ultrasonographic findings. Clin Exp Obst Gyn 31:34–38

Villalba ML, Huynh B, So M et al (2005) An ovary with a twist: a case of interesting sonographic findings of ovarian torsion. J Emerg Med 29:443–446

Wilkinson C, Sanderson A (2012) Adnexal torsion—a multimodality imaging review. Clin Radiol 67:476–483

Complications of Urachal Remnants 15

Maria Elena Latini, Sara Riccioni, Nicola Recchia, Maria Napoletano, and Michele Scialpi

15.1 Definition

The term urachal remnants (URs) refers to a series of anomalies due to the partial or total failure of the urachus obliteration.

15.2 Epidemiology

URs are usually diagnosed in children, while they are rare in adults. The incidence ranges from 1:150,000 among the infants to 1:5,000 in the adult population (Jeong-Sik et al. 1999). They are sometimes associated with other anomalies such as hypospadias, meatal stenosis, bladder-ureteral reflux, renal ectopia, umbilical and inguinal hernias, cryptorchidism, anal atresia, and omphalocele.

URs are almost twice as likely to be diagnosticated in men as in women.

15.3 Physiopathology

Urachus is an embryological remnant of the allantois, which originates from the yolk sac, and of the cloaca, which is the cephalic extension of the urogenital sinus. Between the fourth and the fifth month of gestation, the fetal bladder tends gradually to descend toward the pelvis, and its apical portion creates the urachus, an epithelialized fibromuscular strand. Its length varies from 3 to 10 cm and its diameter from 8 to 10 mm. Its lumen is lined by transitional epithelium in 70 % of cases and by columnar epithelium in the remaining 30 %. The epithelium is surrounded by submucosal connective tissue and smooth muscle tissue, the latter in continuity with the detrusor muscle. This tubular structure, extending from the anterosuperior surface of the bladder toward the umbilicus, connects the bladder dome with the umbilical cord and is located behind the transversalis fascia and anterior to the peritoneum, in the space of Retzius. During the descent of the bladder into fetal life, the urachus obliterates itself, becoming a residual fibromuscular cord: the median umbilical ligament (Jeong-Sik et al. 1999; Bertozzi et al. 2009).

Its persistence over intrauterine life can be manifested with different pathologies, known as urachal remnants. Various URs are due to the different levels of the incomplete regression of the urachus.

Patent urachus, or bladder-umbilical fistula (50 % of cases), comes with a full communication between the bladder and the navel (Fig. 15.1). The urachal cyst (30 %), most frequently in the lower third of the urachus, is a cystic mass that may be encountered frequently in infectious

M.E. Latini (✉) • S. Riccioni • N. Recchia
M. Napoletano • M. Scialpi
Division of Radiology, Department of Surgical and Biomedical Sciences, S. Maria della Misericordia Hospital, S. Andrea delle Fratte, Perugia, Italy
e-mail: elenalatini@hotmail.com

V. Miele, M. Trinci (eds.), *Imaging Non-traumatic Abdominal Emergencies in Pediatric Patients*,
DOI 10.1007/978-3-319-41866-7_15

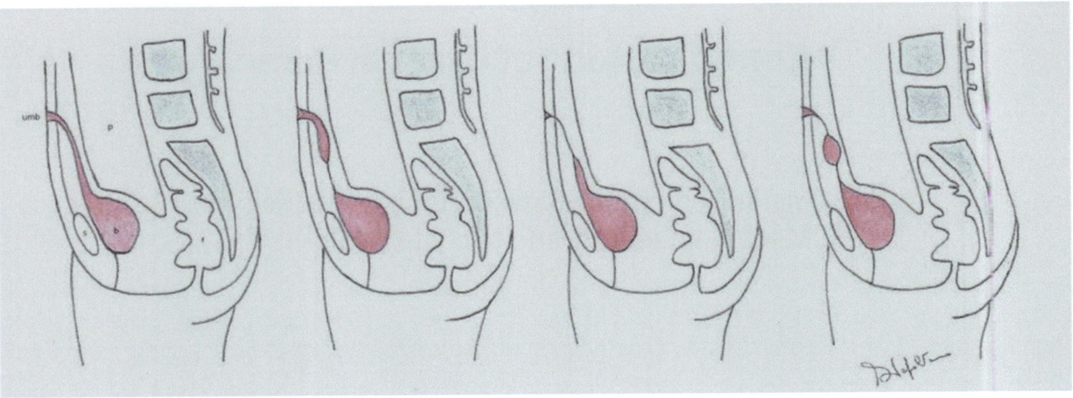

Fig. 15.1 Patent urachus, urachal sinus, urachal diverticulum, urachal cyst

processes for contiguity with the bladder or can become infected hematogenously; it rarely can break into the peritoneum causing peritonitis (Fig. 15.1). Urachal sinus (15 %) shows a dead-end cavity which opens in the navel, sometimes secreting bloody or mucinous material (Fig. 15.1). Finally we have the urachal diverticulum (5 %) which develops from the apex of the bladder and is often asymptomatic (Fig. 15.1). Umbilical-urachal sinus, bladder-urachal diverticulum, and urachal cysts tend to obliterate after birth. However they may reopen after acquired complications, among which, the most frequent are infections. These can spread through blood, lymph, or from the bladder.

Occasionally, some complications, as infections and benign or malignant neoplastic transformation, may develop from the original diseases.

15.4 Symptoms/Clinical Features

The majority of patients with URs, except those with patent urachus, are asymptomatic. Sometimes they become symptomatic in association with certain complications, as the infections.

Patients with infection of URs present with dysuria and lower abdominal pain, urinary tract infections, stranguria, and fever, rarely nausea, vomiting, and constipation. Some signs are hypogastric mass; painful palpation of the lower abdomen with muscle guarding; umbilical mucinous, urinary, or bloody discharge; erythema and a tender umbilical mass; hematuria; and pyuria. Blood analysis shows increase in white blood cell count (leukocytosis) and an increase of PCR. Urinalysis reveals some (5–20 or more) white or red cells per high power fields (Bertozzi et al. 2009, 2014; Copp et al. 2009; Naiditch et al. 2013).

These symptoms and signs may be misdiagnosed as appendicitis, urinary tract infection, Meckel's diverticulitis, acute prostatitis, pelvic inflammatory disease, and bladder carcinoma.

Each anomaly has some particular symptom or sign (Jeong-Sik et al. 1999; Bertozzi et al. 2015).

Patients with patent urachus often present urine leakage from the umbilicus during the neonatal period. Sometimes they are asymptomatic, but an acquired obstructive lesion of the distal urinary tract may result in umbilical-urinary fistulas.

Patients with urachal sinus usually present a small opening of this anomaly into the umbilicus, and this may result in a periodic discharge of bloody or mucinous material. In addition, this anomaly is often associated with infections.

Urachal diverticulum is often asymptomatic and is usually discovered accidentally. In fact, this anomaly is discovered in patients with urinary tract infections, due to stone formation in the diverticulum, in subjects with urinary outflow obstruction, and does not be underestimated because of the risk of evolution (1 %) toward urachal cancer.

Urachal cysts are usually discovered accidentally, or when they increase in size. Also in this case, infections are most commonly associated complications. Superinfected urachal cysts occur with fever, ipogastric pain, abdominal palpable mass, and abdominal tenderness. Sometimes they can break leading to peritonitis.

From the above it is clear how URs are subject to infectious complications. The route of infection may be hematological, lymphatic, or the urinary tract through the bladder. A broad spectrum of bacteria can be the cause, both gram positive and gram negative. Drainage of infected fluids may be either to the bladder (urachal diverticulum), toward the umbilicus (urachal sinus), or in both directions (patent urachus and urachal cysts) In each of these conditions, US, CT, or MRI are useful for the diagnosis. These can be associated with percutaneous drainage purposes, both diagnostic and therapeutic. In most cases of infected URs, the surgical removal of the cyst wall is essential due to the potential risk of reinfection and neoplasm development in unresected or incompletely resected URs. Surgical intervention should be avoided for the patient under 1 year of age because URs might spontaneously disappear (Bertozzi et al. 2009, 2014).

Benign urachal neoplasms, including adenoma, fibromas, fibroadenomas, fibromyomas, and hamartomas, are extremely rare. Malignant urachal neoplasms are less than 1 % of the bladder cancer cases. Urachal carcinoma predominantly manifests as adenocarcinoma (90 %), and the prognosis is considerably worse than that of primary bladder adenocarcinoma. Urachal tumors are typically silent because of their extraperitoneal location, and the majority of patients exhibit local invasion or metastatic disease at presentation. These tumors are most commonly seen in patients aged over 50 years, mostly males, although patients as young as 15 years old have been documented (Jeong-Sik et al. 1999).

However, despite the risk that the urachal remnant develops malignancy is relatively low, it is important that patients with a urachal remnant are aware of the risk they are in. In particular the decision is usually postponed to the parents after properly consulting with the pediatrician, radiologist, and the pediatric surgeon.

It is very important to remove the infected URs due to the infection recurrence risk and the risk of malignant evolution of the urachal epithelium (Bertozzi et al. 2009, 2014).

15.5 Imaging

In most cases of emergencies related to complications of the URs ultrasound study, it is sufficient to obtain optimal imaging of the case. Only in certain cases of particular complexity, it can be useful deepening by CT or MRI study.

15.5.1 US Protocol and Features

US study involves the use of both convex and linear probes, which is associated with the possibility of Color Doppler imaging to assess any hyperemic conditions. To better understand the emergency imaging, we observe how URs present in the absence of complications.

URs usually appear as thread-like formations, hypoechoic below the alba line, which start below the umbilicus and come up to the bladder, sometimes not pervious and sometimes with increased caliber and tubular morphology (patent urachus, Fig. 15.2) Ueno et al. (2003). Other times, the URs appear as hypoechoic

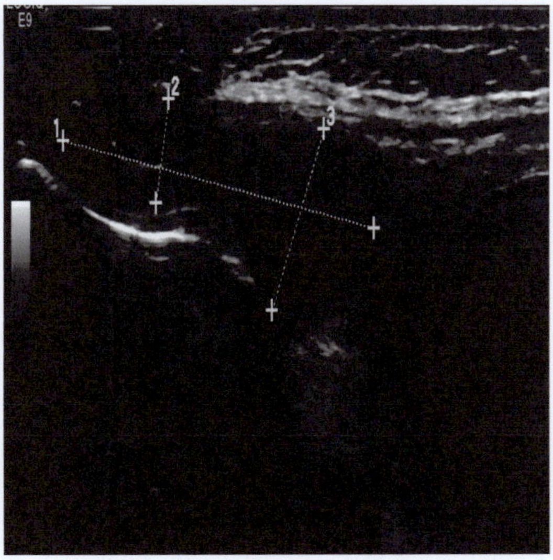

Fig. 15.2 Ultrasound shows a patent urachus with at least two cystic dilations along its course

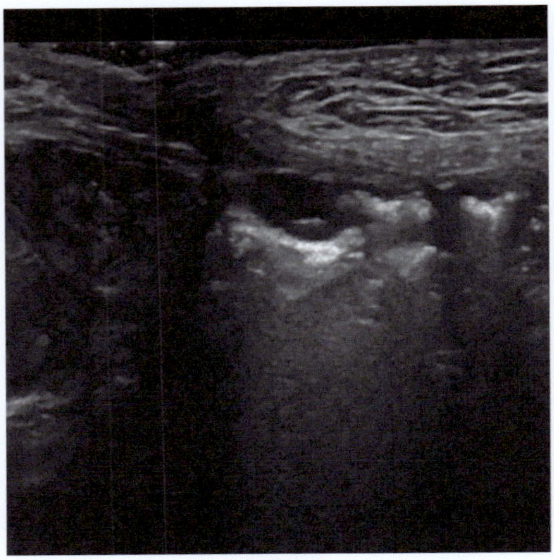

Fig. 15.3 US shows a urachal sinus as hypoechoic tubular formations, starting from the umbilicus, developing behind the anterior abdominal wall, along the mid-paramedian line, to finish dead end

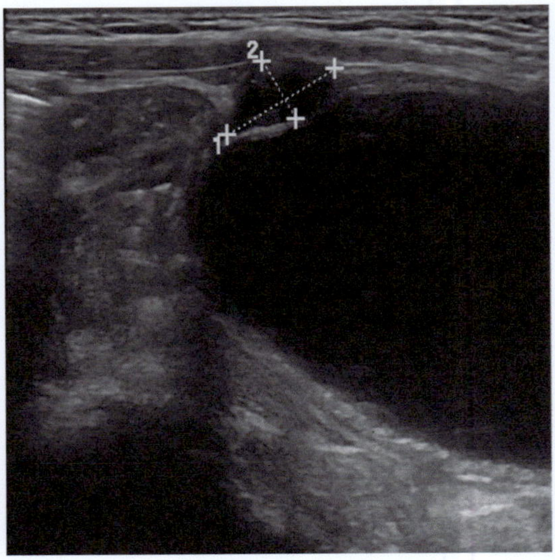

Fig. 15.4 Ultrasound shows a urachal cyst as oval formations at the level of the mid-paramedian line, hypoechoic, that do not break the bladder parietal line

tubular formations, starting from the umbilicus, developing behind the anterior abdominal wall, along the mid-paramedian line, to finish dead end (urachal sinus, Fig. 15.3). More rarely URs look like diverticular eversion that, from the bladder dome, projected toward the umbilicus along the median line ending in a dead end (urachal diverticulum). Frequently the URs are also presented as oval formations, mainly in correspondence of the front bladder wall, at the level of the mid-paramedian line, hypoechoic, which does not break the bladder's parietal line (urachal cyst, Fig. 15.4) (Bertozzi et al. 2009).

In case of inflammatory complications, the above-described signs are enriched with signs that may suggest inflammation in place, and in these cases US is usually sufficient to diagnose infected URs (Figs. 15.5 and 15.6).

One of the first signs is the increase in size of the URs, which is associated with a heterogeneously hypoechoic appearance of the content. The walls appear thickened, irregular, and nuanced. Internal septa may appear, often hyperemic, with pluri-concamerate aspect of the collection. Some associated signs are an increase in size of the adjacent lymph nodes, which may develop purulent complications and appear with polycyclic margins, a heterogeneously hyperechoic structure, and a reduced peripheral vascularity (Donnelly and Frush 2001; Widni et al. 2010; Di Giacomo et al. 2015).

It may present fluid layers into Retzius space, into Douglas space, and between intestinal loops with associated heterogeneously hyperechoic appearance of perilesional adipose tissue (Donnelly and Frush 2001; Widni et al. 2010).

In the case of infected urachal sinus, it can appear as a hypoechoic and hyperemic umbilical scar, which is associated with a heterogeneously hypoechoic formation, with cerebriform morphology, which extends along the linea alba, outlining the framework of an omphalitis with sub-umbilical abscess (Di Giacomo et al. 2015).

15.5.2 Multidetector-row computed tomography (MDCT) Protocol and Features

MDCT for its wide dissemination, is a common method of second instance for the study of the URs. It offers a wide anatomical multiplanar view of the inflammatory condition. In particular, in scans without contrast, it shows the presence of a thick-walled cystic mass superior to the dome of the bladder diffusely contiguous with the anterior

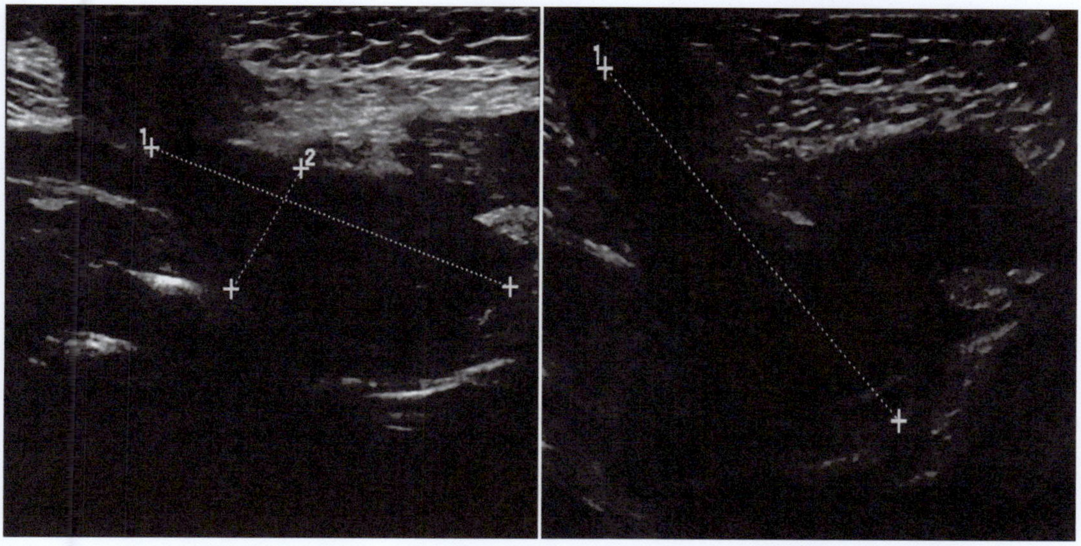

Fig. 15.5 Ultrasound shows a urachal sinus abscess: hypodense collection that is projected along the central line, in continuity with the umbilical scar

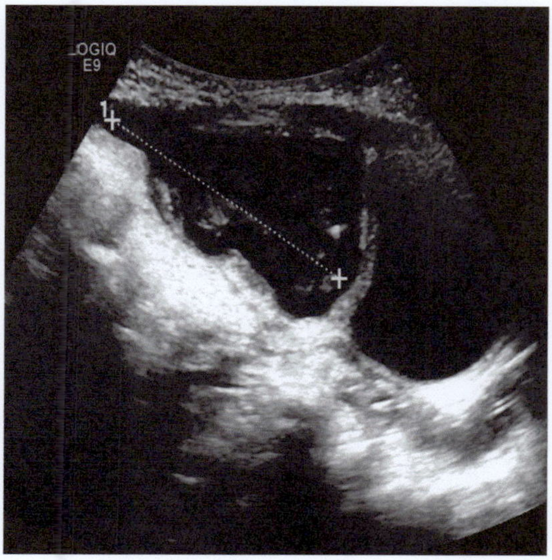

Fig. 15.6 US shows an infected cyst as a heterogeneously hypoechoic collection whose wall appear thickened, irregular, and nuanced; the collection imprints the bladder dome

abdominal wall. This collection has a heterogeneously hypodense lumen with a hyperdense wall. The wall can show a positive CE after MDC injection. This method may show infiltration of perilesional adipose tissue and reactive lymphadenopathy of abdominal-pelvic lymph nodes. It can show also free peritoneal fluid in the abdomen (Jeong-Sik et al. 1999; Donnelly and Frush 2001; Nimmonrat et al. 2008).

15.5.3 MRI Protocols and Features

MRI is performed with multiplanar T2 and axial T1 sequences (Fig. 15.7).

This method, where available, is an excellent alternative to CT, especially in pediatric patients that need to be preserved from the radiation exposure.

The examination, in case of the URs inflammation associated with collection, shows expansive formation, with ovular morphology, behind the anterior abdominal wall, in the median-paramedian. Sometimes there is a continuity with the umbilical scar (sinus with inflammation, Fig. 15.8), sometimes not (cysts with inflammation, Fig. 15.9), or a contact with the bladder dome.

The lesion appears pluri-concamerate, with walls hyperintense on T2 and hypointense on T1, sometimes with polylobulated appearance. The content is dishomogeneous, hyperintense in T2 and hypointense with hyperintense septa on T1.

There may be associated fluid flaps in the pelvic recesses and between intestinal loops and thickening of perilesional adipose tissue and of periumbilical subcutaneous tissue.

In case of perivesical collection, MRI shows wall thickening and a multilayered look as widespread inflammation. In more advanced cases, it may present continuity solutions between the collection and the bladder dome.

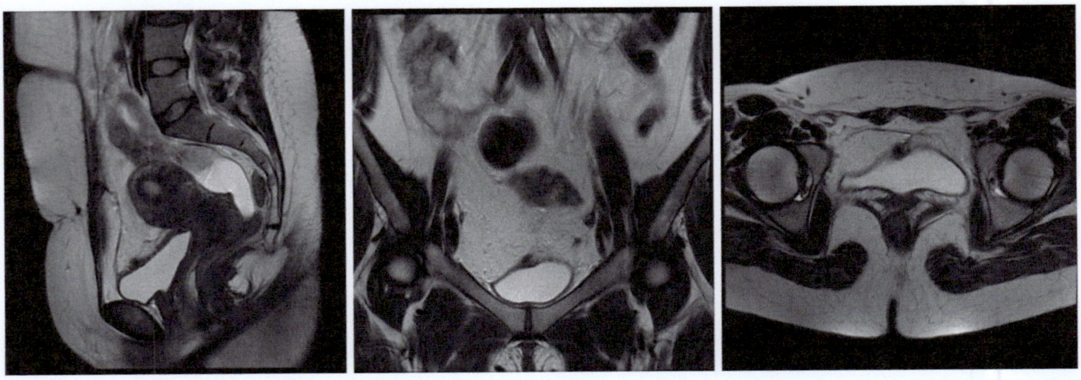

Fig. 15.7 MRI shows a urachal cyst in the paramedian, in contact with the bladder dome; there are no signs of disruption of the bladder wall

In conclusion, US is the first choice and decisive method in the diagnosis of emergencies associated with URs. If a more detailed diagnosis is needed, CT and MRI represent a great depth instrument, bearing in mind that the latter preserves the young patient from exposure to the radiation. For such reason and given their excellent imaging, US and MRI offer alternative radiation-free options that, where available, have almost completely replaced CT in the URs setting in pediatric patients.

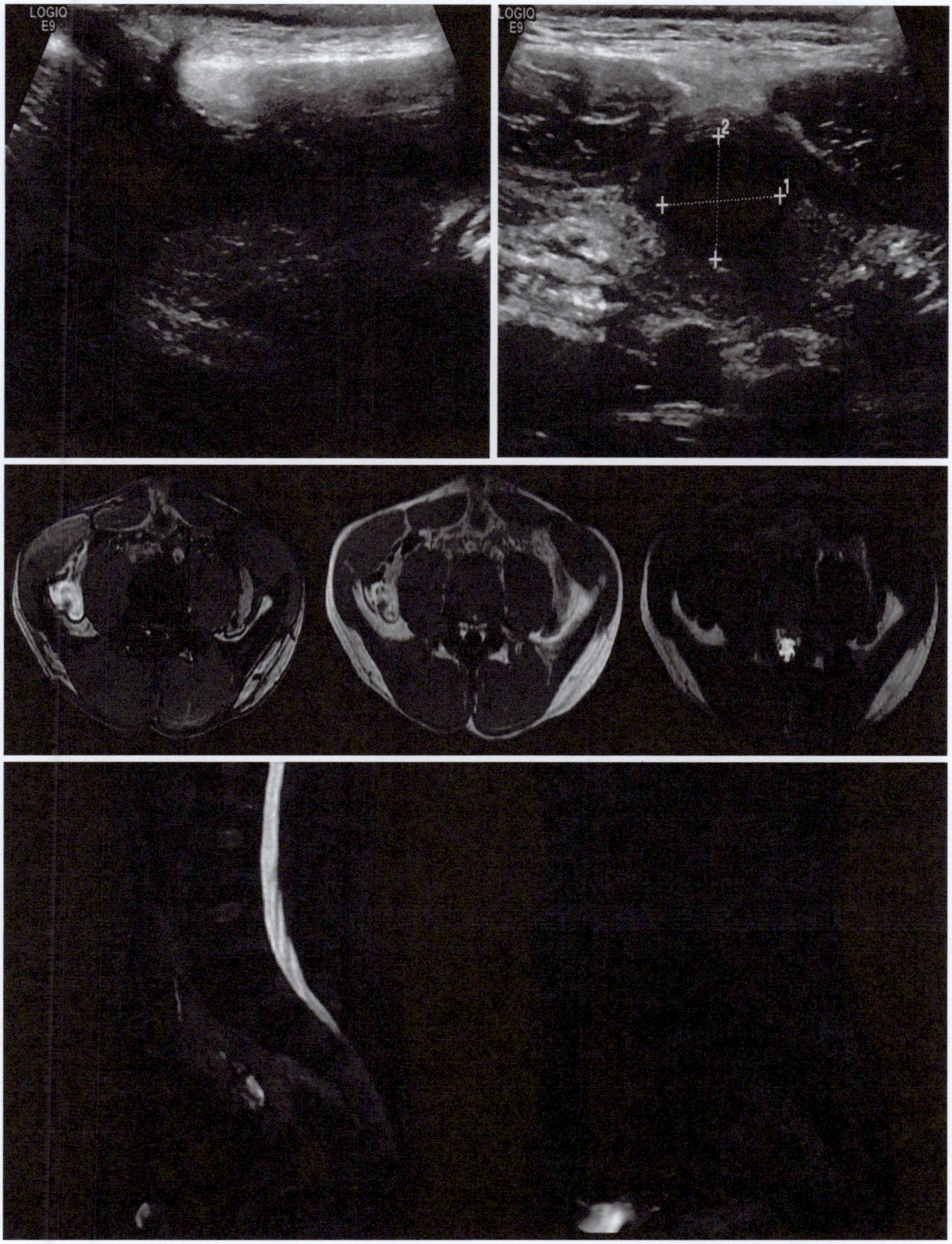

Fig. 15.8 The first two ultrasound images show, in the context of the subcutaneous tissue in the lower periumbilical, a corpuscular anechoic mass, surrounded by fatty tissue dimly hyperechogenic (urachal complicated cysts). The diagnostic study continues through MRI T1-weighted sequences in phase and out of phase and T2-weighted axial and coronal: hypointense on T1 collection, heterogeneously hyperintense on T2, with wall thickened hyperintensely on T1 and slightly hyperintense on T2

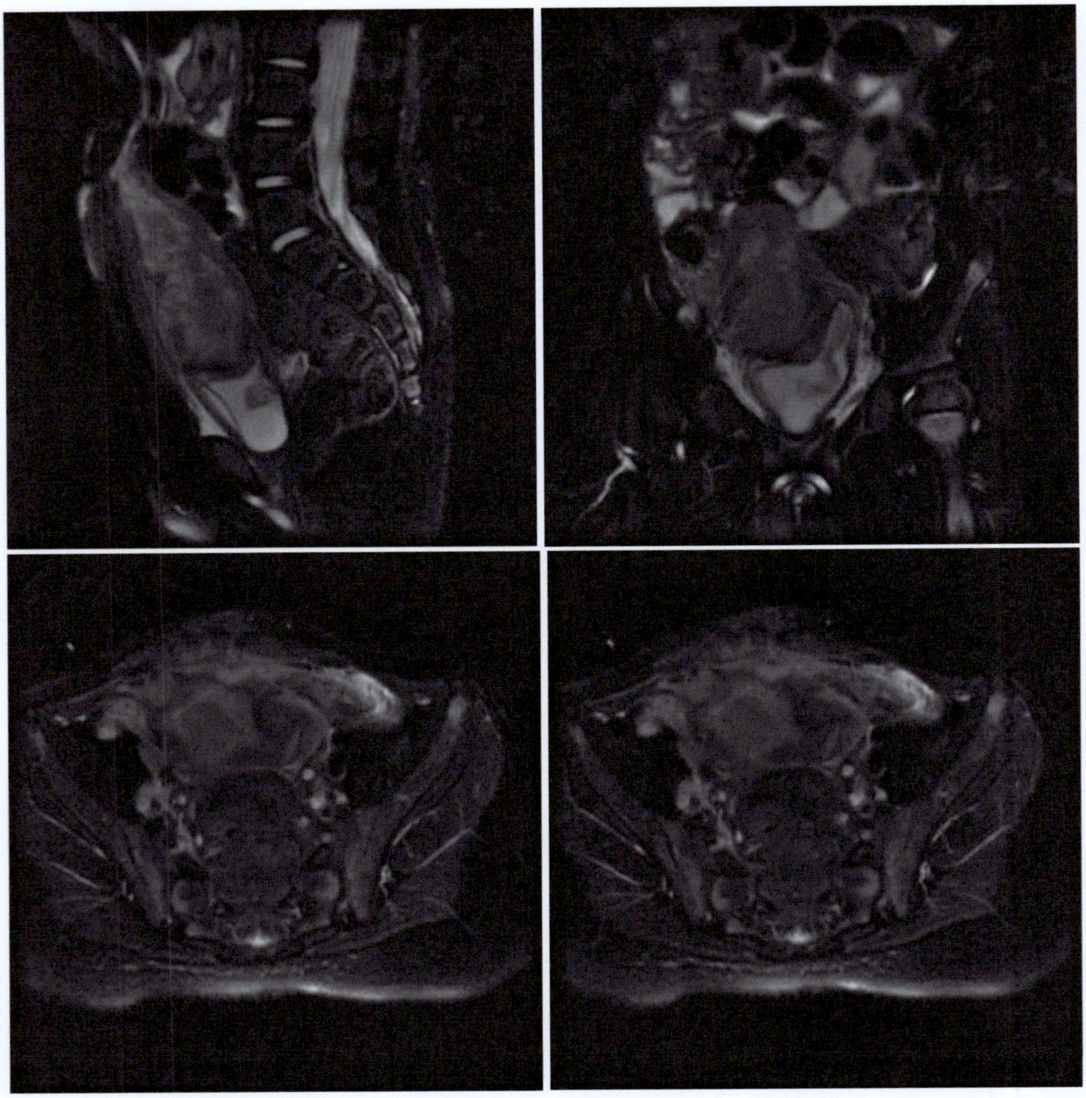

Fig. 15.9 MRI shows an expansive formation, with ovular morphology, behind the anterior abdominal wall, in the median-paramedian. The collection appears pluri-concamerate, with walls hypointense on T2 and hypointense on T1, sometimes with polylobulated appearance. The content is dishomogeneous, hyperintense in T2 and hypointense with hyperintense septa on T1

References

Bertozzi M, Nardi N, Prestipino M, Magrini E, Appignani A (2009) Minimally invasive removal of urachal remnants in childhood. Pediatr Med Chir 31:265–268

Bertozzi M, Riccioni S, Appignani A (2014) Laparoscopic treatment of symptomatic urachal remnants in children. J Endourol 28:1091–1096. doi:10.1089/end.2014.0203. Epub 2014 Jun 3

Bertozzi M, Verrotti A, Di Cara G, Riccioni S, Rinaldi VE, Magrini E, Appignani A (2015) Massive pyuria as an unusual presentation of giant infected urachal remnant in a child. Ann Pediatr Surg 11:244–246

Copp HL, Wong IY, Krwashnan C, Malhotra S, Kennedy WA (2009) Clinical presentation and urachal remnant pathology: implications for treatment. J Urol 182(4 Suppl):1921–1924. doi:10.1016/j.juro.2009.03.026. Epub 2009 Aug 20

Di Giacomo V, Trinci M, Van der Byl G, Catania VD, Calisti A, Miele V (2015) Ultrasound in newborns and children suffering from nontraumatic acute abdominal pain: imaging with clinical and surgical correlation. J Ultrasound 18:385–393. doi:10.1007/s40477-014-0087-4. Epub 2014 Apr 9

Donnelly LF, Frush DP (2001) Cross-sectional imaging of abnormalities of the abdominal wall in pediatric patients. AJR Am J Roentgenol 176:1233–1239

Jeong-Sik Y, Ki Whang K, Hwa-Jin L, Young-Jun L, Choon-Sik Y, and Myung-Joon K (1999) Urachal remnant diseases: spectrum of CT and US findings. Presented as a scientific exhibit at the 1999 RSNA scientific assembly. Received March 21, 2000; revision requested June 8 and received June 28; accepted June 29

Naiditch JA, Radhakrishnan J, Chin AC (2013) Current diagnosis and management of urachal remnants. J Pediatr Surg 48:2148–2152. doi:10.1016/j.jpedsurg.2013.02.069

Nimmonrat A, Na-ChiangMai W, Muttarak M (2008) Urachal abnormalities: clinical and imaging features. Singap Med J 49:930–935

Ueno T, Hashimoto H, Yokoyama H, Ito M, Kouda K, Kanamaru H (2003) Urachal anomalies: ultrasonography and management. J Pediatr Surg 38:1203–1207

Widni E, Michael E, Höllwarth ME, Haxhija EQ (2010) The impact of preoperative ultrasound on correct diagnosis of urachal remnants in children. J Pediatr Surg 45:1433–1437. doi:10.1016/j.jpedsurg.2010.01.001

Nephro-urolithiasis

16

Francesca Pancrazi, Giulia Angelini, Laura Turturici, Laura Tasciotti, Claudio Defilippi, and Michele Tonerini

16.1 Introduction

Nephro-urolithiasis is increasingly diagnosed in children, and it is an important cause of morbidity worldwide. Most common risk factors are infection and metabolic diseases.

Its clinical presentation varies, and in young children, we do not observe the classic acute onset of flank pain commonly seen in adults, but vague abdominal pain, hematuria, and urinary tract infection are more common.

As a result, children are frequently evaluated for other conditions before the diagnosis of nephrolithiasis is made. However a prompt diagnosis in an acute phase is crucial to exclude subsequent complications including renal failure.

At imaging examinations calculi are usually visible on plain radiographs, but sometimes they cannot be identified, either because they are radiolucent or obscured by overlying bowel gas or feces. Ultrasound (US) is the first imaging modality in children with suspected renal tract calculosis. Complications such as obstruction and subsequently dilatation of the proximal upper tract might be visible at US. In children presenting with symptoms suggestive of urolithiasis and a negative US, plain film radiographs or an unenhanced computed tomography (CT) should be performed for confirmation or exclusion. This latter examination might be especially useful for the diagnosis of very small calculi and calculi with poor radiographic density, but should be considered as the last choice due to higher radiation exposure.

16.2 Epidemiology

In pediatric age, nephro-urolithiasis is a worldwide problem and is the result of a multifactorial process. It affects children of all ages with a wide range of incidence and prevalence. According to age, gender, location, and stone composition, it is related to climatic, genetic, dietary, and socioeconomic factors too.

In the developed European countries, the overall incidence of stones in children is reported to be less than two per one million total population, and in the United States, stone disease accounted for 1 in 7600–1000 hospital admissions in children (Lima and Manzoni 2015). Advances in imaging techniques, improved socioeconomic conditions, obesity, and increased consumption

F. Pancrazi • G. Angelini • L. Turturici
Department of Diagnostic and Interventional Radiology, University of Pisa, Pisa, Italy

L. Tasciotti • C. Defilippi
Pediatric Radiology, Meyer University Children's Hospital, Florence, Italy

M. Tonerini (✉)
Department of Emergency Radiology, Cisanello University Hospital, Pisa, Italy
e-mail: m.tonerini@tiscali.it

V. Miele, M. Trinci (eds.), *Imaging Non-traumatic Abdominal Emergencies in Pediatric Patients*,
DOI 10.1007/978-3-319-41866-7_16

of protein-rich diets and dairy products are some of the factors contributing to the increased incidence of this disease in the Western countries.

On the other side, a geographical "stone belt" is described extending from the Balkans across Turkey, Pakistan, and Northern India which is characterized by a high incidence of endemic bladder stones in children due to a chronically inadequate dietary intake of protein and relative dehydration associated with the climate and diarrheal illness (Lima and Manzoni 2015). These data confirm the studies reporting a prevalence of upper tract stones in the developed world and lower tract stones in the developing world.

In the recent decades, studies have shown an age stratification with more kidney stones in younger boys and greater proportions of urolithiasis in adolescent girls (Hernandez et al. 2015).

16.3 Pathogenesis, Etiology, and Risk Factors

Stone formation is a multifactorial process that involves both the patient's underlying metabolic background and the environmental conditions. Multistep pathogenesis includes supersaturation of lithogenics (calcium, oxalate, and phosphate), nucleation, crystal growth, crystal aggregation, and crystal retention (Sas 2011). The supersaturation (crystallization) of certain ions in the urine is the core basis for the formation of calculi. Urine solubility depends on total urine volume, urine pH, and concentration of stone-forming ions, of inhibitors of crystallization, and of promoters of crystallization. Over the past decade and as a result of improvement in the diagnosis and treatment of urinary tract infections, the etiology of pediatric nephrolithiasis has shifted from predominantly infectious to metabolic causes. Nowadays metabolic disorders account for 50 % of all pediatric nephrolithiasis, while infections only for 10 % (especially in developing countries and younger children). Other causes are urinary tract abnormalities (20 %), idiopathic (15 %), and 5 % for cystic fibrosis, surgically augmented bladders, and other pathologies (Kaplan and Meyers 2004; Calisti et al. 2008).

- *Metabolic disorders*. When a metabolite is excreted in high concentrations and its saturation point in the urine is exceeded, crystal deposition occurs, progressing to stone formation. Different disorders of metabolites excretion might occur such as hypercalciuria, hyperoxaluria and oxalosis, cystinuria, and hyperuricosuria.
  - *Hypercalciuria* is the most common metabolic cause of pediatric urinary calculi (up to 25 % of patients) and is usually due to many different causes. In most cases it is idiopathic, with two subtypes described: the first with an enhanced gastrointestinal absorption of calcium and the second with a reduced renal tubular reabsorption of calcium from the glomerular filtrate. Urinary calcium excretion is much higher in infants than in older children. Most children who have hypercalciuria and urolithiasis have normal serum calcium concentrations.
  - *Hyperoxaluria and oxalosis*. Hyperoxaluria is observed in 2–20 % of children and adolescents with urolithiasis. The primary hyperoxalurias, types I and II, are rare autosomal recessive disorders caused by defects in specific hepatic enzymes that result in overproduction of oxalate. Secondary hyperoxaluria occurs with an excessive intake of oxalate precursors, increased absorption of oxalate (inflammatory bowel disease, extensive bowel resection), or deficiency of cofactors in oxalate metabolism. Diets low in calcium predispose to hyperoxaluria due to reduced binding of oxalate to calcium in the intestinal lumen, leaving oxalate free to be absorbed. Abnormalities of the intestinal tract that result in malabsorption of fat typically result in enhanced absorption of oxalate, referred to as "enteric hyperoxaluria."
  - *Cystinuria* accounts for 2–8 % of stones in children and adolescents. An inherited defect in the renal tubular reabsorptive transport of cystine and the dibasic amino acids accounts for the high concentrations of cystine in the urine of patients with this disorder. The only clinical manifestations

of cystinuria are recurrent nephrolithiasis and its complications.
- *Hyperuricosuria* is found in 2–10 % of children with urolithiasis. It may be idiopathic or due to a defect in renal tubular transport of uric acid, high purine intake, uricosuric drugs, renal tubular disorders, cyanotic congenital heart disease, hemolysis, and myeloproliferative disorders, massive cell breakdown (after cytotoxic treatment).

- *Urinary tract infection*. Improvements in healthy conditions, medical treatments, and urologic surgical options for children have reduced the incidence of stones due to urinary tract infections. Specific infective agents like *Proteus* sp., *Providencia* sp., some strains of *Klebsiella* sp., *Pseudomonas* sp., and enterococci are strongly associated with stones due to the consequent elevation of the urinary pH and precipitation of ammonium salts. The association with urine urease – a bacterial product not present in sterile urine – creates a unique urinary milieu that is highly favorable to struvite (magnesium ammonium phosphate) stone formation. Struvite stones containing carbonate apatite tend to branch and enlarge, often filling the renal calyces and producing a "staghorn" appearance. Nowadays it has been reported that most struvite calculi develop from metabolic abnormalities; in particular 30–60 % of patients with infection stones can be demonstrated to have metabolic factors predisposing to stone formation.
- *Anatomical abnormalities of the urinary tract* can be identified in approximately 20–30 % of children with urinary calculi, a far higher data than in adults. More common predisposing urological abnormalities are primary pelviureteric junction obstruction, megaureter, horseshoe kidney or polycystic kidney, hydronephrosis, duplex ureter, posterior urethral valves, and bladder exstrophy and vesicoureteric reflux. Stasis of urine within an obstructed or dilated urinary tract creates an environment in which stone-forming substances are more likely to precipitate.
- *Prematurity*. Ex-premature children (born at less than 37 completed weeks' gestation) are at much greater risk of nephrocalcinosis and nephrolithiasis. The risks are increased with increasing prematurity of birth, decreasing birth weight, comorbidity, and the use of furosemide, thiazides, and other drugs.
- *Diet* plays an important role in pathogenesis of pediatric urolithiasis; in particular one major risk factor is inadequate fluid intake that results in low urine volume which increases the relative supersaturation of uric acid that thereby promotes nucleation, growth, and aggregation of calcium oxalate and uric acid in urine. The risk of stone formation may be further exacerbated by an excessive sugary drink consumption that increases urinary excretion of calcium and oxalate. Sodium intake increases calciuria due to competition between sodium and calcium for passive reabsorption along the nephron, so daily sodium intake less than 2–3 mEq/kg for young children is recommended for patients with hypercalciuria or calcium-based stones. Low-protein diet is not recommended in children because they are still growing, rather than adults in whom it is used to decrease stone risk (Tasian and Copelovitch 2014).

16.4 Stone Composition

Stones are composed of a combination of crystals (both inorganic and organic) and proteins. Crystals in the urine usually form on the surface of a nidus that allows nucleation, growth, and aggregation of a stone particle. As the crystals aggregate, they fuse into plaques in the interstitium and finally extrude through the uroepithelium of the renal papillae (Copelovitch 2012).

Calcium-based stones (calcium oxalate monohydrate, calcium oxalate dihydrate, and calcium phosphate stones) account for 70–80 % of upper urinary tract stones. Struvite stones (infectious calculi) account for 5–15 % of stones and are composed of magnesium ammonium phosphate. Uric acid stones account for 5–10 % of stones and occur in acidic urine (pH <5.8). Other stones, including cystine, xanthine, and protein matrix stones, as well as drug (triamterene, indinavir)-induced calculi, account for less than 5 % of stones.

Stone composition differed according to sex and age of patients. In children younger than 5 years, carbapatite is the main component, predominantly in boys. Struvite is present in 40 % of stones in boys and in 25 % in girls, but it is the main component in only 5 % of all calculi. Calcium oxalate is significantly less frequent in boys. Purines are found in about 10 % of cases in both sexes, essentially as ammonium urate. The proportion of calcium phosphate stones was especially high in infants of both sexes. In patients older than 5 years, calcium oxalate is the main component in about 50 % of cases in both sexes. Struvite, carbapatite, and purine stones are less frequent. In all, calculi of metabolic origin are more frequent in children older than 5 years. In recent years, the proportion of calcium phosphate stones related to metabolic disorders, especially hypercalciuria, has increased, and infectious stones are less frequent than observed at the beginning of the 1990s (Lima and Manzoni 2015).

Infective struvite stones initially comprise a combination of magnesium, ammonium phosphate, and glycoprotein matrix in varying proportions. Calcium phosphate and other inorganic constituents then become incorporated into the expanding stone mass. Their consistency is variable, with areas of hard calcified material embedded within softer, less densely calcified matrix. The descriptive term "staghorn" refers to an infective calculus that has adopted the configuration of the renal pelvis and calyces. Conversely, metabolic stones of cystine and xanthine are predominantly crystalline and correspondingly harder (Thomas et al. 2008).

16.5 Clinic

The clinical presentation of nephrolithiasis in the pediatric population is fairly heterogeneous. In infants, urinary tract infections and passing of stones in diapers are the usual manifestations. The classic renal colic of the adult is uncommon in younger children, who may present with isolated microscopic hematuria, pyuria, and irritability, less frequent with nausea, vomiting, abdominal pain, or urinary tract infection. Patients also may be asymptomatic, with nephrolithiasis incidentally discovered in an imaging study conducted for other indications. Older children and adolescents can better localize pain to the flank or groin area and have an increased chance for spontaneous stone passage. Recurrent stone disease frequently occurs in children and adolescents with nephrolithiasis, but the recurrence risk is lower than in adults.

About 15–20 % of our pediatric stone patients present with renal dysfunction. There are two patient groups: calculus oligo-anuric with two good kidneys (children <5 years) and chronic calculus renal failure (children >5 years). The majority of these patients are from poor socioeconomic backgrounds, coming from rural areas, and live far away from our health facility.

16.6 Diagnosis

In pediatric patients with suspected nephrolithiasis, the evaluation includes a complete medical history and physical examination, complemented by appropriate laboratory and imaging studies. A prompt evaluation is needed to rule out urinary tract obstruction and urinary tract infection.

Laboratory tests such as urine analysis provide information regarding urine pH, hematuria, or pyuria. Tubular dysfunction may be present if the results of urine analysis show glucosuria and proteinuria.

Urine culture is essential, and kidney stone material has to be retrieved and analyzed whenever possible. Kidney stone composition can narrow the differential diagnosis and help tailor evaluation and management especially in cases of metabolic diseases.

Microscopic analysis can demonstrate the presence of cystine crystals in cystinuria, xanthine and dihydroxyadenine crystals (present in case of adenine phosphoribosyltransferase deficiency), and uric acid stone (rare in children and due to inborn errors of purine metabolism).

Metabolic evaluation should incorporate measurement of electrolyte levels, including

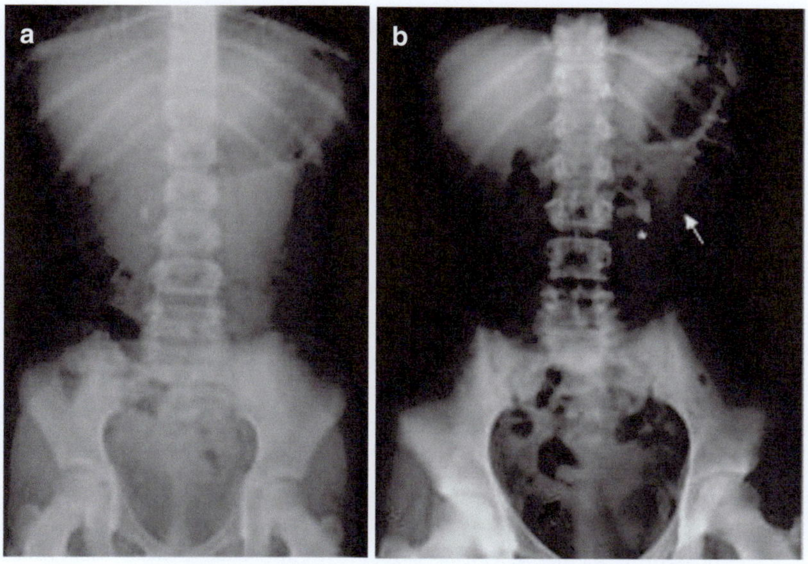

Fig. 16.1 (**a**) Abdominal radiography of the kidney, ureters, and bladder (KUB) shows a radiopaque stone projecting on the right kidney (*arrow*). (**b**) A KUB demonstrates a large radiopaque stone projecting laterally to the left transverse process of L3, on the upper third of the ureter (*asterisk*). In the same patient, the KUB shows also tiny and poor radiopaque opacities in the lower calyces (*white arrow*) of the left kidney and in the lower third of the right ureter (*white arrow*)

calcium, magnesium, and phosphorous. Creatinine levels should be measured to assess overall renal function. Since children with kidney stones have a high risk of recurrence associated with metabolic abnormalities, 24-h urine collection is the mainstay of the workup for pediatric nephrolithiasis, as it is in adults. Because of significant intraindividual variability related to diet and environment, two 24-h urine collections are recommended. Urinary excretion of calcium, oxalate, uric acid, citrate, magnesium, phosphorus, sodium, and potassium should be assessed. Valuable information that can be obtained from the urine collection also includes pH, volume, sulfate, urea nitrogen levels, and supersaturation. When patients are unable to give 24-h urine samples, spot urine samples can be collected, especially in young patients who are not toilet trained.

Imaging evaluation is necessary in the acute onset of a suspected renal urolithiasis in children, and radiologists have to take care in minimizing children's radiation exposure.

External radiation delivered to children should be a constant concern and limited to the as low as reasonably achievable (ALARA) principle, considering that patients with urolithiasis may repeat imaging procedures even after the acute onset during treatment and follow-up (Lima and Manzoni 2015).

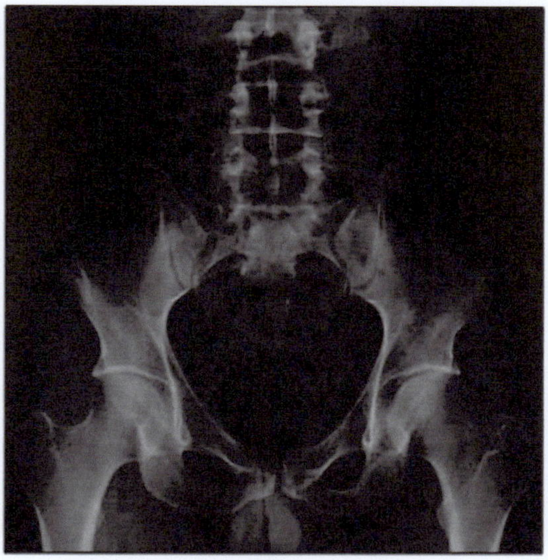

Fig. 16.2 KUB demonstrates a round calcification in the right pelvis with a relatively radiolucent center related to a phlebolith that may mimic a stone (*arrow*)

When a stone is suspected, the combination of an abdominal plain X-ray (kidney, ureter, and bladder [KUB]) and urinary tract US allows the diagnosis in most cases (Fig. 16.1). Most calculi are radiopaque and visible on the plain X-ray; however, not all opacities projecting on the expected location of the urinary tract are stones (Fig. 16.2), not all stones are radiopaque, and a stone can be missed in case of bowel distension, often associated with renal colic (Palmer and Palmer 2014).

The purposes of imaging modalities in the acute suspected cases of nephrolithiasis are the following: to exclude or substantiate the diagnosis; to determine the presence, size, location, and composition of a stone; to assess eventual complications and consequences of obstruction to the urinary tract; to estimate the likelihood of stone passage and the presence of anatomic abnormalities that may coexist with stone formation; and in recurrent cases, to perform the correct therapy, helping to guide the timing of intervention if necessary (Palmer and Palmer 2014; Kambadakone and Eisner 2010; Strohmaier 2015; Dhar 2009).

The possibility to image a stone depends upon its composition and its location.

The majority of stones in children are calcium based (specifically calcium oxalate and/or calcium phosphate) and thus opaque when using X-ray, so easily detectable on both abdominal radiography and unenhanced CT (Palmer and Palmer 2014).

Uric acid and xanthine stones are radiolucent and therefore not visible on abdominal radiography; they may be seen as low-density structures on unenhanced CT. Struvite and cystine stones are of intermediate density and may be difficult to be detected on abdominal radiography. Drug stones (indinavir, ceftriaxone, sulfadiazine) and matrix/protein stones have variable densities and may be indistinguishable from surrounding tissue and not visible even on unenhanced CT.

The location of the stone will also affect how it is seen on various imaging modalities. US often fails to identify ureteral stones, particularly if the ureter is not dilated or if there is overlying bowel gas which prevents penetration of the ultrasound beam. Identifying stones on CT, on the other hand, is unaffected by stone location or bowel gas.

Plain X-ray exposes children to a minimal radiation dose and is quick, easy, and readily accessible. However, there are major limitations to this kind of examination: only radiopaque stones can be seen on radiographs; small radiopaque stones (<3 mm) may be obscured by overlying soft-tissue densities (i.e., colonic stool or superimposed bony structures). Considering this abdominal radiographs only have a sensitivity of 62 % and specificity of 67 % in stone diagnosis (Fig. 16.3). At X-ray examination, pelvic phleboliths and appendicoliths might be confused for distal ureteral stones. Another problem is that classical radiography offers no information about obstruction. For this reason, abdominal radiographs is not the first radiological examination to be performed in the acute evaluation of a kidney stone in children (Kaplan and Meyers 2004; Türk et al. 2015).

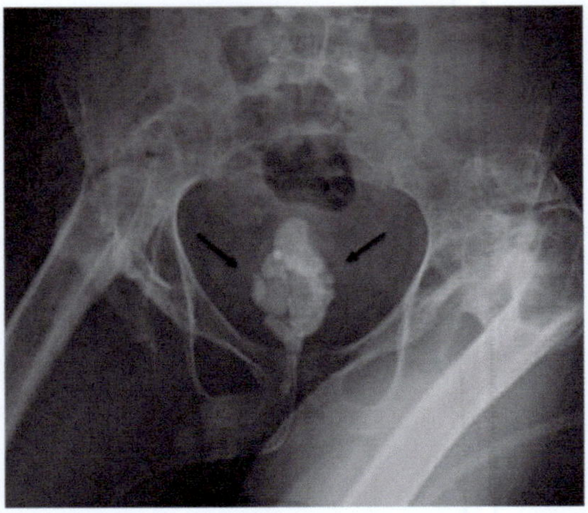

Fig. 16.3 A pelvic plain film displays multiple large radiopaque bladder stones (*arrows*) in an 18-year-old male patient with vesical catheter and bilateral hip dysplasia

US has the advantages of being easily available, noninvasive and avoiding radiation, lower in cost than CT, not requiring sedation, and performed portably allowing bedside evaluation of sick patients. On the other hand, it is limited by its high dependence on the skills of the operator and by the lack of kids' compliance (Strohmaier 2015).

US has to be considered the initial modality of choice in evaluating a pediatric patient with suspected urolithiasis and abdominal or flank pain (Türk et al. 2015).

Its limitations may be the patient's body habitus, interposed bowel gas, or known abnormalities of the renal tract, when the anatomy is too complex to examine with US (such as crossed fused ectopic kidneys, congenital duplications, and other anomalies).

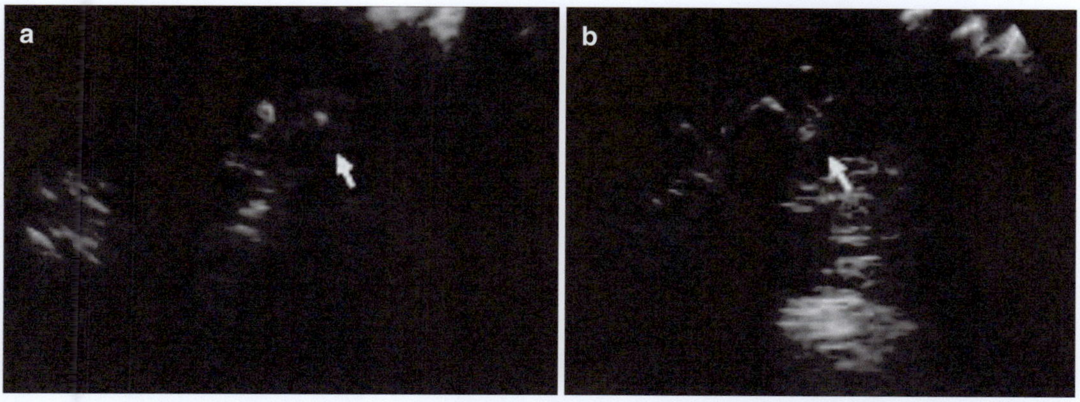

Fig. 16.4 (**a**, **b**) Axial (**a**) and sagittal (**b**) US scans reveal renal stones characterized by increased echogenicity and posterior acoustic shadowing (*arrows*)

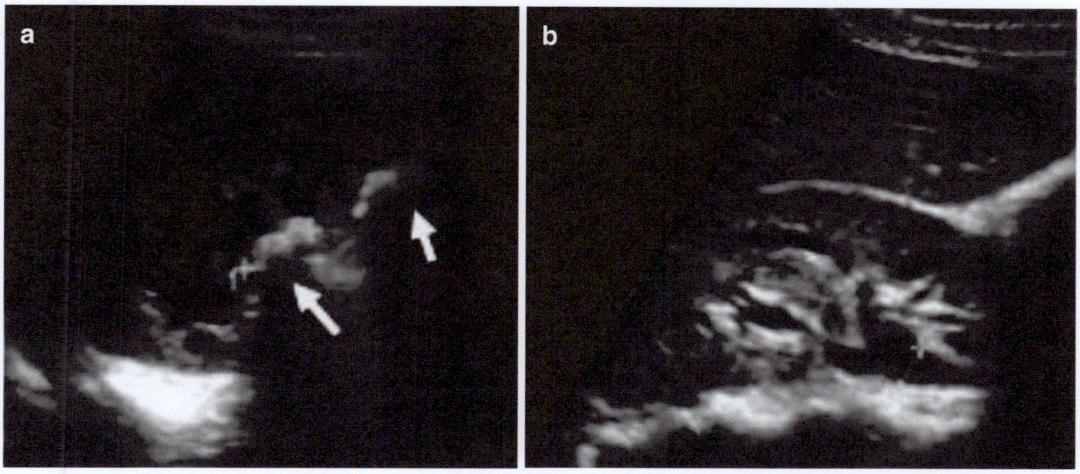

Fig. 16.5 (**a**, **b**) The US examination shows multiple left renal stones characterized by increased echogenicity and posterior acoustic shadowing (calipers and *arrows* in **a**) and a mild dilatation of the right renal pelvis and of the proximal ureter without identification of a stone in a 14-year-old female patient with a history of cystinuria (calipers in **b**)

As regards to US technique, children should be as well hydrated as is feasible. A curvilinear and subsequently linear high-resolution probe must be used. They should be scanned both in supine and in prone position. After a routinary scanning of the kidneys and bladder, particular attention should be paid in visualizing as much of the ureter as possible (Hiorns 2008).

US might directly demonstrate renal stones that typically appear as a very bright or echogenic, rounded structure with a "posterior acoustic shadowing," and it is due to the calculi's high density, resulting in the blocking of penetration of the US beam (Figs. 16.4, 16.5, 16.6, 16.7, 16.8, 16.9, and 16.10).

US also provides information about the renal parenchyma and the eventual enlargement of the collecting system (Lima and Manzoni 2015). In case of ureteral stones, US might be helpful, rather than Rx, in evaluating obstruction, hydroureter, or hydronephrosis, easily depicted as fluid distension of the renal pelvis and calices (Fig. 16.11).

US sensitivity and specificity in case of renal stones are approximately 61–93 % and 95–100 %, respectively; its accuracy in pediatric ureteral

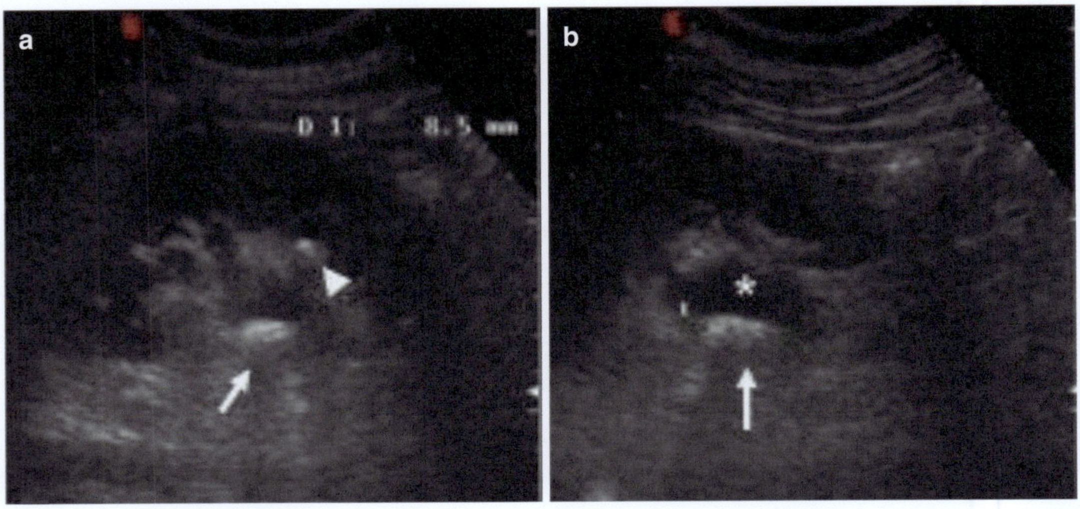

Fig. 16.6 (**a**, **b**) US sagittal (**a**) and axial (**b**) scans show a small stone in the lower calyceal system (*arrowhead* in **a**) and an 8.5 mm hyperechoic pelvic stone (*arrows* in **a** and **b**) with hydronephrosis (*asterisk* in **b**)

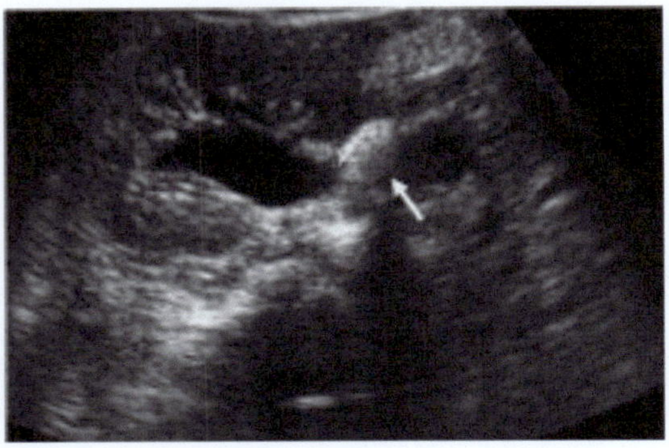

Fig. 16.7 US scan shows a large hyperechoic renal stone with calyceal dilatation (calipers and *arrow*)

lithiasis is also quite variable (Strohmaier 2015; Kokorowski et al. 2010). The ureteral stones could not be easily visible if there is overlying bowel gas or surrounding soft tissue which obscures the ureter. If the dilated ureter at the level of obstruction can be seen, then the stone may be visible. Hydronephrosis may suggest a ureteral stone, but even in the presence of hydroureter, it is often difficult to see the ureteral stone. Ureteral calculi are more easily visible at proximal and distal extremities (Lima and Manzoni 2015).

A special feature of US is the artifact created by color Doppler imaging of a rough reflective surface, known as "twinkling." The "twinkling sign" is a color Doppler artifact appearing as rapidly alternating color pixels, a multicolor signal, behind a strongly reflecting medium, simulating turbulence, being located where one would expect to find an acoustic shadow. This can be used as a supportive evidence when diagnosing stones by US.

Color Doppler US shows differences in the urine jet at the vesicoureteric junction and resistive index of the arciform arteries of both kidneys, which are indicative of the grade of obstruction, improving US examination (Jandaghi et al. 2013) (Fig. 16.12).

Despite all of these considerations, US fails to identify stones in >40 % of pediatric patients and provides no information on renal function.

Confirmatory low-dose unenhanced CT is advocated after high clinical suspicion with a negative US, an equivocal US, or after a positive US to evaluate further calculi, stone location, and burden for appropriate planning of an intervention while accepting the radiation dose penalty to achieve a definitive diagnosis (Hiorns 2008).

CT is typically used in the adult emergency setting due to its speed and high sensitivity/specificity. The matter in children is that CT utilizes significantly more ionizing radiation than the other imaging modalities; the effective dose of an

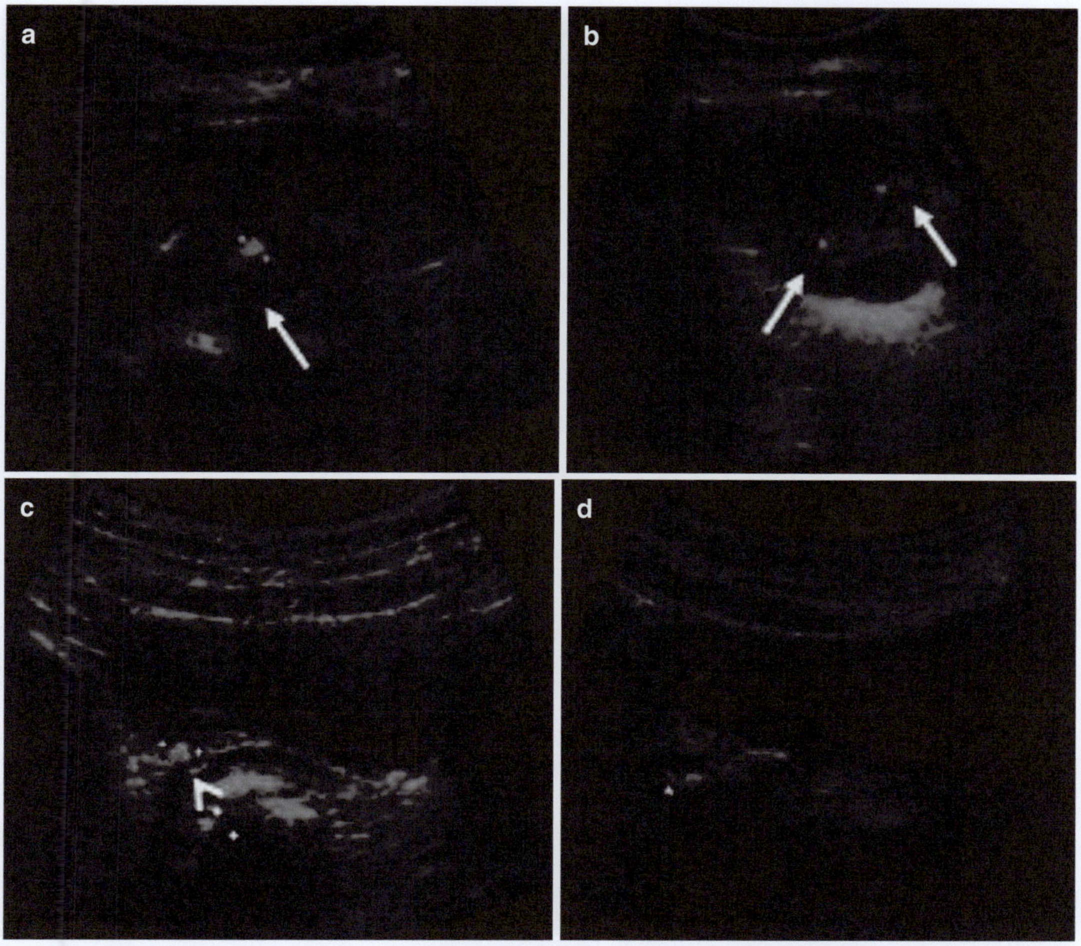

Fig. 16.8 (**a**–**d**) US scans demonstrate multiple renal stones (calipers and *arrows* in **a** and **b**) and an obstructing stone in the right ureterovesical junction (*dotted arrow* in **c**) with mild ureteral dilatation (*asterisk* in **d**)

abdominal/pelvic CT is 4.3–8.5 mSv as compared to an abdominal radiograph which is 0.2–0.7 mSv (Türk et al. 2015).

During the last decade, examination protocols with lower radiation doses have been developed (so-called ultra-low-dose unenhanced CT). Using those protocols, such as tube current modulation, low-voltage protocols, and other adjustments to alter image acquisition and reconstruction, radiation dose can be reduced to approximately 1–2.2 mSv (Strohmaier 2015; Eisner et al. 2009; Hoppe and Kemper 2010), but still being significantly higher than conventional radiology.

Diagnostic accuracy has been shown to be maintained with low-dose protocols, however. The principle of as low as reasonably achievable (ALARA) should always be observed (Türk et al. 2015). Considering the fact that there is no threshold under which radiation is safe, CT has not to be performed as the automatic first choice of imaging in the pediatric population and should be thoughtfully used in these patients who may require multiple imaging procedures in the future.

The only way to most effectively decrease the amount of radiation to which a patient is exposed is to choose nonionizing studies when possible (i.e., US). If CT has to be employed, use it sparingly and limit the scan to only the area of interest.

CT acquisition in case of suspected renal and ureteral stones does not firstly require IV contrast because contrast enhancement of the renal

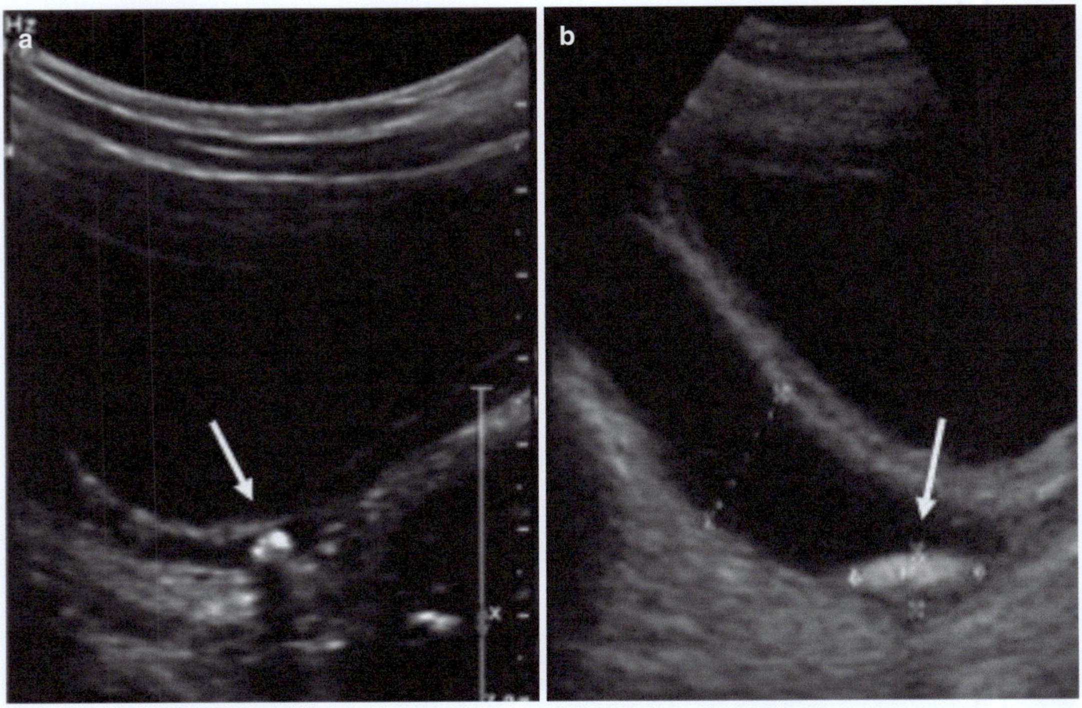

Fig. 16.9 (**a**) US scan shows a stone in the right ureterovesical junction with mild urethral dilatation; (**b**) US scan shows a large hyperechoic stone in the right ureterovesical junction with severe urethral dilatation (caliper)

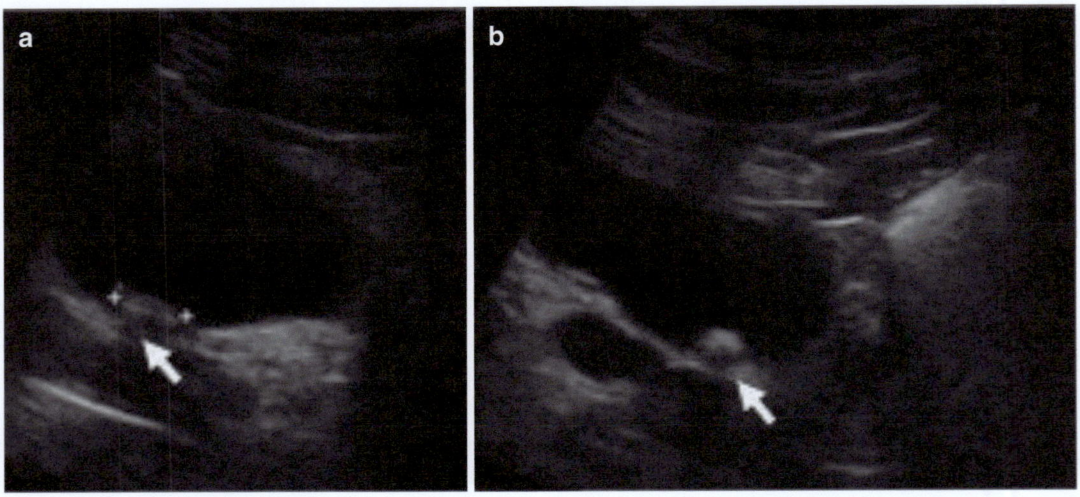

Fig. 16.10 (**a**, **b**) US images show a bladder stone (*arrows*) in supine position (**a**) and left-side decubitus (**b**)

parenchyma and excretion of contrast into the collecting system may obscure small stones. Utilization of thin layers (<5 mm) helps in detecting small concretions (Strohmaier 2015).

In adults CT has a sensitivity of 94–100 % and specificity of 92–100 %. In children, only 5 % of stones escape detection by unenhanced CT, and sedation or anesthesia is rarely needed with modern high-speed CT apparatus (Türk et al. 2015).

Unenhanced CT – with all of the concern about exposure – is overall considered the gold standard imaging technique for urolithiasis and is

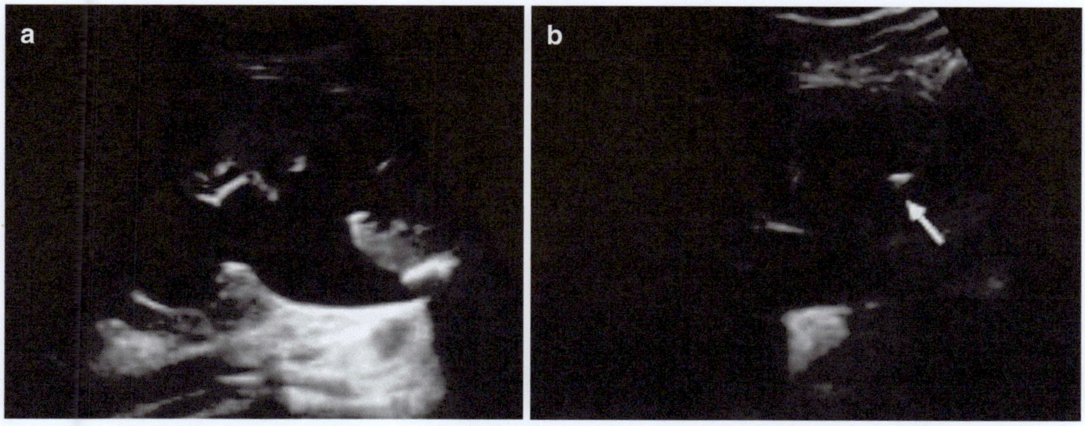

Fig. 16.11 (**a**) US sagittal scan shows a large proximal ureteral stone with hydronephrosis (*asterisk*), (**b**) US axial scan shows a small stone in a lower calyces (*arrows*)

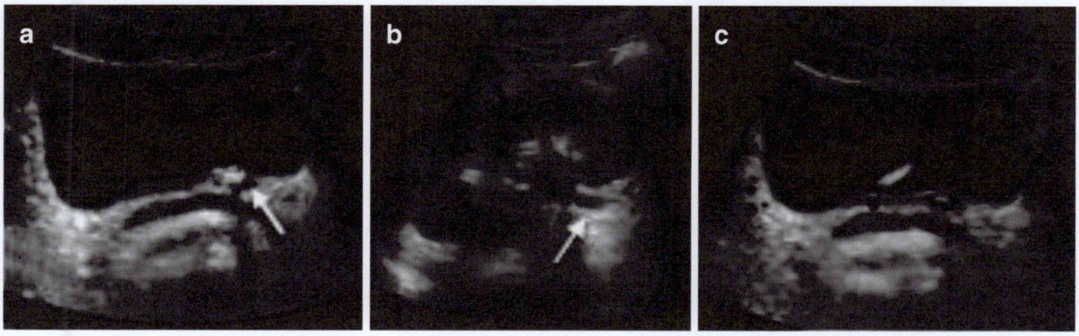

Fig. 16.12 (**a**–**c**) US scans show a hyperechoic stone in the left ureterovesical junction with acoustic shadowing (in **a**) and mild hydrouretheronephrosis (*arrow* in **b**). The color Doppler image (**c**) demonstrates a normal ureter jet only on the right side (*asterisk*)

superior to other imaging modalities in diagnosing and confirming stone disease; it provides accurate information regarding location and size of the stone and relevant surrounding anatomy (Fig. 16.13). It can detect even very small and ureteral stones (Kaplan and Meyers 2004).

Unenhanced CT helps to rule out other pathology or differential diagnoses, but some studies demonstrate that it overestimates stone size by 30–50 % (Van Appledorn et al. 2003).

Virtually all stones are visible at unenhanced CT, including those that are radiolucent on conventional radiographs, such as uric acid, xanthine, and cystine stones. These calculi have an attenuation value (>200 HU) greater than that of the surrounding soft tissue, and multidetector CT helps accurately localize a stone within the renal pelvicalyceal system or ureter. The only stones that are difficult to visualize at CT are pure matrix stones and stones made of pure indinavir (a protease inhibitor used in the treatment of human immunodeficiency virus infection). These stones have soft-tissue attenuation (15–30 HU) and are likely to be missed at unenhanced CT. However, the distinctive clinical manifestation of renal colic in a patient receiving indinavir therapy for human immunodeficiency virus infection, along with the presence of obstructive features at CT, usually helps clinch the diagnosis.

The measurement of stone density might provide preliminary information regarding stone composition, and is useful for therapeutic planning. Each type of stone has its own density (e.g., cystine 100–300 UH, calcium salts 400–600 UH)

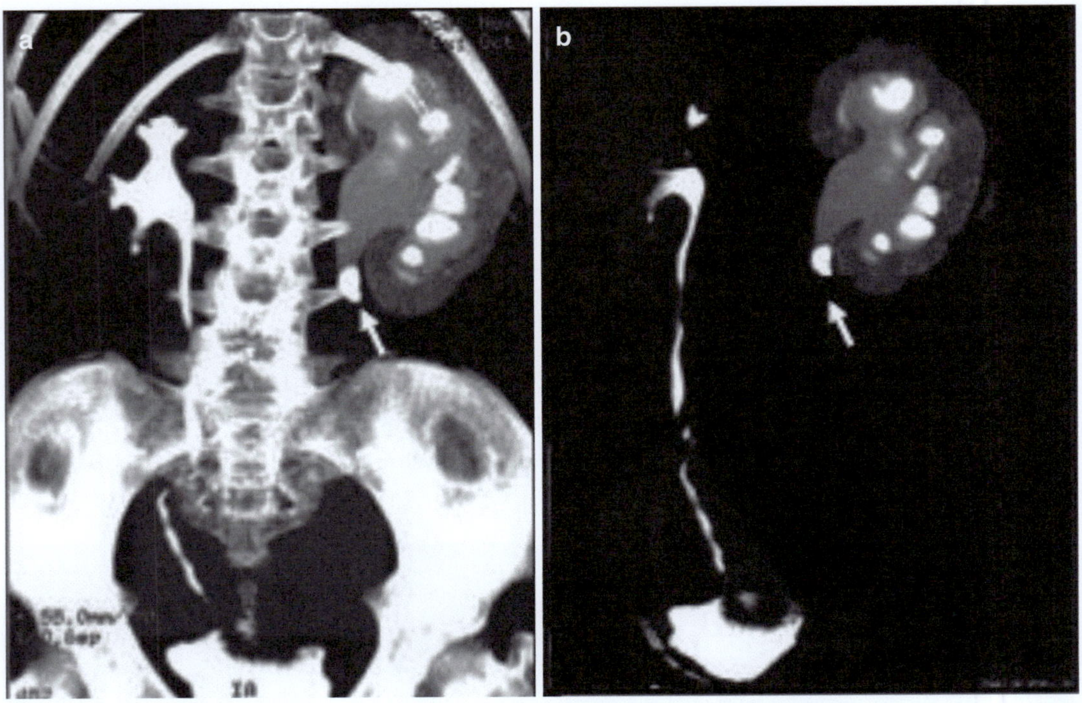

Fig. 16.13 (**a**, **b**) 3D MIP CT reconstructions show a large stone obstructing the left ureteropelvic junction with proximal hydronephrosis and an absence of urinary tree contrast opacification distally to the stone (*arrows*)

measured using bone window settings (1120/300) (Kambadakone and Eisner 2010; Strohmaier 2015; Eisner et al. 2009).

Secondary signs of ureteral stones can also be seen on CT, such as hydroureter, hydronephrosis, unilateral renal enlargement, proximal ureteral dilatation, decreased renal attenuation due to edema, perinephric stranding, and perinephric or periureteral edema.

If multidetector CT demonstrates unilateral ureteral dilatation and perinephric stranding, and a thorough search fails to reveal a stone, two possibilities are likely: either the patient has recently passed the stone, or the stone is present but not of sufficient size or attenuation to be visible (Kambadakone and Eisner 2010).

When obstruction of the urinary tract is suggested by symptoms but is not confirmed on US or noncontrast studies, or when renal colic is suggested by symptoms but a responsible stone is not identified, repeat imaging following administration of a contrast agent should be considered. Confirmation of partial or complete obstruction by a urinary tract stone, as well as detailed anatomic information regarding the structure of the urinary tract, is provided by CT urography (Kaplan and Meyers 2004). In these cases, contrast material administered intravenously and then excreted by the kidneys into the collecting system may be required in order to create a "filling defect" whereby the radiopaque contrast is displaced by the low-density stone in the renal pelvis, ureter, or bladder.

Follow-up examinations. Principally, it is possible to perform follow-up examinations of ureteral colic with all the imaging techniques we are going to describe. Radiological dose and availability are significantly problematic regarding CT. It could be shown that about 80 % of stone patients initially diagnosed by unenhanced CT scan will receive further CT scans for follow-up (Strohmaier 2015).

Intravenous pyelography/urography has been largely replaced with more precise and efficient techniques such as CT urography and is not commonly performed anymore where other modalities are available. However, it still plays a role in some specialist centers for delineating calyceal anatomy in children with known stones who are being worked up for percutaneous nephrolithotomy (PCNL) or lithotripsy and should now only be performed on a case-by-case basis and in conjunction with the urologist who is planning the treatment. In this context images should be taken only after compression applied to the child's abdomen for maximal pyelocalyceal distension and a full exposure only acquired at optimal opacification.

16.6.1 Magnetic Resonance Imaging

Magnetic resonance imaging (MRI) has the benefit of lacking ionizing radiation. Its use in patients with urolithiasis, however, is limited because it is expensive, unable to directly visualize stones (presenting as signal voids), not readily available, especially in the emergency departments, and requires sedation for most young children. It should be considered in children who are able to have the examination without the need for general anesthesia (Hiorns 2008). MRI might provide detailed anatomical information about the urinary collecting system, renal parenchymal morphology, and the location of an obstruction or stenosis in the ureter (Türk et al. 2015, Hiorns 2008).

Nuclear scintigraphy. DMSA scintigraphy (dimercaptosuccinic acid renal scintigraphy) is able to distinguish obstructive hydronephrosis from nonobstructive urinary tract dilation in a pediatric patient with a possibly obstructing stone or to confirm a concomitant anatomical anomaly such as ureteropelvic junction obstruction. Additionally functional imaging is performed in chronic stone disease to guide management and treatment (i.e., remove a stone versus remove the kidney, PCNL, lithotripsy, or open surgery). Functional information concerning the affected kidney and contralateral kidney are important for the final treatment decision (Lima and Manzoni 2015). The kidney must not be removed if it has been established that the kidney has an acceptable level of function (usually greater than 10%).

16.6.2 Differential Diagnosis

The main pathologies that have to be differentiated from nephrolithiasis alone are nephrocalcinosis and medullary sponge kidney. Medullary sponge kidney is a congenital disorder representing as a developmental defect affecting the formation of collecting tubules and results in cystic dilatation of medullary and papillary portions of collecting ducts. It is associated with nephrocalcinosis and nephrolithiasis due to hypercalciuria and hypocitraturia.

Nephrocalcinosis can cause microscopic or gross hematuria, sterile leukocyturia, and pain. Differently from nephrolithiasis (discrete stone formation in the collecting system), nephrocalcinosis is the diffuse deposition of calcium in the kidneys with the greatest concentration found at the tips of the pyramids. The deposition can lead to nephrolithiasis when calcium aggregates form and become large enough to perforate the calyceal epithelium, resulting in a nidus for stone formation in the renal collecting system.

Nephrocalcinosis is best viewed with US, considering the degree of echogenicity, might be classified in medullary, cortical, or diffuse, due to calcium deposition. Medullary nephrocalcinosis is the commonest form, characterized by increased echogenicity in the area of the medulla with posterior acoustic shadowing (echogenic medullary pyramids); this is in contrast to normal renal pyramids which are hypoechoic as compared to the cortex (Hoppe 2010) (Fig. 16.14).

At plain X-ray and CT, clusters of pyramidal medullary calcification are characteristic.

Medullary pyramids of the kidney can be seen normally on unenhanced CT scans and Rx as high-attenuation structures and this is known as the "white pyramid sign,"; this might be a pitfall in diagnosis due to the fact that bilateral high-attenuation renal pyramids are an occasional incidental normal finding. Unilateral appearance of white pyramids is a subtle secondary sign suggestive of contralateral urinary tract obstruction.

In order to differentiate ureteral stones from phleboliths, unenhanced CT demonstrates three typical signs:

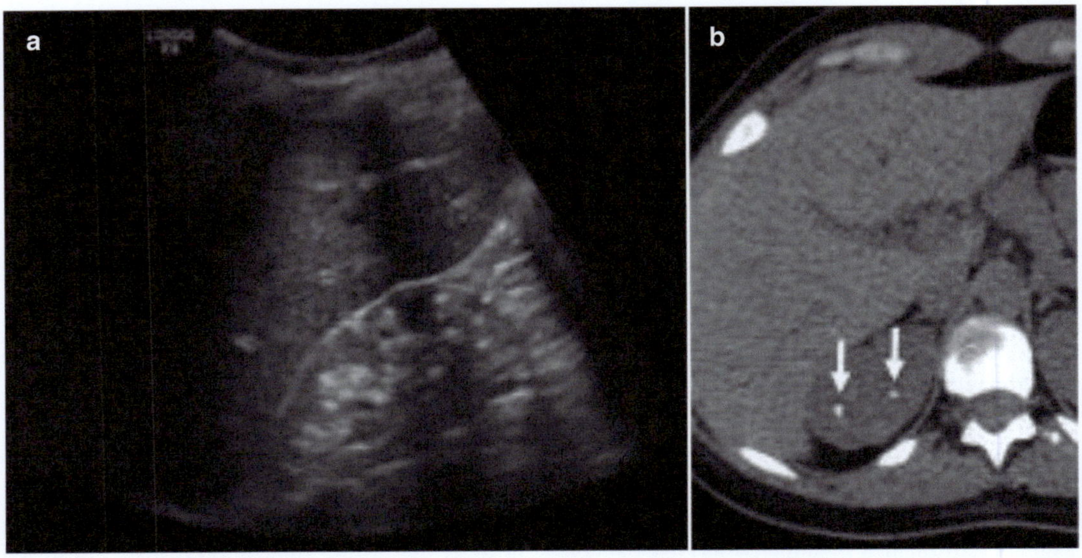

Fig. 16.14 (**a**) US scan shows cortical and medullary nephrocalcinosis represented by hyperechoic spots diffuse in the renal parenchima; (**b**) CT examination confirms nephrocalcinosis with hyperdense renal pyramids (*arrow* in **b**)

- The "soft-tissue rim sign," a circumferential halo of soft-tissue attenuation, representing the ureter encircling the stone, which is not found with a phlebolith
- The "comet tail sign" present in phleboliths and created by an eccentric, tapering soft-tissue area adjacent to the phleboliths calcification
- The "central lucent area" seen in phleboliths, in contrast to the opacified centers seen in calculi (Kambadakone and Eisner 2010)

16.6.3 Therapy

The composition of the stone as evoked by its appearance on imaging greatly influences the therapeutic choice. Uric acid is dissolved with alkalinization of urine as a first-line treatment, but an eventual calcium shell must be fragmented first by extracorporeal shock wave lithotripsy (ESWL). Stone composition affects the efficacy of extracorporeal SWL: brushite, cystine, and calcium oxalate monohydrate stones are hard and more resistant to fragmentation with SWL (Kambadakone and Eisner 2010). The treatment of struvite or calcium phosphate stone must include antibiotic therapy because they are constantly associated with infection (Lima and Manzoni 2015). Many interventional methods (ESWL, ureterorenoscopy, percutaneous nephrolithotomy) are managed with conventional radiology (Strohmaier 2015). Surgical treatment is reserved for stones that do not respond to these therapies.

References

Calisti A et al (2008) The risk of associated urological abnormalities in children with pre and postnatal occasional diagnosis of solitary, small or ectopic kidney: is a complete urological screening always necessary? World J Urol 26:281–284

Copelovitch L (2012) Urolithiasis in children medical approach. Pediatr Clin N Am 59:881–896

Dhar M, Denstedt JD (2009) Imaging in diagnosis, treatment, and follow-up of stone patients. Adv Chronic Kidney Dis 16:39–47

Eisner BH, Kambadakone A, Monga M et al (2009) Computerized tomography magnified bone windows are superior to standard soft tissue windows for accurate measurement of stone size: an in vitro and clinical study. J Urol 181:1710–1715

Hernandez JD, Ellison JS, Lendvay TS (2015) Current trends, evaluation, and management of pediatric nephrolithiasis. JAMA Pediatr 169(10):964–970

Hiorns MP (2008) Imaging of urinary tract lithiasis: who, when and how? Pediatr Radiol 38(Suppl 3):S497–S500

Hoppe B, Kemper MJ (2010) Diagnostic examination of the child with urolithiasis or nephrocalcinosis. Pediatr Nephrol 25:403–413

Jandaghi AB, Falahatkar S et al (2013) Assessment of ureterovesical jet dynamics in obstructed ureter by urinary stone with color Doppler and duplex Doppler examinations. Urolithiasis 41:159–163

Kambadakone AR, Eisner BH (2010) New and evolving concepts in the imaging and management urolithiasis: urologists' perspective. RadioGraphics 30:603–623

Kaplan BS, Meyers KEC (2004) Pediatric nephrology and urology: the requisites in pediatrics. In: Milliner DS (ed) Calculi. Elsevier Mosby, Philadelphia

Kokorowski PJ, Hubert K et al (2010) Evaluation of pediatric nephrolithiasis. Indian J Urol 26:531–535

Lima M, Manzoni G (2015) Pediatric urology: contemporary strategies from fetal life to adolescence. In: Sultan S (ed) Urolithiasis. Springer, Italia

Palmer LS, Palmer JS (2014) Pediatric and adolescent urologic imaging. Springer, New York

Sas DJ (2011) An update on the changing epidemiology and metabolic risk factors in pediatric kidney stone disease. Clin J Am Soc Nephrol 6: 2062–2068

Strohmaier WL (2015) Imaging in pediatric urolithiasis—what's the best choice? Transl Pediatr 4:36–40

Tasian GE, Copelovitch L (2014) Evaluation and medical management of kidney stones in children. J Urol 192:1329–1336

Thomas D, Duffy PG, Rickwood A (2008) Essentials of Paediatric Urology, Second Edition. David F.M. Thomas, Patrick G. Duffy, Anthony M. K. Rickwood

Türk C, Knoll T et al (2015) Guidelines on urolithiasis 81A6U5 European Association of Urology. pp 10–12

Van Appledorn S, Ball AJ et al (2003) Limitations of noncontrast CT for measuring ureteral stones. J Endourol 17:851–854; discussion 854

Acute Pyelonephritis

17

Alessandra Scionti, Piercarlo Rossi, Pietro Gulino, Alessandro Semeraro, Claudio Defilippi, and Michele Tonerini

17.1 Introduction

Pyelonephritis is the inflammation of the upper urinary tract, involving the renal pelvis and parenchyma. Its prompt diagnosis is important in order to avoid both short- and long-term complications such as scarring of the kidneys, hypertension, and in some unfortunate case even chronic renal insufficiency leading to a transplant. In pediatric patients, it usually migrates to the kidney from the bladder, being considered a continuum of disease from the lower to the upper urinary tract, while it is rarely seeded there hematogenously.

In fact, the most frequent pathogens are the same causing infection of the lower tract; in particular *Escherichia coli* is responsible in over 80 % of urinary tract infections (UTIs) in children. Other common pathogens are *Klebsiella*, *Proteus*, *Enterobacter*, *Streptococcus B*, *Enterococcus*, and occasionally *Pseudomonas*. Mycotic infections are rarer in children than in adults (Bhat et al. 2011). The vast majority is maintained by gram-negative bacterial organism since they produce a virulent endotoxin causing inhibition of ureteral peristalsis by blocking the adrenergic nerves of the smooth muscle and thus facilitating their ascent to the kidney with adhesion fimbria, even in the absence of reflux (Goel et al. 2015). When the pathogen gets to the kidney, it causes a focal or diffuse acute inflammation of the tubules and the interstitium with consequent debris formation within the tubules that might result in impaired renal function.

17.2 Risk Factors

Some children are more susceptible than others to UTI, and subsequently they might be more prone to develop pyelonephritis, recurrence, or complication. Their vulnerability might be due to anatomic or functional factors. Generally, in the first months of life, it is easy for neonates to contract UTI due to the immature immune system; after 6 months of age, girls have a higher risk of infections than boys because of anatomic characteristics, while debate has long been ongoing on circumcised males even if in 2012 the American Academy of Pediatrics (AAP) clearly stated the risk reduction of UTI after circumcision. Anatomic issues increasing the risk of UTI and

A. Scionti • P. Rossi
Department of Diagnostic and Interventional Radiology, University of Pisa, Pisa, Italy

P. Gulino • A. Semeraro • C. Defilippi
Pediatric Radiology, Meyer University Children's Hospital, Florence, Italy

M. Tonerini (✉)
Department of Emergency Radiology, Cisanello University Hospital, Pisa, Italy
e-mail: m.tonerini@tiscali.it

V. Miele, M. Trinci (eds.), *Imaging Non-traumatic Abdominal Emergencies in Pediatric Patients*,
DOI 10.1007/978-3-319-41866-7_17

pyelonephritis are the ones causing obstruction to urine flow, consequent urinary stasis, and inadequate clearance of pathogens leading to bacterial overgrowth. Examples are urethral stricture, posterior urethral valves, and ureterocele. Vesicoureteral reflux (VUR) consequent to chronically elevated bladder pressure can also increase the risk of pyelonephritis. Difficult bladder voiding can also be due to dysfunctional elimination syndrome or congenital and acquired neurogenic defects of the spinal cord such as spinal dysraphism (Bhat et al. 2011; Goel et al. 2015; Becknell et al. 2015).

17.3 Symptoms

While for UTI the clinical presentation may be age dependent, for pyelonephritis, the diagnosis is usually more clear and patient's condition might be severe. Before the onset of pyelonephritis symptoms of UTI prevails. In newborns and infant, the manifestation of UTI can be subtle, vague, and nonspecific, such as with poor feeding, decrease urinary output, lethargy or irritability, increased sleeping, vomiting, failure to thrive, and jaundice. Due to their inability to complain in a proper way or to articulate their discomfort, diagnosis of UTI in neonates can be challenging. That is why AAP recommends that all children between 2 months and 2 years with fever of unknown source be screened for UTI. It is also important to keep in mind that the presence of another cause justifying fever, such as gastroenteritis, bronchiolitis, respiratory infection, or otitis media, does not exclude UTI completely since they can be concomitant. In toddlers and older children, clinical onset might still be unspecific, but in the vast majority of cases, they present with the classic symptoms of the adult, such as dysuria, frequency, abdominal or flank pain, regression of incontinence (often nocturnal) in previously toilet-trained children, and fever. Clinical diagnosis gets easier in older verbal children, even if laboratory test are mandatory. Clinical findings of ascending infection are high fever with abrupt onset of chills, back and/or uni-/bilateral flank pain with costovertebral tenderness, vomiting, nausea, diarrhea, or other gastrointestinal symptoms that can contribute to make diagnosis more difficult. As the inflammation progresses, pyelonephritis can lead to bacteremia, with systemic inflammatory response or septic shock (urosepsis) (Bhat et al. 2011; Goel et al. 2015; Becknell et al. 2015).

17.4 Diagnosis

Diagnosis of UTI and acute pyelonephritis is based on clinical findings, physical examination, and laboratory data.

According to the most recent AAP guidelines, standard laboratory findings indicating UTI are pyuria and bacteriuria, so diagnosis requires both urinalysis and urine culture. Demonstrating the presence of >50,000 colony forming units/mL of a single uropathogen, urine culture is the gold standard to confirm the suspicion. To collect urine, Italian guidelines suggest the clean catch method for young children (<2 years), as it is noninvasive or traumatic for the child, but in other countries, the transurethral bladder catheterization or the suprapubic aspirate is recommended since these collection methods are less likely to yield a contaminant (Bhat et al. 2011). It is important to distinguish a true febrile UTI indicative of pyelonephritis from a simple cystitis, and early identification is pivotal in order to avoid permanent renal damage, but imaging is still not routinely required for uncomplicated infections.

Indications for imaging examinations are the following: suggestion of obstruction, no clinical improvement after 72 h of appropriate antibiotic therapy (5 % of cases), rapid recurrence after therapy, and diabetic patients, because they have a higher incidence of complicated urinary tract infections.

The logic behind imaging is to identify patients with high risk of pyelonephritis recurrence and patients at risk for renal scar development and consequently permanent renal damage and possibly chronic renal failure (Bocquet et al. 2015; Yu et al. n.d.; Shaikh et al. 2010; Calisti et al. 2008).

In this setting, imaging is used to identify patient with anatomic or functional genitourinary tract abnormalities that might place the patient at risk for recurrence and subsequently needing a surgical correction and to identify patients with risk factors or with parenchymal damage. The diagnosis of UTI in a child often triggers further evaluation: in the past, the traditional algorithm was to obtain a renal ultrasound to detect anatomic abnormalities, followed by voiding cystourethrography or radionuclide cystography to detect any VUR in all infants under 2 years of age diagnosed with UTI. This approach was due to the fact that VUR was considered the main risk factor and that renal scarring the first step for a progressive and irreversible damage leading to chronic insufficiency. So until now the role of radiologist was to identify children with VUR, to confirm the parenchymal injury, and to identify patients who could benefit from a prophylactic antibiotic therapy or a surgical intervention. As a matter of fact, nowadays the traditional approach has been questioned and there is not a unique consensus on when to image, who to image, and with what, and different guidelines are available. The more recent recommendation subdivides children in two groups based on the age. Imaging in the acute phase is recommended just for infants with an "atypical" presentation, independently from the age. Atypical presentation includes severely ill children, poor urine flow, elevated creatinine, abdominal mass, sepsis, failure to respond to antibiotic therapy in 48 h, or infection with organisms other than *E coli*. In this group of patients, US should be performed in a few days and radionuclide cystography within 4–6 months from the acute episode. If the patient is older than 6 months, no other examinations are required, whereas if the patient is younger than 6 months and any anomaly in the previous exams was found, a voiding cystourethrography should also be executed. In patients with typical UTI symptoms, no imaging examinations are required in the acute phase, especially if there is a good response to treatment within the first 48 h, but if the patient is younger than 6 months, a US within 6 weeks is advised. In case of anomalies found at the US, a voiding cystourethrography should be done. Patients younger than 6 months of age with a history of at least a previous UTI should undergo a US examination in the acute phase of the infection, a radionuclide cystography within 4–6 months, and after that a voiding cystourethrography. If the patient is older than 6 months, the US should be performed within 6 weeks and the radionuclide cystography within 4–6 months (Bocquet et al. 2015; Yu et al. n.d.; Shaikh et al. 2010; Calisti et al. 2008) (Tables 17.1 and 17.2).

Table 17.1 Flowchart showing the current approach for UTI management at its first episode

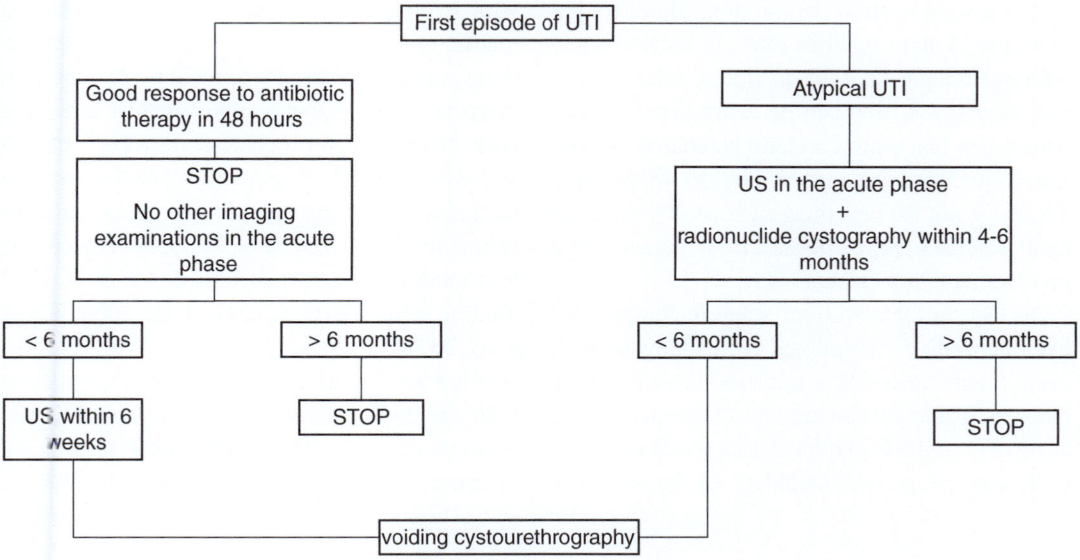

Table 17.2 Flowchart showing the current approach for UTI management at its recurrence

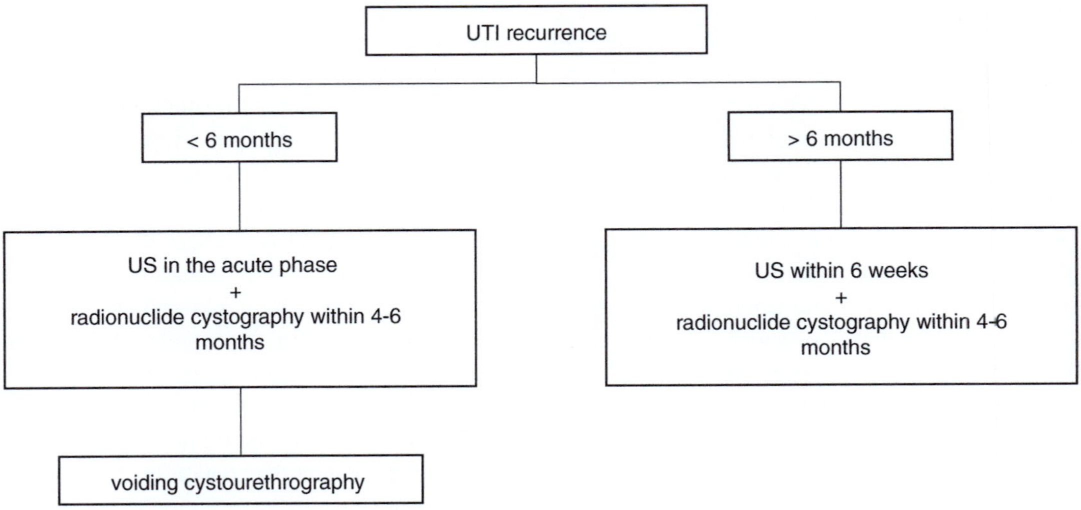

17.5 Ultrasound Sonography

US is usually the first imaging modality used to approach the pediatric patients. As children usually have a small size, it can be possible to use high-frequency probes that allow a better spatial resolution. The same technique is used for the adult but not to the children with poor thickness of the dorsal muscles and to their relative copious abdominal meteorism; the posterior approach is recommended to study the kidney.

US is used to study morphological congenital or acquired abnormalities that can be associated with pyelonephritis, such as kidney enlargement, hydronephrosis (that can be caused by bacterial endotoxins that inhibit ureteral peristalsis), duplicated collecting system, or bladder diverticula, while it is not the best imaging modality to detect renal scarring from prior UTIs or parenchymal involvement with current UTI.

In fact, in the setting of acute uncomplicated pyelonephritis, US findings are usually normal, even if sometimes (25 % of cases) there might be nonspecific changes in kidney echogenicity, such as focal or multifocal hypoechoic area with hypoperfusion at power Doppler, or hyperechoic hemorrhagic region (Fig. 17.1), or loss of renal sinus fat and corticomedullary differentiation because of the edema.

In case of a global involvement of the kidney, the pyelonephritis can be micronodular, with multiple small foci of inflammation or abscess that cause an increase in echogenicity, even if sometimes a reduction in echogenicity might be seen due to the generalized edema. On the other hand, kidney involvement might also be macronodular; in this case, there is a total inhomogeneity of the kidney echostructure, with hypoechoic non-defined areas of inflammation mixed with areas of hyperechoic hemorrhagic infarction. In case of focal pyelonephritis, there is a single hypoechoic or anechoic area with "increased through transmission" artifact and well-defined margins that usually involves the kidney from the medullary to the renal capsule (Fig. 17.2). This area is hypoperfused due to edema and vasoconstriction (Yu et al. n.d.; Shaikh et al. 2010; Calisti et al. 2008; Craig et al. 2008).

Bladder should always be screened together with the kidney: parameters that should raise concern are increased wall thickness, residual volumes of urine in the bladder after voiding,

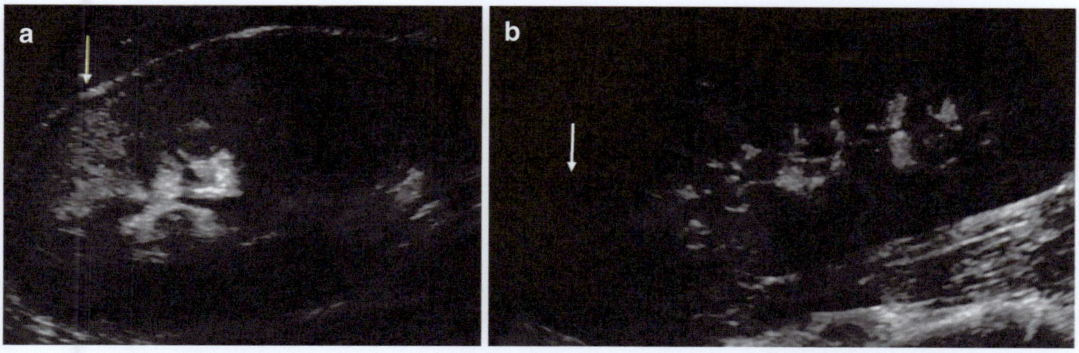

Fig. 17.1 (**a**, **b**) A US sagittal scan of a 15-year-old boy with a focal hyperechoic region of pyelonephritis in the upper pole of the right kidney (*arrow* in Fig. 17.3, **a**). A US sagittal scan of an 18-year-old girl with a hypoechoic area in the upper pole of the right kidney, suggestive for acute pyelonephritis (*arrow* in Fig. 17.3, **b**)

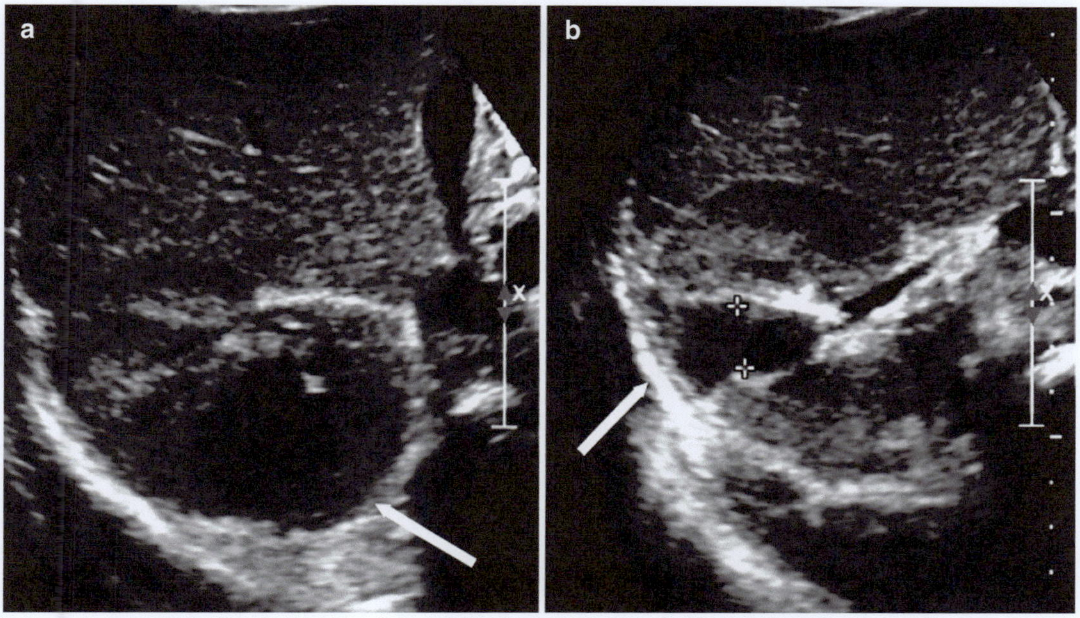

Fig. 17.2 (**a**, **b**) Axial US scans of focal hypoechoic area of pyelonephritis extending from the medullary to the renal capsule in a 5-year-old boy (*arrow* in Fig 17.4, **a**; *arrow* and calipers in Fig. 17.4, **b**)

and heterechoic urine, characterized by mobile echogenic particles floating freely within the bladder (Fig. 17.3) (Craig et al. 2008). To be noted is that bladder wall in newborns is physiologically thicker than in children and adults, both before and after voiding (Fig. 17.4). US is also used as a first imaging examination in the suspicion of complication such as abscess formation.

17.6 Radionuclide Cystography

Radionuclide studies are performed with technetium-99m dimercaptosuccinic acid (DMSA) or other tubular radiotracers, so called because they are retained for a long time in the renal parenchyma (tubular storage) and they are consequently excreted by means of tubular secretion. DMSA accumulates slowly in the proximal tubular cells,

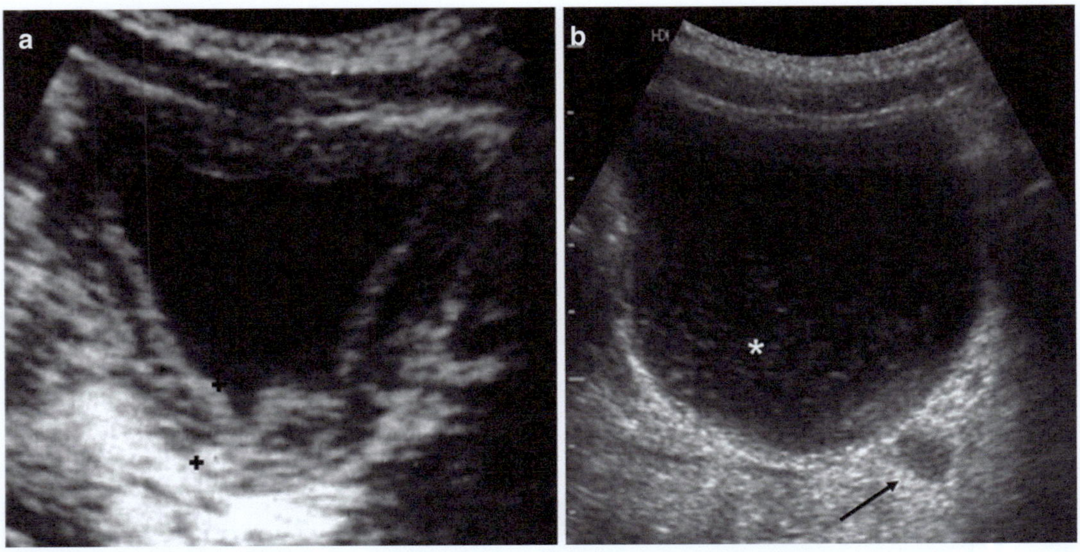

Fig. 17.3 (**a**) A 12-year-old boy with increased thickness of the bladder wall (caliper). (**b**) An 8-year-old boy with mobile echogenic particles floating within the bladder (*). Also a mild ureteral ectasia is visible in the distal portion (*arrow*)

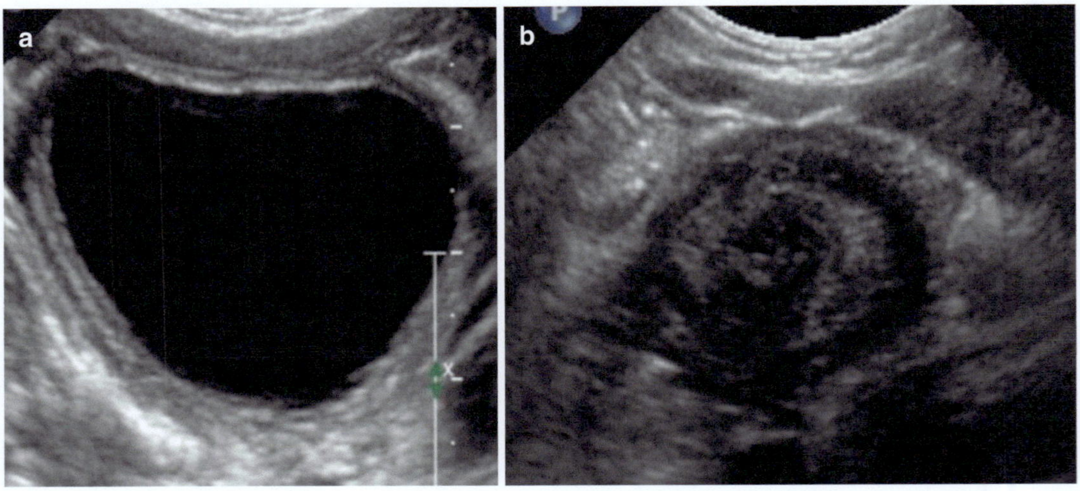

Fig. 17.4 Bladder of a newborn before (**a**) and after (**b**) voiding. The *thickness* of the bladder wall is normally superior than in older children

between 6 and 9 h after injection. Three planar images are usually obtained: posterior and left and right posterior oblique. In infants a pinhole collimated image of each kidney may be used to improve the resolution.

There are, as yet, no generally accepted criteria for the interpretation of the DMSA scintigraphy images. The appearance (size, shape, contour, and tracer distribution) of the kidney is often only subjectively described, with comparison with the contralateral kidney.

Radionuclide studies unify high-resolution morphological and functional information (Fig. 17.5), providing both qualitative and quantitative images of the renal cortex after an acute episode of pyelonephritis allowing to determine if the disease is stable, progressing, or resolving. In fact, the poor or totally failed

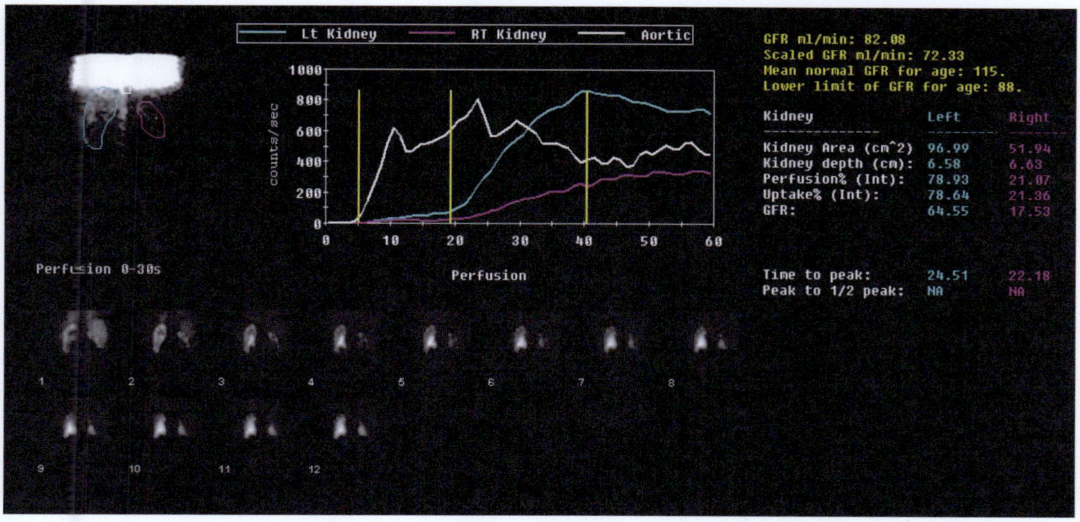

Fig. 17.5 Radionuclide cystography of a young boy who had recurrent episodes of pyelonephritis in the past, showing reduction of the renal function. Stasis of the radionuclide is seen bilaterally. Glomerular filtration rate is around 18 ml/min for the right kidney and 64 ml/min for the left one. Total glomerular filtration rate is 82 ml/min

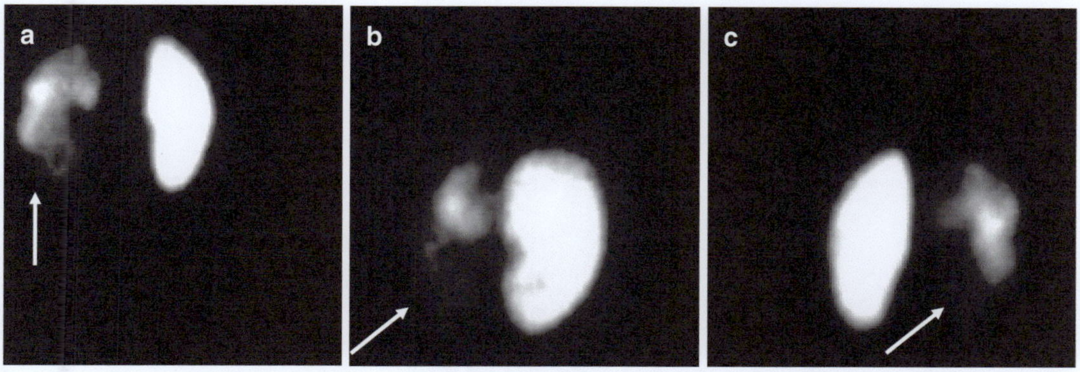

Fig. 17.6 (**a–c**) Poor uptake (*arrow*) of the radiotracer in the right kidney, identifying malfunctioning parenchyma

uptake of the radiotracer in a focal area or in the global kidney identifies areas of mal-/nonfunctioning parenchyma (Fig. 17.6). The agent is normally retained only from the vital and functioning renal parenchyma, so normal kidneys have a homogeneous uptake, with a corticomedullary ratio of 20:1. In case of pyelonephritis, findings change accordingly to the phase of the disease: in the acute setting, the involved kidney presents a round- or wedge-shaped region of failed uptake which appears bigger than the real injury due to the associated edema and the reversible tubular dysfunction caused by the direct action of the bacteria. After 6 months, a most accurate quantitative characterization of the lesion can be made. Renal scarring remains visible as photopenic defect of the renal cortex associated with an irregularity of the kidney outline (Craig et al. 2008).

17.7 Voiding Cystourethrography

Indication and execution modalities of voiding cystourethrography are better described in the following chapter. In case of pyelonephritis, its primary purpose is to identify the presence of a VUR or posterior urethral valves since they have been considered to be a risk factor facilitating UTI and infection recurrence.

17.8 Computed Tomography

CT is not usually performed in the setting of pyelonephritis. However, when CT is executed, focal pyelonephritis is characterized by an ill-defined striated wedge-shaped or rounded mass-like area of decreased enhancement. This region typically creates what is called a "striated nephrogram": an area of alternating hypoattenuate and hyperattenuate rays, radiating from the papilla to the cortex following the direction of the excretory tubules (Figs. 17.7 and 17.8). The appearance reflects the decreased flow and consequent hyperconcentration of the contrast in the infected tubules, which is due to obstructed renal tubules by inflammatory debris and to the impaired function from tubular ischemia. However, the striated nephrogram is not pathognomonic and can also be seen in other conditions such as renal vein thrombosis, ureteric obstruction, and contusion. Focal pyelonephritis might mimic a neoplasm. Diffuse pyelonephritis may cause a global enlargement of the kidney and a poor enhancement of the whole parenchyma, together with absent excretion of contrast. Other nonspecific radiological signs that might be present are the perinephric stranding, thickening, and mucosal enhancement of the urothelium, inflammatory changes in Gerota fascia and/or the renal sinus, and fluid collections/effusions. Non-contrast CT images may be normal or the affected kidney may be enlarged (Craig et al. 2008; Das et al. 2014).

17.9 Complications

Acute pyelonephritis complications include renal scar, abscess, pyonephrosis, papillary necrosis, acute kidney injury, renal infarction, and urosepsis.

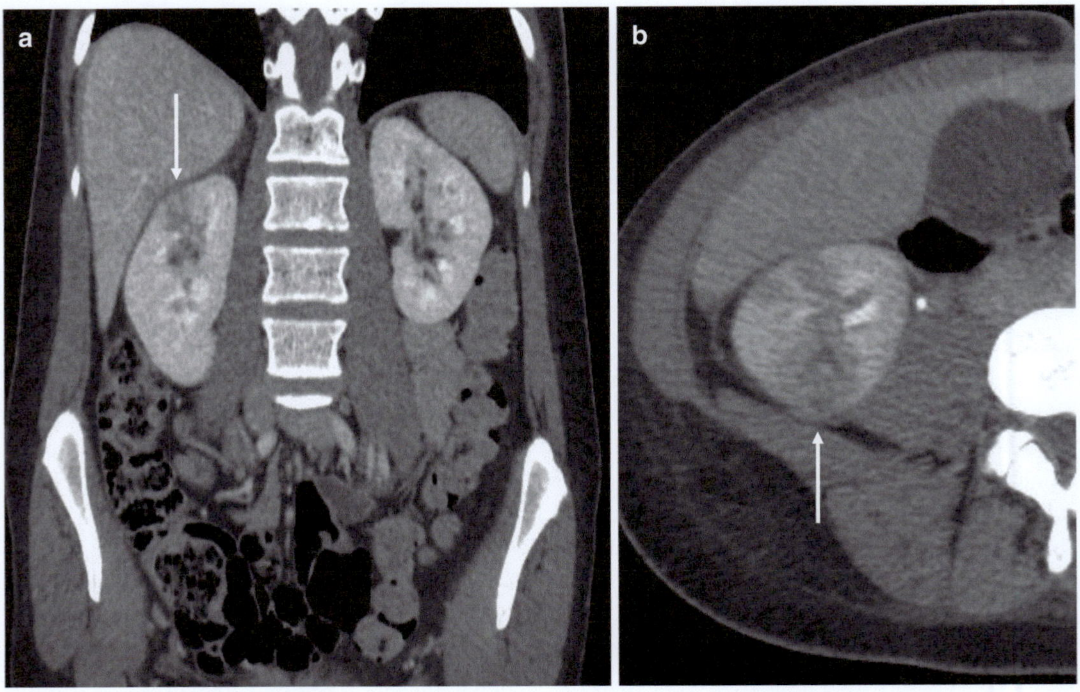

Fig. 17.7 (**a**, **b**) CT coronal view (**a**) and axial view (**b**) of a 12-year-old patient with acute pyelonephritis: a mass-like area of decreased enhancement is present on the right kidney (*arrow*)

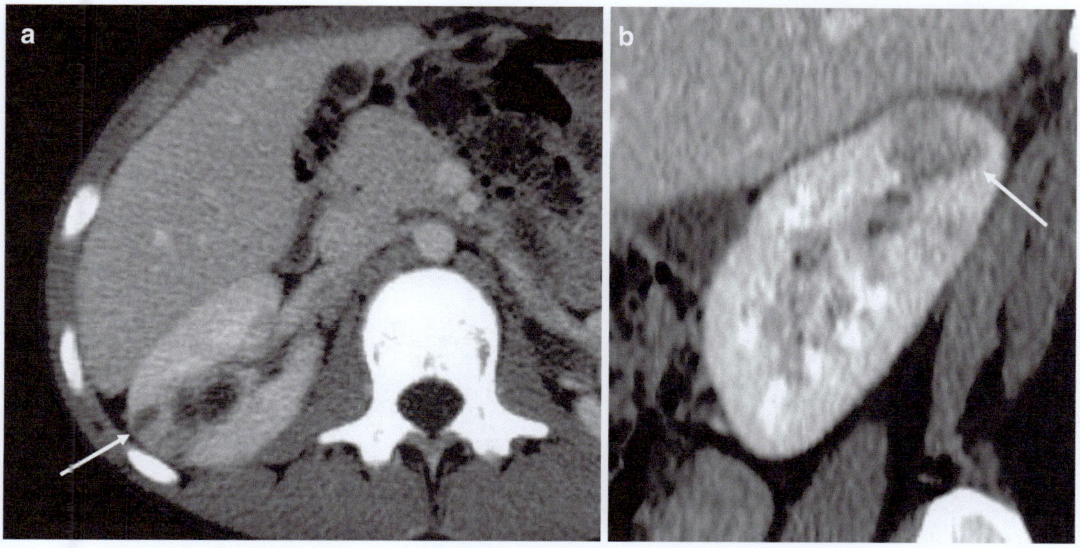

Fig. 17.8 (**a**, **b**) Young girl showing a wedge-shaped hypoattenuating area (*arrow*) of acute pyelonephritis

17.9.1 Renal Scar

Renal scarring is a frequent consequence of pyelonephritis. It is defined as a reduction in cortical thickness, often irregular and asymmetric, associated with deformation of the cups and the overlying parenchyma. Its pathogenesis involves alteration of urinary tract urodynamics and intrarenal reflux (pyelotubular backflow). Multiple scarring may lead to renal failure and hypertension. Compound papillae (fused papillae which drain two or more renal lobes) are more prone to scar than the simple papilla, and they are usually located in the polar regions of the kidneys, explaining why scars are frequently located within these regions. Multifocal scarring leads to a small contracted kidney, with focal areas of compensatory hypertrophy giving the organ an irregular appearance (Fig. 17.9). If scarring is combined with gross reflux or obstruction, generalized calyceal deformation and more general parenchymal reduction may occur. Radiological features visible at US or CT include localized narrowing of the renal parenchyma, deformation of adjacent calyx, and reduced size of the kidney (Fig. 17.10) (Wikstad et al. 1979; Alon et al. 1986; Jakobsson et al. 1992; Gordon et al. 1992; Rink 2011). DMSA shows a reduced uptake of radiotracer, secondary to locally reduced blood flow and disturbed transport mechanism. Its higher sensitivity in renal scar detection is with a delay of at least 3 months after infection (Jakobsson et al. 1992; Gordon et al. 1992).

17.9.2 Renal Abscess

Renal abscess is the collection of infective fluid into the kidney. It represents the most common complication of acute pyelonephritis, and it is the consequence of the severe vasospasm and the inflammation, resulting in colliquative necrosis and abscess formation. Abscesses may be either intraparenchymal, originating in the corticomedullary portion, in the renal cortex, within layers of Gerota's fascia, or extraparenchymal (perinephric abscess). Children may present with persistent high fever, lethargy, and flank pain, associated with leukocytosis, elevated serum erythrocyte sedimentation rate (ESR), or C-reactive peptide (CRP). Dysuria and unpleasant urine smelling are rare; urine cultures can be negative. The distinction between uncomplicated acute pyelonephritis and abscess is important, because the former is treated with antibiotics, whereas an abscess may require drainage (Fig. 17.11). At US typical abscess appears as a hypoechoic/anechoic, septated

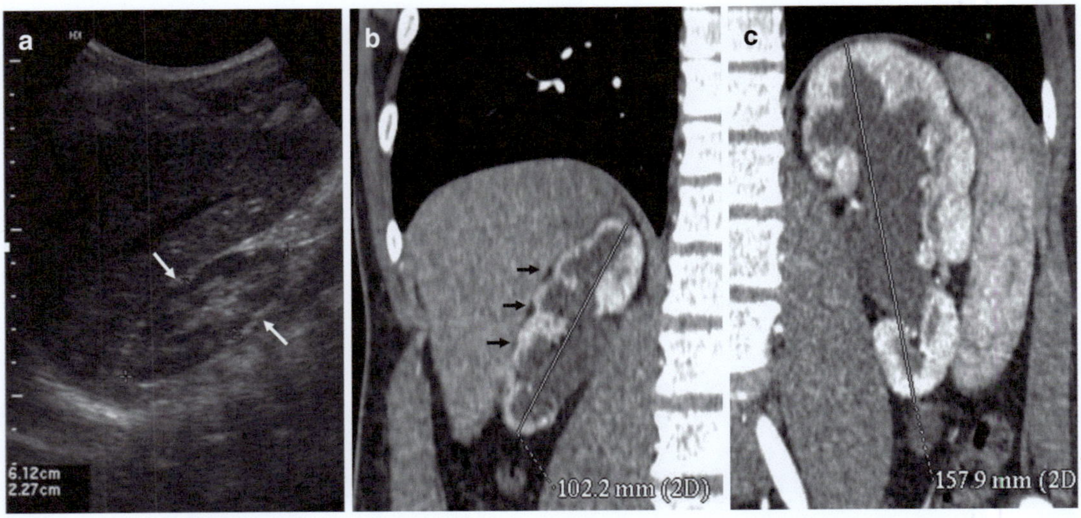

Fig. 17.9 (**a–c**) Two young boys with multiple episodes of acute pyelonephritis in the past. US (**a**) shows reduction of the size of the right kidney, associated with reduction in parenchymal *thickness*, renal calyx corticalization, irregularity of renal profile, and multiple scars (*white arrow*). CT images (**b**, **c**) show the difference in the size and morphology of a pyelonephritic kidney (**b**) and its contralateral (**c**) with compensatory overgrowth. The small kidney also presents reduction of the cortical *thickness* and renal scars (*black arrow*)

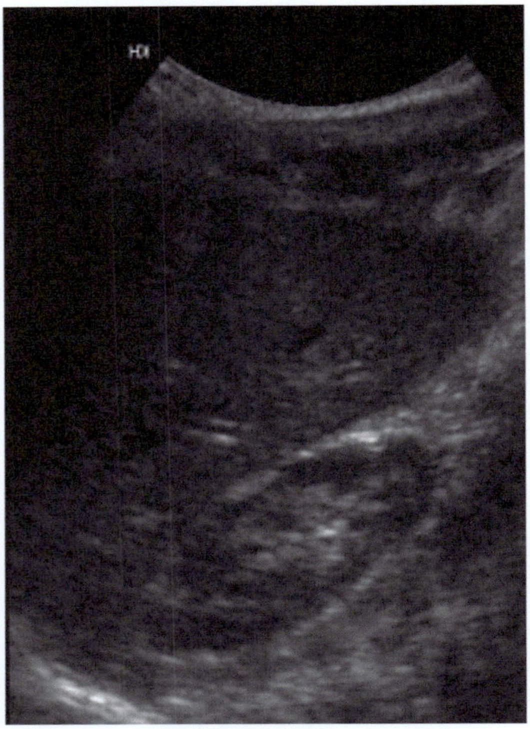

Fig. 17.10 Narrowing of the renal parenchyma and reduced size of the kidney of a 13-year-old boy who suffered from acute pyelonephritis

"mass" within the cortex or in the parenchyma, lacking internal flow at color Doppler (Wippermann et al. 1991). Occasionally, mobile debris or gas may be noted within the collection. US is also the main tool used for follow-up and to determine abscess resolution (Fig. 17.12). CT is not usually necessary for diagnosis, but if performed abscesses typically appear as a well-defined round low-attenuation mass, with a thick enhancing irregular wall (pseudocapsule), although the lesion itself does not enhance. Gas within the collection strongly suggests abscess diagnosis. Surrounding renal parenchyma appears hypoenhancing during nephrographic phase and hyperattenuating in delayed images. Abscess may be associated with perinephric collections and fascial and septal thickening (Rink 2011; Rote et al. 1978). MRI, when performed, shows an enhancing pseudocapsule surrounding a central, low intensity in T1w sequences, high intensity in T2w sequences, and non-enhancing cystic area. Hyperintensity on diffusion-weighted sequences in pyelonephritis and renal abscess results primarily from cytotoxic edema and tubular concentration of inflammatory cells.

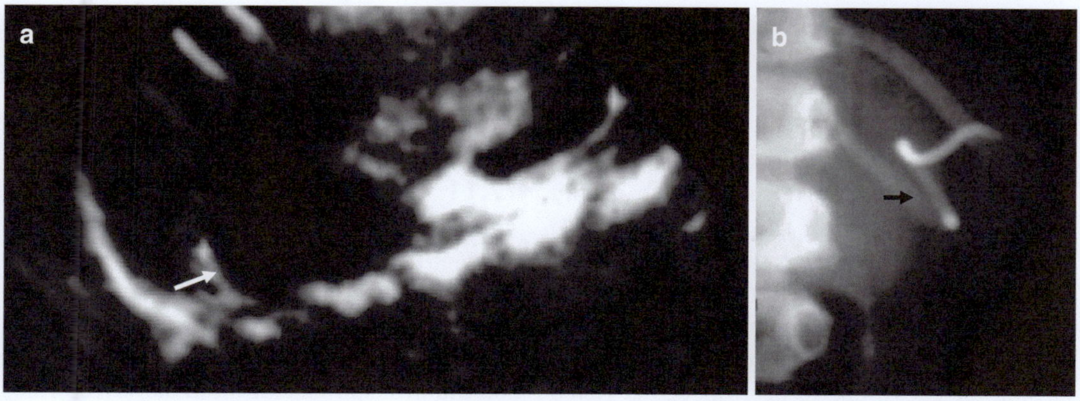

Fig. 17.11 (**a**, **b**) US (**a**) shows a renal abscess (*white arrow*) of the upper pole requiring drainage. An abdominal plain film (**b**) is required to check for drainage positioning (*black arrow*)

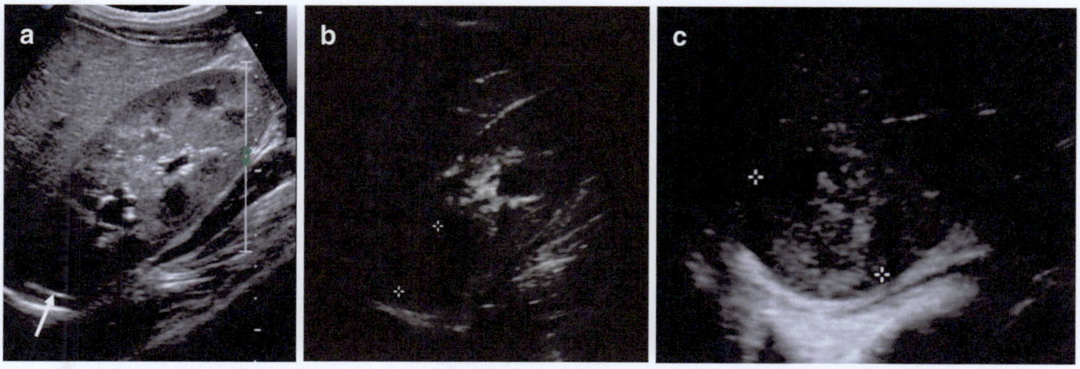

Fig. 17.12 (**a**–**c**) US shows three different phases of evolution of a renal abscess. Image (**a**) shows a focal pyelonephritis (*arrow*) at the *upper pole* of the right kidney, while (**b**) and (**c**) an abscess with necrotic and pyogenic content (caliper)

Because abscesses contain a viscous fluid consisting of water, inflammatory cells, necrotic tissue, and proteinaceous exudates, water proton mobility is very restricted, resulting in a very low signal hypointensity in ADC maps. However, acute or subacute hemorrhage within the collecting system or a renal cyst may also produce high signal intensity on diffusion-weighted sequences potentially mimicking purulent material (Wippermann et al. 1991).

17.9.3 Papillary Necrosis

Acute pyelonephritis may cause renal papillary necrosis as a consequence of the impairment of vascular supply leading to focal or diffuse ischemic necrosis of the distal segments of the renal pyramids, which are particularly vulnerable because the papillary tip receives only a marginal blood supply from the vasa recta. In an early phase, radiological findings are usually normal; afterward multiple poorly marginated, hypoattenuated lesions in the papillary regions can be observed at CT (Bittar and Misanik 1963). In the advanced stage, there are three types of deformity: medullary, papillary, and in situ. In the medullary form, necrosis takes place at the tip of the pyramid, starting in the central part of the calix, creating a round cavity. In the papillary form, necrosis of a larger portion of the papilla occurs. The detachment of necrotic papillae usually begins at the caliceal fornices, and the resulting defect is triangular (lobster claw). In this phase, contrast-enhanced excretory phase CT images show clefts filled with urine and contrast material extending from the fornices to pyramid tip. In the in situ form, necrotic papilla remains attached, shrinks, and may calcify, creating pitfalls at CT, because papillary calcifications may be misinterpreted as small stones (Dyer et al. 2004). During healing phase, shrinkage of the kidney may occur with reduction of parenchymal thickness, due to necrosis of the Henle loops. Loss of renal cortex is associated with hypertrophy of Bertin columns, creating a triangular area of hypoattenuation.

17.9.4 Pyonephrosis

Pyonephrosis is the infection spread to the upper collecting system. Further details on this topic are discussed in the following chapter.

17.9.5 Urosepsis

Urosepsis is the most severe clinical manifestation of acute pyelonephritis, with a mortality rate higher than 40 %. Patients may present with multi-organ dysfunction, hypoperfusion, hypotension, fever, tachypnea, tachycardia, respiratory alkalosis, and pulmonary and abdominal infections.

Its incidence is higher in patients with genitourinary abnormalities or in diabetic and immunosuppressed children.

Whenever complicated urinary infection and urosepsis are suspected but urological abnormalities have not been defined, imaging exam may help in the diagnosis and in the localization of sepsis cause (Kalra and Raizada 2009).

17.10 Acute Kidney Injury

Acute kidney injury (AKI) is defined as an abrupt or rapid decline in renal filtration function. Acute pyelonephritis may rarely be the cause of severe AKI, requiring dialysis in children with an anatomically normal urinary tract and no other predisposing conditions (Nahar et al. 2004).

17.11 Emphysematous Pyelonephritis

Emphysematous pyelonephritis is a life-threatening, rapidly progressive, necrotizing infection of the kidneys that results in gas formation within or surrounding the kidneys. According to literature, *E. coli* or *Enterobacter cloacae* seems to be the most common cause of infection in children. Symptoms are often nonspecific: fever associated with flank pain, nausea, and vomiting. Laboratory findings include leukocytosis, pyuria, elevated creatinine level, hyperglycemia, and thrombocytopenia.

Plain abdominal radiography shows either streaking gas in the renal fossa or crescentic collections of gas within the Gerota fascia (indicative of infection extending into the perinephric space).

Ultrasound shows an enlarged kidney with high-amplitude echoes within the renal parenchyma or collecting system. The echogenic foci show distal ring-down artifact and reverberations; US may demonstrate low-level echoes. Adjacent bowel gas and renal lithiasis may lead to false-positive diagnosis (Päivänsalo and Hellström 1989).

Emphysematous pyelonephritis is classified based on CT configuration as type 1 or type 2. Type 1 is more aggressive, leading to death shortly if not treated immediately. CT shows renal parenchymal destruction manifesting with streaky or mottled areas of gas, with the absence of renal or extrarenal fluid collections.

Type 2 is characterized by gas in the pelvicalyceal system or ureter, associated with renal or extrarenal fluid collections (Huang and Tseng 2000).

17.12 Renal Infarction

Renal infarction is a very rare complication of acute pyelonephritis, presenting as a main differential diagnosis because clinical and laboratory presentations may be undistinguishable. It results from the discontinuation of the normal arterial blood supply or venous drainage to the part of or to the whole kidney. Similar to pyelonephritis, infarcted areas appear as wedge-shaped hypoechoic regions at US, with no flow at color Doppler examination and with no enhancement at CT. However, in approximately 50 % of cases, CT shows a thin rim (2–4 mm) of cortex enhancing normally (cortical rim sign) due to collateral capsular perfusion. This sign is usually absent immediately after infarction, presenting normally 8 h after occlusion, specific of renal infarction (Bourgault et al. 2013). Another specific CT sign is the presence of a region of hypoenhancement on early phases becoming hyperattenuating on delayed imaging (flip-flop enhancement) sign of ischemia rather than true infarction. Moreover, the normal and homogeneous appearance of the perirenal fat, with no stranding or fluid collections throughout the perinephric space, should discourage the diagnosis of acute pyelonephritis (Dalla Palma et al. 1997; Suzer et al. 2002).

17.13 Differential Diagnosis

Differential diagnosis includes renal infarction, renal lymphoma, sarcoidosis, tuberculosis, malacoplakia, renal location of Kawasaki disease, and Castleman disease.

The most common extrapulmonary tuberculosis location is the urinary tract; due to its nonspecific symptoms, CT is essential in the diagnosis showing thickening, distortion, ulceration, and fibrosis, often with stricture formation of the collecting system. Other CT signs are papillary necrosis and calcification. The combination of two of these radiological signs highly suggests diagnosis of tuberculosis, even in the absence of pulmonary findings (Wang et al. 1997).

Malacoplakia (meaning "soft plaque") is an uncommon chronic granulomatous inflammatory disease related to an abnormal host response to chronic infection, usually affecting urinary bladder, but any urothelial organs may be involved. Clinical symptoms are nonspecific similar to those of an acute pyelonephritis. At US malacoplakia lesions appear as poorly defined, hypoehoic masses within an enlarged, deformed kidney. CT shows an enlarged kidney with hypovascular masses, ranging from few mm up to 3–4 cm. At MRI the lesions appear hypointense both in T1- and T2-weighted sequences, with delayed enhancement due to the presence of fibrous tissue (Dobyan et al. 1993).

Extrathoracic involvement in sarcoidosis is not uncommon, occurring in up to 30 % of patients. Renal disease often causes nephrocalcinosis or glomerular nephritis from direct infiltration. Granulomatous pseudotumors are rare presentation of renal sarcoidosis. Nodules are hyperechoic at US and hypoenhancing on contrast-enhanced CT. MRI shows poor circumscription of the nodules form renal parenchyma, indicating interstitial infiltration. On T1- and T2-weighted imaging, lesions remain isointense to the surrounding renal parenchyma and hypointense after contrast administration (Heldmann et al. 2005).

Renal lymphoma rarely may be seen as primary disease. Ultrasound shows single or multiple hypoechoic lesions within renal parenchyma with internal vascularity.

CT reveals single or multiple, homogeneous, hypodense masses.

At MRI renal lymphoma appears hypointense to renal parenchyma on T1-weighted sequences and hyperintense on T2-weighted sequences, showing poor enhancement after contrast administration (Sheth et al. 2006).

References

Alon U, Pery M, Davidai G, Berant M (1986) Ultrasonography in the radiologic evaluation of children with urinary tract infection. Pediatrics 78:58–64

Becknell B et al (2015) The diagnosis, evaluation and treatment of acute and recurrent pediatric urinary tract infections. Expert Rev Anti-Infect Ther 13:81–90

Bhat RG et al (2011) Pediatric urinary tract infections. Emerg Med Clin North Am 29:637–653

Bittar EE, Misanik L (1963) Renal necrotizing papillitis. Am J Med 34:82–87

Bocquet N et al (2015) Imaging strategy for children after a first episode of pyelonephritis. Arch Pediatr 22:547–553

Bourgault M, Grimbert P, Verret C et al (2013) Acute renal infarction: a case series. Clin J Am Soc Nephrol 8:392–398

Calisti A et al (2008) The risk of associated urological abnormalities in children with pre and postnatal occasional diagnosis of solitary, small or ectopic kidney: is a complete urological screening always necessary? World J Urol 26:281–284

Craig WD et al (2008) From the archives of the AFIP. Pyelonephritis: radiologic-pathologic review. RadioGraphics 28:255–276

Dalla Palma L, Pozzi Mucelli R, Pozzi Mucelli F (1997) Delayed CT in acute renal infarction. Semin Ultrasound CT MR 18:122–128

Das CJ et al (2014) Multimodality imaging of renal inflammatory lesions. World J Radiol 6:865–873

Dobyan DC, Truong LD, Eknoyan G (1993) Renal malacoplakia reappraised. Am J Kidney Dis 22:243–252

Dyer RB, Chen MY, Zagoria RJ (2004) Classic signs in uroradiology. RadioGraphics 24(Spec Issue):S247–S280

Gearhart JG, Rink RC, Mouriquand PDE (2011) Pediatric urology

Goel RH et al (2015) Acute urinary tract disorders. Radiol Clin N Am 53:1273–1292

Gordon I, Anderson PJ, Lythgoe MF, Orton M (1992) Can technetium-99m-mercaptoacetyltriglycine replace technetium-99m-dimercaptosuccinic acid in the exclusion of a focal renal defect? J Nucl Med 12:2090–2093

Heldmann M, Behm W, Reddy MP, Bozeman C, Welman G, Abreo F, Minagar A (2005) Pseudotumoral renal sarcoid: MRI, PET, and MDCT appearance with pathologic correlation. AJR Am J Roentgenol 185:697–699

Huang JJ, Tseng CC (2000) Emphysematous pyelonephritis: clinicoradiological classification, management, prognosis, and pathogenesis. Arch Intern Med 160:797–805

Jakobsson B, Nolstedt L, Svensson L, So'derlundh S, Berg U (1992) 99mTechnetium-dimercaptosuccinic acid scan in the diagnosis of acute pyelonephritis in children: relation to clinical and radiological findings. Pediatr Nephrol 6:328–334

Kalra OP, Raizada A (2009) Approach to a patient with urosepsis. J Global Infect Dis 1:57–63

Nahar A, Akom M, Hanes D, Briglia A, Drachenberg CB, Weinman EJ (2004) Pyelonephritis and acute renal failure. Am J Med Sci 328:121–123

Päivänsalo M, Hellström P, Siniluoto T et al (1989) Emphysematous pyelonephritis. Radiologic and clinical findings in six cases. Acta Radiol 30: 311–315

Rote AR, Bauer SB, Retik AB (1978) Renal abscess in children. J Urol 119:254–258

Shaikh N et al (2010) Risk of renal scarring in children with a first urinary tract infection: a systematic review. Pediatrics 126(6):1084–1091

Sheth S, Ali S, Fishman E (2006) Imaging of renal lymphoma: patterns of disease with pathologic correlation. Radiographics 26:1151–1168

Suzer O, Shirkhoda A, Jafri SZ, Madrazo BL, Bis KG, Mastromatteo JF (2002) CT features of renal infarction. Eur J Radiol 44:59–64

Wang LJ, Wong YC, Chen CJ, Lim KE (1997) CT features of genitourinary tuberculosis. J Comput Assist Tomogr 21:254–258

Wikstad I, Aperia A, Broberger O, Ekengren K (1979) Vesicoureteric reflux and pyelonephritis. Long time effect on area of renal parenchyma. Acta Radiol Diagn 20:252–260

Wippermann C, Schofer O, Beetz R, Schumacher R, Schweden F, Riedmiller H et al (1991) Renal abscess in childhood: diagnostic and therapeutic progress. Pediatr Infect Dis J 10:446–450

Yu M, Robinson K, Siegel C, Menias C. Complicated Genitourinary Tract Infections and Mimics. Curr Probl Diagn Radiol 2016 Feb 11 [Epub ahead of print]

18 Hydronephrosis and Pyonephrosis

Silvia Lorenzi, Francesca Fanti,
Giacomo Aringhieri, Marco Di Maurizio,
Claudio Defilippi, and Michele Tonerini

18.1 Introduction

Urinary tract infections (UTIs) are a frequent clinical problem in infants and children, and they may develop into serious complications with long-term sequelae. Their prevalence varies according to age and sex: males are more interested in the neonatal period and in the first year of age, while females are more involved after that time. The clinical outcome and the severity of UTIs depend on many risk factors including urinary tract malformations and dysfunctions, virulence and properties of the pathogen, host response to the infection, and promptness of diagnosis and management.

Febrile UTIs usually are the result of a pyelonephritis, but more serious and uncommon presentation such as renal abscess and a pyonephrosis may occur and they are clinically indistinguishable from pyelonephritis. Various manifestations sometimes coexist and represent different expressions of the same infectious process that may evolve from a mild infection to dangerous complications, like emphysematous pyelonephritis. The pyonephrosis is included in this inflammatory spectrum especially in the presence of obstructed and/or dilated collecting systems (Bitsori et al. 2015).

18.2 Hydronephrosis and Pyonephrosis

A pyonephrosis is associated with dilation and obstruction of the collecting system and is defined as an infected hydronephrotic kidney, which results in the accumulation of pus in the upper excretory pathways.

It is a severe and aggressive infection originated in the enlarged pelvicalyceal system that causes destructive changes of renal parenchyma and inflammatory reactions in the perirenal tissues; in cases of delayed diagnosis, it may determine sepsis and irreversible renal function deterioration. The purulent exudate is composed of sloughed urothelium, bacteria, debris, and inflammatory cells; the amount of pus varies depending on the type of infection and severity of the inflammatory process and can become obstructive or worsen a prior obstructive condition with consequent hydronephrosis. The pathogenesis of pyonephrosis implies infection

S. Lorenzi • F. Fanti • G. Aringhieri
Department of Diagnostic and Interventional Radiology, University of Pisa, Pisa, Italy

M. Di Maurizio • C. Defilippi
Pediatric Radiology, Meyer University Children's Hospital, Florence, Italy

M. Tonerini (✉)
Department of Emergency Radiology, Cisanello University Hospital, Pisa, Italy
e-mail: m.tonerini@tiscali.it

V. Miele, M. Trinci (eds.), *Imaging Non-traumatic Abdominal Emergencies in Pediatric Patients*,
DOI 10.1007/978-3-319-41866-7_18

(almost always ascending dissemination), obstruction, and stasis as trigger mechanisms. The bacterial spectrum responsible for this pathological entity does not differ from that of other forms of UTIs; the vast majority of etiological agents derives from the intestinal flora, including *E. coli*, *Klebsiella*, *Proteus*, and *Enterobacter* species between the most frequent. Pyonephrosis may occur as a complicated evolution of pyelonephritis or represent the clinical manifestation of a superimposed infection developed on a preexisting hydronephrosis; the latter needs further investigations to diagnose the underlying cause, once the acute phase has been solved and the child has recovered. Pediatric hydronephrosis is classified as obstructive and nonobstructive; the most common causes are vesicoureteral reflux (VUR) and pelviureteric junction obstruction, while less frequent are ureteral duplication, ureterocele, ectopic ureter, and posterior urethral valves (Sharma et al. 2004; Patel et al. 2013).

Obstructive uropathy secondary to lithiasis has already been treated in Chap. 16.

18.2.1 Diagnosis

The clinical manifestations of pyonephrosis may range from asymptomatic bacteriuria to frank sepsis. In the older children, the presentation is similar to that of the adults: a history of high-grade fever, chills, flank pain, and tenderness is very suspicious for a patient affected by upper UTIs. Neonates and younger children are not able to describe their clinical condition and may present nonspecific symptoms like fever, lack of appetite, lethargy, irritability, vomiting, or diarrhea. At physical examination, the child manifests pallor, dehydration, abdominal distension, and loose of bowel motion; rarely, a palpable abdominal mass is appreciable in the site of the hydronephrotic kidney. Laboratory studies include blood and urine exams. Hematology results show raised white cell count, C-reactive protein, urea, and creatinine; blood culture is needed in case of suspected sepsis. Urine analysis reveals bacteriuria with leukocytes and nitrites; pyuria may be present; urine culture must be obtained in order to guide antibiotic therapy (Bitsori et al. 2015; St Lezin et al. 1992).

All these clinical and laboratoristic features are not specific for pyonephrosis and have to be associated with the evidence of obstruction, hydronephrosis, and suppurative infection in order to support the diagnosis; these findings are shown by imaging investigations, especially ultrasound (US) that represents the first-level examination.

18.2.2 Imaging Findings

US provides a sensitivity of 90 % and specificity of 97 % in the diagnosis of pyonephrosis versus simple hydronephrosis, by showing in addition to pelvicalyceal dilation the following findings: lack of a completely anechoic collecting system due to echogenic debris, representing the most reliable signs of pyonephrosis, internal echoes dispersed or stratified with evidence of fluid-debris levels, and echogenic foci with acoustic shadowing corresponding to gas within the pelvis, secondary to gas-forming organisms (Fig. 18.1). These findings are specific and their absence excludes pyonephrosis with a high degree of accuracy (Craig et al. 2008; Subramanyam et al. 1983; Jeffrey et al. 1985).

The associated dilation of upper excretory system is commonly evaluated basing on the hydronephrosis grading system represented in Table 18.1 (Figs. 18.2, 18.3, and 18.4) (Riccabona et al. 2008; Schlomer et al. 2014).

Depending on the variable nature of the purulent exudate, occasionally pyonephrosis may be totally anechoic simulating uncomplicated hydronephrosis, and US may only demonstrate nonspecific findings like nephromegaly and/or increased parenchymal echogenicity. In these cases, clinical manifestation and laboratory analysis support the diagnosis when upper UTI is strongly suspected (Schneider et al. 1989).

Computed tomography (CT) is quite rarely performed in pediatric patients, usually in cases of emergency and complicated form of pyelonephritis. Considering that infants have higher radiation sensitivity, it obviously requires

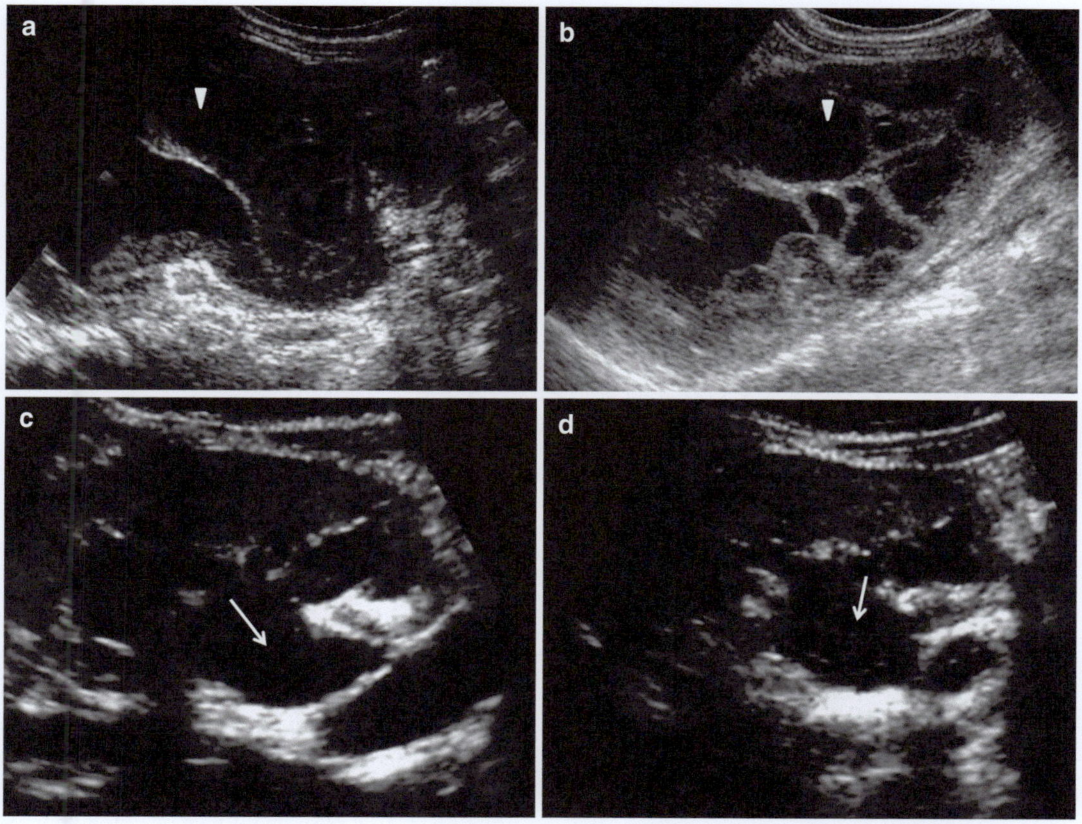

Fig. 18.1 (**a**–**d**) Hydropyonephrosis at US. Dilated and enlarged pelvicalyceal system with lack of normal anechoic aspect due to accumulation of inflammatory material in the excretory pathway: the exudate is well detected by revealing the presence of internal echoes that may appear stratified with evidence of fluid-debris levels (*arrowhead* in **a** and **b**) or dispersed as echogenic foci with acoustic shadowing (*arrow* in **c** and **d**)

Table 18.1 Grading systems of hydronephrosis

Grade 0	Normal examination with no dilation of the renal pelvis
Grade 1	Mild dilation of renal pelvis only (axial diameter less than 5–7 mm), without dilation of the calyces
Grade 2	Moderate dilation of the renal pelvis (axial diameter between 7 and 10 mm) including a few calyces with normal forniceal shape
Grade 3	Marked dilatation of the renal pelvis (larger than 10 mm) and all the calyces with reduced forniceal and papillary differentiation, normal renal parenchyma
Grade 4	Gross dilatation of the collecting system, parenchymal atrophy seen as thinning of the renal cortex

Adapted from the Society of Fetal Ultrasound classification for postnatal use Riccabona et al. (2008)

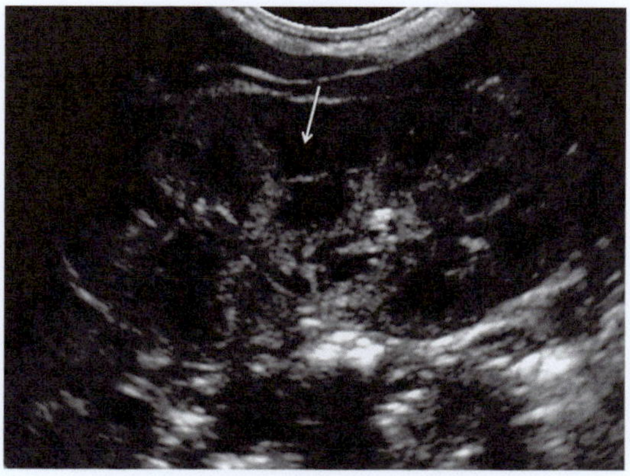

Fig. 18.2 Normal pediatric kidney at US. The aspect of a healthy kidney especially in neonates is characterized by a physiological increased echogenicity of the renal parenchyma with hypo-/anechoic pyramids that are therefore more evident and may resemble dilated calyces, being wrongly diagnosed as hydronephrosis

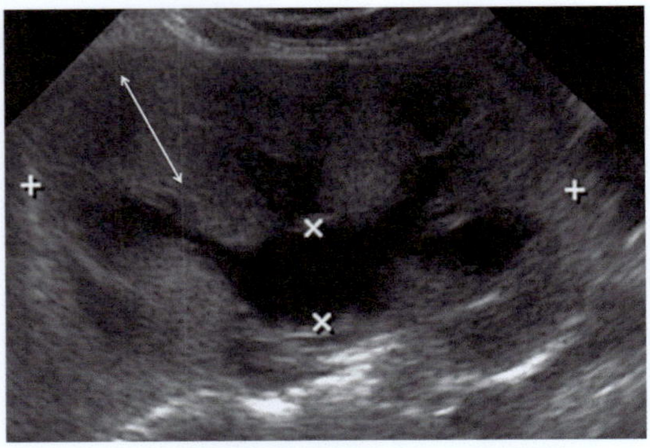

Fig. 18.3 Hydronephrosis: grade 3. Marked dilation of the renal pelvis and calyces with normal thickness of renal parenchyma that is still preserved (*doublehead arrow*)

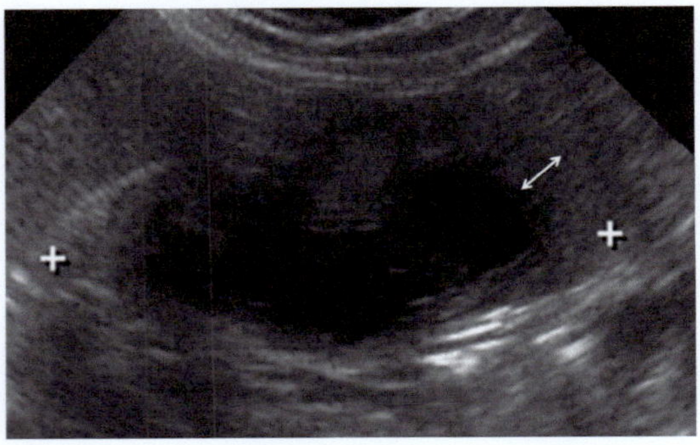

Fig. 18.4 Hydronephrosis: grade 4. Marked dilation of the collecting system with reduced thickness of the renal parenchyma seen as thinning of the renal cortex (*double-head arrow*)

dedicated age- and weight-adapted protocols for exposure parameters and contrast medium, and it may be performed in case of correct indications and after accurate evaluation of the diagnostic advantages (Riccabona 2009).

Actually CT cannot always reliably differentiate an uninfected hydronephrotic kidney from pyonephrosis, especially only on the base of fluid attenuation measurements within the pelvis that should result superior to the water density value (>10–20 Hounsfield unit). In addition to obstruction and dilatation of the collecting system, CT findings suggesting pyonephrosis include thickening of the renal pelvic wall (>2 mm), renal and perirenal inflammatory changes, and layering of contrast material above the purulent debris on excretory study (Craig et al. 2008; Fultz et al. 1993).

The added value of CT consists of showing perinephric findings (such as fat stranding and thickening of the renal fascia), evaluating the nephrogram appearance to reveal the parenchymal involvement, confirming the presence of gas in the collecting system (the strongest indicator for pyonephrosis on CT), and ruling out abscesses or stone disease. Furthermore, CT is relevant when a complicated evolution is suspected especially because a different and more aggressive treatment may be required.

18.2.3 Treatment and Prognosis

The treatment of choice is represented by percutaneous nephrostomy in combination with appropriate antibiotics and other supportive therapy. Nephrectomy is exceptional and limited to complicated cases (Roebuck 2011; Ng et al. 2002).

The prognosis is good in most patients who receive prompt diagnosis and treatment. Pyonephrosis should be diagnosed as soon as possible in order to avoid a rapid decline in renal function risking permanent loss of kidney parenchyma and development of septic shock with severe systemic complications.

UTIs, especially when recurrent, remain a frequent indication for further imaging evaluation of the pediatric urinary tract, and once the acute phase of the infectious disease is solved, potential predisposing factors must be investigated. The goal is early recognition of urinary tract malformations and VUR, in order to improve outcome and prevent end-stage renal failure due to late or inappropriate treatment. Indeed, in spite of prenatal US screening, a number of urinary tract malformations are only detected after symptomatic clinical presentation. On the other hand, in a child with known normal anatomy and a clinically evident diagnosis, additional imaging may be unnecessary.

Second-level investigations include cystourethrography for VUR assessment and morphological evaluation, bladder function studies, dimercaptosuccinic acid (DMSA) scintigraphy, and magnetic resonance imaging (MRI) to evaluate renal parenchymal involvement and scars.

18.3 Vesicoureteral Reflux

The VUR is one of the most important risk factors for recurrent UTIs in children, although VUR itself does not represent the direct cause of infections or renal damage and it may be associated with bladder dysfunction. VUR refers to the retrograde flow of urine from the urinary bladder into the ureter and often to the calyces (Bates and Riccabona 2013). It is an anatomic and functional disorder with potentially serious consequences, such as recurrent febrile UTI and renal parenchymal scars (Altobelli et al. 2014).

VUR is detected in 0, 4–1, and 8 % of normal population without complaints (Eccles and Jacobs 2000; Mak and Kuo 2003; Lama et al. 2000). Its prevalence is probably underestimated because reflux is diagnosed in those patients who are symptomatic. In newborns, VUR is more prevalent in males, but female-to-male ratio of reflux in children over 3 years old seems to be of 2:1 (Altobelli et al. 2014; Chand et al. 2003). White children are affected ten times more than black ones, in particular red-hair children seems to have an increased risk of VUR.

In the population with UTIs, the incidence varies from 30 % to 50 % depending on age and gender. The reported prevalence of VUR in siblings (27 %) and in offspring (36 %) suggested that there is a genetic component, still undefined, but supposed to be dominant with variable penetrance (Skoog et al. 2010; Kelly et al. 2005).

Approximately 20–30 % of children with VUR present with renal lesions: despite neonatal VUR, there is a high percentage of spontaneous resolution (30–40 % of grade 4–5 VUR can resolve within 2–6 years of age); nevertheless this population have high risk of acute pyelonephritis, hypertension, and chronic renal failure during the first months of life (Lama et al. 2000; Caione et al. 2004). In children and young adults who need substitutive renal therapy, VUR incidence is about 6 % and it represents the fifth most common cause of chronic renal insufficiency (CRI) (Ardissino et al. 1995). However, the severity of VUR greatly varies and thus may affect patients differently, and some patients seem to have a genetic predisposition to renal injury (Bates and Riccabona 2013). Hypertension develops in 10 % of children with unilateral scars and in 18.5 % with bilateral scars. Approximately 4 % of children with VUR progress to end-stage renal failure (Ardissino et al. 2004).

VUR is associated with anomalies of the ureterovesical junction (UVJ), and it is often seen in patients with other urinary tract anomalies (Knudson et al. 2007a). UVJ anomalies consist in excessive lateralization, larger dimensions, shorter length of submucosal ureteral tract, or deficiency in longitudinal muscular fibers of the terminal ureter (Bates and Riccabona 2013).

Congenital or primary VUR may be caused by a sort of immaturity of UVJ, which spontaneously solves in large percentage within the first year of life. Secondary VUR is a functional disorder found in patients with bladder outlet obstruction or neurogenic bladder disease, which lead to thinning and weakening of the UVJ musculature and increased intravesical pressure (Bates and Riccabona 2013).

Two types of urine may flow back to the calyces: infected or sterile urine. Intrarenal reflux of infected urine seems to be the cause of renal damage, whereas intrarenal reflux of sterile urine (under normal intrapelvic pressure) has not been identified as responsible for clinical significant renal scars. Thus, renal lesions seem to develop only in the setting of intrarenal reflux in combination with UTIs, except in patients with neurogenic bladder disease (Knudson et al. 2007b). In this condition also reflux of sterile urine may lead to renal damage in association with the highly pressurized system, especially in high grade of reflux (Knudson et al. 2007b). In children, high intravesical pressure may be sustained by overactive bladder (e.g., detrusor hyperreflexia, detrusor instability), aggravating a preexisting primary VUR or causing secondary VUR.

Historically, VUR is classified by the International Reflux Committee into five grades (Table 18.2), based on the degree of retrograde filling and dilatation of the renal collecting system seen on voiding cystourethrogram (VCUG) (Figs. 18.5, 18.6, 18.7, 18.8, and 18.9) (Lebowitz et al. 1985). Higher grades of reflux are associated with decreased self-resolution rate, which is

Table 18.2 VUR classification into 5° on VCUG by the International Reflux Committee (Knudson et al. 2007b)

Grade 1	Urine backs up into the ureter only, and the renal pelvis appears healthy, with sharp calyces
Grade 2	Urine backs up into the ureter, renal pelvis, and calyces; the renal pelvis appears healthy and has sharp calyces
Grade 3	Urine backs up into the ureter and collecting system; the ureter and pelvis appear mildly dilated, and the calyces are mildly blunted
Grade 4	Urine backs up into the ureter and collecting system; the ureter and pelvis appear moderately dilated, and the calyces are moderately blunted
Grade 5	Urine backs up into the ureter and collecting system; the pelvis is severely dilated, the ureter appears tortuous, and the calyces are severely blunted

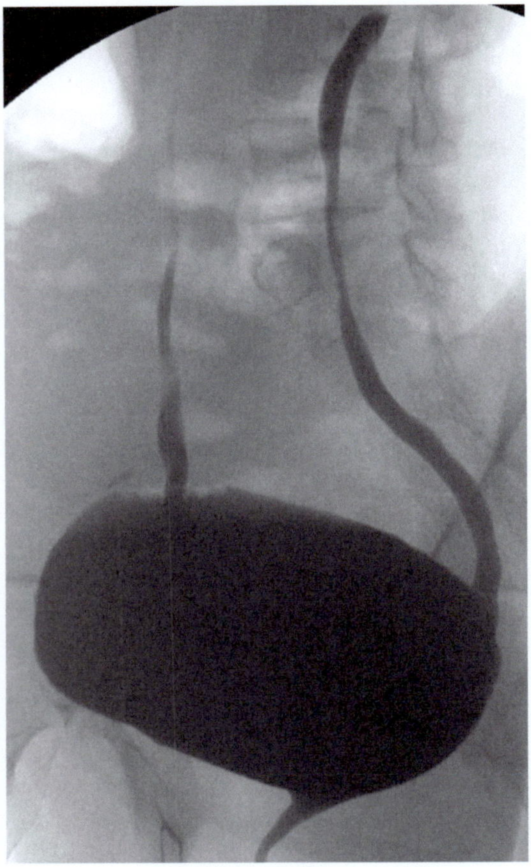

Fig. 18.5 VCUG: vesicoureteral reflux, grade 1. Retrograde filling of contrast medium into the ureters only that are not dilated

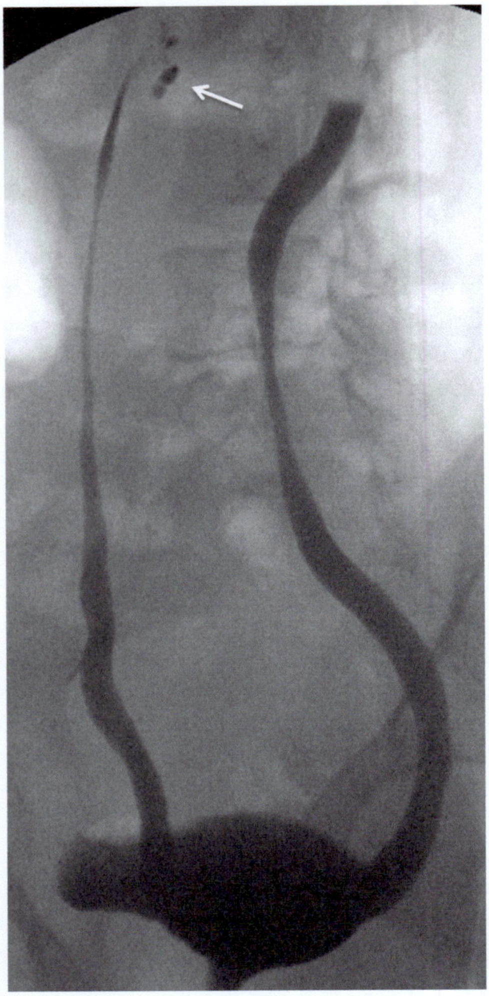

Fig. 18.6 VCUG: vesicoureteral reflux, grade 2. Retrograde filling of contrast medium into the ureters bilaterally and until the pelvis and calyces on the right side (*arrow*), without dilation

also related to some other factors such as age presentation, gender, laterality, bladder volume, and pressure at the onset of reflux, voiding dysfunction, history of UTI, ureteral anatomy, and prevalence of renal scars (Bates and Riccabona 2013).

VUR may be diagnosed in the prenatal period at sonographic examination when transient dilatation of the upper urinary tract is noted in conjunction with the bladder emptying in late gestation (>28 weeks). Approximately 10 % of neonates diagnosed prenatally with dilatation of the upper urinary tract will be found to have reflux postnatally (Ylinen et al. 2003). In neonates

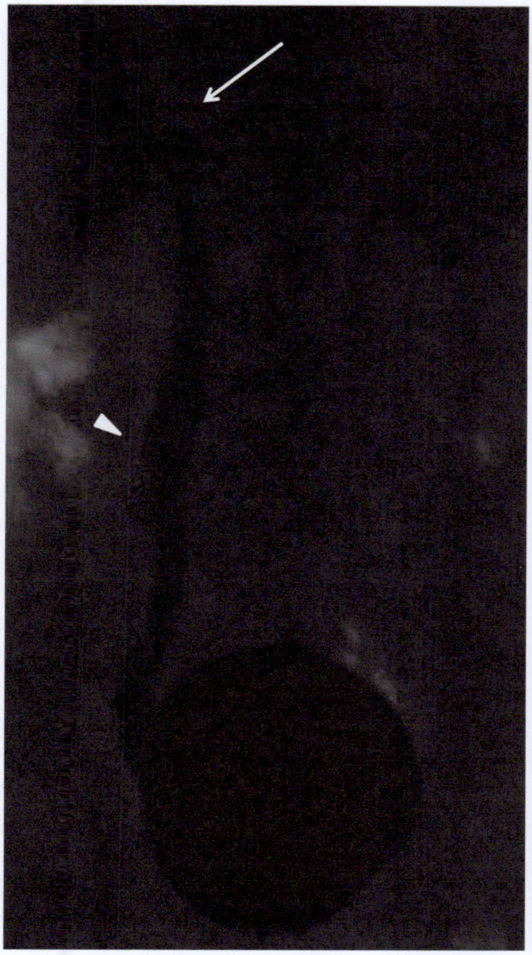

Fig. 18.7 VCUG: vesicoureteral reflux, grade 3. Retrograde filling of contrast medium until the pelvis and calyces bilaterally, with mild pelvis (*arrow*) and ureter (*arrowhead*) dilation on the right side

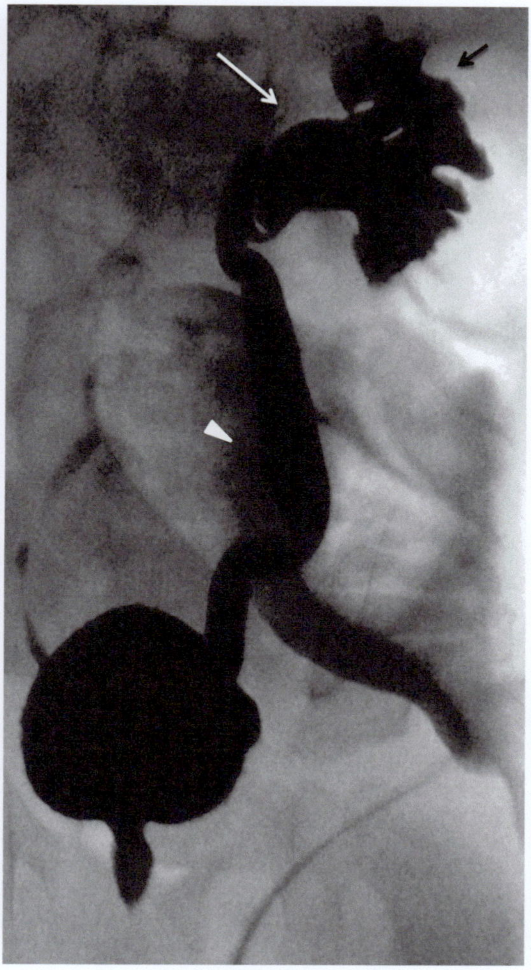

Fig. 18.8 VCUG: vesicoureteral reflux, grade 4. Retrograde filling of contrast medium until the pelvis and calyces on the left side, with dilation of the ureter (*arrowhead*) and pelvis (*white arrow*) and moderate blunted aspect of the calyces (*black arrow*)

clinical presentation is characterized by respiratory distress, persistent vomiting, failure to thrive, renal failure, flank masses, and urinary ascites, and VUR may subsequently be diagnosed with severe UTI. Recurrent febrile UTIs are the most important and common presentation.

In the past, Academy of Pediatrics guidelines recommended renal-bladder US and VCUG for any child from 2 to 24 months of age who presented with their first febrile UTI. After a revision in 2011, only US is recommended after first episode of UTI (Roberts 2011). To evaluate secondary VUR caused by bladder/bowel dysfunction, recent studies have identified specific voiding patterns during urodynamic study in children with voiding dysfunction without anatomical and/or neurological abnormalities (Altobelli et al. 2014).

US is necessary to examine the upper urinary tract morphology, dilatation, parenchymal thickness, and echogenicity (Altobelli et al. 2014). US can identify indirect signs of VUR, such as uroepithelial thickening of the ureter or renal pelvis, changing diameter of the pelvicalyceal system and ureter, quick refilling of the bladder after voiding, asymmetric ureteral inflow jets, and a lateralized position or unusual shape of the ure-

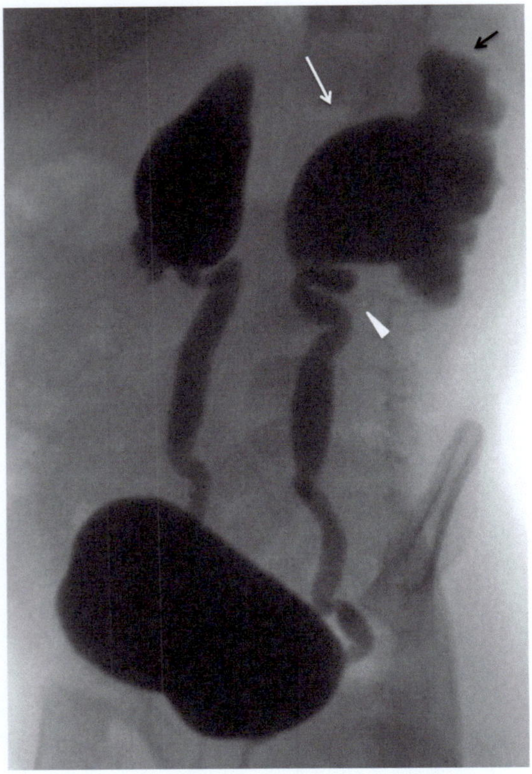

Fig. 18.9 VCUG: vesicoureteral reflux, grade 5. Bilateral retrograde filling of contrast medium until the pelvis and calyces, with severe dilation of the pelvis (*white arrow*) and ureter that is tortuous (*arrowhead*); severe blunted aspect of the calyces (*black arrow*)

teral ostium (Bates and Riccabona 2013). Great dilatation of the whole collective system, with clubbing of the calyces and elongated and tortuous ureters, is typical of severe VUR. These signs are often associated with poor ureteral peristalsis, especially in correlation with high-grade VUR and UTI.

Moreover, VUR may be directly observed by contrast-enhanced voiding ultrasonography (ce-VUS) that consists in a US examination with injection of shaken saline solution with air or commercially available contrast agents via suprapubic or transurethral catheterization till bladder filling (Bates and Riccabona 2013).

Ultrasound techniques such as harmonic imaging, stimulated acoustic emission, or other contrast-specific techniques have further enhanced ce-VUS potential for VUR depiction and grading, resulting in a reported sensitivity and specificity equal to VCUG (Bates and Riccabona 2013; Riccabona 2008).

Nevertheless, VCUG remains the basic imaging technique to detect VUR and to determine its degree (Figs. 18.5, 18.6, 18.7, 18.8, and 18.9). This exam is performed with iodinated contrast medium instilled into the catheterized and emptied urinary bladder, which is filled to near capacity. Bladder capacity is estimated on the basis of weight, multiplied by 7 (mL = kg × 7). Over 1 year of age, it equals age in years plus 2, multiplied by 30 [mL = (age + 2) × 30].

The fluoroscopic observation of the (early) filling phase, the distal ureters (in oblique projections), the renal collecting system, and the urethra during voiding (lateral projection in boys) enables focused imaging of critical areas and conditions such as intrarenal VUR and UVJ anatomy (Bates and Riccabona 2013). VUR is not always well depicted in the first fill and void; in order to avoid missing significant VUR, VCUG should be repeated cyclically.

The appearance of refluxing ureters and pelvicalyceal systems on VCUG is quite variable, ranging from normal-sized upper tracts to extreme upper tract dilatation and marked ureteral tortuosity (Bates and Riccabona 2013). In some patients, VUR is accompanied by a transient phenomenon depicted as marked ballooning of the pelvicalyceal system in the absence of evidence of ureteropelvic junction (UPJ) obstruction. Sometimes VUR may induce a kink at the UPJ, producing a functional valve-like UPJ obstruction.

When VUR is extended to the calyces, finding an intrarenal reflux is important because of its association with renal scarring. Intrarenal reflux may be depicted as a transient pyelotubular and interstitial reflux of contrast media extending outward in a wedge-shaped pattern from one or more papillae to the renal cortical surface (Fig. 18.10).

The physiopathological basis of intrarenal reflux is supposed to be an abnormal morphology of the opening of the collecting ducts of Bellini on the renal papilla, which appears round, more common at the poles, and therefore less resistant

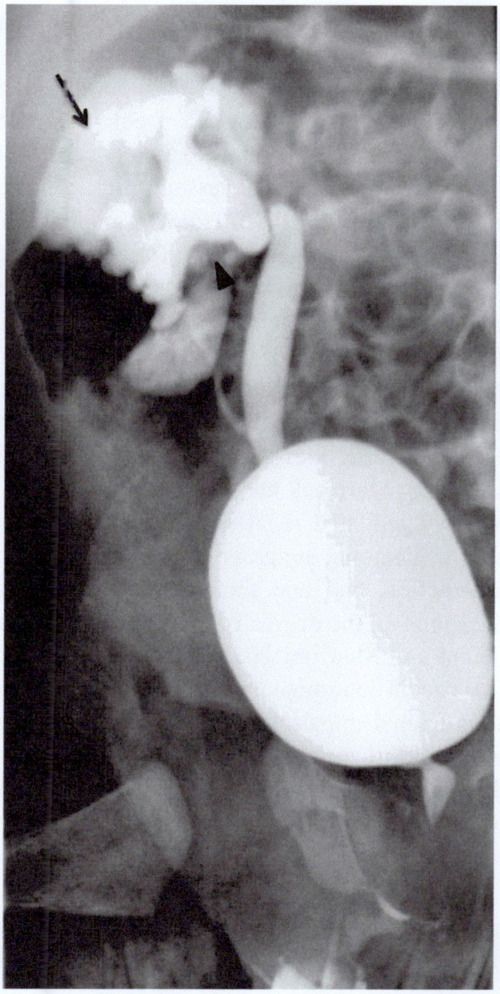

Fig. 18.10 VCUG: intrarenal reflux. Image shows contrast medium reflux until pelvis and calyces extending outward from the papillae to the interstitium of the renal cortex (*arrow*), so that the profile of the kidney results well delineated

to retrograde flow than the slitlike openings of the ducts of simple or conical papillae (Bates and Riccabona 2013).

The study of the renal parenchyma is usually performed by US and by DMSA scintigraphy. US may show parenchymal damage depicted as areas of depression in the outline of the kidney in correspondence of the dilated and distorted calyx. Color Doppler imaging may reveal a focal reduction of peripheral vascularization. Nuclear scintigraphy using DMSA is especially sensitive in detecting renal cortical scars and is considered the gold standard. This technique may reveal the inflammation of acute pyelonephritis or chronic renal scars, evaluating the degree of renal damage, which has main importance during follow-up (Bates and Riccabona 2013).

Other methods for the evaluation of the upper tract are contrast-enhanced CT and MRI, which may become indicated for assessment of complicated disease (Bates and Riccabona 2013).

The European Association of Urology recommends a DMSA scan if VUR is diagnosed on initial VCUG. On the other hand, the American Urological Association recommends the renoscintigraphy study only if an abnormal US is reported during breakthrough UTIs, in children presenting high-grade VUR (grade III–V) or elevated serum creatinine (Peters et al. 2010). This diagnostic approach is "bottom-up" (Altobelli et al. 2014).

The recent National Institute for Health and Clinical Excellence (NICE) guidelines alternatively suggest a "top-down approach" with an initial renal ultrasound or a DMSA scan performed 4–6 months after the infection in order to assess renal scarring rather than pyelonephritis, in children with their first febrile UTI. This approach may avoid unnecessary VCUG in patients with normal DMSA (in 35–60 % of cases), reducing children radiation exposure (Herz et al. 2010; National Collaborating Center for Women's and Children's Health (UK) 2007; Weinberg et al. 2013). This same motivation leads some authors to suggest also the use of ce-VUS with endovesical instillation (Piaggio et al. 2003). This is the main advantage of the recent "top-down approach" (Altobelli et al. 2014).

18.4 Ureteropelvic Junction Obstruction

The UPJ obstruction is the most common cause of hydronephrosis in neonatal age, and it is usually due to an intrinsic cause (a short stenotic segment at the UPJ) or less commonly to an extrinsic compression secondary to bands, kinks, or aberrant vessels (Dewan et al. 1998). Obstruction can be also determined by a high insertion of the UPJ on the dilated renal pelvis, but the UPJ displacement could be an effect rather than a cause. Aberrant or crossing lower pole vessels are found in more than 30 % of older children and adults undergoing pyeloplasty for this cause, while they are present in less than 5 % of infants with prenatally detected UPJ obstruction; they are incidental to an intrinsic obstruction in the latter, but in older patients, they are the cause of the obstruction.

The male-to-female ratio is approximately equal and the left kidney is more commonly affected than the right. The condition usually occurs on a sporadic basis, but familial inheritance has been reported. UPJ obstruction is more common in children with other urinary tract anomalies such as multicystic dysplastic kidneys and the VACTERL spectrum of anorectal and vertebral anomalies (Thomas et al. 2008).

With the development of antenatal ultrasound, UPJ obstruction is now diagnosed more during the perinatal period in asymptomatic infants (Grignon et al. 1986); however, UPJ obstruction may go unnoticed antenatally and present in emergency settings with a palpable mass or abdominal distension in neonates, or with severe abdominal pain, urinary tract infection, or hematuria in older children. Intermittent pain associated with vomiting is also recognized (Marincek and Dondelinger 2007). Unlike nonspecific abdominal pain, the symptoms arising from an obstructed kidney usually last for several hours or several days. Although the pain is typically sited in the region of the loin, it may be experienced predominantly in the central quadrants of the abdomen, with possible diagnostic difficulties (Thomas et al. 2008).

Current assessment of the child with apparent UPJ obstruction rests upon a determination of structure and functional studies. Typically, the sequence comprises ultrasound followed by ^{99m}Tc mercaptoacetyltriglycine (MAG3) dynamic renography. The use of DMSA scintigraphy or ^{99m}Tc DMSA scintigraphy is reserved for poorly functioning obstructed kidneys.

US is the initial imaging of choice used in children with suspected urinary tract obstruction. It shows dilated renal pelvis communicating with dilated calyces in the absence of visualization of the distal ureter (Fig. 18.11). The renal cortex may appear thin, and a crossing blood vessel at the UPJ may be visualized on color Doppler ultrasound. In older children, the concern for a crossing lower pole renal vessel is higher than in infants, so occasionally CT or MR angiography is sometimes obtained to look for these vessels (Fig. 18.12). Occasionally, the distal ureter appears dilated due to associated vesicoureteric reflux or to a more distal cause of obstruction. The UPJ obstruction must be distinguished from a multicystic kidney; the latter appears as non-communicating area of cystic dilation of variable size (Marincek and Dondelinger 2007). A massively dilated renal pelvis without significant caliectasis suggests a lesser degree of obstruction, and one should not base clinical decisions on the degree of pelvic dilation alone (Lima and Manzoni 2015). A similar obstruction can be determined by a retrocaval ureter, by a functional impairment of the peristaltic contraction of the ureter, by secondary obstruction due to gross VUR, and by distortion of the ureter in a horseshoe kidney, so all this conditions must be excluded.

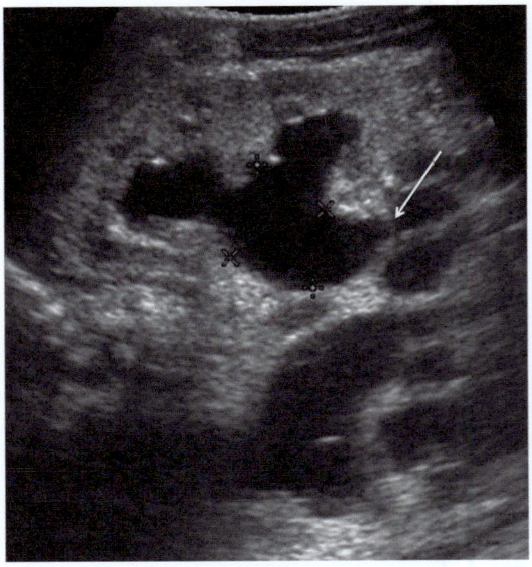

Fig. 18.11 UPJ obstruction. Longitudinal US scan shows dilated renal pelvis communicating with dilated calyces and a sudden narrowing in the site of the ureteropelvic junction (*arrow*). The distal ureter is not visualized

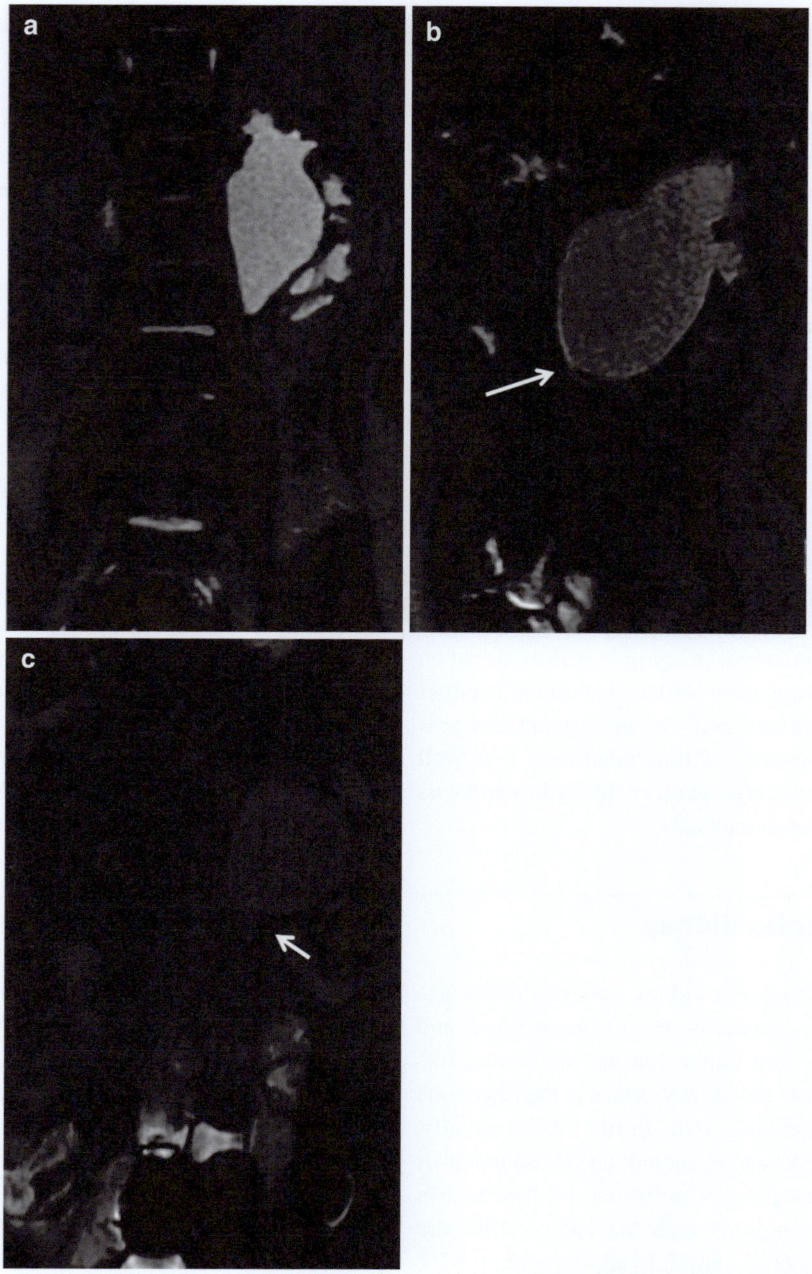

Fig. 18.12 UPJ obstruction at MRI: T2-weighted single-shot fast-spin-echo (SSFSE) images. Coronal SSFSE (**a**) shows severe dilation of the pelvis and calyces with associated thinning of the renal cortex. Sagittal SSFSE (**b**) and coronal fat saturated SSFSE (**c**) better highlight the site of the obstruction and the distal ureter with normal caliber (*white arrows*). In this case, a crossing blood vessel at the UPJ was not identified

The most reliable current method of assessing relative renal function is the diuretic renogram (DR), a functional study using ^{99m}Tc MAG3 performed to assess the renal drainage and compare the function of the kidneys (Stauss et al. 2003). The UPJ obstruction is confirmed by showing dilatation of the upper urinary tract, failure of tracer washout after diuretic administration, and gradually rising activity on the time-activity graph. The greatest value of the DR and washout curve is to monitor the status of the kidney over time, particularly when an observational approach is taken. This is though a burden on families and includes increased radiation. The child with more severe dilation and more delayed washout is more likely to not improve spontaneously or to deteriorate. As long as the family is aware of this and is reliable to return for follow-up, observation is the advisable approach (Thorup et al. 2003).

If the ureter is dilated or the bladder wall is thick, a VCUG is indicated to exclude vesicoureteric reflux and urethral valves.

The goal in diagnosing and treating UPJ obstruction is to prevent ipsilateral renal function loss and minimize associate comorbidities, like UTIs and urolithiasis.

Acute management of a UPJ obstruction is usually the placement of a percutaneous nephrostomy, and functional imaging is performed when acute symptoms have settled. Treatment is either conservative (wait and see) or surgical, depending on the severity of functional loss. It is well established that after surgery the hydronephrosis can resolve spontaneously.

18.5 Duplex Kidney

A duplex kidney is a kidney with two pelvicalyceal systems, generally referred to as upper and lower poles. The upper pole normally accounts for one third of the kidney, whereas the lower one for the remaining two thirds. Anatomically, duplex systems can be incomplete (bifid pelvis or ureter) or complete. The former are four to five times more common than the latter, which are most common in females. In approximately 40 % of cases, the condition is bilateral. Partial duplications will have convergence of the ureters into a single system prior to its entry into the bladder.

When the separate buds incorporate into the bladder, the more cranial bud terminates in a location more caudal and medial than expected. Conversely, the most caudal bud ends more cranial and lateral. This phenomenon is known as the Weigert-Meyer rule and has only rare exceptions (Mackie and Stephens 1975; Jain et al. 2008). The lower pole ureter tends to have a shorter course within in the bladder wall due to its lateral positioning, predisposing it to VUR, whereas the upper pole ureter with a long course within the bladder wall is more often associated with obstruction or ureterocele. In addition, ureteral ectopia is more common in the upper pole, whereas UPJ obstruction in the lower pole (Whitten and Wilcox 2001). Upper pole UPJ obstruction and primary upper pole VUR are rare for anatomical and embryological reasons.

Uncomplicated duplex system anomalies often go undiagnosed for the whole life. In contrast, complicated ureteral duplications are often associated with other urological anomalies and more easily present themselves with different symptoms.

Febrile UTIs are the most common presenting symptoms. They occur more commonly when a VUR is associated with the condition in any of the moieties or with hydroureteronephrosis (Lima and Manzoni 2015). Risk of infection might be higher in case of ureterocele, although it is still unclear whether this is due to the ureterocele itself or to the fact that VUR is often associated (Castagnetti et al. 2012).

Basic diagnostic workup in patients with a complicated duplex system should generally undergo US of the upper urinary tract and bladder and a renal nuclear scintigraphy. A VCUG should be considered if a dilated ureter is visible on US. Additional imaging may be useful when anatomical information is necessary.

The US of the urinary tract is generally the first investigation. Sonographically, duplicated systems will have an intervening bar of renal parenchyma separating the upper and lower poles. This parenchyma is more evident in the presence of hydronephrosis (Fig. 18.13). The US should define the laterality of the condition and identify the moieties that are dilated; the degree of the dilatation, whether or not ureteral dilatation is associated; and the aspect of the bladder including the presence of a ureterocele.

Since duplication is often associated with VUR, VCUG should always follow but in suspicion of lower pole UPJ obstruction (Kim et al. 2001). VUR into a lower pole ureter may displace

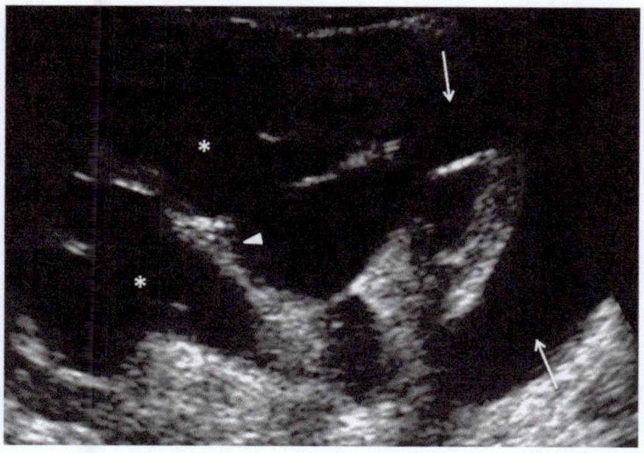

Fig. 18.13 Hydronephrotic duplex kidney. Longitudinal US scan shows two dilated pelvicalyceal systems (*asterisks*), with interposed renal parenchyma (*arrowhead*) separating the upper and lower poles. Ureteral dilation of both the excretory system is associated (*arrows*)

the lower pole downward and outward, with the renal pelvis and calyces appearing like a "drooping lily." In order to rule out the presence of a ureterocele, a picture should be taken after injection of few cc of contrast into the bladder, at low-volume bladder filling, to prevent ureterocele collapse.

Finally, an assessment of moiety function should be achieved by nuclear scintigraphy. The dynamic ^{99m}Tc MAG3 scintigraphy allows for simultaneous assessment of cortical function and upper tract drainage: the information necessary for the decision-making is the gross presence of any function in the moiety or its complete absence. Patients with primary lower pole VUR are the only exception, in which using a static ^{99m}Tc DMSA scintigraphy can be useful to search for parenchymal scars. It is recommended, however, also a MAG3 scan if any trapping of contrast in the upper tract is seen on the VCUG, in order to rule out any concomitant obstruction that might contraindicate the injection of bulking agent as treatment of reflux, should recurrent febrile UTIs occur (Othman et al. 2012).

If additional imaging is required, i.e., for massive nonrefluxing dilatation of both upper and lower ipsilateral moieties or for incongruence in the basic assessment tests, uro-MRI allows for simultaneous optimal anatomical definition and functional assessment (Grattan-Smith and Jones 2006).

Treatment of duplications is conservative in the majority of cases, surgical only in the presence of severe complications or concomitant pathology.

18.6 Ureterocele

A cystic dilation of the distal ureter where it inserts into the bladder or urethra is called a ureterocele.

Ureteroceles are most commonly associated with the upper pole in a duplex kidney and occur more frequently in females (Shokeir and Nijman 2002a). The reported incidence of ureteroceles is 1 in every 1,000 births (Palmer and Palmer 2014). The risk of UTI in children with ureteroceles may be as high as 50% (Besson et al. 2000). Ureteroceles are classified as intravesical (or orthotopic) if they are entirely within the bladder and as ectopic if part of the ureterocele extends into the bladder neck or into the urethra. The exact embryologic explanation for ureteroceles is unknown, but one popular theory is that there is a membrane between the mesonephric duct and the ureteric bud that does not completely break down and leads to a stenotic ureteral orifice and obstruction (Palmer and Palmer 2014).

Single-system ureteroceles are most common in boys and usually incidentally found during sonographic examinations, but they can present with acute signs of UTI or lithiasis. Upper tract dilatation is absent or of mild to moderate severity and renal function is normally preserved. They usually lie entirely within the bladder (orthotopic ureteroceles).

Duplex system ureteroceles are associated with the upper pole ureter and can cause reflux or obstruction in the ipsilateral lower pole and, being more often ectopic, can cause bladder outlet obstruction. They can alter the function of the whole bladder, because of the trigone development already being partly abnormal due to the presence of two ipsilateral ureters (Lima and Manzoni 2015). Dysplasia of the upper pole parenchyma is the rule with duplex system ureteroceles, usually to the extent that the upper pole has little if any useful function. Often this correlates with dilatation of the upper pole ureter. Clinical presentation of ureteroceles in a duplex system is typically with UTI, occasionally with Gram-negative septicemia, acute urinary retention, or, in females, with a vaginal mass determined by urethral prolapse of the ureterocele.

Most ureteroceles are diagnosed by ultrasonography that demonstrates a thin-walled cystic mass within the posterior wall of the bladder and potentially hydroureteronephrosis (Fig. 18.14). Attention should be paid to the degree of bladder fullness during the exam, as ureteroceles can collapse and be overlooked in a full bladder. Conversely, if the bladder is too empty, the ureterocele can easily be lost among the folds of the bladder wall. Pseudoureteroceles (the dilated distal ureter pressing on the bladder wall) can be differentiated from real ureteroceles by the thickness of their walls: thin-walled for a true ureterocele and thicker bilaminar bladder wall for a pseudoureterocele. Upper pole dysplasia can be seen as hyperechoic parenchyma and smaller relative size with varying degrees of thickness.

A VCUG is generally performed as well because of the increased incidence of ipsilateral lower pole reflux in duplex systems. Reflux into both poles is usually indicative of incomplete duplication. Contralateral reflux can also be seen.

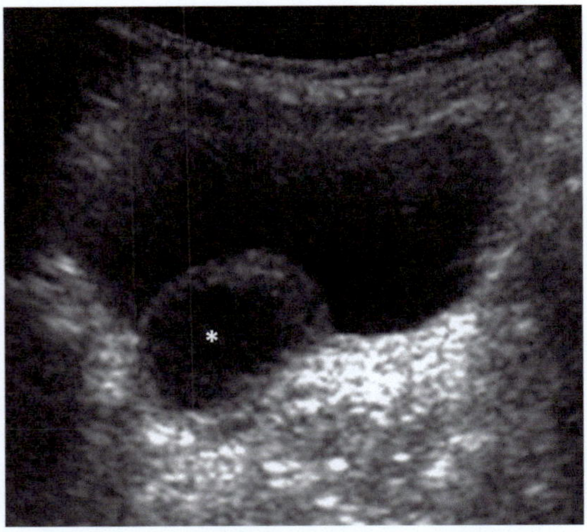

Fig. 18.14 Ureterocele. Axial US scan of the pelvis shows a thin-walled cystic dilation (*asterisk*) within the posterior wall of the bladder

Early images of the bladder with the VCUG will often demonstrate the ureterocele as a large, smooth, filling defect on the posterior wall/trigone. Once the bladder is full, the ureterocele may evert to look like a diverticulum with its location at the bladder base as the only indication of being a ureterocele. During the voiding phase, prolapse of a large ureterocele can be demonstrated with movement of it into the urethra.

Cystoscopy is routinely advisable for the assessment of duplex system ureteroceles, principally in order to determine if the lesion is orthotopic or ectopic (Shokeir and Nijman 2002b).

MRI has the potential to clarify anatomy and provide functional information without exposure to radiation. The major disadvantage is the requirement for general anesthesia or sedation in children to ensure they remain still while the scan is being performed.

Ureteroceles are treated to prevent or reduce UTI and to prevent renal damage. It is generally agreed upon that all children with a ureterocele should be on prophylactic antibiotics to prevent UTI and urosepsis (Husmann et al. 1995). The treatment for a child with a ureterocele and sepsis, unresponsive to antibiotics, is urgent endoscopic decompression via transurethral incision.

Indications to surgery are febrile UTIs and bladder outlet obstruction (Shokeir and Nijman 2002b).

18.7 Ectopic Ureter

An accessory bud that arises from the mesonephric duct in a more cephalic position than the normal site and which drains the upper renal pole will come to enter the urinary tract in a distally ectopic location, as said before. It may drain into either the bladder, the urethra, or the urogenital sinus. In females, such ectopic ureters may be sited above the sphincter mechanism (suprasphincteric), close to or at the level of the striated sphincter (although usually below the bladder neck), or distal to the sphincter (infrasphincteric), either at the introitus or in the distal vagina. In males, the termination is always suprasphincteric (because mesonephric duct derivatives are all proximal to the external urethral sphincter), connecting with the ductus deferens, the seminal vesicle, or, most often, the ejaculatory duct.

Ureteric ectopia is usually associated with a dysplastic renal pole, while the ureter itself is frequently dilated, either as a consequence of reflux, obstruction, or dysmorphism. Even in the absence of dysplasia, the affected pole typically exhibits some degree of dilatation, the only common exception being in some girls with infrasphincteric ectopia.

Ectopic ureter is rare, affecting some 0.01 % of individuals, mostly females.

Clinical presentation of suprasphincteric ectopic ureters is almost invariably with urinary infection, which, in males, may manifest as epididymo-orchitis. Rarely it can present with an abdominal palpable mass, represented by the hydronephrotic kidney. Urinary incontinence and hematuria can be typical of infrasphincteric ectopia. This incontinence is very specific, with a constant dribbling of urine superimposed upon an otherwise normal pattern of micturition, a clinical picture that distinguishes it from all other causes of incontinence (Thomas et al. 2008).

In cases where an ectopic ureter is suspected, radiological evaluation begins with a renal and bladder US. The greater the degree of ureteral dilatation, the easier it is to determine the site of ectopic insertion. The location of the ectopic ureter insertion is often not determinable. The dilated distal ureter can be visualized behind the bladder (Fig. 18.15). Often hydronephrosis of the upper renal pole is visible. If the ectopic ureteral orifice is in the external urethral sphincter, a unique situation can occur where an obstructed, refluxing megaureter is found. In some girls with infrasphincteric ectopia, the upper renal pole is not hydronephrotic but is small and dysplastic (and can be ectopic) and consequently difficult or impossible to detect by ultrasonography (cryptic duplication). When visible the upper pole can have hyperechoic parenchyma and thinning as a result of the hydronephrosis and high association with renal dysplasia.

VCUG in suprasphincteric ectopia demonstrates reflux to the upper pole only during voiding, when the external sphincter is relaxed. In patients with an ectopic ureter at the bladder neck (Fig. 18.16), it is not unusual that the catheter inserted in the urethra for the VCUG instead of entering the bladder goes straight into the ectopic ureter. The injection of contrast actually results in a retrograde pyelography of the upper pole moiety.

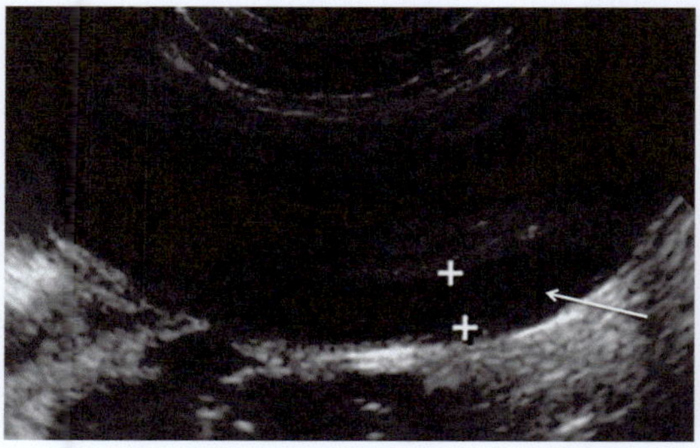

Fig. 18.15 Ectopic ureter. US scan of the pelvis shows a dilated distal ureter (*arrow*) behind the bladder, suggesting an ectopic insertion; the exact location is not easy to visualize and often not determinable on US examination

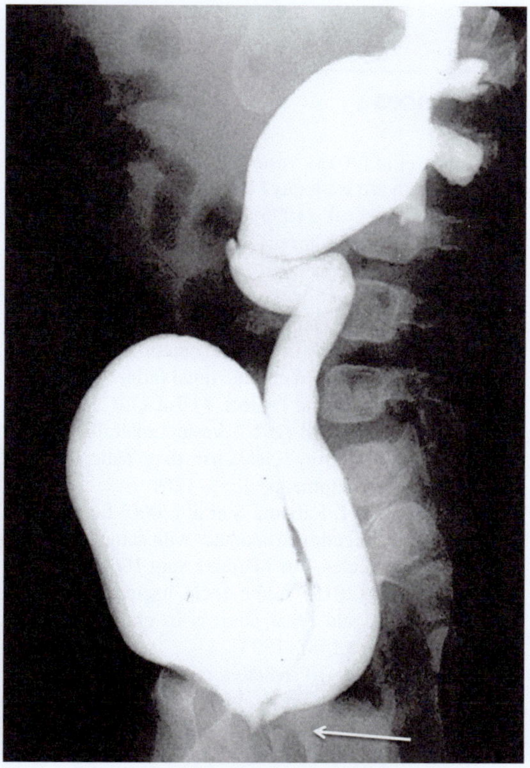

Fig. 18.16 VCUG: ectopic ureter associated with high-grade VUR. Left ectopic ureteral insertion (*arrow*) at the bladder neck with retrograde filling of contrast medium until the pelvis and calyces that appear severely dilated

MRI is excellent in showing the location of the orifice (Krishnan and Baskin 2005; Wille et al. 2003), especially with sagittal views. No contrast is needed and ionizing radiation is absent. T2-weighted images are excellent at delineating fluid-filled structures such as an ectopic ureter. In most cases, utilizing MRI for young children has required sedation in some form for optimal imaging. This fact, along with the increased cost, has limited MRI to equivocal cases in need of definition of anatomy rather than as a screening modality.

DMSA radionuclide scans remain the gold standard to determine renal function and to guide surgical plan.

Treatment of suprasphincteric ectopic ureters requires reimplantation of the ureters into the bladder, plus augmentation cystoplasty when the bladder is small. The only treatment for infrasphincteric ectopic ureters is the exeresis of the related small dysplastic kidney (Thomas et al. 2008).

References

Altobelli E et al (2014) Vesicoureteral reflux in pediatric age: where are we today? Urologia 81(2):76–87

Ardissino GL et al (1995) For the Italian Registry of Childhood Chronic Renal Insufficiency in Conservative Treatment (ITALKID): population-based registry of childhood chronic renal insufficiency on conservative treatment. Pediatr Nephrol 9:C69

Ardissino G et al (2004) Long-term outcome of vesicoureteral reflux associated chronic renal failure in children. Data from the ItalKid Project. J Urol 172(1):305–310

Bates DG, Riccabona M (2013) Vesicoureteral reflux. In: Coley B (ed) Caffey's pediatric diagnostic imaging. Elsevier, Philadelphia, pp 1253–1261

Besson R, Ngoc BT, Laboure S et al (2000) Incidence of urinary tract infection in neonates with antenatally diagnosed ureteroceles. Eur J Pediatr Surg 10(2):111–113

Bitsori M et al (2015) Acute focal bacterial nephritis, pyonephrosis and renal abscess in children. Pediatr Nephrol 30(11):1987–1993

Caione P et al (2004) Predictive risk factors for chronic renal failure in primary high grade vesicoureteric reflux. BJU 93:1309–1312

Castagnetti M, Cimador M, Esposito C et al (2012) Antibiotic prophylaxis in antenatal nonrefluxing hydronephrosis, megaureter and ureterocele. Nat Rev Urol 9(6):321–329

Chand DH et al (2003) Incidence and severity of vesicoureteral reflux in children related to age, gender, race and diagnosis. J Urol 170:1548–1550

Craig WD et al (2008) Pyelonephritis: radiologic-pathologic review. RadioGraphics 28:255–276

Dewan PA1, Ng KP, Ashwood PJ (1998) The relationship of age to pathology in pelviureteric junction obstruction. J Paediatr Child Health 34(4):384–386

Eccles MR, Jacobs GH (2000) The genetics of primary vesicoureteric reflux. Ann Acad Med Singap 29: 337–345

Fultz PJ et al (1993) Computed tomography of pyonephrosis. Abdom Imaging 18:82–87

Grattan-Smith JD, Jones RA (2006) MR urography in children. Pediatr Radiol 36(11):1119–1132

Grignon A, Filion R, Filiatrault D et al (1986) Urinary tract dilatation in utero: classification and clinical applications. Radiology 160(3):645–647

Herz D et al (2010) 5-year prospective results of dimercapto succinic acid imaging in children with febrile urinary tract infection: proof that the top-down approach works. J Urol 184:1703–1709

Husmann DA, Ewalt DH, Glenski WJ et al (1995) Ureterocele associated with ureteral duplication and a nonfunctioning upper pole segment: management by partial nephroureterectomy alone. J Urol 154(2 Pt 2):723–726

Jain P, Parelkar S, Shah H et al (2008) Uncrossed complete ureteral duplication with dysplastic lower moiety: a violation of the Weigert-Meyer law. J Pediatr Urol 4(5):404–406

Jeffrey RB et al (1985) Sensitivity of sonography in pyonephrosis: a reevaluation. AJR 144:71–73

Kelly H et al (2005) Uroplakin III is not a major candidate gene for primary vesicoureteral reflux. Eur J Hum Genet 13:500–502

Kim YS, Do SH, Hong CH et al (2001) Does every patient with ureteropelvic junction obstruction need voiding cystourethrography? J Urol 165(6 Pt 2):2305–2307

Knudson MJ et al (2007a) Computational model for predicting the chance of early resolution in children with vesicoureteral reflux. J Urol 178:1824–1827

Knudson MJ et al (2007b) Predictive factors of early spontaneous resolution in children with primary vesicoureteral reflux. J Urol 178:1684–1688

Krishnan A, Baskin LS (2005) Identification of ectopic ureter in incontinent girl using magnetic resonance imaging. Urology 65(5):1002

Lama G et al (2000) Primary vesicoureteric reflux and renal damage in the first year of life. Pediatr Nephrol 15:205–210

Lebowitz RL et al (1985) International system of radiographic grading of vesicoureteric reflux. International reflux study in Children. Pediatr Radiol 15:105–109

Lima M, Manzoni G (2015) Pediatric urology. Springer, Milan

Mackie GG, Stephens FD (1975) Duplex kidneys: a correlation of renal dysplasia with position of the ureteral orifice. J Urol 114:274–280

Mak RH, Kuo HJ (2003) Primary ureteral reflux: Emerging insights from molecular and genetic studies. Curr Opin Pediatr 15:181–185

Marincek B, Dondelinger RF (2007) Emergency radiology – imaging and intervention. Springer, Heidelberg

National Collaborating Center for Women's and Children's Health (UK) (2007) Urinary tract infection in children: diagnosis, treatment and long-term management. RCOGPress, London
Ng CK et al (2002) Outcome of percutaneous nephrostomy for the management of pyonephrosis. Asian J Surg 25(3):215–219
Othman S, Al-Hawas A, Al-Maqtari R (2012) Renal cortical imaging in children: 99mTc MAG3 versus 99mTc DMSA. Clin Nucl Med 37(4):351–355
Palmer LS, Palmer JS (2014) Pediatric and adolescent urological imaging. Springer Science+Business Media, New York
Patel R et al (2013) Primary neonatal MRSA pyonephrosis. Int Urol Nephrol 45:939–942
Peters CA et al (2010) Summary of the AUA guideline on management of primary vesicoureteral reflux in children. J Urol 184:1134–1144
Piaggio G et al (2003) Cystosonography and voiding cystourethrography in the diagnosis of vesicoureteral reflux. Pediatr Nephrol 18(1):18–22
Riccabona M (2008) The ureter and vesicoureteral reflux. In: Slovis T (ed) Caffey's pediatric diagnostic imaging, 11th edn. Mosby, Philadelphia
Riccabona M (2009) Urinary tract imaging in infancy. Pediatr Radiol 39(Suppl 3):S436–S445
Riccabona M et al (2008) Imaging recommendations in paediatric uroradiology: minutes of the ESPR workgroup session on urinary tract infection, fetal hydronephrosis, urinary tract ultrasonography and voiding cystourethrography, Barcelona, Spain, June 2007. Pediatr Radiol 38:138–145
Roberts KB (2011) Urinary tract infection: clinical practice guideline for the diagnosis and management of the initial UTI in febrile infants and children 2 to 24 months. Pediatrics 128:595–610
Roebuck D (2011) Genitourinary intervention in children. Pediatr Radiol 41:17–26
Schlomer B et al (2014) Renal imaging: congenital anomalies of the kidney and urinary tract. In: Palmer LS, Palmer JS (eds) Pediatric and adolescent urologic imaging. Springer-Verlag New York; CRC Press Boca Raton, Florida, pp 174–175
Schneider K et al (1989) Pyonephrosis in childhood – is ultrasound sufficient for diagnosis? Pediatr Radiol 19:302–307
Sharma S et al (2004) Neonatal pyonephrosis – a case report. Int Urol Nephrol 36:313–316
Shokeir AA, Nijman RJ (2002) Ureterocele: an ongoing challenge in infancy and childhood. BJU Int 90(8):777–783
Skoog SJ et al (2010) Pediatric vesicoureteral reflux guidelines panel summary report: clinical practice guidelines for screening siblings of children with vesicoureteral reflux and neonates/infants with prenatal hydronephrosis. J Urol 184:1145–1151
St Lezin M et al (1992) Pyonephrosis: diagnosis and treatment. Br J Urol 70(4):360–363
Stauss J, Connolly LP, Connolly SA et al (2003) Dynamic renal scintigraphy in children with vesicoureteral reflux and suspected coexisting ureteropelvic junction obstruction. J Urol 170(5):1966–1970
Subramanyam BR et al (1983) Sonography of pyonephrosis: a prospective study. AJR 140:991–993
Thomas DFM, Duffy PG, Rickwood AMK (2008) Essential of pediatric urology, 2nd edn. Informa UK Ltd. Springer-Verlag New York; CRC Press Boca Raton, Florida
Thorup J et al (2003) The results of 15 years of consistent strategy in treating antenatally suspected pelviureteric junction obstruction. BJU Int 91(9):850–852
Weinberg AE et al (2013) Current management of vesicoureteral reflux in pediatric patients: a review. J Pediatr Health Med Ther 4:1–12
Whitten SM, Wilcox DT (2001) Duplex systems. Prenat Diagn 21(11):952–957
Wille S, von Knobloch R, Klose KJ et al (2003) Magnetic resonance urography in pediatric urology. Scand J Urol Nephrol 37(1):16–21
Ylinen E et al (2003) Risk of renal scarring in vesicoureteral reflux detected either antenatally or during the neonatal period. Urology 61:1238–1243

Posterior Urethral Valves

19

Cinzia Orazi, Antonio Maria Zaccara,
Massimiliano Silveri, and Paolo Maria Schingo

19.1 Introduction

Lower urinary tract obstruction (LUTO) includes a heterogeneous group of congenital anomalies. Posterior urethral valves (PUVs) represent the most common cause of LUTO in males, with incidence ranging from 1:5.000 to 1:8.000 live births, according to most of the series (Nasir et al. 2011; Malin et al. 2012; Gharpure 2013; Thakkar et al. 2014; Keihani and Kajbafzadeh 2015). However, the true incidence remains difficult to assess and is probably underestimated due to fetal or perinatal demise and, on the other hand, to delayed diagnosis in milder forms (Caione and Gerocarni Nappo 2011). PUVs represent a congenital phenomenon mostly occurring sporadically, although familial forms have rarely been reported (Kajbafzadeh 2005). The classic form of PUVs is in the prostatic urethra, below or after the verumontanum (Kajbafzadeh 2005). They consist of abnormal mucosal folds between the urethral wall and the distal end of the verumontanum (Dacher 2008) and present with a spectrum of severity, from mild to lethal forms, depending on the configuration of the obstructive membrane inside the urethra and on the degree of obstruction (Nasir et al. 2011; Mirshemirani et al. 2013). Most of the obstructive forms are usually detected by prenatal sonography, although one-third of the cases still present postnatally with urinary sepsis, abdominal distention, abdominal mass, or poor urinary stream in infancy. Newborns may occasionally present with respiratory distress due to pulmonary hypoplasia and renal failure. Late presentation during infancy or even childhood with urinary incontinence and urinary tract infections (UTI) does not always correlate with better outcome. Also urinary upper tract consequences are extremely variable (from no alteration in mild forms to severe renal impairment associated with bladder dysfunction in severe cases). The most severe forms with oligohydramnios exit in stillborn fetuses with Potter's syndrome (Hutton 2004; Dacher 2008; Sudarsanan et al. 2009; Malin et al. 2012).

C. Orazi (✉) • P.M. Schingo
Diagnostic Imaging Department, Children's Hospital Bambino Gesù, Rome, Italy
e-mail: cinzia.orazi@opbg.net

A.M. Zaccara
Urology Department, Children's Hospital Bambino Gesù, Rome, Italy

M. Silveri
Surgery Department, Children's Hospital Bambino Gesù, Rome, Italy

19.2 Historical Background

Giovanni Battista Morgagni, an Italian anatomist, was the first to describe congenital obstruction of the posterior urethra in 1717 (Morgagni 1769).

V. Miele, M. Trinci (eds.), *Imaging Non-traumatic Abdominal Emergencies in Pediatric Patients*,
DOI 10.1007/978-3-319-41866-7_19

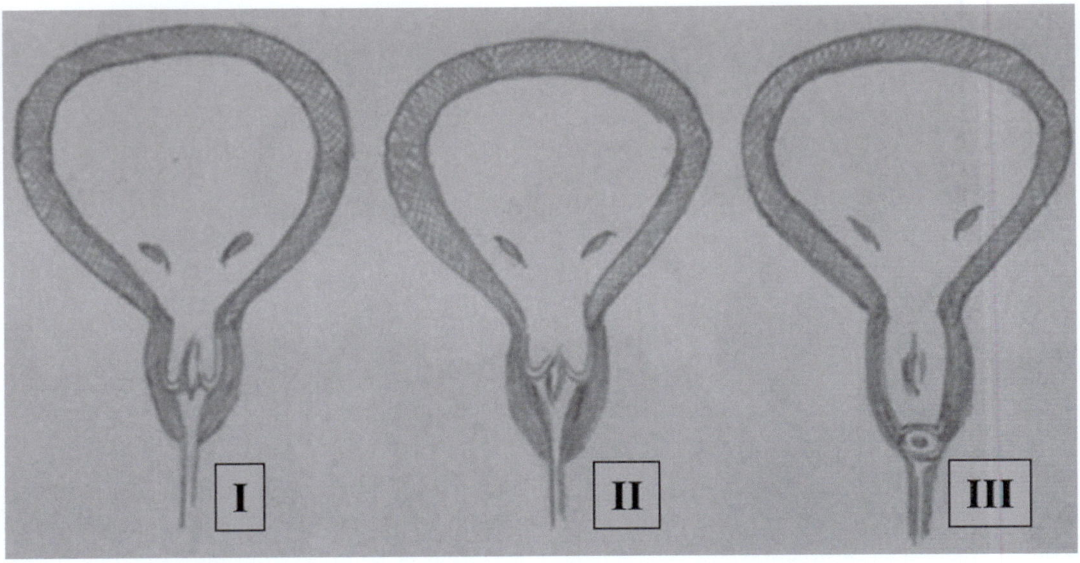

Fig. 19.1 Types of posterior urethral valves: Young's classification

In 1802 Langenbeck reported valve-like urethral folds in autopsy specimens in his monograph on stone disease (Langenbeck 1802).

Velpeau, in 1832, coined the term "valves" because folds resembled cardiac valves and inferred its clinical relevance as an obstructive condition (Velpeau 1832).

Budd, in 1840, presented the case of a young sailor who died because of uremia and hydronephrosis with a membranous fold or valve in the posterior urethra and secondary changes in the bladder (Budd 1840).

A comprehensive description, including an embryological theory, was made in 1870 by Tolmatschew, who defined the valves as "overgrowths of the normally present anatomical folds and ridges in the urethra," so a hypertrophy of the urethral mucosal folds. Urine flow from the bladder caused swelling of the membranes and obstruction of the lumen, preventing the bladder from emptying (Tolmatschew 1870).

Bazy suggested the theory of the persistence and continuation of the urogenital membrane in 1903 (Bazy 1903).

In 1914 Lowsley proposed that PUVs were, instead, due to an anomaly of the Wolffian or Müllerian duct origin (Lowsley 1914).

In 1921 Watson hypothesized that PUV formation occurred because of an arrest of normal development, with persistent attachment of the verumontanum to the posterior urethral roof epithelium (Watson 1921). Finally, PUVs were described as a clinical and pathological condition in a seminal article by Young, who presented a retrospective series of 12 patients with urethral valves, together with a review of cases from the literature, in 1919 (Young et al. 1919). Based on autopsy findings, he subdivided PUVs in three types, depending on the orientation of the valves and their relationship to the verumontanum (Fig. 19.1). Type 1, the most common, were composed of a ridge coursing anterior from the distal verumontanum, dividing into two separate leaflets, attaching to the anterolateral walls of the urethra. Type 2, the most rare, extended from the proximal verumontanum toward the bladder neck. Type 3 valves consisted of a diaphragm with a central perforation, attached to the entire circumference of the urethra, distal or proximal to the verumontanum. In 1955 Stephens considered PUVs as a result of abnormal integration of the Wolffian ducts into the urethra, causing an abnormally obstructing membrane that would normally be seen as nonobstructing "fins" radiating distal from the verumontanum in the unaffected infant (Stephens 1955). In 1965 Williams and Eckstein supported the theory of Tolmatschew that valves represented an exaggeration of normal folds first seen in the urethra, with no relation to Wolffian duct structures (Williams and Eckstein 1965). The study of Robertson and Hayes in 1969 as well as that of Lowsley supported the hypothesis of an extraurethral or Wolffian origin of PUVs (Robertson and Hayes 1969). This also raised the question as to whether they should be called valves at all since they perhaps actually were made up of a single membranous structure, instead of the bicuspid morphology proposed in 1919 by Young. However, the nomenclature of PUVs remained unchanged up to the early 1990s, with the series of Dewan et al. (1992, 1994) who considered the term valves incorrect because the obstruction of the posterior urethra was caused by a single membrane and coined the term COPUM (congenital obstructive posterior urethral membrane). Moreover, types 1 and 3 valves of Young had to be considered the same, being either mistaken one for the other during endoscopy, because of the angle of visualization, or being type 3 modified in type 1 by prior urethral instrumentation (Dewan et al. 1992; Dewan and Goh 1995). According to Dewan, there are two distinct entities with two distinct embryological origins, causing obstruction in the posterior urethra, namely, COPUM and Cobb's collar. COPUM is an oblique membrane associated to the distal verumontanum, while the Cobb's collar (or congenital urethral stricture) is a transverse membrane located distal to the external urethral sphincter, with no relation to the verumontanum (Cobb et al. 1968; Dewan et al. 1992; Dewan and Goh 1995). He believes in the theory of Watson for COPUM and persistence of the urogenital membrane for Cobb's collar (Watson 1921).

19.3 Anatomy and Embryology

The normal male urethra extends from the bladder neck to the external urethral meatus and is anatomically divided into the posterior urethra (with the prostatic and membranous portions) and the anterior urethra (cavernous or spongy portion). The prostatic urethra, extending from the bladder neck to and through the urogenital diaphragm, is the widest portion. Along the posterior urethra, there is a mucosal ridge called urethral crest, which is lined by a dip on each side, the prostatic sinus, with numerous openings of the prostatic ducts. Slightly below there are the openings of the two ejaculatory ducts. The verumontanum (colliculus seminalis) is a bulge on the posterior urethral floor on which the foramen of a small diverticulum of the urethra, the prostatic utricle, opens. The urethral crest continues naturally below the verumontanum with two thin folds (plicae colliculi) that distally attach onto the lateral walls of the urethra (Kajbafzadeh 2005; Benz-Bohm 2008). Stephens believes that these folds represent the embryological integration of the Wolffian ducts into the urethra (Stephens 1983).

The membranous urethra is short and narrow and is surrounded by the urinary sphincter.

The anterior urethra is divided by the suspensory ligament of the penis into a proximal, bulbar urethra and a distal, pendulous, or penile urethra. On the floor of the bulbar urethra, there are the two openings of the ducts of the Cowper glands (Kajbafzadeh 2005; Benz-Bohm 2008).

Embryologically, the cloaca is separated by the urogenital septum into the urogenital sinus and the rectum between the fourth and the sixth weeks of gestation. The most caudal end of the Wolffian duct is absorbed into the primitive cloaca at the site of the future verumontanum in the posterior urethra. The remnants of this process are represented by the posterior urethral folds, called plicae colliculi. PUVs are formed at approximately 4 weeks' gestation, as the Wolffian duct fuses with the developing cloaca (Krishnan et al. 2006; Nasir et al. 2011). The prostatic urethra and membranous urethra are derived from the urogenital sinus, while the bulbar urethra and pendulous urethra are derived from the urethral plate on the ventral aspect of the genital tubercle (Krishnan et al. 2006). Embryology of PUVs, actually, is not well known, but it appears to be a multifactor gene-mediated embryopathy (Nasir et al. 2011). Similarly to plicae colliculi, PUVs also arise at the distal lateral aspect of the verumontanum, but extend more distally in an oblique fashion along the lateral walls of the urethra and continue anteriorly, where they fuse determining obstruction of the lumen. PUVs could be due to abnormally anterior insertion of the mesonephric (Wolffian) duct on the cloaca, prior to its division into the urogenital sinus and the anorectal canal (Verma 2008) preventing normal migration of these ducts, or to abnormal fusion of the ducts, resulting in abnormal ridges or folds (Nasir et al. 2011; Lukong et al. 2014), or a consequence of an abnormality of the cloacal membrane (Steven and Desai 2016).

19.4 Classification of PUVs

The classification created by Young remains commonly used even today (Young et al. 1919; Nasir et al. 2011), though most authors agree that is not completely correct (Caione and De Pasquale 2011) (Fig. 19.1). The three types of PUVs were differentiated on the basis of the orientation of the valves and their relationship to the verumontanum. Type I is the most frequently encountered: abnormal ridges or folds in the posterior urethra originating from the caudal end of the verumontanum and extending distally are believed to be the origin of 95% of PUVs (Elder and Shapio 2005). The membranes arising from the verumontanum and extending toward the bladder neck of type II are actually not considered obstructing valves, but simply hypertrophy of the plicae colliculi. Type III represents the other 5%: the mucosal web with a central defect or circular diaphragm in the region of the caudal end of the verumontanum could be due to incomplete dissolution of the urogenital membrane (Murphy and Gatti 2006; Nasir et al. 2011). This type was later subdivided into type IIIa when the hole is above the verumontanum and type IIIb when it is below the verumontanum (Young et al. 1919; Krishnan et al. 2006; Nasir et al. 2011). This type of obstructive tissue was termed congenital obstructive posterior urethral membrane (COPUM) by Dewan (Dewan et al. 1992; Lukong et al. 2014), on the basis of studies of the pristine uninstrumented posterior urethra of babies with PUVs after suprapubic drainage. He considers the three types of valves, probably representing the same obstructing structure, as a membrane with a central defect, called COPUM (congenital obstructive posterior urethral membrane), which can be modified because of antenatal rupture, but mostly by instrumentation. Instead of a true valve, a persistent oblique membrane could be ruptured by initial catheter placement and, secondary to the rupture, assume a valve-like configuration. Moreover, he regards the type III inframontane obstruction, with a central defect, without attachment to the verumontanum, probably a remnant of the urogenital diaphragm, and reasonably the same as those called Cobb's collar, Moormann's ring, or congenital stricture. Cobb described cases of narrowing in the bulbar urethra which appeared to be congenital, hence the term Cobb's collar, resulting from the persistence of the urogenital membrane, minor or significant and muscular or fibrous (Cobb et al. 1968). Moormann's ring is another term used for congenital narrowing in the bulbar urethra (Dewan 2014). There is a type IV valve associated with prune belly syndrome (Aaronson 1983; Lukong et al. 2014).

19.5 Associated Anomalies

PUVs can be associated with other anomalies of the urinary tract (Piçarro et al. 2016).

The association of PUVs with anterior urethral valves (AUVs), mostly in the bulbar urethra, anyway with a distinct embryological origin, is exceedingly rare (Tran et al. 2014; Keihani and Kajbafzadeh 2015).

The incidence of cryptorchidism is 16-fold higher, and the incidence of inguinal hernia is 7-fold higher in PUV patients than in the normal population (Heikkila 2015).

19.6 Pathophysiology

PUVs cause anatomical obstruction of the urethra, with different degrees from one patient to another, depending on the size of the lumen and the resistance to urine flow (Heikkila 2015).

The importance of PUVs is based on the secondary effects of urinary outflow obstruction of the fetal bladder, and the secondary effects of bladder function on the fetal kidney, as well as its effects after birth or even after elimination of the urethral valves (Kajbafzadeh 2005. Sudarsanan et al. 2009). As a consequence of the obstruction, the posterior urethra elongates and dilates, while the bladder neck hypertrophies. Reflux into the prostatic ducts, seminal vesicles, vasa deferentia, and epididymis as well as to the ureters may also occur. The bladder wall becomes trabeculated and thickens, because of muscular hypertrophy, and diverticula may develop. Consequently, the bladder loses contractile strength and compliance, resulting in high intravesical pressure, which reverberates on the ureterovesical junctions and on the kidneys (Heikkila 2015). In a dynamic process, bladder dysfunction may cause progressive renal deterioration (Bomalaski 2016). Ureteral dilatation may be due to vesico-ureteric junction obstruction, or to inefficient ureteric drainage secondary to high intravesical pressure, or it can be the consequence of vesicoureteral reflux (VUR). VUR can either occur because of an abnormal location of the ureteric bud arising from the mesonephric duct or it can be itself secondary to the high intravesical pressure (Nasir et al. 2011, Caione and De Pasquale 2011). The congenital obstruction of the urinary tract during organogenesis may affect lifelong kidney, ureteral, and bladder function (Bomalaski 2016). Renal damage can be due to the obstructive uropathy, with changes that are potentially reversible, but renal dysplasia can be related to damage in early fetal life or abnormal embryogenesis, with changes that are not reversible and account for long-term renal failure (Nasir et al. 2011). Polyuria results from nephrogenic diabetes insipidus caused by injury to the renal collecting tubules (Dinneen et al. 1995; Naghizadeh et al. 2005). Polyuria and bladder overdistention lead to increased infravesical pressure and upper tract dilatation and renal injury (Koff et al. 2002). In addition, PUV patients may develop reflux nephropathy in the presence of VUR (Heikkila 2015). Renal insufficiency is caused by PUVs in approximately 10–15 % of children undergoing renal transplantation, and approximately one-third of patients born with PUVs progress to end-stage renal disease (ESRD) (Bomalaski 2016).

19.7 Presentation and Diagnosis

19.7.1 Prenatal Presentation

Nowadays, with the widespread use of prenatal ultrasonography and increasing awareness, PUVs are most frequently detected during routine prenatal ultrasound (US). Since the second trimester exams, hydronephrosis, a constantly distended and thick-walled bladder and a dilated prostatic urethra, may become evident (Hodges et al. 2009; Nasir et al. 2011; Heikkila 201), but evidence increases after 28 weeks of gestation (Malin et al. 2012). The peculiar sign is the thick-walled bladder, with the so-called "keyhole sign" in the bladder neck in male fetuses (Fig. 19.2). This sign is due to the distention of both the bladder and the posterior urethra immediately proximal to the obstructing valve. The presence of an echogenic line in the dilated posterior urethra, confirmed postnatally to be a valve, has also been reported (Cohen et al. 1998; Vanderheyden et al. 2003; Dyer et al. 2004; Quintero 2005; Avni et al. 2008; Gharpure 2013; Heikkila 2015).

Secondary pyelocaliceal dilatation with parenchymal thinning and ureteral dilatation may be present (Berrocal et al. 2002; Hodges et al. 2009; Nasir et al. 2011; Malin et al. 2012; Bickle 2016). PUVs are frequently associated with VUR, and the degree of renal dysplasia due to reflux also determines the extent of postnatal morbidity and mortality (Yohannes and Hanna 2002). This disorder may account for up to 10 % of all prenatally detected hydronephrosis (Yohannes and Hanna 2002). Differential diagnoses include prune belly syndrome; megaureter, ureteral duplication; urethral atresia; neurogenic bladder; bilateral vesicoureteric reflux; and, less frequently, the megacystis microcolon intestinal hypoperistalsis disorder (Hutton 2004; Gharpure 2013; Bickle 2016; Steven and Desai 2016). In severe cases, oligohydramnios; renal dysplasia, presenting as increased echogenicity of the kidneys and discrete subcortical cysts; and fetal ascites may be observed (Berrocal et al. 2002; Yohannes and Hanna 2002; Hodges et al. 2009; Nasir et al. 2011; Bickle 2016). Serial monitoring of urinary tract dilatation and amount of amniotic fluid are usually necessary (Sudarsanan et al. 2009). Ascites and perirenal urinoma represent spontaneous forms of urinary tract decompression (Silveri et al. 2002; Caione and De Pasquale 2011). Ascites results from leakage of urine from ruptured pyelocaliceal structures (Mirshemirani et al. 2013). Fetuses with signs of urethral obstruction are grouped under the term "lower urinary tract obstruction" (LUTO). It is

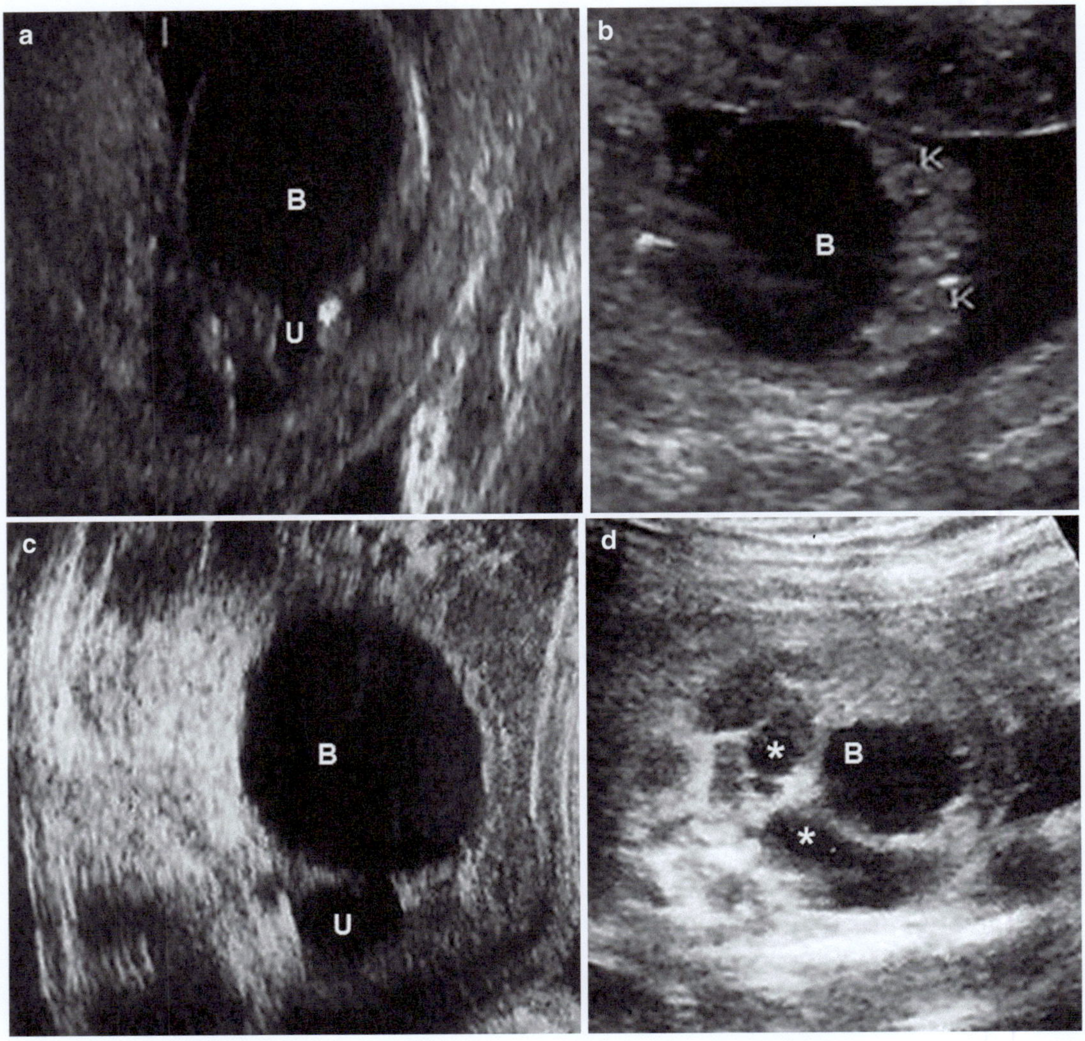

Fig. 19.2 Prenatal US: (**a**, **b**) 14 weeks' gestation, (**c**, **d**) 19 weeks' gestation: enlarged bladder (*B*) and dilated posterior urethra (*U*) ("keyhole sign"); hyperechoic kidneys (*K*); dilated ureters (*)

sometimes difficult to identify the exact cause of urethral obstruction prenatally (Martín et al. 2004; Heikkila 2015; Miller 2015). Definitive diagnosis is made by postnatal voiding cystourethrography (VCUG) and cystourethroscopy. Prenatal imaging is meant to address the diagnosis and ensure proper counseling. MRI offers a valuable aid to US in the evaluation of the fetal urinary tract, especially when resolution is impaired because of severe oligohydramnios (Poutamo et al. 2000; Payabvash et al. 2008; Ruano 2011; Chauvin et al. 2012; Heikkila 2015). The prognosis depends on, gestational age at manifestation, degree of oligohydramnios, hydronephrosis, and parenchymal changes, such as the presence of renal cysts. Poor outcome is predicted by earlier presentation (before 24 weeks' gestation) and by complete bladder outflow obstruction (Hutton 2004; Gharpure 2013). MRI enables evaluation of the amount of amniotic fluid, the status of the renal parenchyma, the presence of macro- or microcystic changes, the size of the kidneys, and the degree of ureteral and bladder distention with thickened walls

(Chauvin et al. 2012). Determination of AFI (amniotic fluid index) represents a prognostic clue in evaluating renal function in fetuses (Zaccara et al. 2005). Depending on the degree of obstruction and renal function, the amniotic fluid may vary from normal to markedly decreased. An appropriate volume of amniotic fluid, produced by the fetal kidneys, is necessary for complete development of the lungs, with normal branching of the bronchial tree and alveoli. If long-standing oligohydramnios is present, the thorax often appears small with hypoplastic lungs, and postnatal pulmonary failure is most likely (Yohannes and Hanna 2002; Chauvin et al. 2012; Miller 2015). Intrauterine interventions such as vesicoamniotic shunting unexpectedly have not improved long-term renal kidney outcome after birth (Biard et al. 2005; Lissauer et al. 2007; Malin et al. 2012; Taskinen et al. 2012; Gharpure 2013; Morris et al. 2013). While vesicoamniotic shunting may modify disease lethality by restoring fluid volume, renal and other genitourinary benefits are minimal or absent, supporting the concept that bladder decompression is being performed after irreversible injury has already occurred (Miller 2015). Elevated fetal urine electrolytes and β2-microglobulin levels are indications of irreversible renal dysfunction (Nasir et al. 2011).

19.7.2 Postnatal Presentation

19.7.2.1 Newborn and Infants

Newborns with prenatal diagnosis of PUVs need to be assessed postnatally, in the first hours of life. These patients and those who are not detected by prenatal US (about one-third of the cases) may present after birth with findings such as delayed voiding or poor urinary stream, abdominal mass, poor feeding, lethargy, urosepsis or urinary ascites, and failure to thrive (Hutton 2004; Nasir et al. 2011). The enlarged bladder with hypertrophic detrusor muscle can be appreciated as a palpable mass in the pelvis. In case of oligohydramnios, the baby can present with Potter facies and limb deformities, skin dimpling, and indentation of the knees and elbows, due to compression within the uterus. In addition, respiratory distress at birth, with poor breathing movements and small chest cavity, due to pulmonary hypoplasia, may be the initial sign of urethral obstruction (Hutton 2004; Nasir et al. 2011). In infants, poor urinary stream and recurrent urinary tract infection are common. Delayed postnatal presentation is often with specific urological symptoms like voiding disturbance, urine retention, and urinary tract infection (UTI). Signs of renal failure or sepsis are not uncommon. Rare presentations include urinary ascites or urinoma, which may occur as a result of spontaneous bladder perforation or fornicial urinary leakage (Nasir et al. 2011).

Ultrasound

Ultrasound (US) is, in most cases, the primary imaging method. Prenatal sonographic findings need to be confirmed, in particular the thickened, trabeculated bladder walls and the elongated and dilated posterior urethra. The "keyhole sign," due to the distention of both the bladder and the posterior urethra, needs to be looked for (Blews 1999; Dacher 2008; Hodges et al. 2009; Nasir et al. 2011; Heikkila 2015; Bickle 2016) (Fig. 19.3).

Examination of the posterior urethra can be performed through the perineum, ideally during micturition at which time the proximal urethra can be seen to dilate. The diameter of the posterior urethra before and after voiding is larger than in normal children (Cohen et al. 1994; Good et al. 1996; Blews 1999; Chowdhury et al. 2002; Schoellnast et al. 2004; Kulshrestha 2006; De Bruyn 2010; Nasir et al. 2011). The valve may actually be seen as an echogenic line floating during voiding inside the posterior urethra (Blews 1999; Bickle 2016) (Fig. 19.4).

A thick-walled bladder on US means a poorly compliant bladder that can lead to obstruction of distal ureters and upper tract damage (Hodges et al. 2009) (Fig. 19.5).

Extended criteria include frequent uni- or bilateral dilatation and tortuosity of the ureter and uni- or bilateral dilatation of the renal pelvis

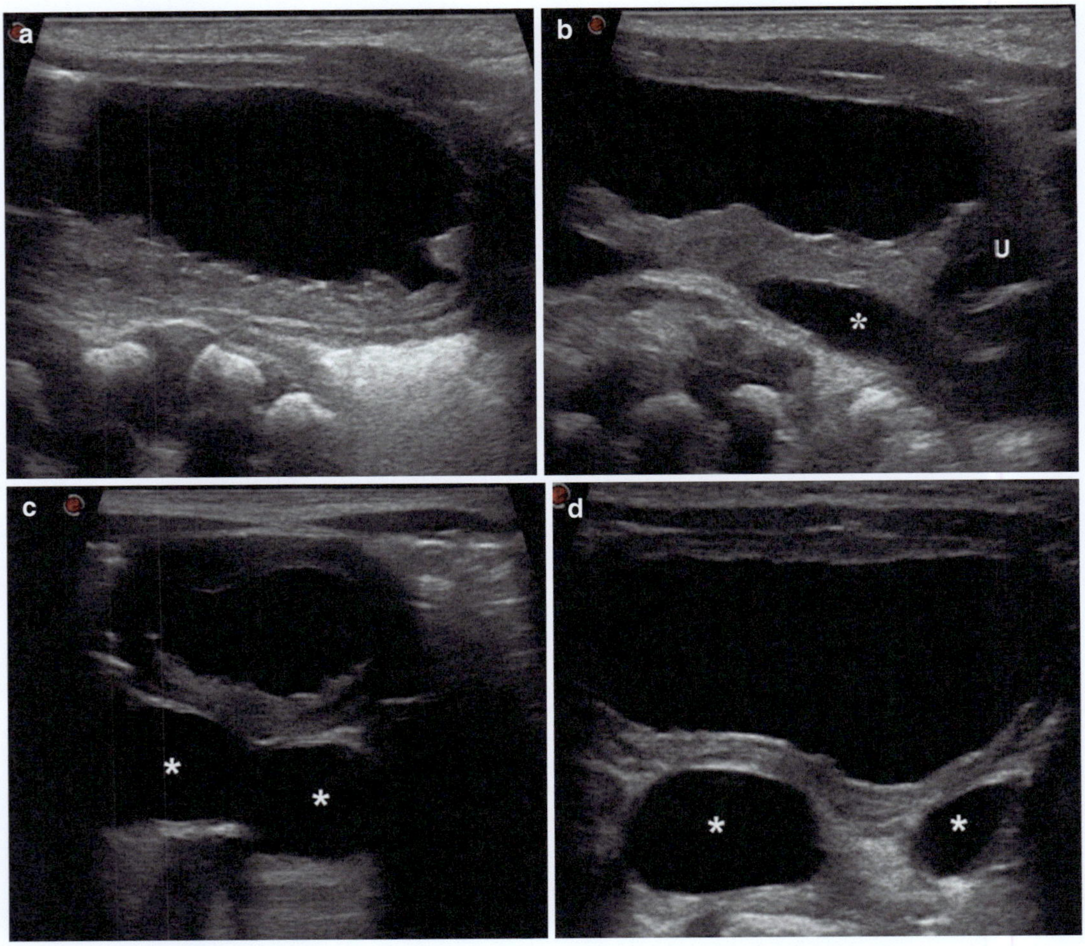

Fig. 19.3 Newborn US: (**a**, **b**) longitudinal scans, (**c**, **d**) transverse scans: enlarged bladder, with thickened and trabeculated walls; dilated posterior urethra (*U*); dilated ureters (*)

(Dacher 2008; Hodges et al. 2009; Nasir et al. 2011; Bickle 2016) (Fig. 19.6).

Because newborns commonly have oliguria during the first few days of life, repeat ultrasound after the first week of life may be necessary if previous findings are normal in a child with prenatal diagnosis of hydronephrosis, before assuming that hydronephrosis has resolved.

Renal parenchyma needs to be evaluated as to thickness, echogenicity, corticomedullary differentiation, and subcortical cysts, though it is not possible to exactly infer renal function (Dacher 2008; Hodges et al. 2009; Heikkila 2015) (Fig. 19.7).

Renal dysplasia seems to depend on the gestational age and the presence/absence of protective factors such as VUR and urinoma.

Perirenal urinoma, large bladder diverticula, ascites, or even hydrothorax may be present, as a consequence of increased pressure and ruptured calyceal fornices (Figs. 19.8 and 19.9). They have been described as the "pop-off" mechanism (Rittenberg et al. 1988). However, the presence or absence of urinoma does not clearly correlate with renal function impairment (Dacher 2008; Hodges et al. 2009; Nasir et al. 2011; Bickle 2016).

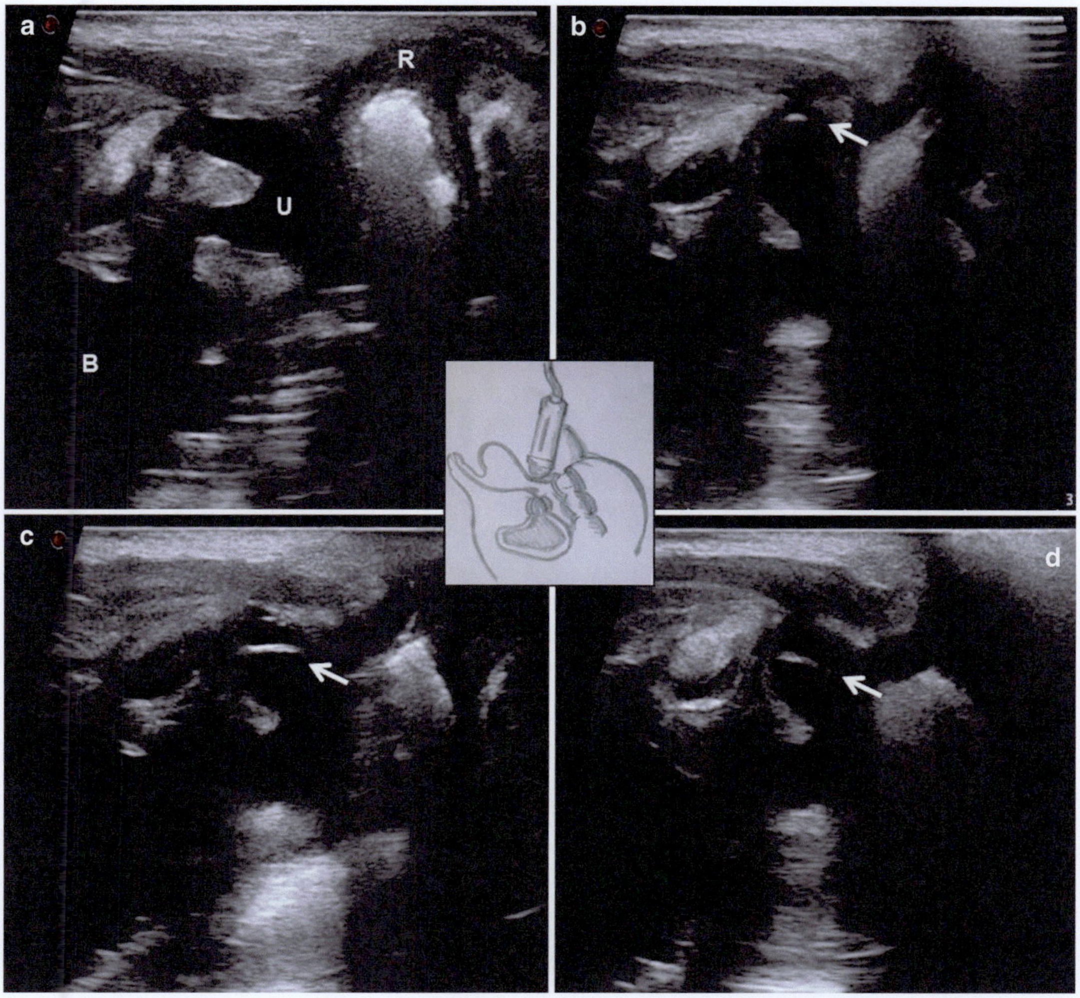

Fig. 19.4 Newborn US: (**a–d**) transperineal longitudinal scans: dilated posterior urethra (*U*) with valve leaflets floating inside (*arrows*), *B* bladder, *R* rectum

Voiding Cystourethrography

Voiding cystourethrography (VCUG) is the most valuable radiological examination and the method of choice to image the bladder and the neck, so it is the only direct means of diagnosing PUVs, before cystoscopic evaluation (Hutton 2004; Hodges et al. 2009; Sudarsanan et al. 2009; Gharpure 2013; Heikkila 2015; Bickle 2016; Bomalaski 2016).

VCUG can be performed after suprapubic puncture, in premature babies, or in rare cases in which it is not possible to catheterize the bladder (Gharpure 2013) (Figs. 19.10 and 19.11).

Mostly VCUG is performed by retrograde opacification. Valves produce only one-way obstruction; however, sometimes it can be difficult to pass through the bladder neck because the catheter is retained in the dilated posterior urethra (Dacher 2008). VCUG will demonstrate dilatation and elongation of the posterior urethra (similar to the US "keyhole sign"), occasionally a linear radiolucent band corresponding to the valve, thickened bladder walls with sacculations, trabeculations, and diverticula (Dacher 2008; Hodges et al. 2009; Gharpure

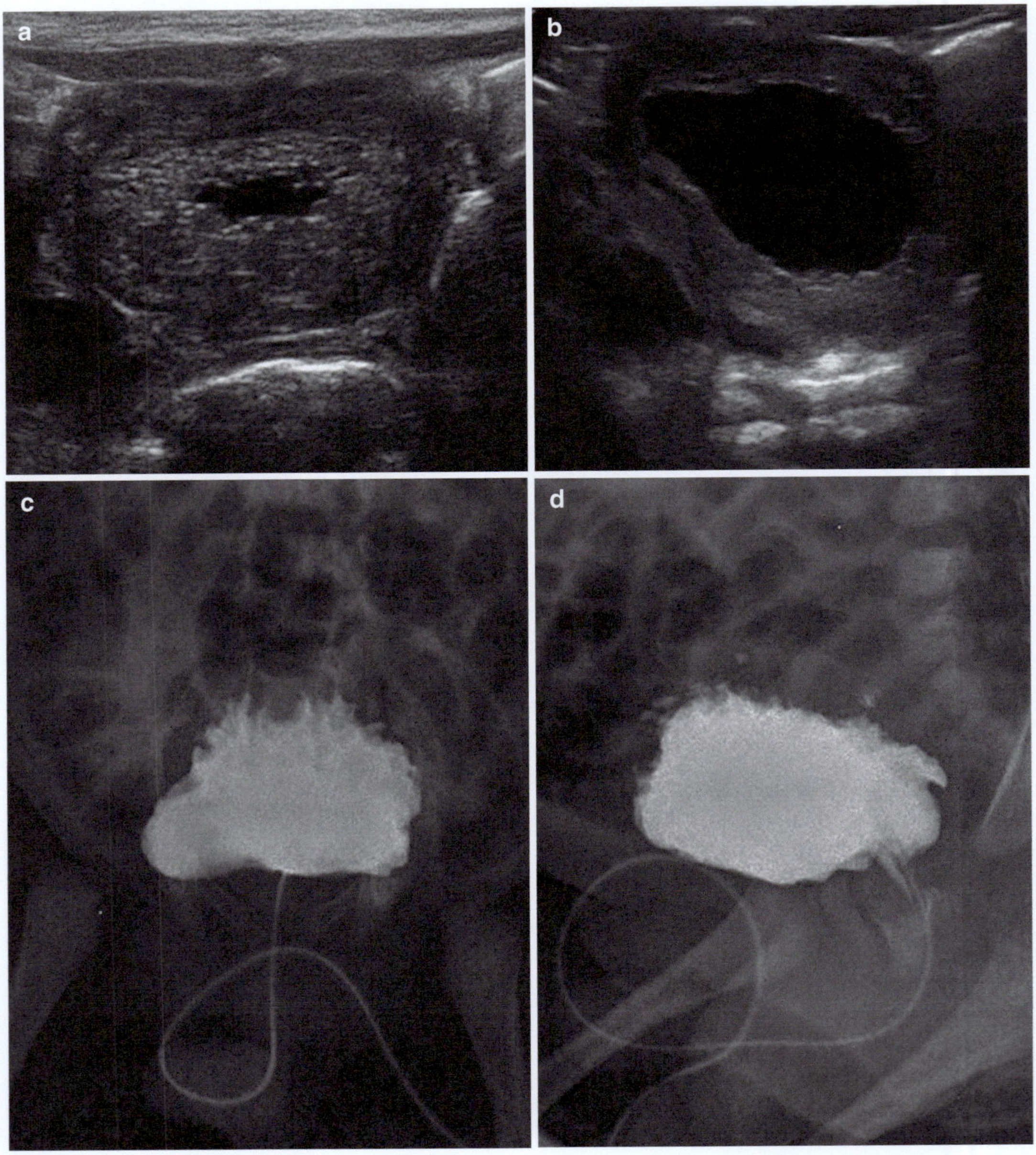

Fig. 19.5 US: (**a**, **b**) transverse scans VCUG: (**c**) anteroposterior view (**d**) oblique view: thick-walled trabeculated bladder

2013; Bickle 2016; Bomalaski 2016). The bladder neck becomes hypertrophic and appears narrow in relation to the dilated posterior urethra (Berrocal et al. 2002; Bomalaski 2016). There appears a circumferential filling defect at the level of the pelvic floor (Nasir et al. 2011). Different degrees of posterior urethra dilatation may be expected in children with PUVs, though a correlation with the severity of obstruction and long-term outcome has not been established (Figs. 19.12 and 19.13).

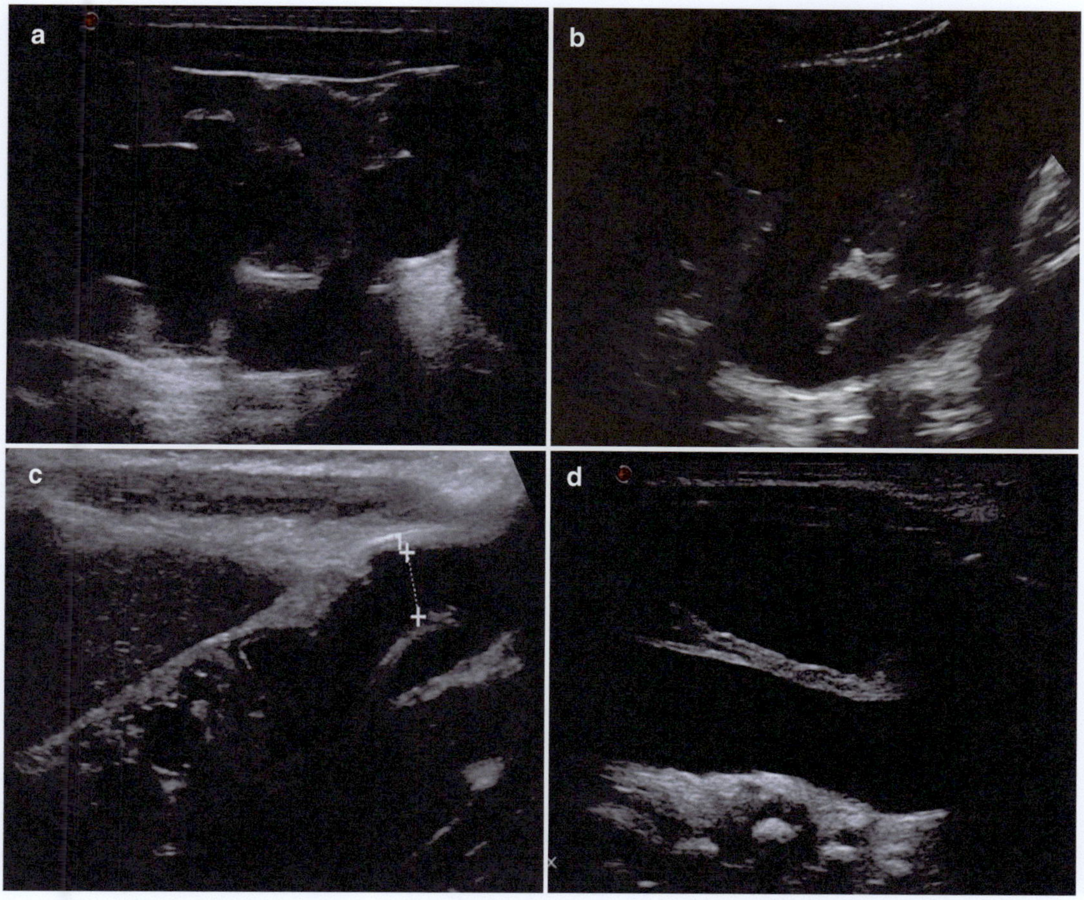

Fig. 19.6 US: (**a**–**d**) longitudinal scans: dilation of the pelvicalyceal system; dilated and tortuous proximal ureter; markedly dilated distal ureter behind the bladder

The voiding phase is an essential diagnostic step – and it is important to obtain it with the catheter removed – since it shows the discrepancy between the posterior and anterior segments of the urethra with a posteriorly located orifice (Dacher 2008; Hodges et al. 2009; Gharpure 2013; Steven and Desai 2016).

In Young type I PUVs, the "sail in the wind" sign and, in Young type III PUVs, the "wind in sock" sign can be appreciated. However, these different patterns are more likely to be the consequence of endourethral procedures rather than different diseases (Lissauer et al. 2007). Differentiating the type of valve is not always possible on VCUG (Yohannes and Hanna 2002). Anyway, the classification of PUVs has no clinical value with regard to treatment and prognosis, and the clinical symptoms are not related to the valve type (Kajbafzadeh 2005). Occasionally reflux into the prostatic ducts, ejaculatory ducts, seminal vesicles, and vasa deferentes, secondary to the elevated bladder and urethral pressures, may also be present (Kwong et al. 2013; Bomalaski 2016) (Fig. 19.14). VCUG also identifies preobstructive secondary changes in the urinary tract and detects and grades VUR (Heikkila 2015) (Figs. 19.15 and 19.16). VUR is frequent and can be unilateral or bilateral (Hutton

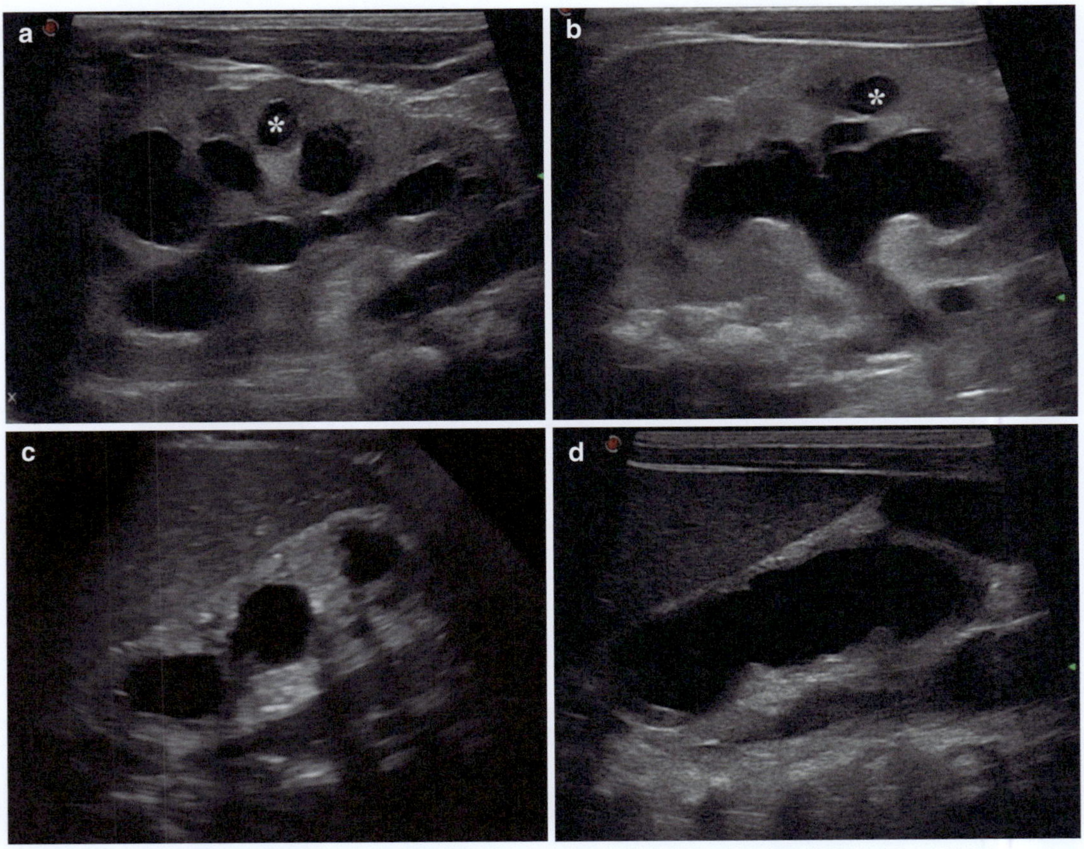

Fig. 19.7 US: (**a–d**) longitudinal scans: various degrees of pelvicalyceal dilatation; proximal ureterectasis (**b**); thinned and hyperechoic renal parenchyma; reduced corticomedullary differentiation with cortical cysts (*) (**a**, **b**); severely thinned renal parenchyma, loss of corticomedullary differentiation (**c**, **d**)

2004; Kibar et al. 2011). It occurs in about one-half to two-thirds of children with PUVs, of whom approximately two-thirds have unilateral reflux (Bates 2013). The incidence of VUR is variably reported and ranges from 26 % to 72 % according to Dinneen (Dinneen and Duffy 1996) and from 37 % to 67 % according to Hutton (2004). It was 60 % in the series by Priti et al. (2004) and 64 % in the series by Heikkila (2015) and Heikkila et al. (2009). Approximately 50 % of patients with PUVs have VUR according to Berrocal, Nasir, Steven, and Blicke (Berrocal et al. 2002; Nasir et al. 2011; Steven and Desai 2016; Bickle 2016). VUR is believed to be secondary to the bladder outflow obstruction and coexistent bladder dysfunction (Hassan et al. 2003; Heikkila et al. 2009; Steven and Desai 2016), but can also be due to the abnormal location of the ureteric bud arising from the mesonephric duct (Nasir et al. 2011). Following valve ablation, the severity of VUR may decrease or resolve completely in 25–50 % of cases (Johnston and Kulatilake 1971; Johnston 1979; Heikkila et al. 2009; Steven and Desai 2016). The incidence of disappearance of reflux is even higher in other series, 29–64 % according to Farhat et al. (2000) and 78.94 % in the study by Priti et al. (2004). Kidneys with refluxing ureters have worse primary function than the contralateral kidneys (Heikkila et al. 2009). Reflux is the

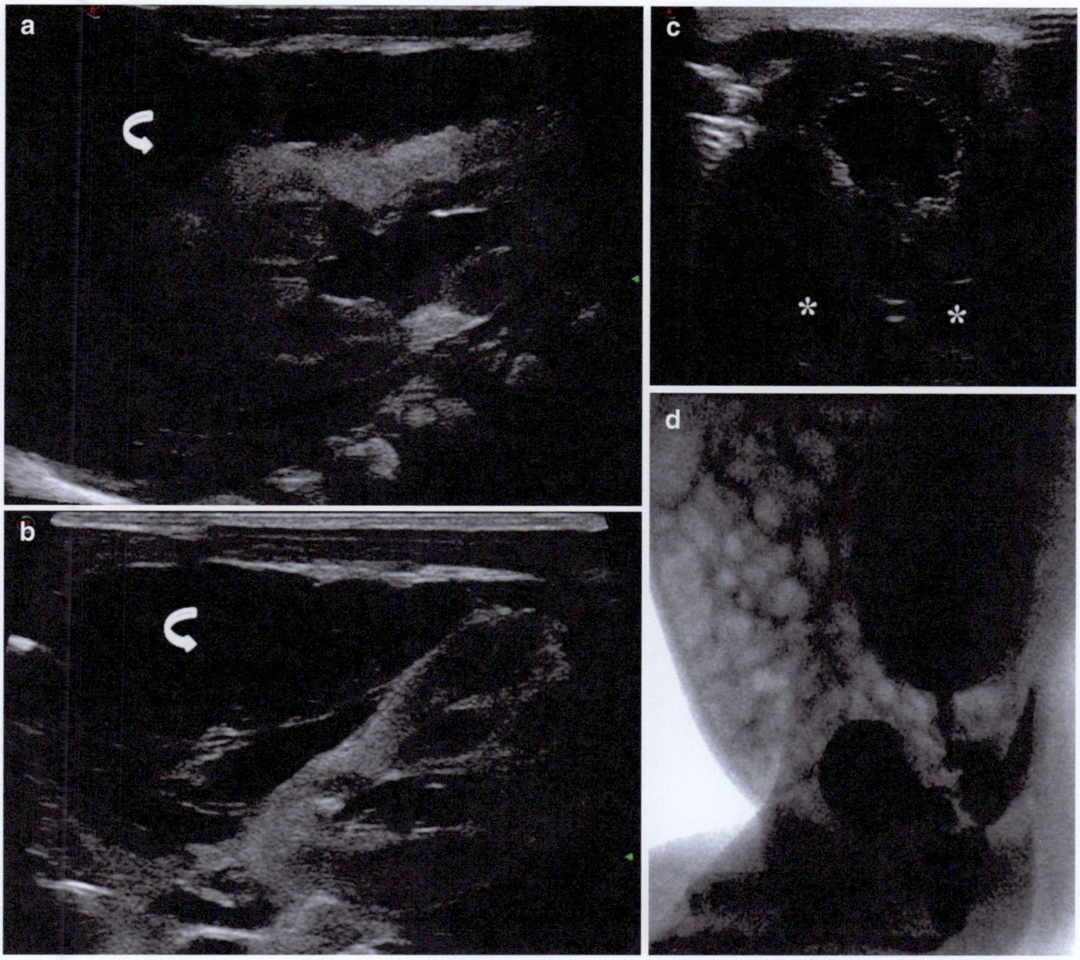

Fig. 19.8 US: (**a**) longitudinal scan (**b**, **c**) transverse scans: perinephric subcapsular fluid collection due to a urinoma (*curved arrows*); mild dilatation of the intrarenal collecting system, partially decompressed into the subcapsular space; thickened bladder walls; dilated ureters (*) VCUG: (**d**) lateral view: posterior urethral valves, vesicoureteral reflux, transparenchymal flow of contrast medium into the subcapsular space

major cause of postnatal renal damage in PUVs, and persistent reflux is associated with poor outcome (Parkhouse et al. 1988; Priti et al. 2004). Bilateral reflux, especially if persistent, is associated with decreased overall renal function outcome (Hassan et al. 2003; Ziylan et al. 2006; Heikkila et al. 2009; Nasir et al. 2011; Steven and Desai 2016). If the VUR is high grade and unilateral, a "pop-off" mechanism may allow selective dissipation of back pressure, resulting from urethral obstruction (Steven and Desai 2016). VURD (valves unilateral reflux and renal dysplasia) syndrome is the combination of persistent unilateral VUR associated with an ipsilateral dysplastic, poorly functioning kidney in patients with PUVs. Generally, contralateral renal function in patients with unilateral reflux into a nonfunctioning kidney is preserved (Bomalaski 2016). The concept of pressure "pop-offs" in the posterior urethral valves was

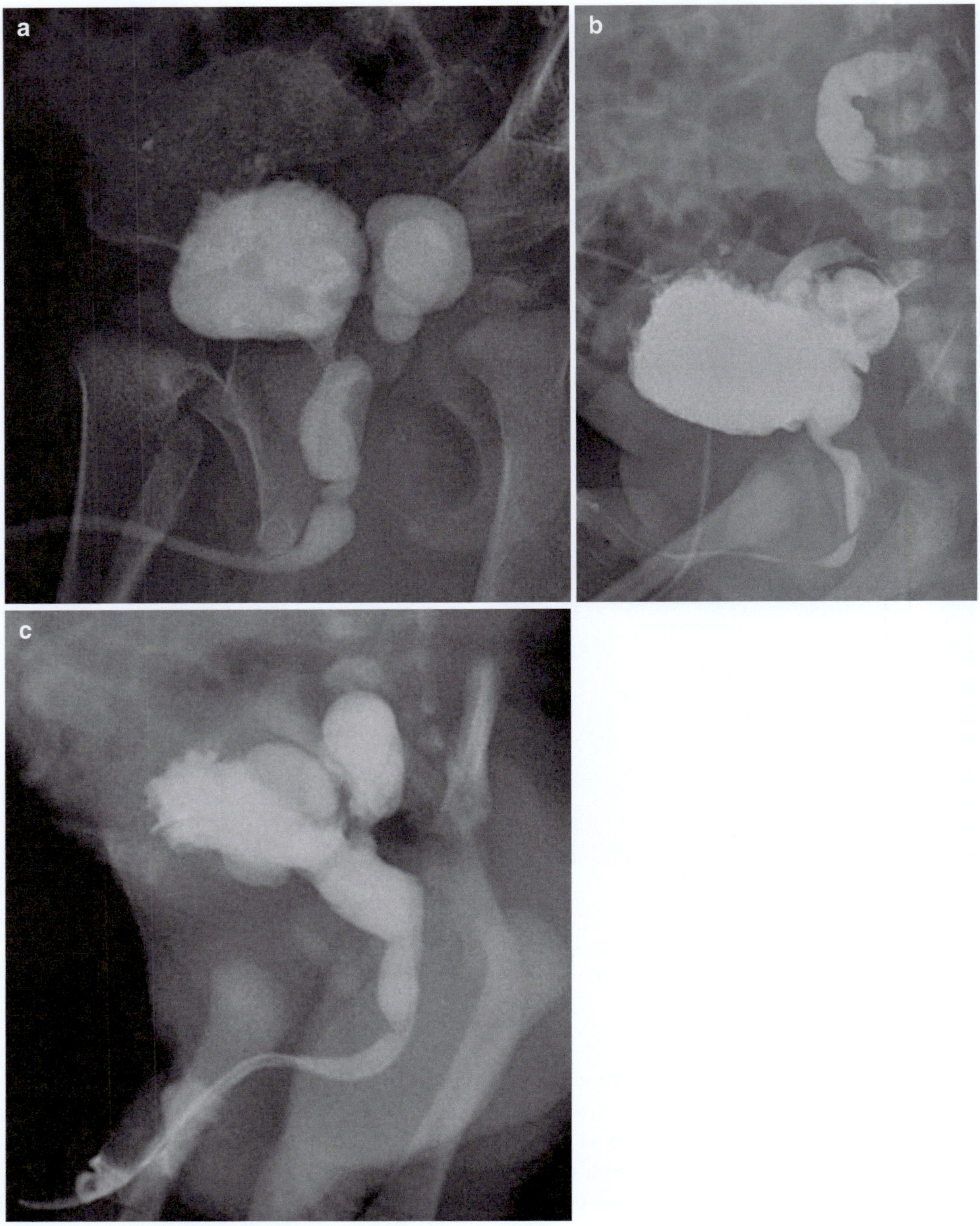

Fig. 19.9 VCUG: (**a**–**c**) oblique views: posterior urethral valves, trabeculated bladder with cellulae and sacculi; huge bladder diverticula: left-sided diverticulum (**a**); left-sided diverticulum with associated right-sided vesicoureteral reflux (**b**) bilateral diverticula (**c**)

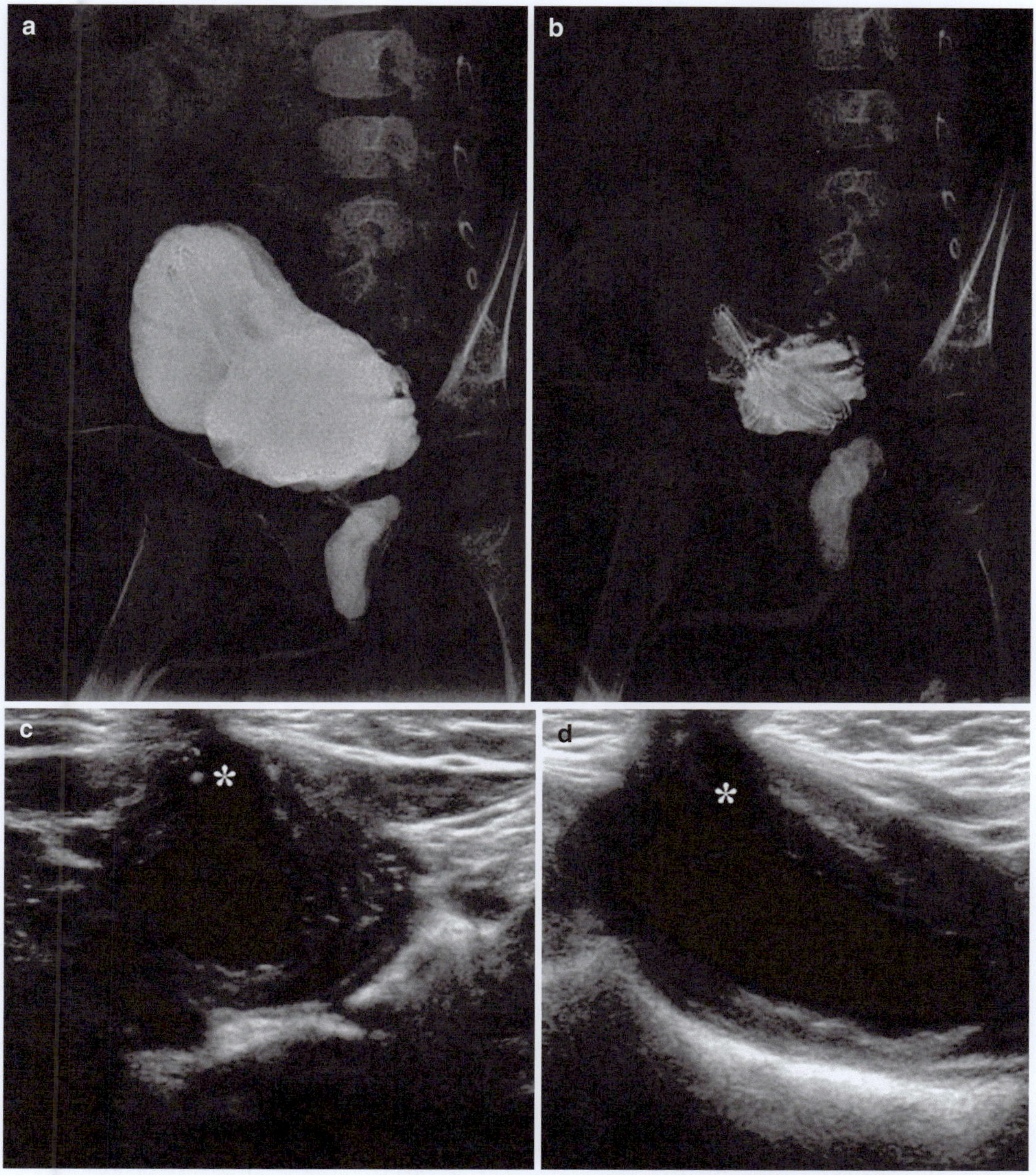

Fig. 19.10 Epicystostomy VCUG: (**a**, **b**) oblique views: posterior urethral valves, thick-walled trabeculated bladder US: (**c**) transverse scan (**d**) longitudinal scan: thick-walled trabeculated bladder; insertion of the catheter (*)

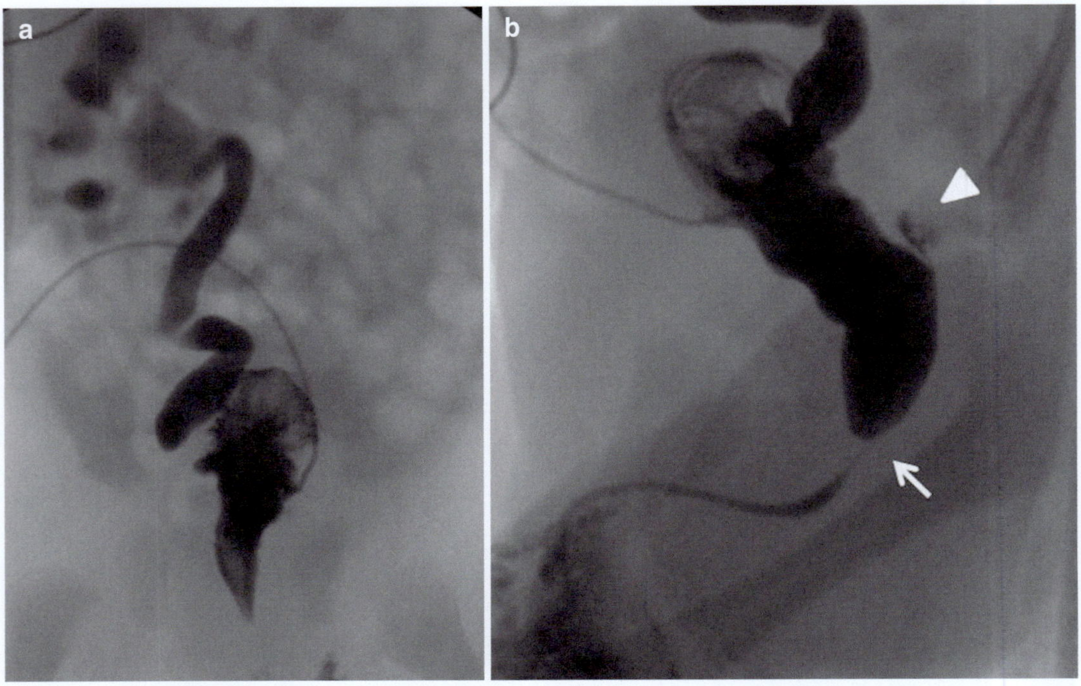

Fig. 19.11 Epicystostomy VCUG: (**a**) anteroposterior view, (**b**) steep oblique view voiding cystourethrograms: poorly distensible bladder with thickened and irregular walls, right-sided vesicoureteral reflux, posterior urethral valves, dilated posterior urethra, minimal reflux into the prostatic ducts (*arrowhead*), filling defect (*arrow*) and abrupt transition at the level of valves to a narrow anterior urethra

defined in 1988 and included the VURD syndrome, large congenital type bladder diverticula, and urinary extravasation with or without urinary ascites (Rittenberg et al. 1988). The high-grade VUR into a nonfunctioning kidney had been already thought to act as a protective factor with a pop-off mechanism, leading to dissipation of pressure into the dilated nonfunctioning system, preserving contralateral renal function (Hoover and Duckett 1982). This phenomenon is commonly known as the VURD syndrome. However, in the long run, the VURD syndrome may not have the favorable outcome it was once thought to have, with no statistical significance between the presence and absence of these pop-off mechanisms and final renal outcome (Sarhan et al. 2011; Bomalaski 2016). So, in the long term, renal function may be affected all the same, with hypertension, proteinuria, and renal failure (Narasimhan et al. 2005).

19.7.2.2 Presentation in Older Boys

Late presentations are rare nowadays (Mahadik et al. 2012). The main clinical complaints in older children are usually dysuria, bladder retention and storage and emptying symptoms, pain or dysfunction on voiding, decreased force of urinary stream, diurnal and nocturnal incontinence, recurrent UTI, or less commonly hematuria (Bomalaski et al. 1999; Hutton 2004; Dacher 2008; Hodges et al. 2009; Kanaroglou et al. 2011; Nasir et al. 2011; Mahadik et al. 2012; Steven and Desai 2016).

PUVs are sometimes discovered during evaluation of an abdominal mass or renal failure or conditions of proteinuria (Hodges et al. 2009; Kanaroglou et al. 2011; Bomalaski 2016).

Late presentation does not always correlate with better long-term prognosis (Bomalaski et al. 1999; Hutton 2004), and renal impairment can occur at any age (Kanaroglou et al. 2011).

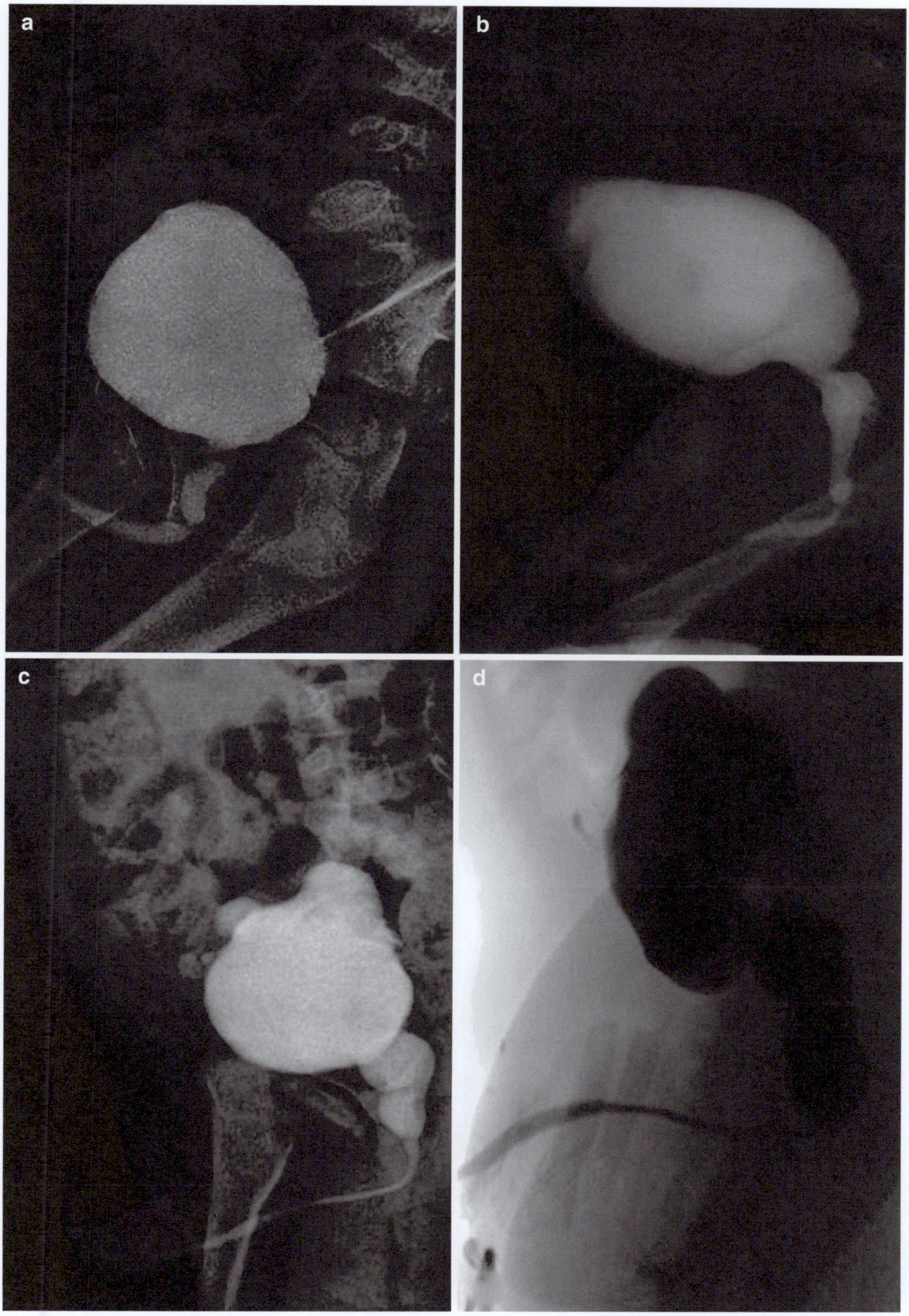

Fig. 19.12 VCUG: (**a–d**) oblique view voiding cystourethrograms: posterior urethral valves with progressively increasing degree of dilatation and elongation of the posterior urethra and progressively abrupt transition at the level of valves to the narrow anterior urethra; thickened and irregular bladder walls

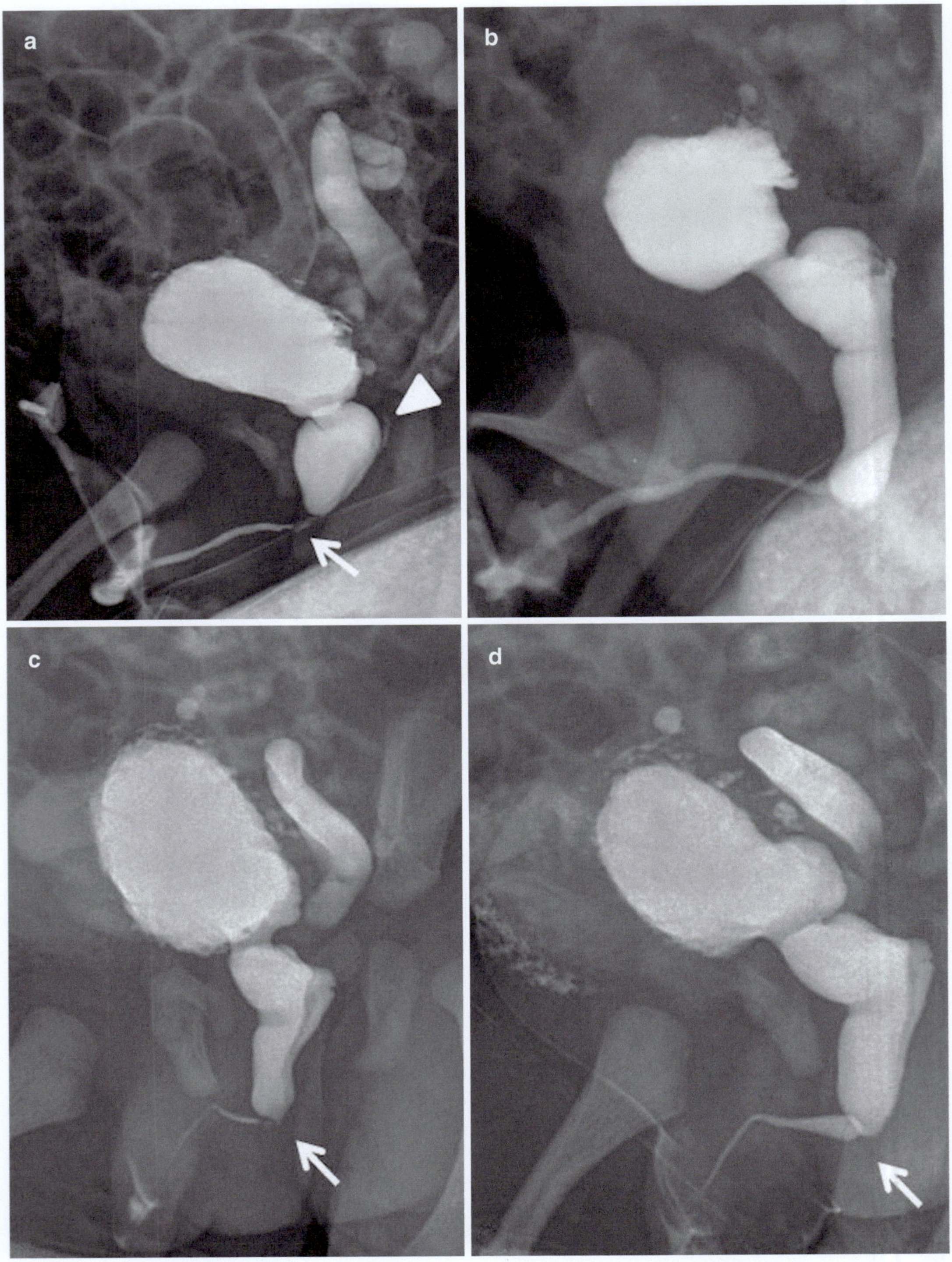

Fig. 19.13 VCUG: (**a**–**d**) oblique view voiding cystourethrograms: elongated and dilated posterior urethra with filling defect (*arrows*) and a marked decrease of urethral caliber at the level of the defect, followed by transition to the narrow anterior urethra; thickened and irregular bladder walls with cellulae and sacculi; right-sided vesicoureteral reflux (**a**, **c**, **d**); minimal reflux (*arrowhead*) into the seminal vesicles (**a**)

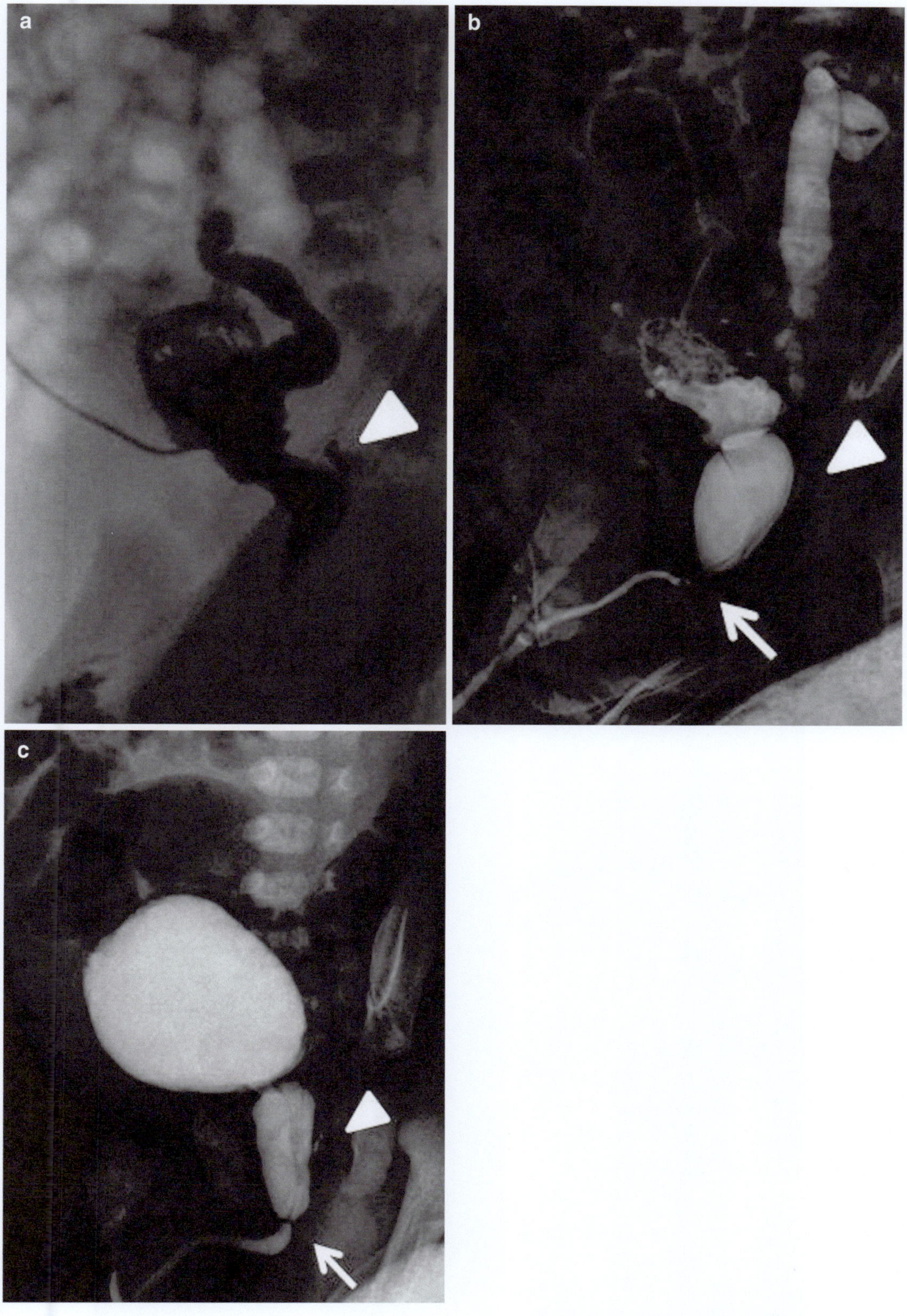

Fig. 19.14 VCUG: (**a**–**c**) oblique view voiding cystourethrograms: elongated and dilated posterior urethra, posterior urethral valves, filling defect (*arrows*), and marked decrease of urethral caliber at the level of the defect, transition to the narrow anterior urethra; thickened and irregular bladder walls; minimal reflux (*arrowheads*) into the prostatic ducts (**a**) and seminal vesicles (**b**, **c**); right-sided vesicoureteral reflux (**b**)

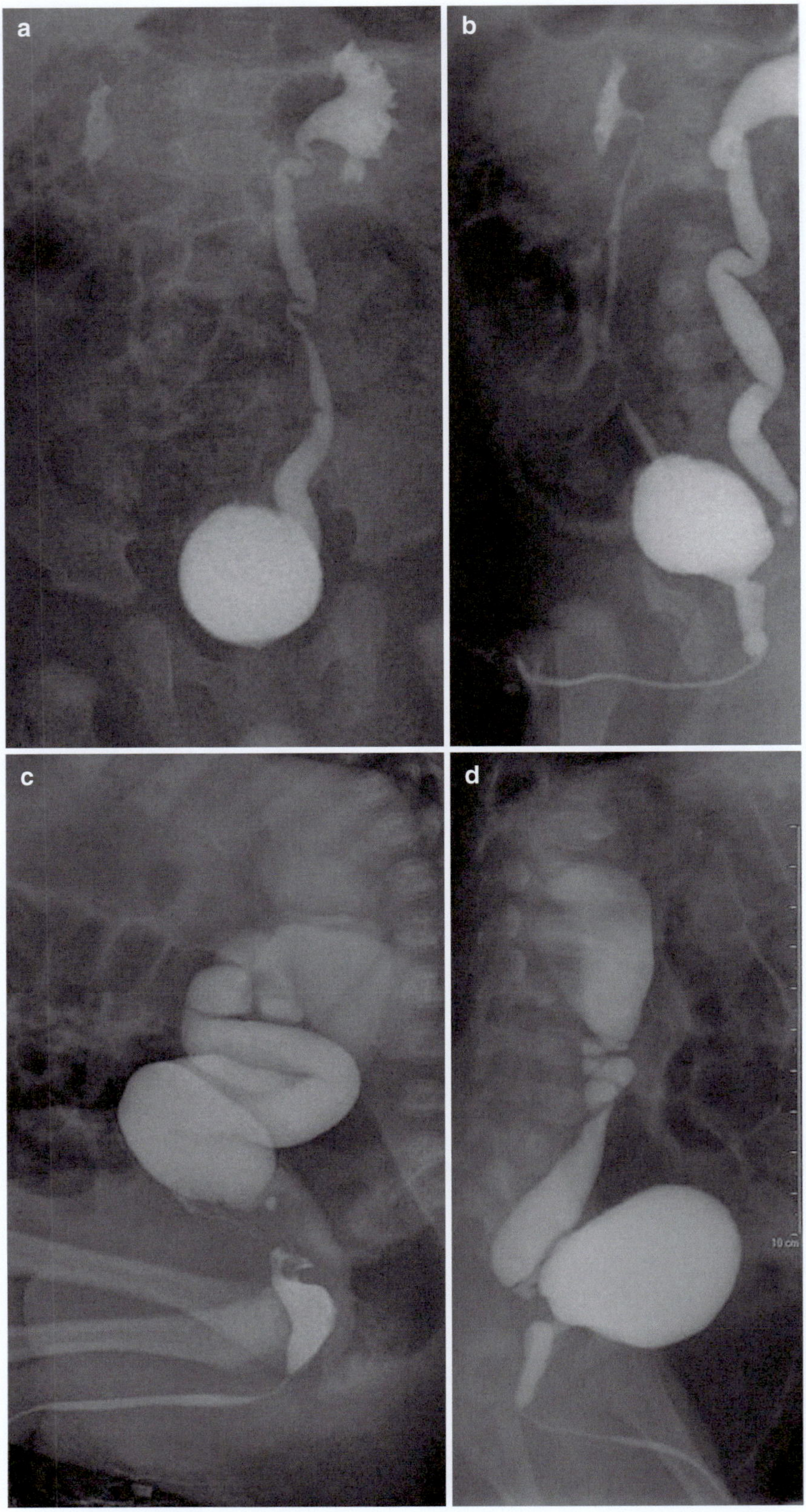

Fig. 19.15 VCUG: (**a**) anteroposterior postvoiding (**b**–**d**) oblique view voiding cystourethrograms: posterior urethral valves; bilateral refluxes (**a**, **b**), right-sided reflux (**c**, **d**)

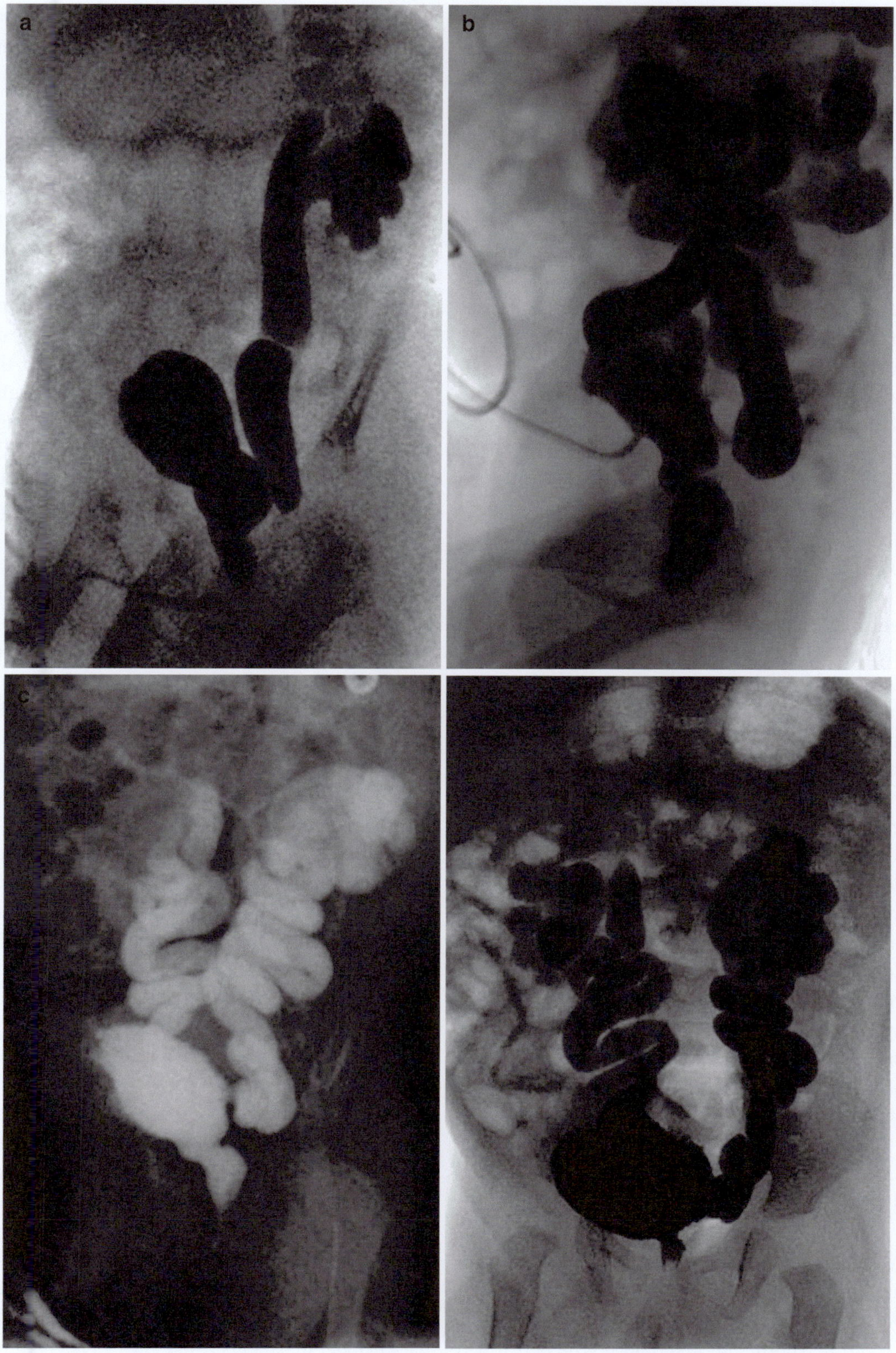

Fig. 19.16 VCUG: (**a–c**) oblique view (**d**) anteroposterior view voiding cystourethrograms: posterior urethral valves; left-sided reflux (**a**) bilateral high-grade refluxes (**b–d**)

19.8 Treatment

Treatment of PUV is long established. The mainstay of treatment is resolution of urethral obstruction which has long been undertaken by electrofulguration of the valves by Bugbee electrode or, alternatively, by neonatal resectoscope. Use of electrical current, however, is a very delicate procedure in a thin and narrow urethra like the one of a neonate; even in experienced hands, it is not exempted from risks of late-onset urethral strictures and stenosis, which may be very difficult to treat (Warner et al. 2015). In this respect, laser ablation has proven as a valid alternative with significantly fewer complications (Palminteri et al. 2014; Pagano et al. 2015) both in the short and in the long term. Not infrequently, a "second look" may be required later for residual valve tissue ablation. In some cases exhibiting persistent impairment of renal function or recurrent UTI, urinary diversion may be required during the first few months of life (nephrostomy/ureterostomy/vesicostomy) with direct valve ablation being deferred to a later date. However, optimal diversion is not straightforward and studies comparing different techniques in the long run are lacking. While there is evidence that vesicostomy affects bladder contractility later in life, effects of higher diversion on the upper and lower urinary tract have not been studied in details. At follow-up patients treated with temporary vesicostomy had comparatively higher end filling detrusor pressure, decreased bladder capacity, poor compliance, and increased serum creatinine than those treated with initial valve ablation. Thus, when primary ablation is possible, it is the preferred postnatal treatment of infants with PUVs (Podesta et al. 2002).

19.9 Radionuclide Studies

Although not necessary in every child, renal scintigraphy may be helpful in some cases. Functional imaging of the upper tract is usually not necessary in newborn, and it should not be performed in that period, because of kidney's immaturity that does not allow a correct evaluation of renal function, so it is usually deferred to at least about 4 weeks of age (Nasir et al. 2011; Gharpure 2013; Bomalaski 2016).

Radionuclide studies are useful when renal parenchyma is thinned or abnormal and when postoperative US examination shows no improvement (Nasir et al. 2011). Diethylenetriaminepentaacetic acid (DTPA) or mercaptoacetyltriglycine (MAG3) are sensitive to renal dysplasia and scarring and also allow dynamic studies. These tracers are taken up by the kidney and excreted into the urine. DTPA is excreted primarily by glomerular filtration. MAG3 is excreted principally through tubular secretion. The renal extraction of MAG3 is greater than that of DTPA, so it represents the isotope of choice in infants with a relatively large extracellular space and a low glomerular filtration rate (Fig. 19.17a).

Differential renal function (DRF) and drainage are evaluated. In the presence of dilatation. T he excretory phase can demonstrate the degree of obstruction, through the time/intensity curve, also with the use of diuretics (furosemide) (Fig. 19.17b–d).

A static scan using dimercaptosuccinic acid (DMSA) can evaluate DRF and focal parenchymal defects (Nasir et al. 2011; Heikkila 2015).

Radionuclide cystography (RNC) is usually reserved for follow-up studies of VUR, because it is sensible to detect VUR, but it does not allow the evaluation of morphological changes in the urinary tract (Cooper 2009; Heikkila 2015) (Fig. 19.17e, f).

19.10 Urodynamic Studies

Urodynamic evaluation provides information about bladder storage and emptying. Normal bladder should store urine at a low pressure and then completely empty at appropriate pressures. Patients with PUVs have a spectrum of urodynamic abnormalities (Nasir et al. 2011; Bomalaski 2016). There are three main clinical patterns of urinary bladder in patients with PUVs: (1) hypertonic

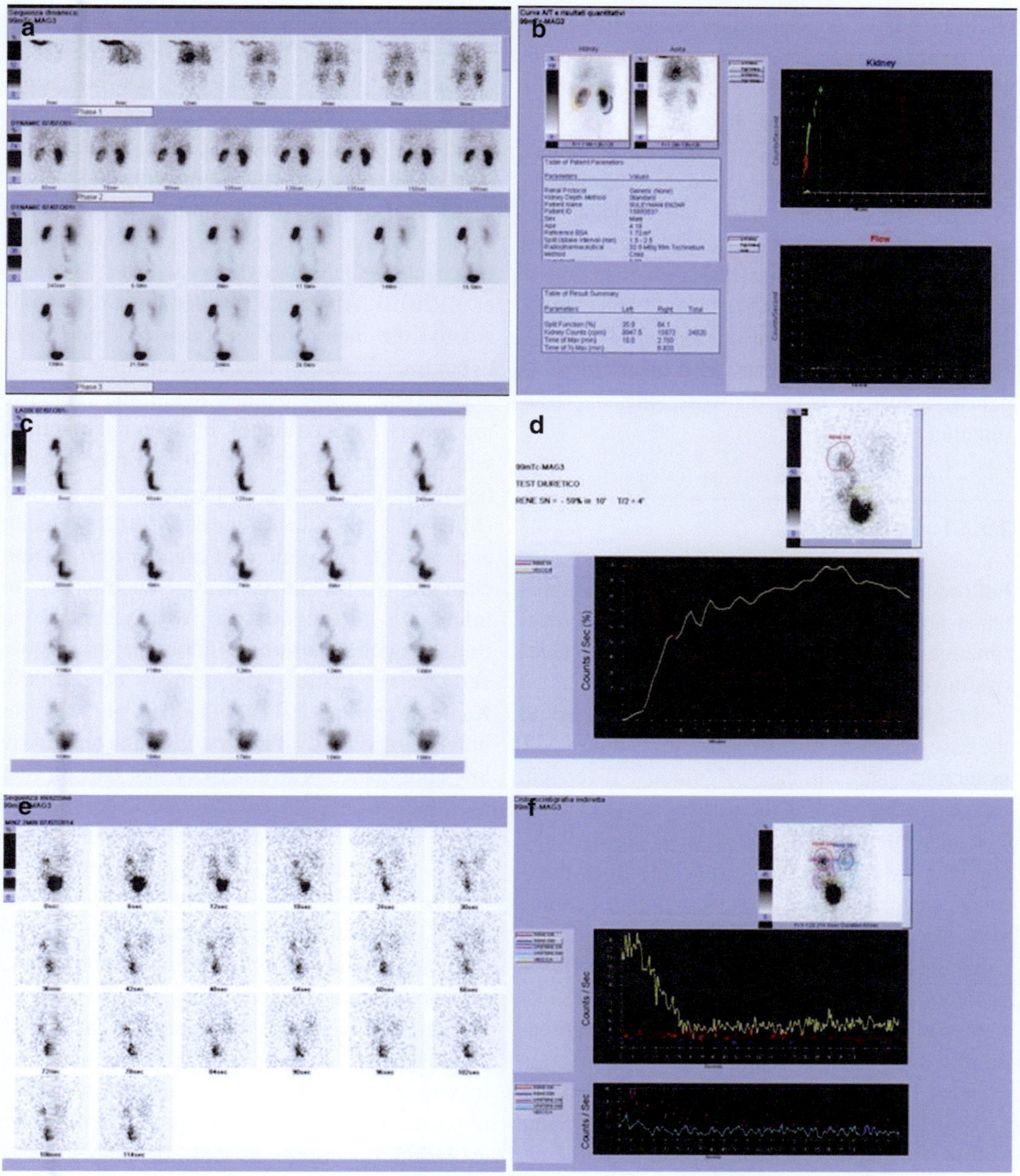

Fig. 19.17 99mTC-MAG3 renal scintigraphy: (**a**) Dynamic scan (**b**) Differential renal function (DRF) (**c**, **d**) Diuretic test (furosemide) (**e**, **f**) Voiding radionuclide cystography: Hypofunction of the left kidney with nonobstructive pelvicalyceal and ureteral urinary stasis; morphofunctionally normal right kidney; no demonstration of refluxes on voiding cystography

low complaint, small capacity bladder; (2) hyperreflexic bladder with uninhibited contractions; and (3) myogenic failure with Valsalva voiding and overflow (Thomas 2010).

Urodynamic investigations are not usually performed in the neonatal age or before valve ablation, while this exam should be an essential component of follow-up of patients with PUVs, after valve ablation, especially in case of persistent or recurrent hydronephrosis, UTI, incontinence, or persistent reflux, so as to address the type of bladder therapy (Hassan et al. 2003; Caione and De Pasquale 2011; Nasir et al. 2011). Noninvasive urodynamic studies (flowmetry, evaluation of bladder capacity and residual volume) should be preferred in the evaluation of these patients with sensate urethra, who often require repeated examinations (Capitanucci et al. 2012). Invasive studies in this subset of patients should be reserved to cases with severe incontinence, recurrent UTI, or worsening of renal function.

19.11 Follow-Up

Follow-up in PUV boys is of paramount importance and has the purpose of preserving renal function, preventing UTI, and managing bladder dysfunction (Steven and Desai 2016).

In this respect, imaging follow-up is based on the association of nuclear medicine studies, MR urography, and, in case of urinary diversion, direct opacification of the urinary tract. In addition, as mentioned, noninvasive urodynamic studies play a pivotal role especially in addressing bladder therapy after valve ablation (Caione and De Pasquale 2011; Nasir et al. 2011; Capitanucci et al. 2012). Continence is often a problem in children and adolescents with a history of PUVs. Urodynamic studies are sometimes helpful to evaluate vesical and sphincter function (Dacher 2008). In mild incontinence, urotherapy (pelvic floor rehabilitation, biofeedback, double voiding) can help in achieving complete dryness. Serial assessments of the urethral caliber by perineal ultrasound might perhaps be useful not only for the diagnosis in neonates and male infants but also in the long-term follow-up in patients with residual incontinence.

The use of drugs in PUVs patients has long been a matter of contention: on the one side, the use of oxybutynin to reduce involuntary contractions and to improve continence is long established; on the other side, alphalitic drugs to overcome obstruction induced by hypertrophied bladder neck are far from being straightforward.

The vast majority of selective antimuscarinic drugs such as solifenacin and darifenacin are not approved for use in children, so that valid therapeutic alternatives to oxybutynin are still lacking.

Bladder dysfunction is common in boys post-valve ablation and seems to evolve with age (Mitchell 1982; Kanaroglou et al. 2011; Mahadik et al. 2012). Abnormal bladder function is considered the most important cause of persistent upper tract dilatation after valve ablation (Hutton 2004). The "valve bladder syndrome" actually represents a spectrum of bladder dysfunction, which occurs in about 38–70 % of boys with neonatal diagnosis and treatment for PUVs (Mitchell 1982; Kanaroglou et al. 2011; Mahadik et al. 2012). The pattern of bladder dysfunction changes from unstable/hypercontractile in infancy, to hypocontractile in childhood, to a true myogenic failure in adolescence, despite early valve ablation (De Gennaro et al. 2000; Kanaroglou et al. 2011; Mahadik et al. 2012). In infancy, bladder dysfunction is characterized by low compliance or overactivity, but later in life, the bladder tends to enlarge and become difficultly emptying. So the bladder changes from poorly compliant or overactive in infancy to poorly emptying in adolescence (Taskinen et al. 2012). Polyuria, which is a result of a prenatal damage to renal collecting tubules (nephrogenic diabetes insipidus), determines progressive distention of the bladder (Dinneen et al. 1995; Naghizadeh et al. 2005). On the other hand, the hypertrophic bladder neck causes secondary obstruction, leading to myogenic failure and evolution in time toward decompensation, despite early correction of obstruction (Holmdahl et al.1996; Androulakakis et al. 2005; Taskinen et al. 2012,). Overall long-term outcome after valve ablation in older patients is variable (Mahadik et al. 2012). Usually, if renal function quickly improves immediately after obstruction relief, then renal deterioration develops slowly in the following years (Drozdz et al. 1998). End-stage renal disease (ESRD) can occur in about one-third of patients born with PUVs, by their lifetime (Bomalaski 2016). In adulthood, one-third of the patients who were operated on for PUVs still have moderate or severe lower urinary tract symptoms (LUTSs), including urinary incontinence in up to 15% of the cases (Bomalaski 2016). Risk factors for sexual dysfunction, in a minor number of patients, are represented by the abnormal posterior urethra, cryptorchidism, and recurrent epididymo-orchitis, besides chronic renal failure. Overall, fertility is similar to the normal, healthy population (Heikkilä et al. 2008; Taskinen et al. 2012).

References

Aaronson IA (1983) Posterior urethral valve masquerading as the prune belly syndrome. Br J Urol 55:508–512

Androulakakis PA, Karamanolakis DK, Tsahouridis G, Stefanidis AA, Palaeodimos I (2005) Myogenic bladder decompensation in boys with a history of posterior urethral valves is caused by secondary bladder neck obstruction? BJU Int 96:140–143

Avni FE, Maugey-Laulom B, Cassart M, Eurin D, Massez A, Hall M (2008) The fetal genitourinary tract. In: Callen PW (ed) Ultrasound in obstetrics & gynecology, 5th edn. Saunders, Philadelphia

Bates DG (2013) Bladder and urethra. In: Coley BD (ed) Caffey's pediatric diagnostic imaging, 12th edn. Saunders, Philadelphia, pp 1262–1273

Bazy F (1903) A propos du diagnostic de lesions renales unilaterales. Bull Mem Soc Chir Paris 29:101

Benz-Bohm G (2008) Anomalies of kidney rotation, position and fusion. In: Fotter R (ed) Pediatric uroradiology, 2nd edn. Springer, Berlin, pp 81–88

Berrocal T, Lopez-Pereira P, Arjonilla A, Gutierrez J (2002) Anomalies of the distal ureter, bladder, and urethra in children: embryologic, radiologic, and pathologic features1. RadioGraphics 22:1139–1164

Biard JM, Johnson MP, Carr MC, Wilson RD, Hedrick HL, Pavlock C, Adzick NS (2005) Long-term outcomes in children treated by prenatal vesicoamniotic shunting for lower urinary tract obstruction. Obstet Gynecol 106:503–508

Bickle I (2016) Posterior urethral valves. http://radiopaedia.org

Blews DE (1999) Sonography of the neonatal genitourinary tract. Radiol Clin N Am 37:1199–1208

Bomalaski MD (2016) Posterior urethral valves in Medscape reference updated Feb 16, 2016. http://emedicine.medscape.com/article/1016086overview#showall

Bomalaski MD, Anema JG, Coplen DE, Koo HP, Rozanski T, Bloom DA (1999) Delayed presentation of posterior urethral valves: a not so benign condition. J Urol 162:2130–2132

Budd G (1840) Case of extraordinary dilatation of the kidneys, ureters, and bladder, in consequence of a membranous fold in the urethra, which acted as a valve, and prevented the free escape of the urine from the bladder. Lancet 1:767–769

Caione P, De Pasquale V (2011) Posterior urethral valves. In: Puri P (ed) Newborn surgery, 3rd edn. Hodder Arnold, London, pp 916–933

Caione P, Gerocarni Nappo S (2011) Posterior urethral valves: long-term outcome. Pediatr Surg Int 27:1027–1035

Capitanucci ML, Marciano A, Zaccara A, La Sala E, Mosiello G, De Gennaro M (2012) Long-term bladder function followup in boys with posterior urethral valves: comparison of noninvasive vs invasive urodynamic studies. J Urol 188:953–957

Chauvin NA, Epelman M, Victoria T, Johnson AM (2012) Complex genitourinary abnormalities on fetal MRI: imaging findings and approach to diagnosis. AJR 199:W222–W231

Chowdhury DN, Kabiraj SP, Kundu AK (2002) Posterior urethral valves: transperineal ultrasonography: a diagnostic tool, pictorial essay. Indian J Urol 18:140–142

Cobb BG, Wolf JA Jr, Ansell JS (1968) Congenital stricture of the proximal urethral bulb. J Urol 99:629–631

Cohen HL, Susman M, Haller JO, Glassberg KI, Shapiro MA, Zinn DL (1994) Posterior urethral valve: transperineal US for imaging and diagnosis in male infants. Radiology 192:261–264

Cohen HL, Zinn HL, Patel A, Zinn DL, Haller JO (1998) Prenatal sonographic diagnosis of posterior urethral valves: identification of valves and thickening of the posterior wall. J Clin Ultrasound 26:366–370

Cooper CS (2009) Diagnosis and management of vesicoureteral reflux in children. Nat Rev Urol 6:481–489

Dacher JN (2008) Abnormalities of the lower urinary tract and urachus. In: Fotter R (ed) Pediatric uroradiology, 2nd edn. Springer, Berlin, pp 123–135

De Bruyn R (2010) The renal tract. In: De Bruyn R (ed) Pediatric ultrasound, how, why and when, 2nd edn. Churchill Livingstone, London, pp 41–114

De Gennaro M, Capitanucci ML, Mosiello G, Caione P, Silveri M (2000) The changing urodynamic pattern from infancy to adolescence in boys with posterior urethral valves. Br J Urol 85:1104–1108

Dewan P (2014) Posterior urethral obstruction: COPUM. Bangladesh J Endosurg 2:29–32

Dewan PA, Goh DG (1995) Variable expression of the congenital obstructive posterior urethral membrane. Urology 45:507–509

Dewan PA, Zappala SM, Ransley PG, Duffy PG (1992) Endoscopic reappraisal of the morphology of congenital obstruction of the posterior urethra. Br J Urol 70:439–444

Dewan PA, Keenan RJ, Morris LL, LeQuesne GW (1994) Congenital urethral obstruction: cobb's collar or

prolapsed congenital obstructive posterior urethral membrane (COPUM). Br J Urol 73:91–95
Dinneen MD, Duffy PG (1996) Posterior urethral valves. Br J Urol 78:275–281
Dinneen MD, Duffy PG, Barratt TM, Ransley PG (1995) Persistent polyuria after posterior urethral valves. Br J Urol 75:236–240
Drozdz D, Drozdz M, Gretz N, Möhring K, Mehls O, Schärer K (1998) Progression to endstage renal disease in children with posterior urethral valves. Pediatr Nephrol 12:630–636
Dyer RB, Chen MY, Zagoria RJ (2004) Classic signs in uroradiology1. RadioGraphics 24:S247–S280
Elder JS, Shapio E (2005) Posterior urethral valves. In: Ashcraft KW, Holcomb GW, Murphy JP (eds) Pediatric surgery, 4th edn. Elsevier Saunders, Philadelphia, pp 781–792
Farhat W, McLorie G, Capolicchio G, Khoury A, Bagli D, Merguerian PA (2000) Outcomes of primary valve ablation versus urinary tract diversion in patients with posterior urethral valves. Urology 56:653–657
Gharpure V (2013) Posterior urethral valves in neonate. J Neonatal Surg 2:37
Good CD, Vinnicombe SJ, Minty IL, King AD, Mather SJ, Dicks-Mireaux C (1996) Posterior urethral valves in male infants and newborns: detection with US of the urethra before and during voiding. Radiology 198:387–391
Hassan JM, Pope JC, Brock JW, Adams MC (2003) Vesicoureteral reflux in patients with posterior urethral valves. J Urol 170:1677–1680
Heikkila J (2015) Posterior urethral valves. Early features and renal outcome. Academic dissertation to be publicly discussed, with permission of the Medical Faculty of the University of Helsinki, in Lecture Hall 2, Haartman Institute, Helsinki on 4th December 2015, at 12 noon. ISBN 978-951-51-1634-5 (pdf) Unigrafia Helsinki 2015
Heikkilä J, Taskinen S, Toppari J, Rintala R (2008) Posterior urethral valves are often associated with cryptorchidism and inguinal hernias. J Urol 180:715–717
Heikkila J, Rintala R, Taskinen S (2009) Vesicoureteral reflux in conjunction with posterior urethral valves. J Urol 182:1555–1560
Hodges SJ, Patel B, McLorie G, Atala A (2009) Posterior urethral valves. Sci World J 9:1119–1126
Holmdahl G, Sillén U, Hanson E, Hermansson G, Hjälmås K (1996) Bladder dysfunction in boys with posterior urethral valves before and after puberty. J Urol 155:694–698
Hoover DL, Duckett JW Jr (1982) Posterior urethral valves, unilateral reflux and renal dysplasia: a syndrome. J Urol 128:994–997
Hutton KAR (2004) Management of posterior urethral valves. Curr Paediatr 14:568–575
Johnston JH (1979) Vesicoureteric reflux with urethral valves. Br J Urol 51:100–104
Johnston JH, Kulatilake AE (1971) The sequelae of posterior urethral valves. Br J Urol 43:743–748
Kajbafzadeh AM (2005) Congenital urethral anomalies in boys. Part I: posterior urethral valves. Urol J 2:59–78
Kanaroglou N, Braga LHP, Massaro P, Lau K, DeMaria J (2011) Lower abdominal mass in a 16-year old adolescent: an unusual presentation of posterior urethral valves. Can Urol Assoc J 5:e1–e3
Keihani S, Kajbafzadeh AM (2015) Concomitant anterior and posterior urethral valves: a comprehensive review of literature. Urology 86:151–157
Kibar Y, Ashley RA, Roth CC, Frimberger D, Kropp BP (2011) Timing of posterior urethral valve diagnosis and its impact on clinical outcome. J Pediatr Urol 7:538–542
Koff SA, Mutabagani KH, Jayanthi VR (2002) The valve bladder syndrome: pathophysiology and treatment with nocturnal bladder emptying. J Urol 167:291–297
Krishnan A, De Souza A, Konijeti R, Baskin LS (2006) The anatomy and embryology of posterior urethral valves. J Urol 175:1214–1220
Kulshrestha R (2006) Posterior urethral valves. In: Kulshrestha R (ed) Common problems in pediatric surgery, 2nd edn. CBS, New Delhi, pp 322–328
Kwong J, Lorenzo AJ, DeMaria J, Braga LHP (2013) Bilateral epididymitis in a child with undiagnosed posterior urethral valves. Urology 82:225–227
Langenbeck CJM (1802) Memorie sur la lithomie
Lissauer D, Rachel KM, Mark DK (2007) Fetal lower urinary tract obstruction. Semin Fetal Neonatal Med 12:464–470
Lowsley OS (1914) Congenital malformation of the posterior urethra. Ann Surg 60:733
Lukong CS, Ameh EA, Mshelbwala PM, Jabo BA, Gomna A, Anumah MA, Nmadu PT, Mfuh AY (2014) Role of vesicostomy in the management of posterior urethral valve in Sub-Saharan Africa. J Pediatr Urol 10:62–66
Mahadik P, Vaddi SP, Godala CM, Sambar V, Kulkarni S, Gundala R (2012) Posterior urethral valve: delayed presentation in adolescence. Int Neurourol J 16:149–152
Malin G, Tonks AM, Morris RK, Gardosi J, Kilby MD (2012) Congenital lower urinary tract obstruction: a population-based epidemiological study. BJOG 119:1455–1464
Martín C, Darnell A, Durán C, Bermúdez P, Mellado F, Rigol S (2004) Magnetic resonance imaging of the intrauterine fetal genitourinary tract: normal anatomy and pathology. Abdom Imaging 29:286–302
Miller RS (2015) Fetal lower urinary tract obstruction: an update. Open Urol Nephrol J 8(Suppl 3: M6):124–135
Mirshemirani A, Khaleghnejad A, Rouzrokh M, Sadeghi A, Mohajerzadeh L, Sharifian M (2013) Posterior urethral valves; a single center experience. Iran J Pediatr 23:531–535
Mitchell ME (1982) Persistent ureteral dilatation following valve resection. Dial Pediatr Urol 5:8–11
Morgagni JB (1769) Seats and causes of diseases investigated by anatomy. In: Millar A, Cadell T (eds) Five books, containing a great variety of dissections with remarks to which are added very accurate and copi-

ous indexes of the principal things and names therein contained. Johnson and Payne, London, pp 540–556

Morris RK, Malin GL, Quinlan-Jones E, Middleton LJ, Hemming K, Burke D, Daniels JP, Khan K, Deeks J, Kilby M (2013) Percutaneous vesicoamniotic shunting versus conservative management for fetal lower urinary tract obstruction (PLUTO: a randomised trial). Lancet 382:1496–1506

Murphy JP, Gatti JM (2006) Abnormalities of the urethra, penis, and scrotum. In: Grosfeld JL, O'Neill JA, Fonkalsrud EW, Coran AG (eds) Pediatric surgery, 6th edn. Mosby Elsevier, Philadelphia, pp 1899–1910

Naghizadeh S, Kefi A, Dogan HS, Burgu B, Akdogan B, Tekgul S (2005) Effectiveness of oral desmopressin therapy in posterior urethral valve patients with polyuria and detection of factors affecting the therapy. Eur Urol 48:819–825

Narasimhan KL, Mahajan JK, Kaur B, Mittal BR, Bhattacharya A (2005) The vesicoureteral reflux dysplasia syndrome in patients with posterior urethral valves. J Urol 174:1433–1435

Nasir AA, Ameh EA, Abdur-Rahman LO, Adeniran JO, Abraham MK (2011) Posterior urethral valve. World J Pediatr 7:205–216

Pagano MJ, van Batavia JP, Casale P (2015) Laser ablation in the management of obstructive uropathy in neonates. J Endourol 29:611–614

Palminteri E, Maruccia S, Berdondini E, Di Pierro GB, Sedigh O, Rocco F (2014) Male urethral strictures: a national survey among urologists in Italy. Urology 83:477–484

Parkhouse HF, Barrat TM, Dillon MJ, Duffy PG, Fay J, Ransley PG, Woodhouse CR, Williams DI (1988) Long-term outcome of boys with posterior urethral valves. Br J Urol 62:59–62

Payabvash S, Kajbafzadeh AM, Saeedi P, Sadeghi Z, Elmi A, Mehdizadeh M (2008) Application of magnetic resonance urography in diagnosis of congenital urogenital anomalies in children. Pediatr Surg Int 24 979–986

Piçarro C, Lazaroni TL, Botelho Filho FM, Miranda ME, Magalhães Victoria A, Cruzeiro PC (2016) Association of posterior urethral valve with congenital lobar emphysema: a case report. Pediatr Urol Case Rep 3:84–88

Podesta M, Ruarte AC, Gargiulo C, Medel R, Castera R, Herrera M, Levitt SB, Weiser A (2002) Bladder function associated with posterior urethral valves after primary valve ablation or proximal urinary diversion in children and adolescents. J Urol 168(4 Pt 2) 1830–1835

Poutamo J, Vanninen R, Partanen K, Kirkinen P (2000) Diagnosing fetal urinary tract abnormalities: benefits of MRI compared to ultrasonography. Acta Obstet Gynecol Scand 79:65–71

Priti K, Rao KLN, Menon P, Singh N, Mittal BR, Bhattacharya A, Mitra SK (2004) Posterior urethral valves: incidence and progress of vesicoureteric reflux after primary fulguration. Pediatr Surg Int 20:136–139

Quintero RA (2005) Fetal obstructive uropathy. Clin Obstet Gynecol 48:923–941

Rittenberg MH, Hulbert WC, Snyder HM, Duckett JW (1988) Protective factor in posterior urethral valves. J Urol 140:993–996

Robertson WB, Hayes JA (1969) Congenital diaphragmatic obstruction of the male posterior urethra. Br J Urol 41:592–598

Ruano R (2011) Fetal surgery for severe lower urinary tract obstruction. Prenat Diagn 31:667–674

Sarhan OM, El-Ghoneimi AA, Helmy TE, Dawaba MS, Ghali AM, Ibrahiem E-HI (2011) Posterior urethral valves: multivariate analysis of factors affecting the final renal outcome. J Urol 185:2491–2496

Schoellnast H, Lindbichler F, Riccabona M (2004) Sonographic diagnosis of urethral anomalies in infants. Value of perineal sonography. J Ultrasound Med 23:769–776

Silveri M, Adorisio O, Pane A, Zaccara A, Bilancioni E, Giorlandino C, De Gennaro M (2002) Fetal monolateral urinoma and neonatal renal function outcome in posterior urethral valves obstruction: the pop-off mechanism. Pediatr Med Chir 24:394–396

Stephens FD (1955) Urethral obstruction in childhood; the use of urethrography in diagnosis. ANZ J Surg 25:89–109

Stephens FD (1983) Congenital intrinsic lesion of the posterior urethra. In: Stephens FD (ed) Congenital malformations of the urinary tract. Praeger, New York, pp 95–125

Steven LC, Desai D (2016) Posterior urethral valves. In: Wilcox D, Godbole P, Cooper C (eds) Pediatric urology book on line. http://www.pediatricurologybook.com

Sudarsanan B, Nasir ARA, Puzhankara R, Kedari PM, Unnithan GR, Damisetti KRP (2009) Posterior urethral valves: a single center experience over 7 years. Pediatr Surg Int 25:283–287

Taskinen S, Heikkilä J, Rintala R (2012) Effects of posterior urethral valves on long-term bladder and sexual function. Nat Rev Urol 2:699–706

Thakkar D, Deshpande AV, Kennedy SE (2014) Epidemiology and demography of recently diagnosed cases of posterior urethral valves. Pediatr Res 76:560–563

Thomas J (2010) Etiopathogenesis and management bladder dysfunction in patients with posterior urethral valves. Indian J Urol 26:480–489

Tolmatschew N (1870) A case of semilunaren flaps of the urethra and vergrosserter vesicula prostatice. Archiv Path Anat 11:348

Tran CN, Reichard CA, McMahon D, Rhee A (2014) Anterior urethral valve associated with posterior urethral valves: report of 2 cases and review of the literature. Urology 84:469–471

Vanderheyden T, Kumar S, Fisk NM (2003) Fetal renal impairment. Semin Neonatol 8:279–289

Velpeau AALM (1832) Urètre et Prostate. Traite Complet Anat Chirurgicale 2:247

Verma A (2008) Posterior urethral valves. In: Verma A (ed) Spotters in pediatrics. Jaypee, New Delhi, pp 121–122
Warner JN, Malkawi I, Dhradkeh M, Joshi PM, Kulkarni SB, Lazzeri M, Barbagli G, Mori R, Angermeier KW, Storme O, Campos R, Velarde L, Gomez RG, Han JS, Gonzalez CM, Martinho D, Sandul A, Martins FE, Santucci RA (2015) A multi-institutional evaluation of the management and outcomes of long-segment urethral strictures. Urology 85:1483–1487
Watson EM (1921) The structural basis for congenital valve formation in the posterior urethra. J Urol 7:371
Williams DI, Eckstein HB (1965) Obstructive valves in the posterior urethra. J Urol 93:236–246
Yohannes P, Hanna M (2002) Current trends in the management of posterior urethral valves in the pediatric population. Urology 60:947–953
Young HH, Frontz WA, Baldwin JC (1919) Congenital obstruction of the posterior urethra. J Urol 3:289–365
Zaccara A, Giorlandino C, Mobili L, Brizzi C, Bilancioni E, Capolupo I, Capitanucci ML, DE Gennaro M (2005) Amniotic fluid index and fetal bladder outlet obstruction. Do we really need more? J Urol 174:1657–1660
Ziylan O, Oktar T, Ander H, Korgali E, Rodoplu H, Kocak T (2006) The impact of late presentation of posterior urethral valves on bladder and renal function. J Urol 175:1894–1897

Acute Scrotum

20

Riccardo Palliola, Antonio Alessandro Pallottino, Michele Galluzzo, Stefania Ianniello, Viola Valentini, and Margherita Trinci

20.1 Introduction

Acute scrotum is a group of clinical manifestations with the same clinical presentation characterized by testicular pain, frequently associated with swelling and inflammation signs; these signs could extend to the near anatomic regions.

Acute scrotum is the second cause of emergency for surgery in pediatric age, preceded only by acute abdomen, which could take to risk of life threatening the patient. Acute scrotum could have important consequences for the fertility and for reproductive organs (DaJusta et al. 2013; Mansbach et al. 2005).

It's important to make diagnosis rapidly to recognize lesions to send to the surgeon and which one needs only medical treatment. After the clinical exam, in an emergency department for a child with a clinical presentation of acute scrotum that has been made by the pediatrician, generally a sonography (best exam in scrotum/testicular evaluation) or a surgery evaluation follows. Pain, redness, and swelling are always typical in lots of scrotal pathologies; the only objective examination, often difficult because of the intensive pain of the patient to the palpation, is not exhaustive and makes it difficult to take a rapid decision.

Ultrasound (US) with color Doppler (CDUS) is the gold standard for the diagnosis, because it gives anatomic and physiologic (vascularization) information about the testicle (Feld and Middleton 1992), and it allows to choose rapidly the correct way to treat the patient (Muttarak 2003); MRI could be used as second-level exam when ultrasound is not exhaustive or when there are conditions as hematomas or bulks; CT is used only in the suspect of the presence of gas in the scrotal tissues, when X-ray exam is not sufficient (Pavlica and Barozzi 2001).

20.2 US Technique

A linear probe (high frequency, generally between 7.5 and 14 Hz) has to be used for a correct examination of the scrotum. The exam is mandatory for both the testicles, beginning from the not hurting one and continuing to the hurting one, using both baseline ultrasound and color Doppler. Both longitudinal and axial scans for imaging acquisition have been made, with a comparison between sonographic and vascular structure of both testicles.

Color Doppler setting has been optimized on the not hurting testicle, identifying the most lower flow with an acceptable signal/noise ratio, the most lower wall kernel, and the most lower

R. Palliola (✉) • A.A. Pallottino • M. Galluzzo
S. Ianniello • V. Valentini • M. Trinci
Department of Emergency Radiology, S. Camillo Hospital, Rome, Italy
e-mail: palliola@libero.it

V. Miele, M. Trinci (eds.), *Imaging Non-traumatic Abdominal Emergencies in Pediatric Patients*,
DOI 10.1007/978-3-319-41866-7_20

speed (PRF between 500 and 1,000 Hz; wall kernel between 25 and 50 Hz; priority filters between 70 % and 90 %; color persistence on) (Aso et al. 2005).

Power Doppler could be useful because it uses information based on red blood cells contained in the volume sample analyzed (analysis of the range of the signal) and it's from three to five times more sensible to lower flows rather than color Doppler (Rubin et al. 1994; Weskott 1997). In the last years, there are studies on the possible applications of contrast-enhanced ultrasound (CEUS), which uses contrast agent which consists of microbubbles containing an inert gas that resonates at low acoustic pressure ranges emitting a specific signal which is possible to detect with a specific software (Moschouris et al. 2009; Farina et al. 2015). CEUS is generally used for the abdominal blunt trauma, as in adults, as in pediatric patients (Pinto et al. 2014, 2015; Sessa et al. 2015; Menichini et al. 2015; Miele et al. 2015, 2016a, b, c); the role in the scrotal pathologies is not yet recognized, but there are many studies about it. Substantially, CEUS could help scrotal imaging because it images blood flow better than color and power Doppler, by overcoming the limitations of these techniques (Cokkinos et al. 2013), being more accurate in the final diagnosis compared to US, and potentially reducing the need for further imaging (Valentino et al. 2011; Miele and Di Giampietro 2014).

20.3 Anatomy

The morphology of the testicles appears oval in longitudinal scans and round in axial ones. Dimensions of the testicles are different and depend from parameters as the age and the build of the patients. The normal dimensions in the adult patients are 35–50 mm for length, 25–35 mm for width, and 15–25 mm for thickness. It's easy to calculate testicular volume as an ellipsoid (*length* × *width* × *thickness* × *0.52*). Testicular volume is considered normal between 12 and 25 ml, at inferior limits of the normal values between 10 and 12 ml, and hypotrophic under 10 ml (Fig. 20.1 and Table 20.1).

Didymal structures are characterized by echoes purposes and thickened with homogeneous pattern.

Sonographic structure changes by age; in the newborn and in the child, the didymus presents itself as hypoechoic, it becomes moderately echoic with sexual maturity, and it tends to become moderately hypoechoic and atrophic in

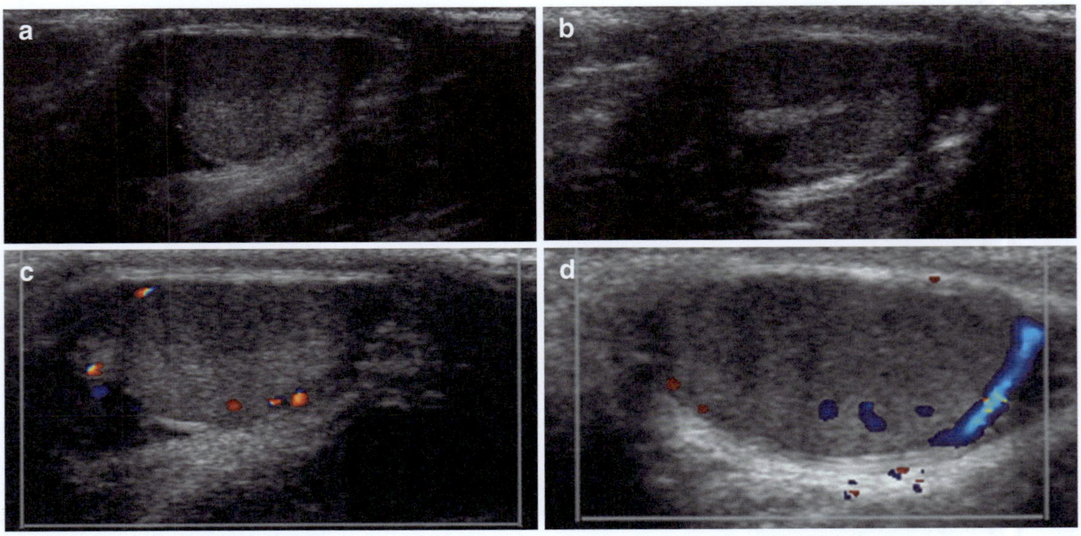

Fig. 20.1 Ultrasound longitudinal scans show the normal anatomy of a 9-year-old child. Note the normal echogenicity of the testis with its Doppler signal (**a**, **c**, **d**), the slight hyperechogenicity of the mediastinum testis (**b**)

Table 20.1 Normal dimensional values depending from the age of the patients

Age	Medium width for length (cm)
Newborn	1.9×1.2
From 1 to 9 years	1.5×1
10	1.8×1.1
11	2×1.4
12	2.3×1.8
13	3×2.3
14	3.4×2.5
15	3.6×2.6
16	3.8×2.7
17	4×2.8

old patients. The thin hyperechoic line recognizable to the didymal surface is the tunica albuginea covered by the visceral vaginal tunic.

Structural homogeneity of didymus is interrupted only from the following structures:

- In the back superior part, there is the mediastinum testis, which is a prolongation of albuginea tunic that appears as a triangular-shaped hyperechoic area which extends into the testis parenchyma (Bree and Hoang 1996).
- Less frequently (35 %) there are transtesticular vessels, which are hypoanechoic linear or curved, easily recognizable to color Doppler examination.
- Rarely (18 % of normal testis) there is "rete testis" which is a hypoanechoic area near mediastinum, or a little serpiginous avascular area, sometimes associated with cysts or spermatocele.

In newborns and children testicle's vascularization, it's difficult to see and always difficult to demonstrate in cryptorchidism. In pediatric age, flow demonstration presents percentage variable between 32 % and 46 % for a testis volume less than 1 ml. The epididymis localizes in medial back posterior position respect of didymus and has elongated shape, and it's formed from three parts: the head (max thickening 10–12 mm in adults), body (max thickening 2–5 mm in adults), and queue (thickening less than 5 mm). The queue continues with deferent duct recognizable to the level of spermatic cord; this last structure has ribbon shape and high echogenicity, broken from vascular striations.

In normal epididymis, because of little dimensions of vessels, flow is not appreciated. Scrotal bag, made from some anatomic structures stratified, presents itself as a structure with average echogenicity, with multiple layers, not clearly differentiable between them.

20.4 Extra and Intravaginal Torsion

Torsion represents the most frequent cause of scrotal pain in the acute scrotum with edema in child and youth people, with high frequency between 15 and 25 years (average 13 years).

The torsion is the most frequent cause; then there are hydatid appendix and inflammatory causes which are most probable than a torsion with the growth.

Diagnosis for testicular torsion has to be quickly to make surgery rapidly (6 h from the onset of symptoms) with the objective of testicle saving; in other causes of scrotal pain, medical therapies are enough. The testicle more frequently affected by torsion is the left; rarely (2 %) the illness is bilateral. Diagnosis is clinical for typical funicular torsion (more frequent), and sonography has to be made only in doubt cases; if sonography is not exhaustive, surgery exploration has to be made.

In 10 % of cases, sonographic diagnosis of torsion isn't reliable because the absence of Doppler signal could be consequent to a disorderly regulation of the sonographic machine or for the difficulty in recognizing blood flow, in the small caliber vessels of the children.

20.5 Extravaginal Torsion

Extravaginal or funicular torsion is caused by a poor fixation of the spermatic cord in the inguinal channel; the scrotal content of the side interested by rotation at the high of inguinal external ring goes to extensive ischemic process. In 21 % of cases, torsions are bilateral and synchronous and

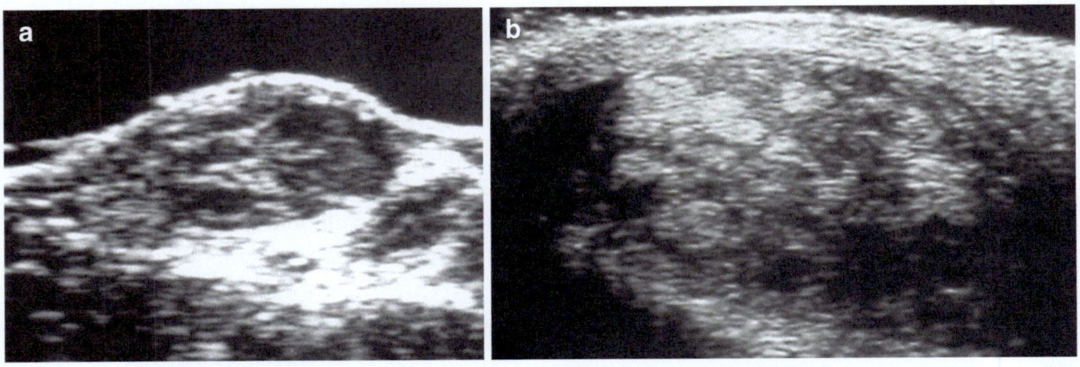

Fig. 20.2 Ultrasound longitudinal scan shows a case of extravaginal torsion in a newborn with a palpable mass above the scrotum without evident acute pain; (a,b) the testicle is swollen and heterogeneouss

only in 3 % of cases bilateral metachronous. This kind of torsion occurs during the intrauterine growth, before the closing of peritoneal-vaginal duct; rarely it occurs in the postnatal period (Kyriazis et al. 2008) (Fig. 20.2).

In the first case, testicle is necrotic at birth, so there aren't possibilities of recovery of surgery that instead there are in cases of extravaginal postnatal birth. In the newborn suckling, the clinical presentation is often sneaky, and the sonographic presentation doesn't differ from the intravaginal torsion, and it changes during the various moments of observation from a red-violaceous swelling to a hard and not transilluminable one.

Testicle generally appears bigger at sonographic exam, with inhomogeneous sonographic structure, with hypoanechoic peripheral or central zones, and without blood signal at color Doppler exam; hydrocele and thickening from the same part are always associated. Testicular swelling in newborn has to be differentiated from meconium peritonitis, from peritoneal hemorrhages with patency of peritoneal-vaginal duct, from testicular tumors, and from incarcerated hernia (which needs surgery). Scrotal hematoma is a rare cause following an adrenal neonatal bleeding: from the adrenal space, the blood goes down opening a way in the peritoneal fat and arriving in the groin region determining an infarction of superficial structure of the scrotal bag (Miele et al. 1997, 2000).

20.6 Intravaginal Torsion

The testis and spermatic cord rotates of 360° determining a stop of the blood flow, before venous, then the arterial one. Intravaginal torsion is frequently on the age around puberty, and it's favored from an abnormal growth of the vaginal tunic. This anomaly, defined also "bell clapper deformity," is characterized from a big vaginal tunic, which involves completely the testis and the epididymis, and it's fixed to the scrotum with a thin meso (Dogra 2003). In these cases the testis presents an abnormal motility at clinical exam, which favors the development of a torsion. Rarely the torsion can accomplish between the testis and the epididymis head, when a long and weary mesorchium is present.

Intense exercise, cold, and injury can be causes of a torsion for the sharp contraction of the cremaster.

When there is high clinical suspicion of testicular torsion, surgery is mandatory because of the possibility of saving the testis is higher than shorter is the time between the onset of symptoms and surgical detorsion (Kapoor 2008). Percentage of therapeutic success is 85–97 % for surgery in the first 6 h, gets off to 55–85 % between 6 and 12 h, and is lesser than 10 % between 12 and 24 h from the onset of symptoms. After 24 h the testis damage is not reversible, and necrotic testis has been removed, because if it's left in, it could have a

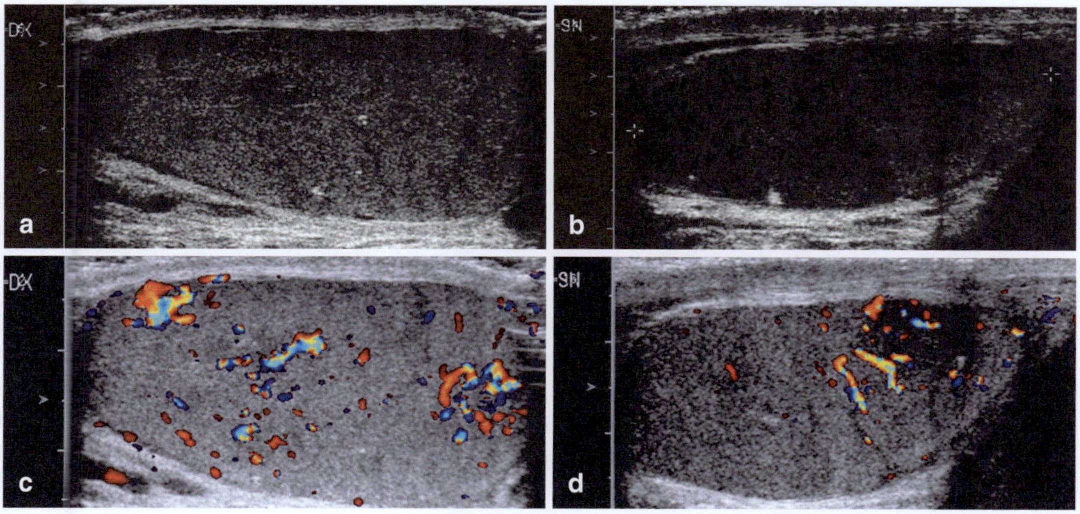

Fig. 20.3 Ultrasound longitudinal scans (A,B) in teenager with pain in the left testicle due to partial left testis torsion. Note the similar echogenicity of the two testicles but the difference of vascularization, normal color Doppler signal (c), and reduced color Doppler signal (d)

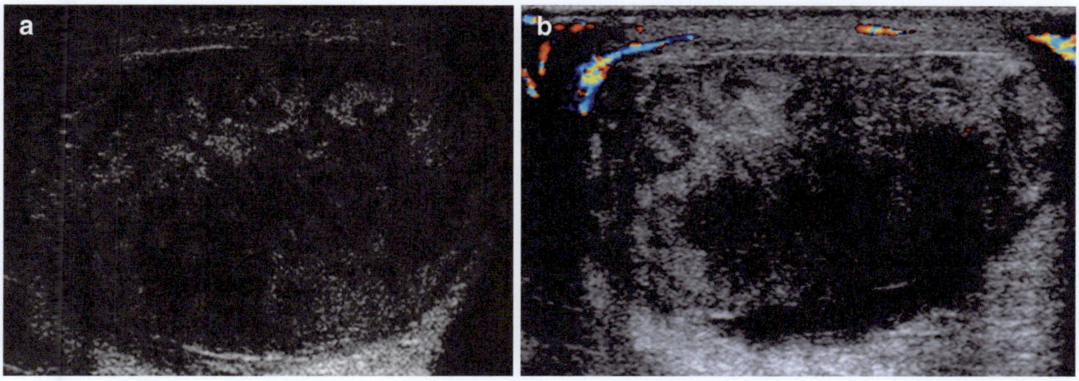

Fig. 20.4 Ultrasound longitudinal scan shows a case of extravaginal torsion in a newborn with a palpable mass above the scrotum without evident acute pain; (a,b) the testicle is swollen and heterogeneous

negative action on the same testis for the production of sperm antibodies (little recognized thesis).

Ischemic damage starts after 4 h for Sertoli cells and after 10 h for Leydig ones. Symptomatology is sudden pain to the emiscrotum interested which radiates to the groin, toward the cord or the inferior quadrants; it associates vomiting, nausea, and shock and can be fever or low-grade fever. Objective exam shows bigger, swelling, flushed, and edematous scrotum, reactive hydrocele, and strained, hardened testis without cremasteric reflex. Imaging methods are generally used in doubt cases or to confirm a torsion after 24 h (Figs. 20.3 and 20.4).

The vascularization of the testis can be difficult to evaluate in pediatric population, in which the flow is slow and near the limit of the instrumental capacity. In these patients it's necessary to set color Doppler parameters to slower speed as possible; power Doppler in these cases is useful for the major sensitivity to slower flows (Ragheb and Higgins 2002).

In the incomplete torsion, it can be also useful to evaluate Doppler spectrum for the flow. A reduced flow in the sore testicle can be the only sign of a torsion. In the intravaginal torsion, sonographic B-mode scene varies in relationship to the moment in which the exam has been made. In the first 2–4 h, changes cannot be appreciated in the normal echogenicity of the testis, while, after 4–6 h the testis appears bigger, with globous appearance and hypoechoic for edema.

With the passage of the hours, echostructure modifies itself and becomes very inhomogeneous for edema, bleeding, ischemia, and necrosis (Lee et al. 1996; Lin et al. 2007).

The enlargement of the testis can interest also the epididymis, which appears hypoechoic and can simulate an epididymitis. The study of cord region is very suggestive, because it allows to see the spiral appearance of the cord structures twisted. It's possible to visualize turns of the coils of the spermatic cord, "the spiral node," with axial and longitudinal scans, at external orifice of inguinal channel, vascularized (incomplete torsion) or not vascularized (complete torsion) at color Doppler. Modest reactive hydrohematocele wrap available and minimum edematous thickness of the scrotal bag are associated.

When the necrotic testis isn't removed, it goes to a progressive dimensional reduction and appears diffusely hypoechoic. Color and power Doppler present advantages with respect to the sonography with gray scale, and they permit a rapid and specific diagnosis because they point out perfusion variation from the first moment. Using high-frequency probe and a correct choice of speed scale, it's possible to see the absence of flow in the symptomatic testis, while the contralateral testis flow is normal and the absence of hypervascularization of the epididymis is observed. In the partial or incomplete torsion, with rotation less of 360°, there's a complete stop of venous circulation, while it's possible to identify an arterial flow. In these cases spectral analysis demonstrates an increase of resistance index, until to an inversion of diastolic flow, which is not detectable only with the color investigation. After 24 h from the starting of the torsion, a clear accentuation of the flow in the soft tissues around the testis is observed, to refer a vascular reactive answer (Lee et al. 1996) with the development of a collateral circle around the testis starting from the cremaster vessels. Hypervascularization on a single testis can depend from a spontaneous or intermittent detorsion, so it can be observed, immediately after the detorsion, a diffuse hyperemia which simulates a phlogosis; it's associated with a reduction of IR, without hypervascularization of the epididymis. It's possible groping a manual derotation if the age is higher than 12 years. Diagnosis of spontaneous detorsion or intermittent torsion has to be suspected when there is an association between acute scrotal pain which resolves spontaneously associated with a unilateral hypoperfusion of the testis visible at color Doppler exam or scintigraphy. Diagnosis of spontaneous detorsion is important, because affected patients have to have surgery though it's not a surgical emergency.

The involved testicle has to be fixed with three stitches (possibly not absorbable) to the dartos (orchidopexy); it's necessary always to explore and fix the contralateral testis. Can we be foreseeing the torsion? The answer is yes if in anamnesis there is remarkable mobility of the testis with particular evidence of cremaster reflex and the precedent suspect of incomplete downhill of the testis. It's necessary to remember that testis pain episodes with spontaneous resolution have to be considered as "intermittent testis torsion"; in 18–36% of cases incomplete torsions precede complete ones.

Particular attention has to be placed for the undescended testicles, because testicular torsion on cryptorchid is a devious form which presents itself as abdominal pain, in particular in iliac fossa. The discovery of an empty bag at clinical exam needs deepening with sonography which shows a bulk in inguinal region, painful at passage of the probe, so a surgical exploration is necessary, to make a detorsion, lowering the testicle and fixing it in a single surgical intervention.

20.7 Testicular Appendix Torsion

Hydatids are present in the major part of the males (diameter 3–5 mm) and represent the residual of Mullerian structures (embryonal tissue which generates female genital organs), which in males don't have any particular function.

20.7.1 Hydatid Scheme

The appendix more frequently involved in the genesis of acute scrotum is the hydatid or Morgagni testis which, turning on the stalk, goes toward ischemic hemorrhage necrosis, determining an inflammatory reaction associated with pain and swelling. Higher incedence is observed in children between 6 and 12 years and is favorite to the pedicle aspect of this appendix. Certainty diagnosis can be posed only at the onset of the torsion, when a blue and pain body is palpable at the superior pole of the testis (blue dot sign). In the hours successive to the clinical onset (Cohen et al. 1992), swelling and thickness of scrotal tissues make taking a differential diagnosis virtually impossible with other responsible pathologies of acute scrotum. The therapy of Morgagni's hydatid torsion, caused from necrosis of appendix which once detached generates a mobile endoscrotal body which with time tends to calcify (scrotolith), is generally conservative with rest, and anti-inflammatory drugs. are enough to determine the disappearance of the pathology, caused from necrosis of appendix which once detached generates a mobile endoscrotal body which with time tends to calcify (scrotolith).

Rarely surgery is used, which consists of its removal, only in the cases of very high pain and in the doubt of a torsion of the testis. Acute torsion of testis' appendix generates a clinical situation similar to the complete torsion of the testis, but the pain is generally localized to the superior pole of the testis and anyway less intense respect to that of funicular torsion.

Sonographic aspect changes in relationship to observation timing (Fig. 20.5). A round formation hyperechoic which is a sign of recent bleeding will be found in the testicular epididymis in the early phases, often associated with a modest reactive hydrocele. With the passage of the time, the hemoglobin absorption will lead to a hypoechoic formation with branches which reduces its volume up to break away and calcify. To color-power Doppler testicular flow, it is preserved, while you may sometimes encounter an increased flow around the appendix twisted at the level of the upper pole (Berman et al. 1996) with the appendix that appears without Doppler signal. It can also be observed a moderate hyperemia of

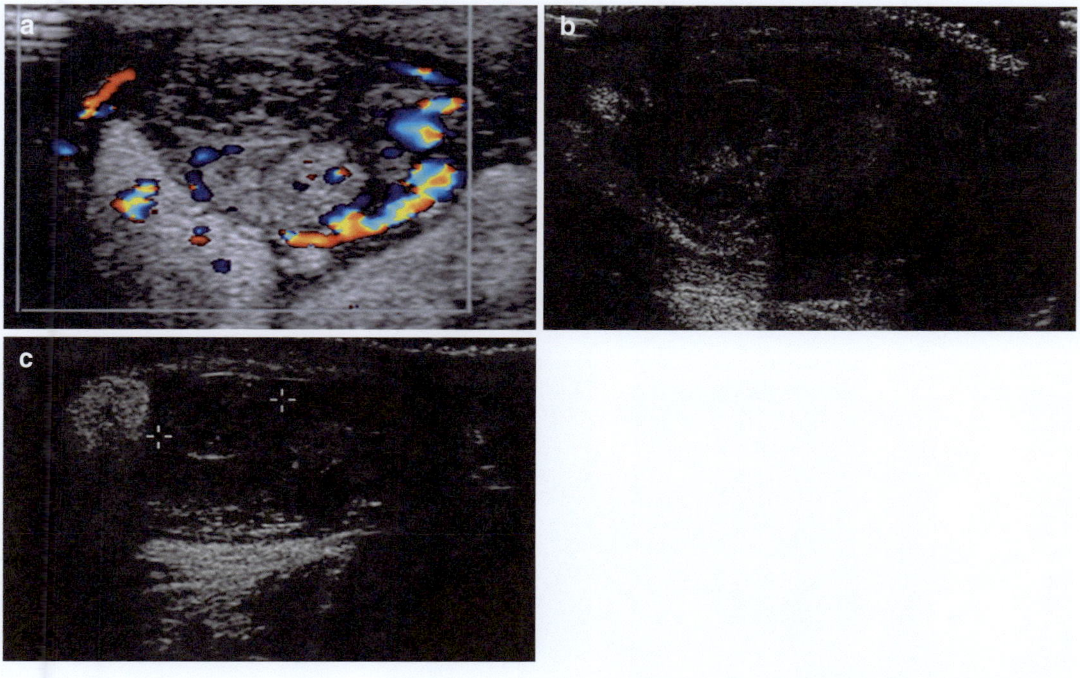

Fig. 20.5 Ultrasound scans in case of hydatid torsion show the enlargement and inhomogeneity of the hydatid that is slightly hyperechoic in the early phases of torsion; note the absence of color Doppler signal (**a**); the hydatid reduces itself with the passage of the time (mildly stage **b** and late stage **c**)

tissues around the testis affected by the twist on the side interested. The differential diagnosis with testicular inflammation epididymis is often very difficult and has to be made on the basis of clinical and laboratory findings.

20.8 Epididymitis and Orchitis

Inflammatory processes affect principally the epididymis and are the most common cause of acute scrotum in the adult; after 30 years the torsion is little frequent. Inflammation processes are very rare in the age around the puberty, because inflammation is caused from germs which transmit toward sexual activity and the onset of an orchi-epididymitis is generally favored from congenital causes predisposing as stenosis outlets or ectopic ureters. Inflammation is generally localized to the epididymis, and only in 20 % of cases is associated with orchitis; unilateral or bilateral isolated orchitis, without epididymis involvement, is always viral and from hematogeneous origin.

Acute epididymitis develops in 24–48 h, generally unilateral, and presents itself with pain (shows itself when scrotum is relieved to symphysis pubis as "positive Prehn sign"), swelling with eventual erythema, and scrotal edema; the presence in 90 % of cases of hydrocele transilluminable in modest quantity; fever (50 %), dysuria (50 %), and pyuria (if well wanted in 90 % of cases).

At sonographic exam the epididymis appears as augmented in size with reduced echogenicity (hypoechogenicity) for edema, and the presence of hemorrhagic hyperechoic or necrotic hypoechoic areas is possible; hydrocele can be associated. The color Doppler shows increased vascularity usually very lively in epididymis which instead normally does not show vascular signals (Figs. 20.6 and 20.7). The inflammation sometimes affects the testicle, who appears as enlarged and hypoechoic with increased color signal and sometimes is associated with a funiculitis (thickness greater than 10 mm) with abnormal enhancement of vascular structures and mild enlargement of deferens ducts (greater than 3 mm).

Semiotics ultrasound is completed with the involvement of the sheaths that appear irregularly thickened. The spectral analysis shows a reduction of the resistance below the value of 0.7 in the epididymis arteries and 0.5 in the arteries of the testis (Suzer et al. 1997). The abscess formation after an acute inflammation is rare and may result in focal orchitis with ultrasound examination characterized by a liquid or markedly hypoechoic lesion with ill-defined limits, surrounded by a hypoechoic halo (hard to differentiate from neoplasia), or a widespread orchitis with increased volume of didymus with echostructure hypoechoic "loose knit" and small areolas hypoanechoic to report to abscesses (Fig. 20.8). The color Doppler shows perilesional hyperemia with no flow within the abscess cavity. The primitive orchitis is rare and, in the great majority of cases of viral origin, associated with the mumps.

Rare complication of the epididymis-orchitis is the widespread testicular ischemia, which results from compression of testicular vessels from the epididymis and spermatic cord magnified. The ultrasound shows a testicle increased in

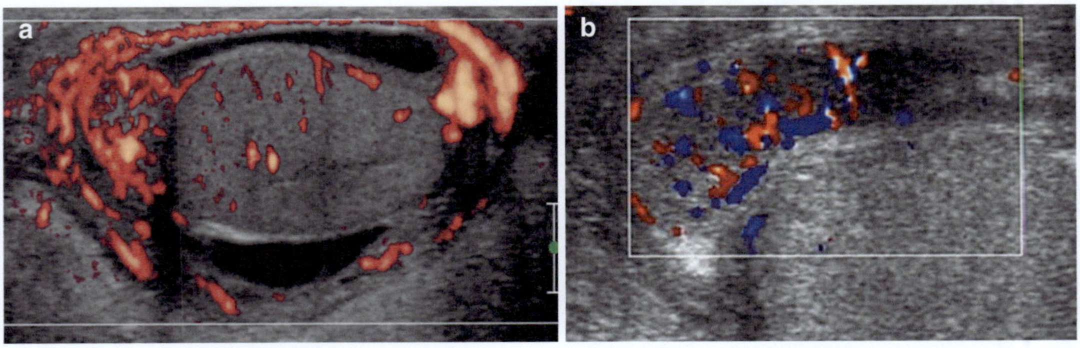

Fig. 20.6 (**a**, **b**) Ultrasound scan in case of epididymitis show the increased vascularity at the level of the epididymis, seen as a higher color Doppler signal. Hydrocele is associated (**a**)

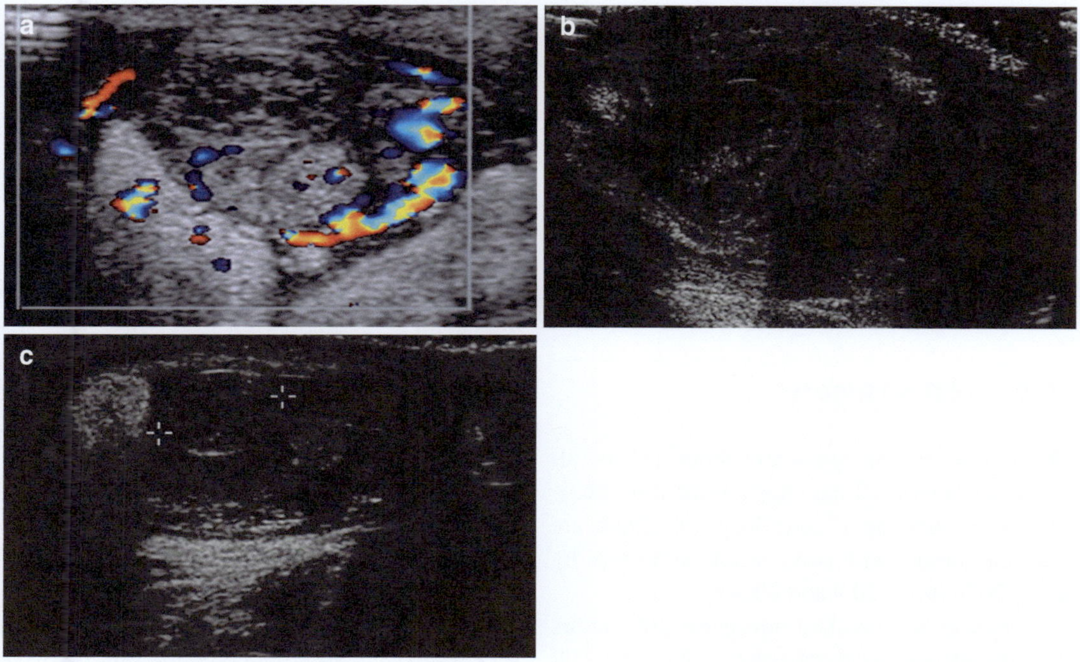

Fig. 20.7 Ultrasound scans in a child with testicular pain and swelling due to an orchiepididymitis. Note the diffuse hyperemia of the testis with a large and widespread Doppler signal (**a**, **b**); note the normal Doppler signal of the contralateral testis (**c**)

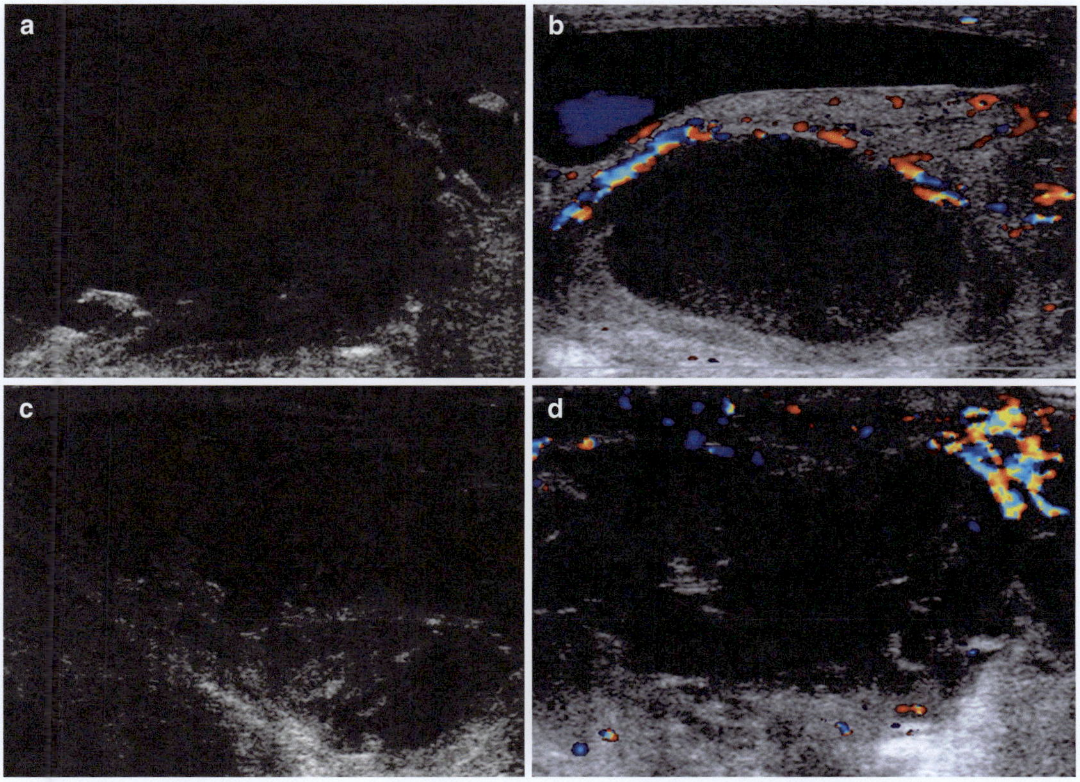

Fig. 20.8 Ultrasound scans in case of testicular abscess; note the widespread lack of homogeneity with anechoic gaps both the testicle that hydrocele (**a**, **c**) and peripheral Doppler signal (**b**, **d**)

size and uneven, with the reduction or absence of arterial flow to the color Doppler, which is opposed to the hyperemia of adjacent epididymis. The spectral analysis shows reduction or reversal of diastolic flow with increased resistive index, expression of obstructed venous outflow. These findings at eco-Doppler exam allow to differentiate the postischemia inflammation from torsion inflammation (Suzer et al. 1997).

20.9 Testis Tumors

The tumors of the testis are about 1 % of all malignant tumors of man and are the most common form between 15 and 34 years. These are treatable tumors with survival rate at 5 years by about 90 % (Figs. 20.9 and 20.10).

They can be classified into germ cell tumors (95 %) and non-germinal (rare). The germ cell tumors include seminoma (50 %) and nonseminomatous (50 %) as the embryonic carcinoma, choriocarcinoma, and teratoma. The non-germ cell tumors, the most rare, are mainly represented by lymphomas and leukemias, in most cases insurgents elsewhere. Usually the patient arrives in the emergency room for the presence of a nonpainful scrotal mass.

However, in 10 % of cases, patients present themselves with acute scrotal symptoms due to hemorrhage or intratumoral necrosis, mimicking a testicular torsion or epididymis-orchitis (Pavlica and Barozzi 2001).

At the US testicular cancer appears as a focal lesion, hypoechoic, with vascularization usually increased, to highlight even with power Doppler. Hemorrhagic or necrotic areas are appreciable with focal alterations of the echogenicity of the mass. The lack of a swelling of the epididymis, thickening of the scrotal sac, and the absence of significant hydrocele must place a testicular cancer suspicion and allows you to discard the hypothesis vascular or inflammatory.

In the suspicion of cancer, it's necessary to research lumbar-aortic lymphadenopathy and seek a possible simultaneous bilateral involvement. In lymphomas and leukemias, the testicular involvement is manifested by an increase of considerable volume and with a hypervascularity similar to that observed in acute orchitis. In children is relatively frequent; the onset of attitude to infiltrative tumors spread through-

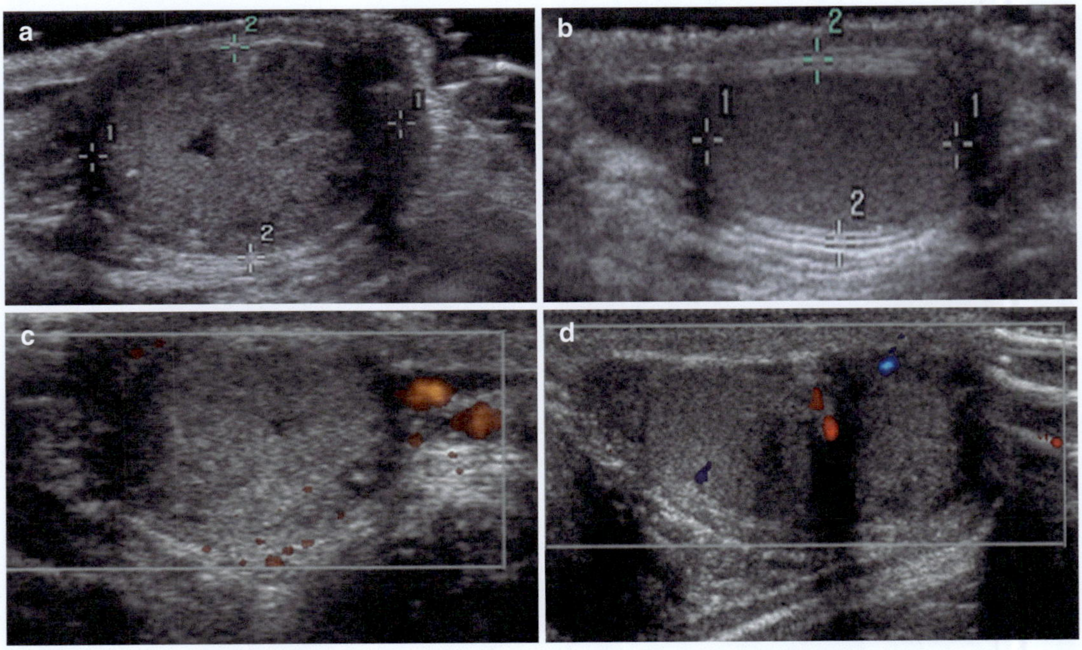

Fig. 20.9 Ultrasound scans in case of testicular tumor; note the oval capsular slightly hyperechogenous formation, with lack of homogeneity and without Doppler flow (**a**, **c**); note the normal testis with normal Doppler signal (**b**, **d**) in a patient 6 years old

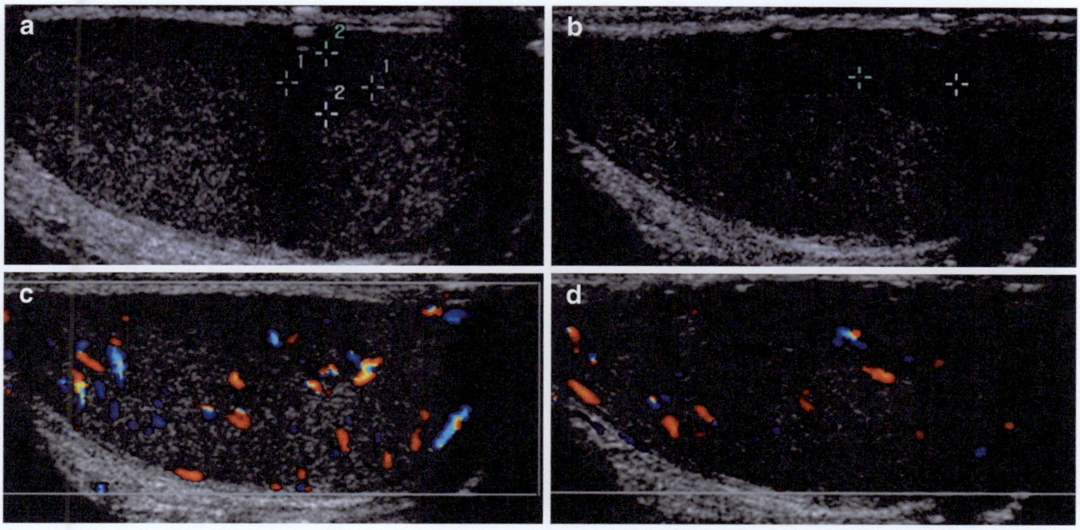

Fig. 20.10 Ultrasound scans in child with incidental finding of testicular tumor. Note the hypoechoic focal lesions (a,b), with irregular shape and margins, peripheral increased color Doppler signal (c,d); sonography shows only two lesions, while a third one was seen in the next MR exam

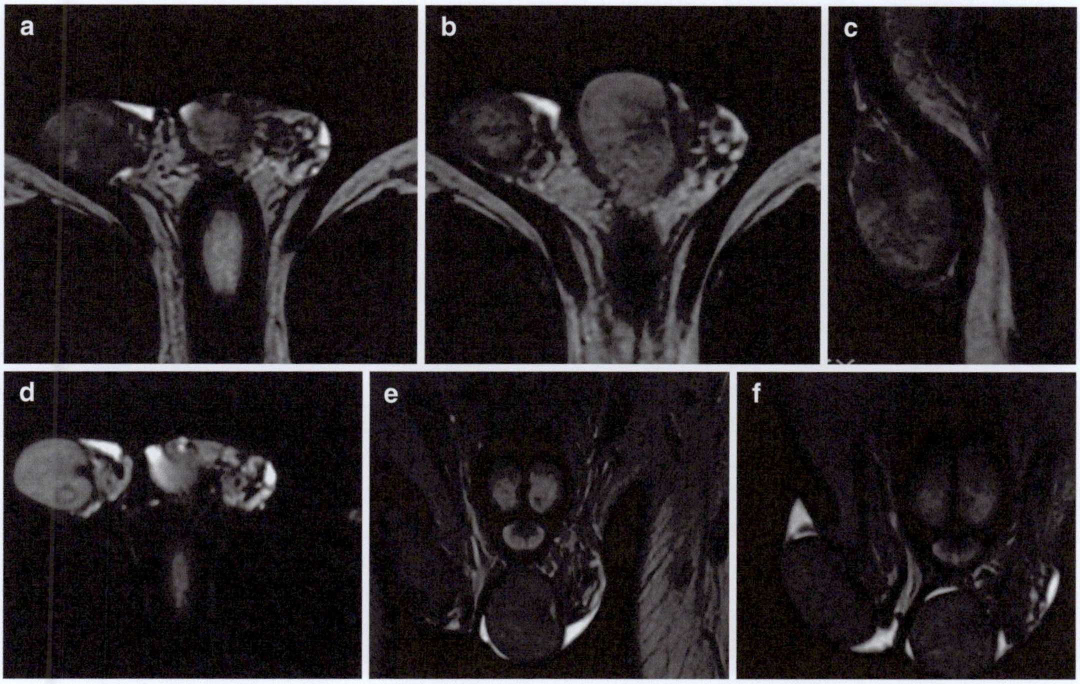

Fig. 20.11 MR in case of testicular tumor (same patient of Fig. 20.10); note the multifocal ovalar circumscribed (A,B,D) little formations of the right testis. The MR exam in coronal (E,F) and sagittal planes (C) shows three lesions, one more than sonography (seen at Fig. 20.10)

out the testicular parenchyma, without deformation of didymus; in the absence of clear data of clinical inflammation, the increasing of vascularization with abnormal spatial distribution of vessels can orient the diagnosis. The reflected ultrasound suspicion of a testicular tumor may require integration with diagnostic MRI (Figs. 20.11 and 20.12).

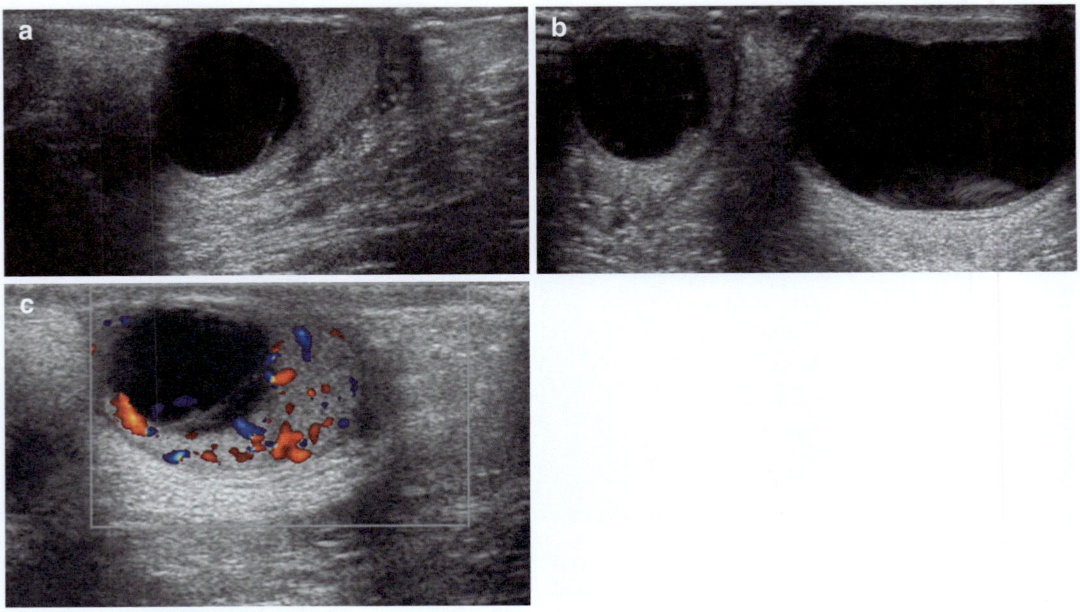

Fig. 20.12 Ultrasound scans in case of testicular tumor; note the ovalar cystic bilateral mass (**a**, **b**), anechogenous and with inner hyperechoic solid septa and only peripheral color Doppler signal (**c**)

20.10 Testicular Trauma

Since the difficulty in collecting the medical history in newborns and children and the impossibility to be aware about any traumas, it is essential to know this pathology in order to establish properly differential diagnosis.

Severe testicular trauma is relatively uncommon (1.5 % of polytrauma), because the testes are protected from injuries by the anterior arch of the pelvis and the root of the thighs. Most of severe traumas are due to work or road accidents, sport injuries, and direct perineal trauma with scrotum compression against the pubis bone.

On the contrary, mild testicular traumas are highly frequent, causing acute and lasting pain. Since clinical examination is often limited by pain and edema, ultrasound examination plays an essential role in establishing the presence of scrotal hematoma, hematocele, testicular hematoma, or testicular rupture (Fig. 20.13).

Prompt testicular rupture diagnosis is important to ensure well-timed surgical treatment with testicular salvage rate of 90 % if it is performed by 72 h. On the other hand, delayed treatment makes orchiectomy unavoidable in about 50 % of cases. Moreover, correct diagnosis prevents atrophy development after testicular injury. This condition may be associated with autoimmune damage of contralateral testes, with subsequent infertility problems. In cases of traumas, ultrasound examination of sheaths shows a hematoma with diffuse and stratified thickening of scrotal layers (greater than 6 mm); hematoma associated with urinoma caused by urethral or bladder rupture will appear stratified as an "onion bulb." Follow-up is recommended until hematocele or hematoma is present because posttraumatic epididymitis or epididymal hematoma may occur (differential diagnosis with preexisting neoplasia).

Surgical treatment of hematocele and intratesticular hematoma without tunica albuginea rupture is usually not indicated unless the uncommon case causes testis compression ischemia. Scrotal hematomas are easy to identify because they cause dissociation of scrotal tunicas and extratesticular fluid collection.

Color Doppler is used to rule out posttraumatic testicular torsion. Hematocele is a blood collection in vaginal cavity and shows different ultrasound features at different examination phases. At early stages, blood usually appears

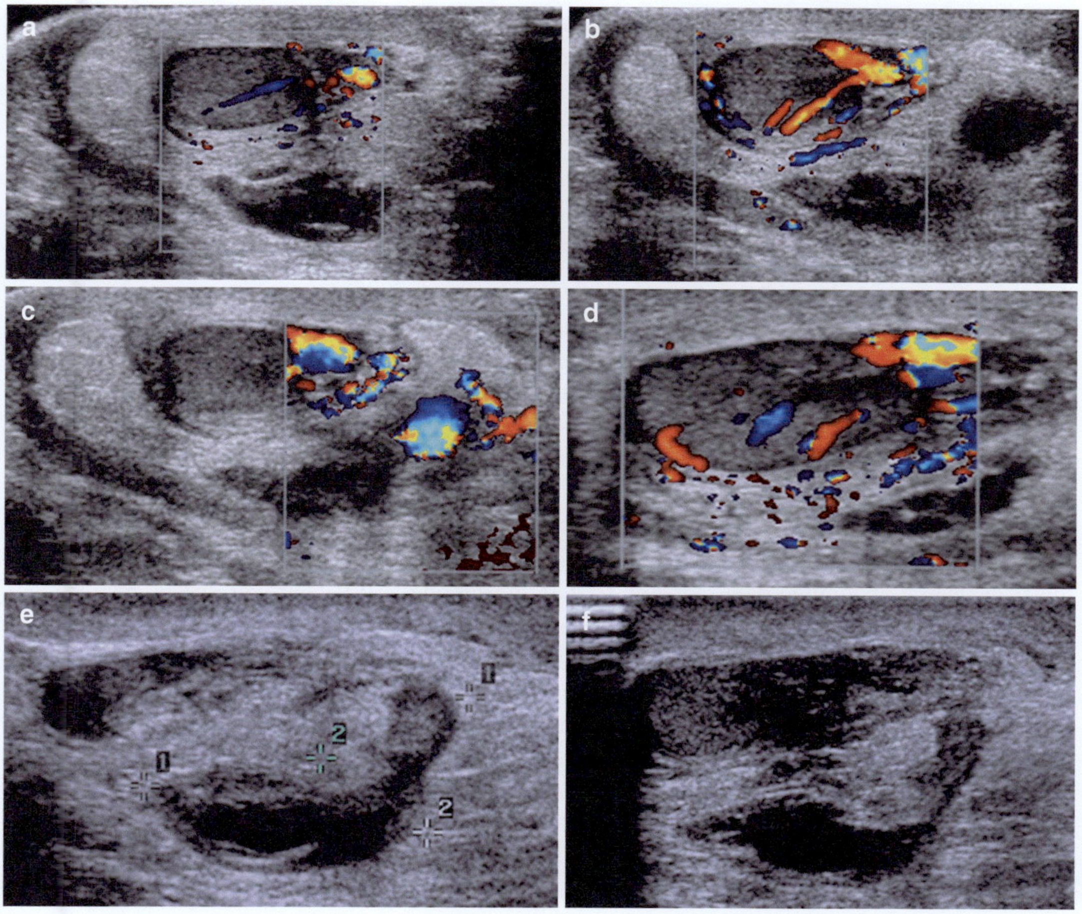

Fig. 20.13 Color doppler scans (A,B,C,D)and ultrasound scans (E,F) in traumatic testicular lesion. Note the hemorrhagic swelling of soft tissues and scrotal bags and the posterior hematoma

hyperechoic, but septa and anechoic areas may develop in following phases. Hematocele may evolve in pyocele. Another complication is dislocation and compression of testes.

Testis damage may be classified into:

- Mild contusion – testicular swelling or interstitial edema which requires conservative treatment.
- Severe contusion – subalbugineal hematoma which may demand drainage.
- Testis and tunica albuginea rupture with blood collection in vaginal cavity (hematocele) which requires prompt surgical treatment.
- Gubernaculum laceration with traumatic testicular dislocation; rare and associated with severe pelvis traumas.
- Posttraumatic testicular torsion.

In mild traumas, testicular swelling and interstitial edema cause global testicular enlargement with hypoechoic appearance "loose knit." Hyperechoic areas may be present in case of intratesticular hematomas and may rapidly become hypoechoic due to clot formation and its retraction. Follow-up is necessary because of similar tumor appearance. Rarely, hypo- or anechoic stripes directed from the testicular convexity to the central zone are detectable caused by testis laceration. Testis rupture is characterized by tunica albuginea interruption with subsequent spreading of testicular tissue in the vaginal cavity or in the scrotal sac. Uncommonly, in extremely severe traumas, shattered parenchyma appears as a complex solid-cystic mass. Color Doppler has a limited role, but may be useful in establishing the degree of viable remnant tissue and to identifying the testicular ischemia caused by compression of spermatic funiculus.

20.11 Extratesticular Causes of Acute Scrotal Pain

Acute scrotal pain may have extratesticular causes due to the innervation shared with other pelvic organs or to the spread of fluid collections through retroperitoneal spaces if process vaginalis is patent.

Most important causes are ureteral colic, rupture and dissection of abdominal aortic aneurysm, strangulated inguinal hernia, or peritonitis. Ureteral colic often manifests as severe flank and lower ipsilateral abdominal pain radiating to the testes, but it may be difficult to diagnose if scrotal pain is the only symptom. Pain is caused by acute ureteral distension due to obstruction that induces hyperperistalsis and smooth muscle spasm. Obstruction usually occurs in the lower ureteral tract and causes irritating bladder symptoms such as a sudden and unstoppable need to urinate (Di Giacomo et al. 2015).

Intrascrotal inguinal hernia sometimes presents as a testicular painful mass. In this case, ultrasound examination can identify the presence of bowel loops in the scrotum, characterized by corpuscular content, excluding a testicular pathology. Uncommonly, hernial sac may contain the appendix, bladder, or colon. If only herniation of the omentum occurs, ultrasound shows a hyperechoic mass without peristalsis.

Acute scrotum may be the clinical presentation of a strangulated hernia. Ultrasound examination shows thickened and hypoechoic bowel loop, without vascularization at color Doppler. The presence of fluid filling the tunica vaginalis and hyperechoic scrotal mass, related to herniated mesenterial fat tissue inflammation, may be observed. In the abdomen, there are associated mechanical bowel obstructions signs and peritoneal effusion.

In perinatal period, meconium periorchitis may occur caused by a mild and self-limiting peritonitis with migration of meconium in the scrotal sac through a patent process vaginalis. In the first month of life, this determines a scrotal mass inducing a foreign body reaction. Ultrasound and radiography may show microcalcifications and soft tissue thickening. Differential diagnosis includes calcified tumors (teratoma, gonadoblastoma) and extravaginalis testicular torsion. Ultrasound may rule out these pathologies demonstrating normal testicular appearance (Aso et al. 2005).

20.11.1 Henoch-Schönlein Purpura

Henoch-Schönlein purpura (HSP) is the most common systemic vasculitis in children. The tetrad of purpura, arthritis, kidney inflammation, and abdominal pain represents the classical manifestation of HSP. However, scrotal involvement, with "acute scrotum" presentation, is observed in 10 % of cases. Histologically, HSP is an arteritis with infarct, hematomas, and aneurysm formation. At ultrasound examination, testes appear enlarged and inhomogeneous, with small, peripheral, hypoechoic foci of infarction, and scrotal layers are thickened and edematous. As shown in literature, the management of "acute scrotum" caused by HSP may be conservative.

20.11.2 Idiopathic Scrotal Edema

Idiopathic scrotal edema (ISE) was first described by Qvist in 1956 and consists of scrotal edema and erythema. Usually ISE is unilateral and is characterized by sudden onset and spontaneous resolution in 1–4 days without effects.

This pathology affects mostly prepubertal children (5–10 years old), and the possible etiology is allergic or hyperergic. In some cases, ISE presents with pain that mimics a testicular torsion, and the diagnosis is made excluding other conditions, since there are no positive laboratory findings. Ultrasound examination shows scrotal wall thickness (sometimes with stratified appearance) without hydrocele or pathologic testis features (Aso et al. 2005). At color Doppler exam, the typical appearance is with the "fountain sign," with color Doppler signal that shows as a fountain (Fig. 20.14).

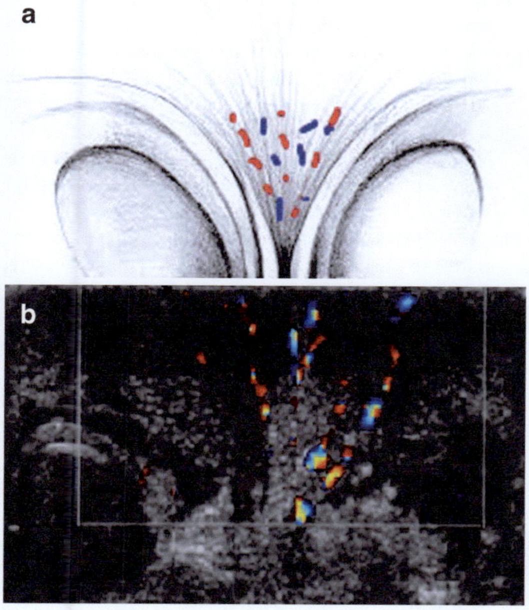

Fig. 20.14 Ultrasound scans in case of idiopathic scrotal edema. Note the scrotal thickness without hydrocele and the color Doppler aspect as a fountain (fountain sign)

20.12 Fournier's Gangrene

Fournier's gangrene or necrotizing fasciitis of the scrotum is an acute obliterans endoarteritis of the external pudendal artery caused by anaerobic infection. This results in a thrombosis of the small vessels that induces necrosis of cutaneous, subcutaneous, and fat tissue. Fournier's gangrene is an uncommon disease that may affect both children and newborns, with 66 % of incidence in babies lesser than 3 months old.

The most common microorganism that causes necrotizing fasciitis is *Clostridium perfringens*, although this is usually found in at least one other anaerobic bacteria. The syndrome is mainly mediated by a lecithinase toxin, which destroys red blood cells (causing hemolysis and hematuria) and induces damage to muscles, cellular membranes, and renal tubules. As a result, severe shock may occur leading to death within 6 h if an appropriate treatment is not undertaken.

Fournier's gangrene clinically manifests with scrotal edema and, if not treated, is associated with a 20 % of mortality. Testes, epididymis, and spermatic cord are rarely involved, because the arteritis did not affect the internal spermatic artery.

Ultrasound is especially useful because it allows to demonstrate the thickness of the scrotal layers that also presents inhomogeneity, stratified appearance, and hyperechoic spots due to gas bubbles. X-ray examination may also show air in soft tissues. Hyperemia with vessel dilatation, usually not detectable, may be observed at color Doppler examination; the testes and epididymis are usually regular.

The therapy consists in high-dose intravenous antibiotic treatment and surgical debridement and removal of necrotic tissues.

References

Aso C, Enriquez G, Fitè M, Toran N, Pirò C, Piqueras J, Lucava J (2005) Gray-scale and color Doppler sonography of scrotal disorders in children: an update. Radiographics 25:1197–1214

Berman JM, Beidle TR, Kunberger LE et al (1996) Sonographic evaluation of acute intrascrotal pathology. AJR Am J Roentgenol 166:857–861

Bree RL, Hoang DT (1996) Scrotal ultrasound. Radiol Clin North Am 34:183–205

Cohen HL, Shapiro MA, Haller JO et al (1992) Torsion of the testicular appendage. Sonographic diagnosis. J Ultrasound Med 11:81.83

Cokkinos DD, Antypa E, Kalogeropoulos I, Tomais D, Ismailos E, Matsiras I, Benakis S, Piperopoulos PN (2013) Contrast enhanced ultrasound performed under urgent conditions. Indications, review of the technique, clinical examples and limitations. Insights Imag 4:185–189

DaJusta D, Granberg C, Villanueva C (2013) Contemporary review of testicular torsion: new concepts, emerging technologies and potential therapeutics. J Pediatr Urol 9:723–730

Di Giacomo V, Trinci M, Van der Byl G, Catania VD, Calisti A, Miele V (2015) Ultrasound in newborns and children suffering from nontraumatic acute abdominal pain: imaging with clinical and surgical correlation. J Ultrasound 18:385–393. doi:10.1007/s40477-014-0087-4, Epub 2014 Apr 9

Dogra V (2003) Bell clapper deformity. AJR Am J Roentgenol 180:1176–1177

Farina R, Catalano O, Stavolo C, Sandomenico F, Petrillo L, Romano L (2015) Emergency radiology. Radiol Med 120:73–84

Feld R, Middleton WD (1992) Recent advances in sonography of the testis and scrotum. Radiol Clin North Am 30:1033–1051

Kapoor S (2008) Testicular torsion: a race against time. Int J Clin Pract 62:821–827
Kyriazis ID, Dimopoulos J, Sakellaris G, Waldschmidt J, Charissis G (2008) Extravaginal testicular torsion: a clinical entity with unspecified surgical anatomy. Int Braz J Urol 34:617–626
Lee FT, Winter DB, Madsen FA et al (1996) Conventional color Doppler velocity sonography versus color Doppler energy sonography for the diagnosis of acute experimental torsion of the spermatic cord. AJR Am J Roentgenol 167:785–790
Lin EP, Bhatt S, Rubens DJ et al (2007) Testicular torsion: twists and turns. Semin Ultrasound CT MR 28:317–328
Mansbach JM, Forbes P, Peters C (2005) Testicular torsion and risk factors for orchiectomy. Arch Pediatr Adolesc Med 159:1167–1171
Menichini G, Sessa B, Trinci M, Galluzzo M, Miele V (2015) Accuracy of contrast-enhanced ultrasound in the identification and characterization of traumatic solid organ lesions in children: a retrospective comparison with baseline-US and CE-MDCT. Radiol Med 120:989–1001
Miele V, Di Giampietro I (2014) Diagnostic Imaging in Emergency. Salute e Società, (2EN):127-138. doi:10.3280/SES2014-002010EN
Miele V, Galluzzo M, Patti G, Mazzoni G, Calisti A, Valenti M (1997) Scrotal hematoma due to neonatal adrenal hemorrhage: the value of ultrasonography in avoiding unnecessary surgery. Pediatr Radiol 27:672–674
Miele V, Galluzzo M, Pedicelli C, Adami A, Calisti A (2000) Neonatal adrenal hemorrhage associated with a scrotal hematoma. Radiol Med 99:299–301
Miele V, Di Giampietro I, Ianniello S, Pinto F, Trinci M (2015) Diagnostic imaging in pediatric polytrauma management. Radiol Med 120:33–49
Miele V, Piccolo CL, Sessa B, Trinci M, Galluzzo M (2016a) Comparison between MRI and CEUS in the follow-up of patients with blunt abdominal trauma managed conservatively. Radiol Med 121:27–37
Miele V, Piccolo CL, Galluzzo M, Ianniello S, Sessa B, Trinci M (2016b) Contrast enhanced ultrasound (CEUS) in blunt abdominal trauma. Br J Radiol 89(1061):20150823. doi:10.1259/bjr.20150823Epub2016Jan8
Miele V, Piccolo CL, Trinci M, Galluzzo M, Ianniello S, Brunese L (2016c) Diagnostic imaging of blunt abdominal trauma in pediatric patients. Radiol Med 121:409–430. doi:10.1007/s11547-016-0637-2, Epub 2016 Apr 13
Moschouris H, Stamatiou K, Lampropoulou E, Kalikis D, Matsaidonis D (2009) Imaging of the acute scrotum: is there a place for contrast-enhanced ultrasonography? Int Braz J Urol 35:692–702
Muttarak M (2003) Anatomy and diseases of the scrotum. In: The asian-oceanian textbook of radiology. Produced by TTG Asia Media, Singapore, pp 809–821
Pavlica P, Barozzi L (2001) Imaging of the acute scrotum. Eur Radiol 11:220–228
Pinto F, Miele V, Scaglione M, Pinto A (2014) The use of contrast-enhanced ultrasound in blunt abdominal trauma: advantages and limitations. Acta Radiol 55:776–784
Pinto F, Valentino M, Romanini L, Basilico R, Miele V (2015) The role of CEUS in the assessment haemodinamically stable patients with blunt abdominal trauma. Radiol Med 120:3–11
Ragheb D, Higgins JL Jr (2002) Ultrasonography of the scrotum: technique, anatomy, and pathologic entities. J Ultrasound Med 21:171–185
Rubin JM, Bude RO, Carson PL, Bree RL, Adler RS (1994) Power Doppler US: a potentially useful alternative to mean frequency-based color Doppler US. Radiology 190:853–856
Sessa B, Trinci M, Ianniello S, Menichini G, Galluzzo M, Miele V (2015) Blunt abdominal trauma: role of contrast-enhanced ultrasound in the detection and staging of abdominal traumatic lesions compared with US and CE-MDCT. Radiol Med 120:180–189
Suzer O, Ozcan H, Kupeli S (1997) Color doppler imaging in the diagnosis of the acute scrotum. Eur Urol 32:457–461
Valentino M, Bertolotto M, Derchi L, Bertaccini A, Pavlica P, Martorana G, Barozzi L (2011) Role of contrast enhanced ultrasound in acute scrotal diseases. Eur Radiol 21:1831–1840
Weskott HP (1997) Amplitude Doppler US: slow blood flow detection tested with a flow phantom. Radiology 202:25–130

Part IV

Critical Issues in Pediatric Emergencies

Abdominal Neoplasm: Clinical Onset in Emergency Setting

21

Barbara Sessa, Roberto Castellucci, Antonio Solazzo, Eugenio Rossi, Massimo Zeccolini, and Sandro Sironi

21.1 Introduction

The diagnosis of abdominal neoplasm in children is often delayed because the presenting symptoms tend to be nonspecific and common with the benign conditions.

The most frequent clinical presentation of paediatric abdominal neoplasm is a palpable mass, frequently in an emergency department as the first access.

When a child arrives in emergency department with a palpable abdominal mass, he requires urgent evaluation to determine if this is malignant, if it compresses vital organs or if it represents an internal haemorrhage.

B. Sessa (✉)
Department of Radiology, Papa Giovanni XXIII Hospital, Bergamo, Italy
e-mail: barbara.sessa@tiscali.it

R. Castellucci
Department of Urology, Humanitas Gavazzeni Clinic, Bergamo, Italy

A. Solazzo
Department of Radiology, Bolognini Hospital, Seriate, BG, Italy

E. Rossi • M. Zeccolini
Department of Pediatric Radiology, Pausilipon Oncologic Pediatric Hospital, Naples, Italy

S. Sironi
Department of Radiology, Papa Giovanni XXIII Hospital, Bergamo, Italy

University of Milano Bicocca, Milano, Italy

Other possible clinical presentation in emergency setting of a child with an unknown abdominal tumour is with genitourinary symptom, gastrointestinal symptom, haemorrhage, infection, anaemia, etc.

The history and physical examination, together with the age of the patient and the help of specific laboratory tests and imaging evaluations, can lead to the diagnosis. Diagnostic imaging in emergency (Miele et al. 2006; Miele and Di Giampietro 2014) plays a main role in identifying and characterizing the abdominal mass. Diagnostic techniques include X-ray studies, ultrasound, CT and MRI.

21.2 The Abdominal Physical Examination

The physical examination of the abdomen is performed with the child in supine position. It is important to note the shape of the abdomen and the position of the umbilicus. In case of a palpable mass, the following should be defined: the location, size, shape, texture, mobility and tenderness. It should be classified as solid, cystic or air filled.

A malignant mass is generally described as a non-tender, nonmobile or firm mass.

Abdominal mass is most often found in children less than 5 years of age, generally with a retroperitoneal location. The most common

V. Miele, M. Trinci (eds.), *Imaging Non-traumatic Abdominal Emergencies in Pediatric Patients*, DOI 10.1007/978-3-319-41866-7_21

malignant abdominal tumour in infants is neuroblastoma followed by Wilms tumour. Other abdominal tumours in this age range include hepatoblastoma, germ cell tumours and soft tissue sarcomas (Golden and Feusner 2002).

After 10 years of age, this tumour became less frequent, but sarcomas, germ cell tumours and abdominal lymphomas increase in incidence (Marten and Kirks 1985).

21.3 Clinical Sign or Symptoms Associated

Other general signs and symptoms associated with malignant abdominal mass in a child are increased abdominal girth, pain with movement or palpation, constipation or decreased urination.

Occasionally it should be associated with weight loss, fever or decreased appetite.

Alarm symptoms, anyway common also in most benign conditions, are fever, lymphadenopathy, vomiting, pallor or localized or generalized lymphadenopathy (Fragkandrea et al. 2013).

Specific symptoms may be associated at different types of neoplasm.

Flushing, sweating and irritability may be associated to neuroblastoma because of the production of catecholamines; also an explosive and secretory diarrhoea may be caused by vasoactive intestinal polypeptides also produced by the tumour.

In Wilms tumour, there could also be possible anaemia caused by bleeding that could be profound; local stimulation of renin can result in hypertension.

Genitourinary symptoms may be associated with rhabdomyosarcoma (RMS) of the genitourinary tract; in bladder RMS, gross haematuria and decreased urinary output may be observed, with a possible progression to anuria, consisting of a genitourinary emergency.

Amenorrhoea and vaginal bleeding could be associated with ovarian germ cell tumour. Ovarian torsion or rupture of the mass could be an emergency presentation of an ovarian mass, which requires a prompt intervention.

Primary malignant tumour in children can also present as an emergency of the gastrointestinal tract; for example, acute lymphoblastic leukaemia, Burkitt lymphoma and hamartoma are often the causes of an intussusception in children more than 2 years of age.

Furthermore, many tumours may be associated with congenital anomalies.

21.4 Laboratory Testing

General laboratory studies routinely performed in emergency setting can give important information about the child's general health. They include a complete blood cell count and chemistry panel (electrolytes, liver transaminases, bilirubin, albumin, etc).

Leucocytosis can suggest a diagnosis of infection; pancytopenia can be caused by a malignant process that infiltrates the bone marrow or by an infection that stresses the marrow; anaemia can be a sign of haemorrhage into the tumour or caused by chronic disease. Thrombocytosis is often found in liver tumours. Coagulation tests are important to check the presence of disseminated intravascular coagulopathy or liver dysfunction.

A baseline urinalysis can detect the haematuria or proteinuria which can suggest a primary renal or bladder tumour. In Wilms tumour when haematuria is present, it is usually microscopic.

Other specific laboratory tests can be performed in following the steps to define, together with other elements, the specific histological characterization of the tumour (tumour markers or specific hormones produced by different tumours as neuroblastoma, phaeochromocytoma, germ cell tumours, liver tumours or teratoma).

21.5 Imaging

If an abdominal mass is suspected by a physical examination in a child who arrives in emergency department, the first imaging approach could be the ultrasound examination.

Paediatric ultrasound imaging of the abdomen is a safe, non-invasive, radiation-free, painless test that uses sound waves, particularly valuable for evaluating abdominal, pelvic or scrotal pain in children. It is also easily available in emergency radiological setting and allows a real-time dynamic optimal visualization of the abdomen, especially in children for the characteristics of the child's body. A linear or convex probe with warmed gel may be used on the basis of the size of the baby.

It can provide detailed information about the mass location, dimensions, nature, tissue components, vascularization and relationship with the adjacent organs. With an adequate bladder distension, it is also allowed to detect the pelvic region in children with high resolution.

With the use of colour Doppler technique, it is possible to detect the mass pattern of flow.

Also contrast-enhanced ultrasound (CEUS) with intravenous injection of microbubble contrast agent could be performed in these cases, providing additional information about the enhancement of the mass and the presence of any neoplastic thrombi of the vessels involved. Despite the use of ultrasound contrast agents in children has not been officially approved since these contrast media are not licensed for paediatric use, a large survey study were carried out, which also included the use of product in intravenous route and responses suggest a favourable safety profile of this second-generation ultrasound contrast agents in children (Menichini et al. 2015).

It is already established the use of CEUS in paediatric abdominal traumatic lesions with the proliferation of a lot of studies in literature, but also in paediatric abdominal oncological emergencies, it may have a crescent role (Pinto et al. 2014, 2015; Sessa et al. 2015; Miele et al. 2015, 2016a, b, c).

When an abdominal tumour is confirmed by ultrasound is recommended a total body staging CT to better define the invasion of vessels or vital organs by the lesions and any lymph node or distant metastasis. MDCT optimization is mandatory in children, including justification for scan, patient preparation, technical and scan parameters with the low-dose CT protocols and contrast administration, with parameters of contrast material volume and flow rate depending on the age and the weight of the baby.

In some cases, it can be useful the use of MR for a more accurate detection and follow-up of oncological disease of some districts (i.e. the female pelvis, liver) or better characterization of tissue component of a detected mass; it is a free radiation exam but often requires a pharmacological sedation in children.

MR is also increasingly used in oncological disease in children, also for the introduction of fast sequences, giving very important information also with the use of new functional imaging techniques such as diffusion-weighted imaging.

When is suspected a gastrointestinal obstruction emergency presentation of the mass, it can be helpful a plain abdominal radiograph.

21.6 The Main Childhood Abdominal Malignancies

21.6.1 Neuroblastoma

It is the most common extracranial solid tumour in childhood and the most common malignancy in infants.

It accounts for about 8 % of all cancers diagnosed in children less than 15 years of age and for 15 % of all cancers in children less than 5 years of age (Matthay 1995).

Neuroblastoma arises from neural crest cells and can arise anywhere along the sympathetic chain, but 75 % of the tumours have an abdominal location and 65 % originate from the adrenal glands (Berthold et al. 1996; Calisti et al. 2012).

The clinical and prognostic behaviour of this tumour is not always predictable: it can regress spontaneously or differentiate into a benign tumour in infants, or it can have a rapidly progressive, metastatic and sometimes fatal course in children over 1 year of age. Fifteen percent of all the cancer-related deaths in children are due to neuroblastoma (Kinnier-Wilson and Draper 1974; Black 1998).

It is a solid, retroperitoneal tumour, generally fixed and unilateral, but it may cross the midline. They are lesions biologically active that produce hormones. In 90 % of patients, the tumour excretes high levels of catecholamines and their metabolites (Graham-Pole et al. 1983; Laug et al. 1978).

21.6.1.1 Clinical Presentation

The clinical presentation is related to the production of specific hormones by the tumour, to its location and the extent of disseminated disease.

The catecholamine production can result in flushing, sweating and irritability; they can produce also vasoactive intestinal polypeptides that may cause watery, explosive, secretory diarrhoea.

Most of these tumours arise from the adrenal gland (35 % of cases), 30–35 % in the extra-adrenal retroperitoneum and 20 % in the posterior mediastinum. Less common sites are the neck (1–5 % of cases) and pelvis (2–3 %) (Morris et al. 1995).

A higher incidence of cervical and thoracic primary tumour is depicted in infants with only 25 % with an abdominal location.

Through haematogenous spread it can do metastases to the bone, bone marrow, liver and skin and in the brain and lungs in end-stage disease (Kramer et al. 2001). Only in 3% of patients there is a pulmonary involvement at the diagnosis and it is an extremely poor prognostic indicator (Kammer et al. 2001). Through lymphatic dissemination, it can affect the regional lymph nodes or nodes in other body cavities.

Abdominal distension is the most frequent presenting symptom.

Other signs and symptoms mostly associated with neuroblastoma are malaise, irritability, weight loss, shortness of breath (if it is a large abdominal tumour) and peripheral neurologic deficit (from neural foraminal invasion and nerve compression by tumour).

Other less common presentations include exophthalmos, ecchymoses, Horner's syndrome, back pain weakness, scoliosis, bladder dysfunction and palpable non-tender subcutaneous nodules.

21.6.1.2 Evaluation

Neuroblastoma, together with rhabdomyosarcoma, lymphoma, Ewing's sarcoma and leukaemia, is considered a "small, round, blue cell tumour".

An international neuroblastoma study group established the minimum criteria required to the diagnosis of neuroblastoma: (1) unequivocal pathologic diagnosis by light microscopy of tumour tissue, with or without immunohistology, or increased urine (or serum) catecholamine or metabolites and (2) bone marrow aspirate or biopsy with unequivocal tumour cells and increased urine or serum catecholamines or metabolites (Brodeur et al. 1988).

Urinary levels of homovanillic acid, vanillylmandelic acid, adrenaline, noradrenaline, dopamine and metanephrines are elevated in 90–95 % of patients with neuroblastoma (Graham-Pole et al. 1983; Laug et al. 1978).

Serum markers, although less sensitive and less specific, include ferritin, NSE and lactate dehydrogenase (LDH). The biologic factors used to stratify risks groups include (1) assessment of an oncogene called n-myc, (2) DNA ploidy and (3) specific histologic characteristics. Amplification of the proto-oncogene n-myc located on the short arm of chromosome 2 is associated with advanced stage disease and poor prognosis (Brodeur 1995; Broduer et al. 1994, 1997).

The DNA content (DNA index or DI) refers to ploidy or the chromosome complement in tumour cells. A normal chromosome number in a somatic cell is diploid (1=46 chromosomes), more is hyperdiploid, >1, and less is aneuploid, <1. A DNA index higher than 1 is associated with a favourable outcome, and an index of 1 or lower has a worse outcome (Seeger et al. 1985).

Two histological classification systems are used in the United States to stratify neuroblastic tumours into risk groups: the Pediatric Oncology Group (POG) classification and the Shimada classification (Joshi et al. 1992; Shimada et al. 1999).

The POG system is based on the degree of differentiation of the histologic elements; in particular neuroblastoma contains less than 50 % differentiated elements. It may be further subclassified as undifferentiated, poorly differentiated or differentiating (Joshi et al. 1992).

The Shimada classification is a morphologic characterization system based on the presence or absence of Schwannian stroma, the age of patient,

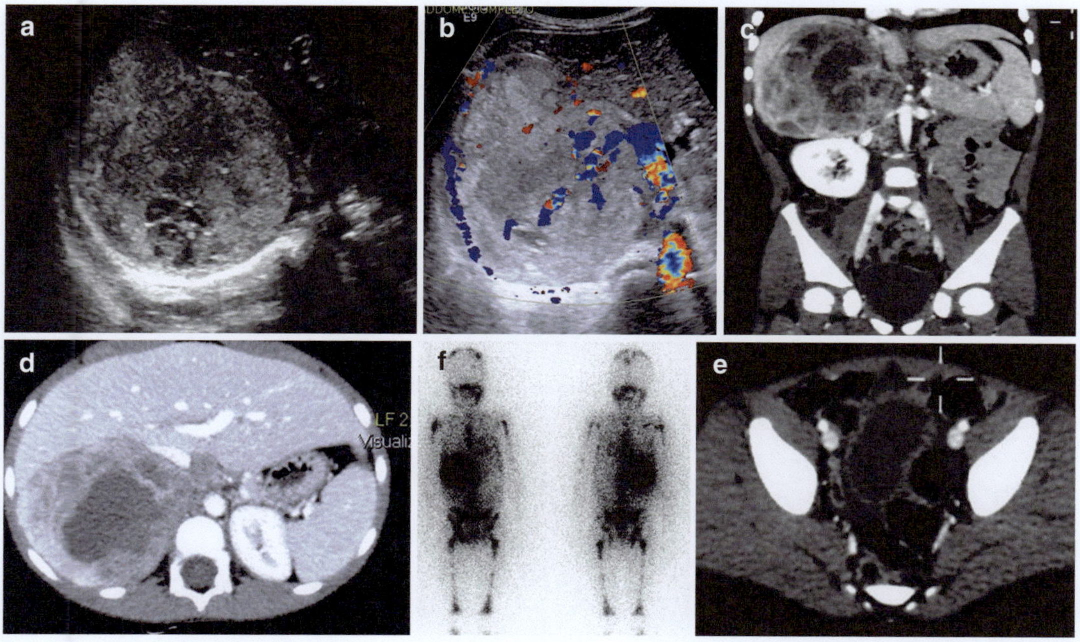

Fig. 21.1 Male, 7 years old. The child went in emergency department with a palpable mass and pain at right abdominal quadrants. Right adrenal gland neuroblastoma was discovered. US (**a**, **b**): a heterogeneously echogenic hypervascular right adrenal mass with hypoechoic area inside was depicted. CT (**c**, MPR coronal reconstruction and **d**): it shows a large and heterogeneous right adrenal mass with low-attenuation areas of necrosis or haemorrhage. Vessels were compressed but not invaded. Celiac lymph node involvement was depicted. The baby has also acute appendicitis (**e**). The 123 MIBG scintigraphy (**f**), in anterior and posterior views, shows the radiopharmaceutical uptake in primary tumours

the degree of cellular maturity and the nuclear characteristic; it is an independent prognostic indicator, either favourable or unfavourable (Shimada et al. 1999).

21.6.1.3 Imaging

Children present in emergency department with abdominal distension, constipation and abdominal pain could be generally investigated with an abdominal plain radiography and/or abdominal ultrasound.

Radiographs may show a posterior retroperitoneal, mediastinal or neck mass. Calcification is evident in at least 30 % of neuroblastoma at plain radiography (Stark et al. 1983).

Posterior mediastinal tumours may cause spreading or erosion of adjacent ribs, and both retroperitoneal and posterior mediastinal tumours may cause pedicle erosion (Miele et al. 1996). Skeletal metastases may also appear as focal lucent (occasionally sclerotic) areas (Stark et al. 1983; Miele et al. 1996; Abramson 1997).

At ultrasonography (US) neuroblastoma is generally heterogeneously echogenic (Figs. 21.1 and 21.2). It should have anechoic areas within the tumour corresponding to haemorrhage or necrosis. Calcifications are common and appear as focal echogenic areas. US may delineate the tumour from adjacent organs such as kidney, making determination of adrenal origin; when the tumour invades the kidney, this is difficult.

US and also CEUS may also evaluate the other organs such as liver, the presence of lymph nodes, the vascular invasion and so on (Stark et al. 1983; Miele et al. 1996; Abramson 1997); however these parameters are better detected by CT or MR imaging.

CT is the most commonly used imaging modality for the assessment of neuroblastoma to evaluate the extent of tumour, organ of origin, regional invasion, vascular encasement, adenopathy and calcification (Figs. 21.1 and 21.3). CT of the chest, abdomen and pelvis is the gold standard technique for all new diagnosed cases.

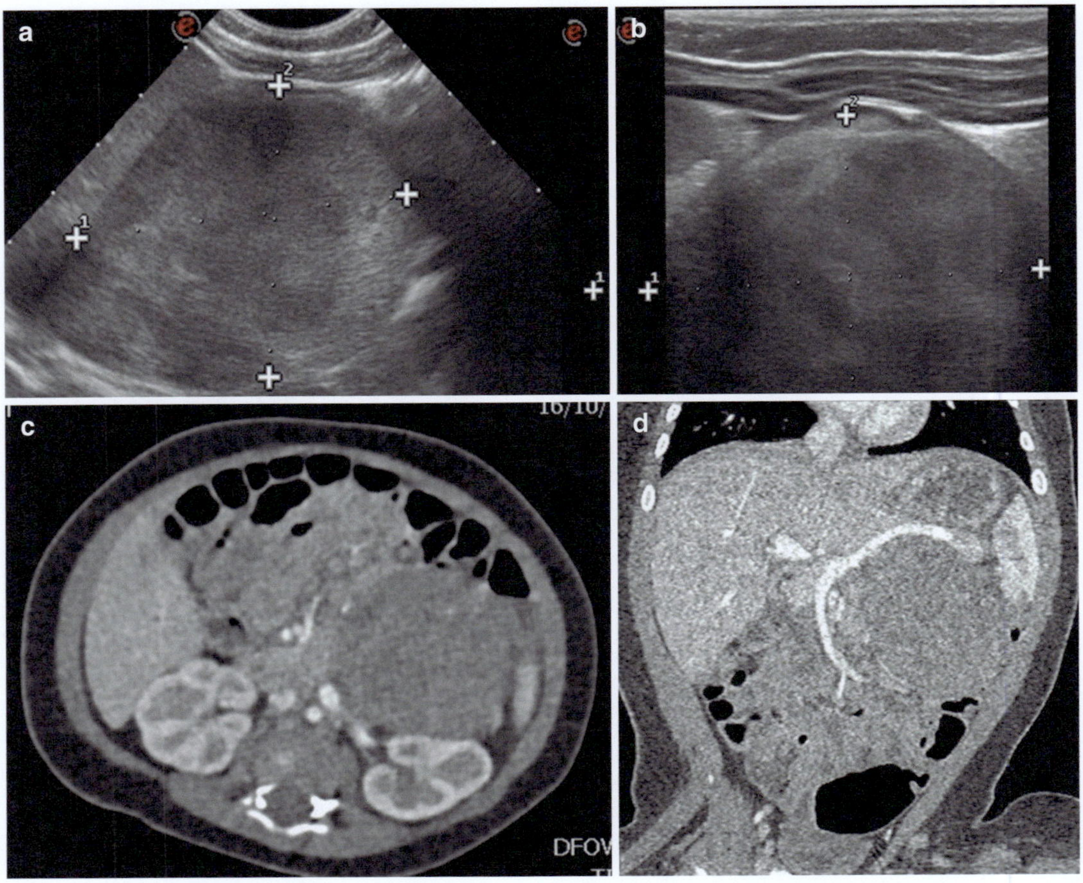

Fig. 21.2 Female, 1 year old. She presents with abdominal distension and nausea. A left adrenal gland neuroblastoma was depicted. US scans (**a**, **b**) show a quite homogeneous echogenic adrenal mass. CT (**c** and d MPR coronal reconstruction): a quite large homogeneous left adrenal mass with regular margins, not invading adjacent structures and vessels

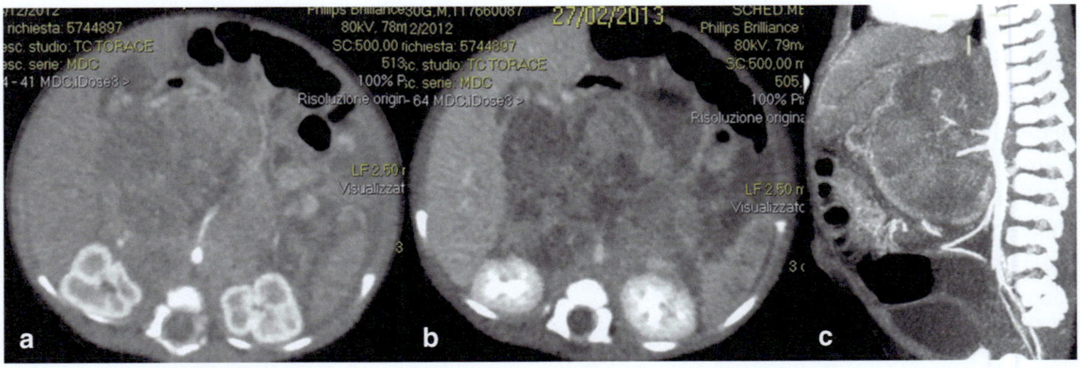

Fig. 21.3 Male, 3 years old with abdominal distension and malaise and weight loss. A retroperitoneal neuroblastoma. MDCT in arterial and venous phase axial scans (**a**, **b**) and MPR sagittal MIP reconstruction (**c**) show a retroperitoneal neuroblastoma. A heterogeneous large retroperitoneal large mass at the level of the celiac vessels was depicted. The sagittal MPR shows the encasement of the celiac tripod and the superior mesenteric artery

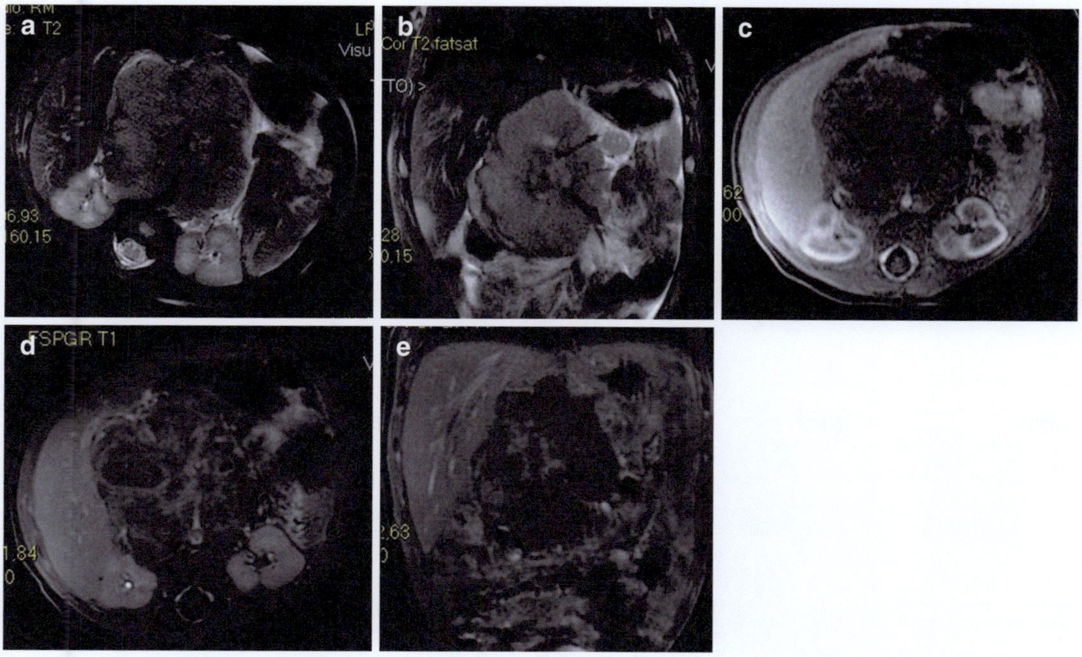

Fig. 21.4 MR exam of the retroperitoneal neuroblastoma at celiac tripod. T2w axial and coronal images (**a**, **b**). T1w axial images in arterial and venous phase and T1w coronal venous phase after Gd administration (**c**–**e**). The large retroperitoneal neuroblastoma at the level of the celiac vessels shows a relatively high signal intensity on T2-weighted images and a heterogeneous CE after Gd injection in arterial and venous phases

Abdominal and pelvic tumours are usually large and heterogeneous; 80–90 % of neuroblastomas demonstrate calcification on CT scans, and low-attenuation areas of necrosis or haemorrhage are frequently depicted (Stark et al. 1983; Miele et al. 1996; Abramson 1997). Small tumours may be homogeneous.

Vascular invasion is rare; vascular encasement and compression of the renal vessels, splenic vein, inferior vena cava, aorta, celiac artery and superior mesenteric artery may occur.

Regional invasion of psoas and paraspinal musculature may also occur, and invasion of the neural foramen into the epidural space is also frequent and better evaluated in MR imaging (Dresler et al. 1979; Aronson et al. 1995; Kenny et al. 1995).

Adenopathy of the renal hilum, porta hepatis and retroperitoneum may be seen.

Metastases at liver or lung are also depicted by CT. Liver metastases may take two forms: diffuse infiltration and focal hypoenhancing masses.

Brain metastases are unusual.

At MR imaging neuroblastoma is typically heterogeneous, variably enhancing and of relatively low signal intensity on T1-weighted images and high signal intensity on T2-weighted images (Fig. 21.4). Calcifications may be difficult to detect at MR imaging. Haemorrhagic areas may be depicted as area of high signal intensity on T1w images and cystic change may appear bright on T2w images (Dietrich et al. 1987).

MR imaging is the better modality to detect intraspinal extension of primary tumour; it should be performed at any patient with a paraspinal tumour (King et al. 1975). MR may also detect marrow disease, appearing as areas of low signal intensity on T1w images and high areas on T2w images (King et al. 1975; Siegel et al. 1986; Couanet et al. 1988).

Finally MR imaging is superior to CT in the detection of diffuse hepatic metastases in infants with stage 4S disease, as areas of high signal intensity on T2w images (Abramson 1997).

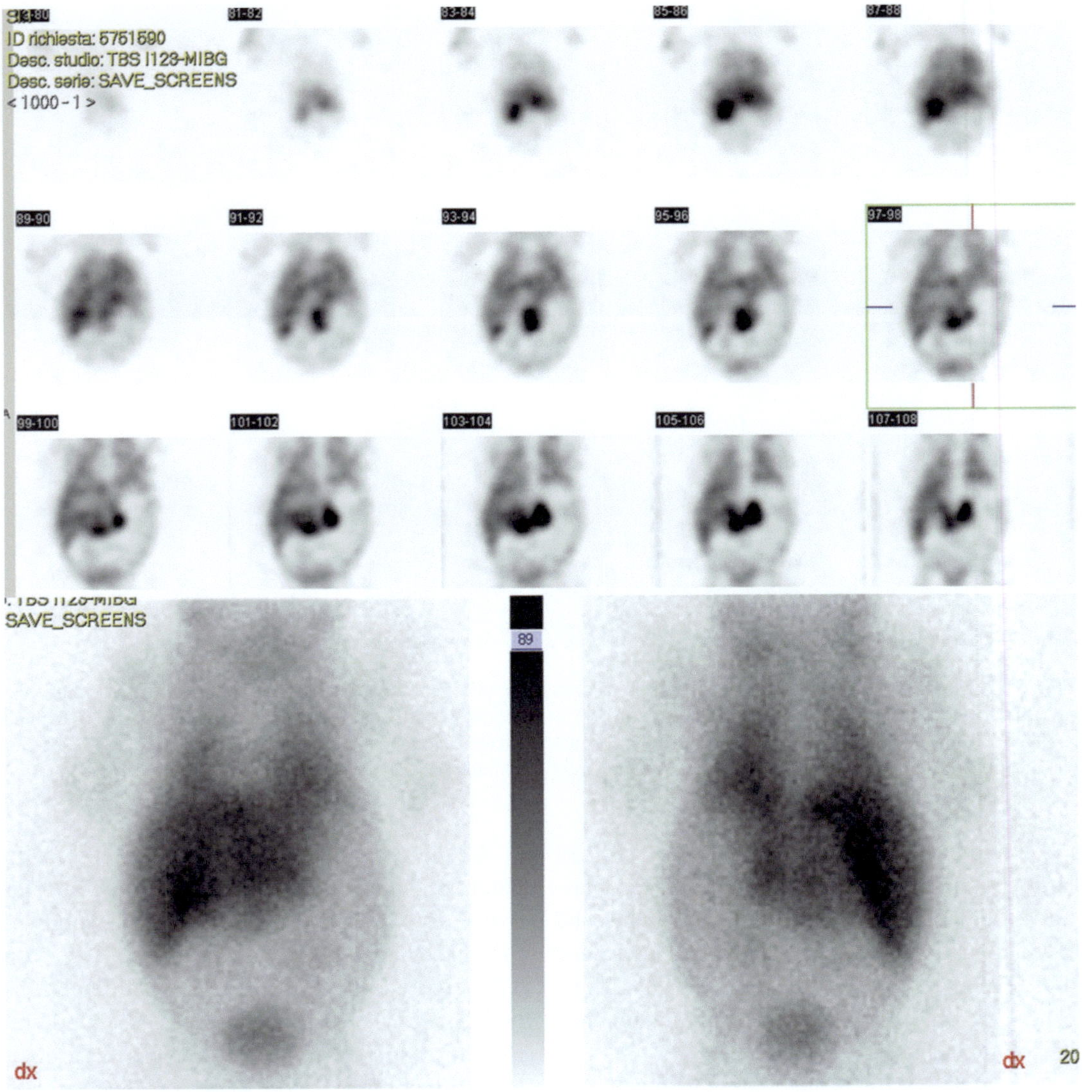

Fig. 21.5 Retroperitoneal neuroblastoma at celiac tripod. I 123 MIBG scintigraphy. The radiopharmaceutical was uptaken by the mass

Scintigraphic evaluation of neuroblastoma may be used to identificate the primary tumour and for metastatic surveillance.

For the first aim, it was performed with either a catecholamine analogue, metaiodobenzylguanidine labelled to iodine-123, referred to as MIBG (Figs. 21.1 and 21.5), or a somatostatin analogue (pentetreotide labelled to indium-11). MIBG is taken by catecholamine-producing tumours but only 70% of neuroblastomas are MIBG positive. When a tumour is evaluated by MIBG scintigraphy and is positive, it gives an excellent map of disease, but it does not allow marrow to be distinguished from cortical disease, which may be important for staging.

The 111 pentetreotide scintigraphy may also demonstrate neuroblastic tumours, but it does not appear to be superior to MIBG scintigraphy (Frappaz et al. 1997; Hattner et al. 1984; Shulkin et al. 1992; Biasotti et al. 2000; Andrich et al. 1996; Shalaby-Rana et al. 1997).

A more commonly performed scintigraphic examination is TC-99 m MDP scintigraphy which is done for evaluation of bone disease, both cortex and marrow.

TC-99 m MDP scintigraphy is initially performed on all patients with neuroblastoma to assess metastatic setting because it is more sensitive than plain radiographs in the detection of bone metastases from neuroblastoma, depicted as focal areas of an increased uptake or an increased uptake at the metaphysis (Gilday et al. 1977; Heisel et al. 1983).

21.6.1.4 Staging

Clinical staging of neuroblastoma is necessary to determine the optimal course of therapy.

The determination of the primary tumour size and the invasion of adjacent structures, the study of the liver and the lymph nodes for metastatic disease and the assessment of tumour resectability detected by CT and MRI are necessary to stage the disease.

The International Neuroblastoma Staging System (INSS) is generally used (Brouder et al. 1993) (Table 21.1).

Tumours that are grossly completely resected and have no adherent positive lymph nodes or metastases are stage 1; tumours that invade one side of the neural canal are stage 2. Tumours that extend across the midline are stage 3. When marrow involvement with tumour cells is less than 10 % of all marrow cells in the biopsy specimen, it is stage 4S; when the tumour cells are greater than 10 % of all marrow cells, the stage is 4 (Brouder et al. 1993).

Table 21.1 Neuroblastoma staging

Stage	Characteristics
Stage I	Localized tumour, complete gross total resection. Microscopic residual disease may be present
Stage IIA	Localized tumour, gross residual disease
Stage IIB	Localized tumour with ipsilateral lymph node involvement whether or not resectable
Stage III	Invasion of tumour across the midline either by direct extension or contiguous lymph node involvement
Stage IV	Disseminated disease with metastases to distant lymph nodes, bone, bone marrow, liver or other organs (except for those patients defined as IVS)
Stage IVS	Limited to age <1 year of age, localized primary (as in stages I, IIA or IIB) with metastases limited to the skin, liver or bone marrow

21.6.1.5 Prognosis and Therapy

Age and clinical stage are the two most important independent prognostic factors. Children less than 1 year of age at diagnosis have a better outcome than those diagnosed later regardless of stage disease.

Patients with localized disease also have a better prognosis. Favourable biologic characteristics include non-amplification of n-myc, a DNA index greater than 1 and a favourable histology by Shimada classification.

Management of patients with neuroblastoma is based on the risk for recurrent disease.

Stage I tumours are low risk and are treated only with surgery and observation, regardless of biologic factors.

Stage IIA-IIB tumour treatment depends on age, n-myc status and histology.

Patients with stage III tumour are treated as intermediate- or high-risk patients on the basis of age and biology.

Stage IV patients under the age of 1 year without n-myc amplification are intermediate risk, all other are high risk.

Stage 4S (special) disease infants have disseminated disease but paradoxically have a favourable prognosis with spontaneous regression. In this group histologic classification and n-myc status are fundamental for therapeutic decision-making; patients with amplification of n-myc need intensive chemotherapy treatment (Evans et al. 1996; Kushner et al. 1996; Matthay et al. 1989; Perez et al. 2000).

Adjuvant therapy is also recommended in patients with life-threatening symptoms such as vascular compromise caused by hepatomegaly, significant respiratory distress renal or bowel ischemia, obstruction of internal organs or coagulopathy (Matthay et al. 1994).

Radiation therapy should be used in the subset of patients with IVS disease that is symptomatic because of spinal cord compression or massive hepatomegaly.

Low-risk patients are treated with surgical excision and then observation.

After a gross total resection, the relapse-free survival is 90 % (Nitschke et al. 1988).

21.6.2 Wilms Tumour

Wilms tumour is the second most common abdominal tumour of childhood, is the most common renal tumour and accounts for approximately 6 % of all childhood cancers. The peak age at diagnoses is 2–3 years; it is rare in infants; a renal mass in a neonate is more likely a congenital mesoblastic nephroma (Crist and Kun 1991).

It is bilateral in 4–13 % of children (Lonergan et al. 1998).

They arise from pluripotent embryonic renal precursor cells; nephrogenic rests are metachronous disease in patients with nephrogenic rests. In only 1 % of cases, it is familial (Breslow et al. 1996; Grundy et al. 1988). It may be associated with congenital disorders and developmental abnormalities: Beckwith-Wiedemann syndrome, Sotos syndrome, Perlman syndrome and Denys-Drash syndrome. Additionally genitourinary anomalies, including hypospadias, cryptorchidism, duplicated collecting system, horseshoe kidney, cystic kidneys and renal dysplasia or aplasia, could be present.

Two loci on chromosome 11 have been implicated in the genesis of a minority of Wilms tumour: locus 11p13, known as the WT1 gene, and locus 11p15, known as WT2 gene.

The WT1 protein is mainly expressed in the development of the kidney, testis, and ovary. Constitutional deletion of this gene is often associated with WAGR syndrome, a syndrome comprising aniridia, genitourinary anomalies and mental retardation, associated with a risk of greater than 30 % for the development of Wilms tumour. WT1 deletion is also associated with sporadic aniridia and a point mutation of this gene is seen with Denys-Drash syndrome.

The other Wilms tumour gene, WT2, is associated with Beckwith-Wiedemann syndrome or hemihypertrophy (Charles et al. 1998).

Screening for Wilms tumour in patients with associated syndromes should be at 6 months of age with initial computed tomography followed by serial ultrasonography every 3 months up to 7 years of age. After the age of 7 years, screening can be discontinued because the risk of developing Wilms tumour decreases significantly (White and Grossman 1991; Beckwith 1998).

21.6.2.1 Clinical Presentation

Wilms tumour most often presents as an asymptomatic mass in the flank. It is generally large at diagnosis without significant impingement of other vital structures because of its retroperitoneal location. Approximately 25 % of patients have associated systemic symptoms or signs as malaise, pain, haematuria or hypertension. Haemorrhage is infrequent but can cause severe anaemia (Ganguly et al. 1973).

The mass is generally large, non-tender, not moving with respiration. Venous obstruction of the spermatic vein can cause varicocele. Acquired von Willebrand's disease is seen in 8 % of patients with Wilms tumour and may cause bruising or mucosae membrane bleeding.

Wilms tumour syndrome in patients with a very large tumour is a constellation of signs and symptoms as hypertension, rapid abdominal enlargement, anaemia and eggshell calcifications (Ganguly et al. 1973).

Initial laboratory evaluation includes a CBC with differential, electrolytes, creatinine, blood urea nitrogen, bilirubin, liver enzymes, serum calcium and phosphorus levels and urinalysis.

21.6.2.2 Imaging

It manifests as a solid intrarenal mass with a pseudocapsule and distortion of the renal parenchyma and collecting system; at histologic analysis, Wilms tumour is composed of variable amounts of blastema, stroma and epithelium.

The tumour typically spreads by direct extension and displaces adjacent structures but does not typically cause encasement or elevation of the aorta, findings characteristic of neuroblastoma. It may cause vascular invasion of the renal vein and inferior vena cava with occasional extension into the right atrium.

Metastases are more common in the lungs (80–85 %), liver (15 % of cases) and regional

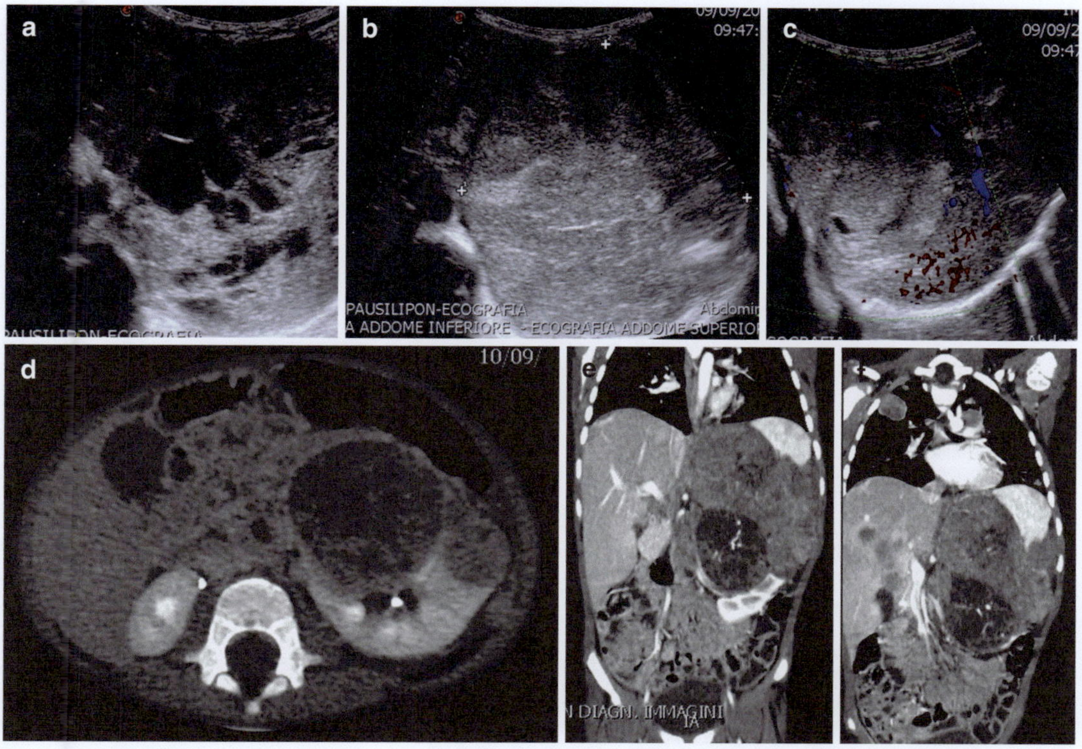

Fig. 21.6 Female, 5 years old with malaise and pain as presenting symptoms. Wilms tumour of the left kidney. US appearance (**a–c**): a heterogeneous echogenicity mass with necrotic areas inside. CT on axial scan (**d**) and MPR coronal reconstructions (**e**, **f**) show a solid heterogeneous intrarenal mass with necrotic areas inside and distortion of the renal parenchyma and collecting system. Also liver and lung metastases are depicted

lymph nodes, with also vascular invasion (Lonergan et al. 1998).

Ultrasound (US) is the initial imaging modality of choice in children that present in emergency department with a mass in the flank. It detects the kidney origin of the mass and quantifies the size. It most often presents as a heterogeneous echogenicity mass (Figs. 21.6 and 21.7) with hemorrhagic, fatty or necrotic areas inside and calcifications (found in only about 5–10% of Wilms tumour, unlike neuroblastoma) (Fishman et al. 1983).

US can detect also the presence and extent of tumour thrombi which could modificate the surgical approach.

CT can better depict the degree of tumour involvement of the kidney and systemic metastases (Miele et al. 1998a) (Figs. 21.6, 21.7, 21.8 and 21.9).

When a renal mass is detected by US, a chest and abdominal CT with intravenous administration of contrast material is mandatory to detect the tumour extension, presence of fat and calcifications, tumour invasion of the renal vein and inferior vena cava, contralateral synchronous tumour, associated nephrogenic rests and pulmonary, hepatic or nodal metastasis and parameters fundamental for the tumour staging.

At magnetic resonance (MR) imaging, Wilms tumour demonstrates low signal intensity on T1w and high signal intensity on T2w images. MR imaging also permits assessment of caval patency and multifocal disease. Wilms tumour is often very large at presentation and can cause severe distortion of adjacent organs, including the inferior vena cava. MR imaging has been reported to be the most sensitive modality for determination of caval patency but it requires sedation.

Wilms tumour is occasionally largely cystic; in these cases there may be difficult differential diagnosis from cystic partially differentiated

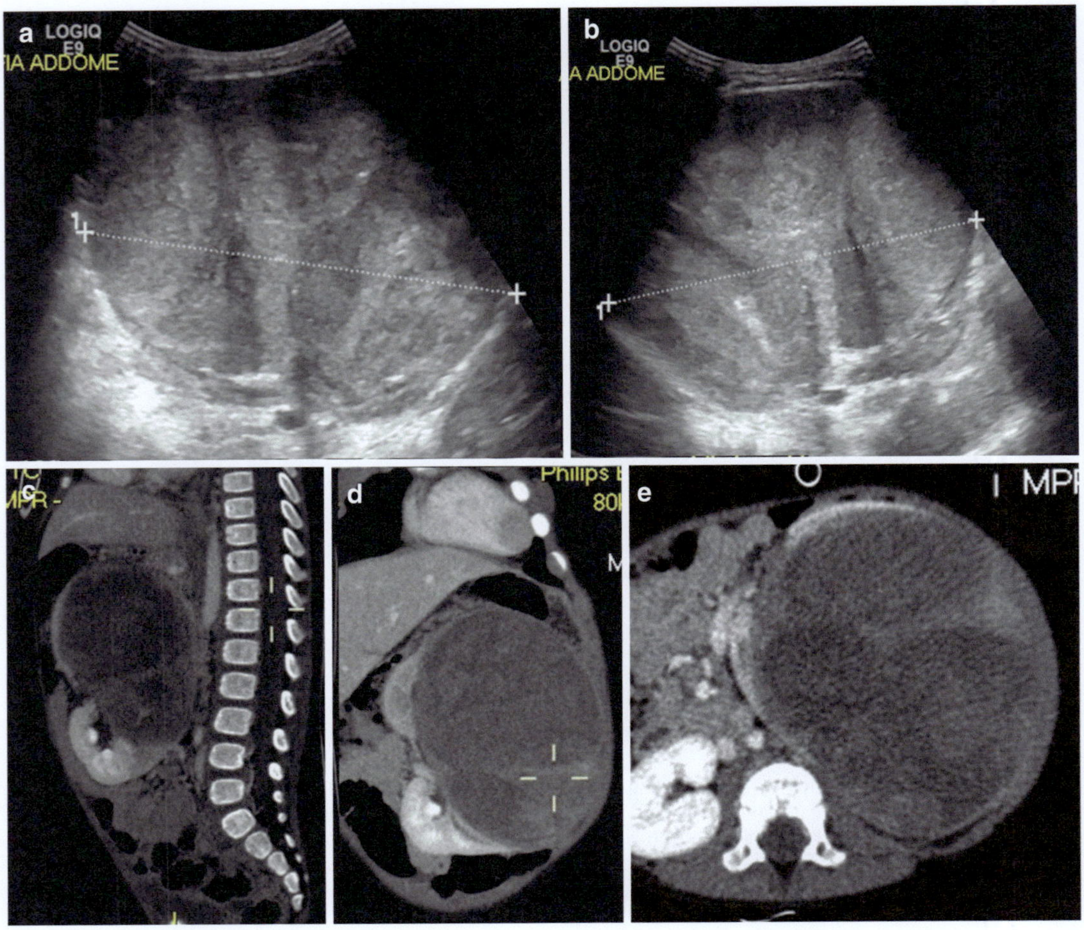

Fig. 21.7 Female, 3 years old. She presents in emergency department with a palpable mass in the left flank. US (**a**, **b**) shows a heterogeneous large predominantly hyperechoic mass with kidney origin. A MDCT (**c**, sagittal MPR reconstruction; **d**, coronal MPR reconstruction; **e**, axial scan) was then performed to better depict the degree of tumour involvement of the kidney. No metastases were depicted

nephroblastoma, a subtype of multilocular cystic nephroma treated in the next session "Neonatal abdominal masses".

21.6.2.3 Staging and Treatment

Staging and therapy for Wilms tumour depend on a timely nephrectomy with accurate surgical staging and determination of specific and biologic characteristics.

Wilms tumour staging is surgical, reported in Table 21.2 (Green et al. 1996).

Unilateral Wilms tumour is generally treated with nephrectomy followed by adjuvant chemotherapy.

Stage I and II tumours with favourable histology are usually treated post-operatively with vincristine and dactinomycin.

Patients with slightly more advanced disease also get a third drug, doxorubicin, and the length of therapy is extended. Patients with diffuse anaplasia are treated with more aggressive chemotherapy including vincristine, doxorubicin, cyclophosphamide and etoposide. In addition to surgery and chemotherapy, abdominal radiation therapy is given to all but the patients with stage I disease and those with stage II disease and favourable histology (Green et al. 1996).

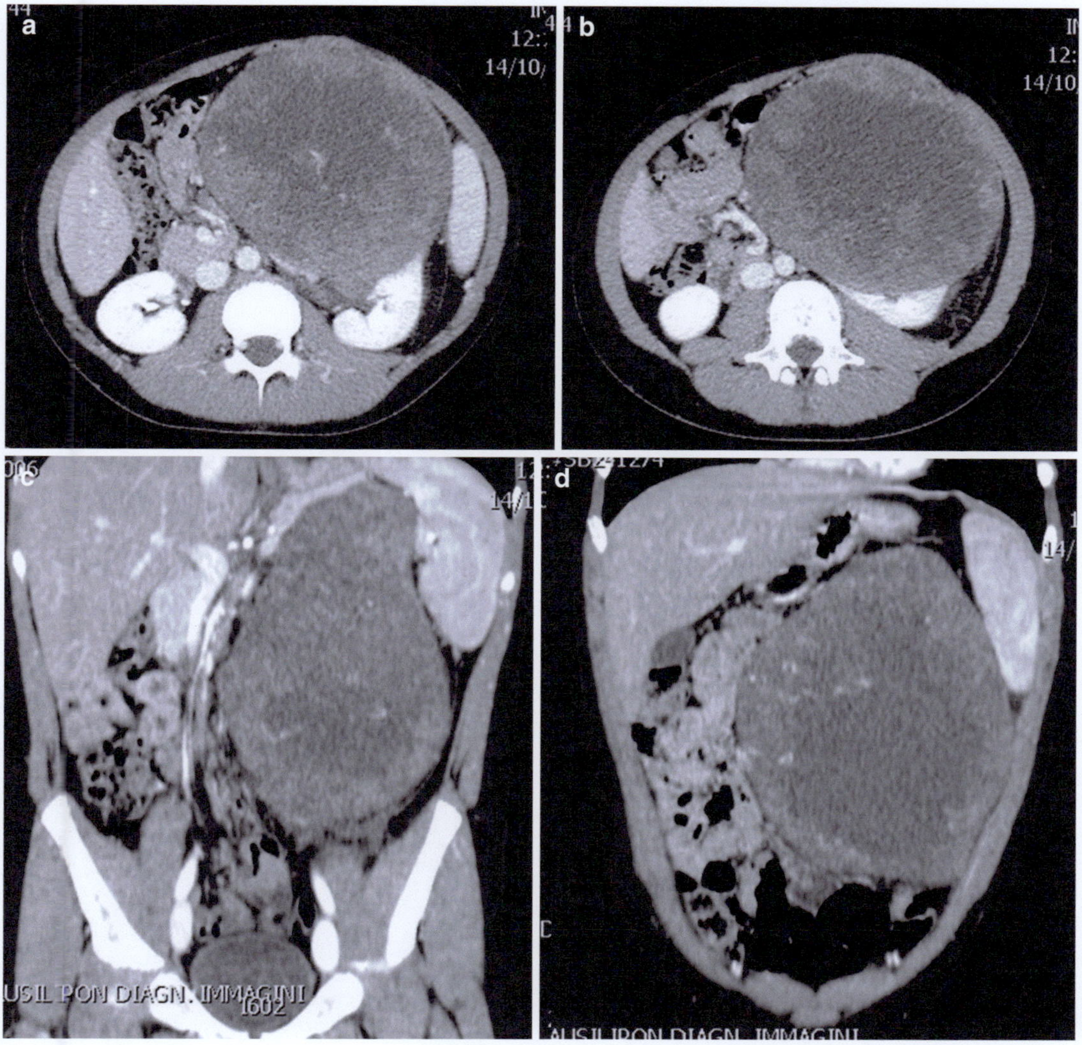

Fig. 21.8 Male, 10 years old. The child has a palpable mass in the left flank and haematuria. MDCT (**a**, **b**, axial scans **c**, **d**, MPR coronal reconstruction) shows a large mass of the left kidney with heterogeneous contrast enhancement. A Wilms tumour at histological exam was found

Patients with pulmonary metastases may receive radiation to the lungs.

21.6.3 Hepatoblastoma

The most significant primary hepatic malignancy in neonates is hepatoblastoma, comprising approximately 1% of paediatric malignancies (Schnater et al. 2003).

The mean age at diagnoses is 1 year, with more of 80% of cases diagnosed before 3 years of age.

Hepatocellular carcinoma is much more rare and occurs in older children and adolescents, with a mean age at diagnosis of 11 years.

Hepatoblastoma may be seen in association with Beckwith-Wiedemann syndrome, with familial adenomatous polyposis (Kingston et al. 1983; Li et al. 1987) and prematurity (Feusner et al. 1997).

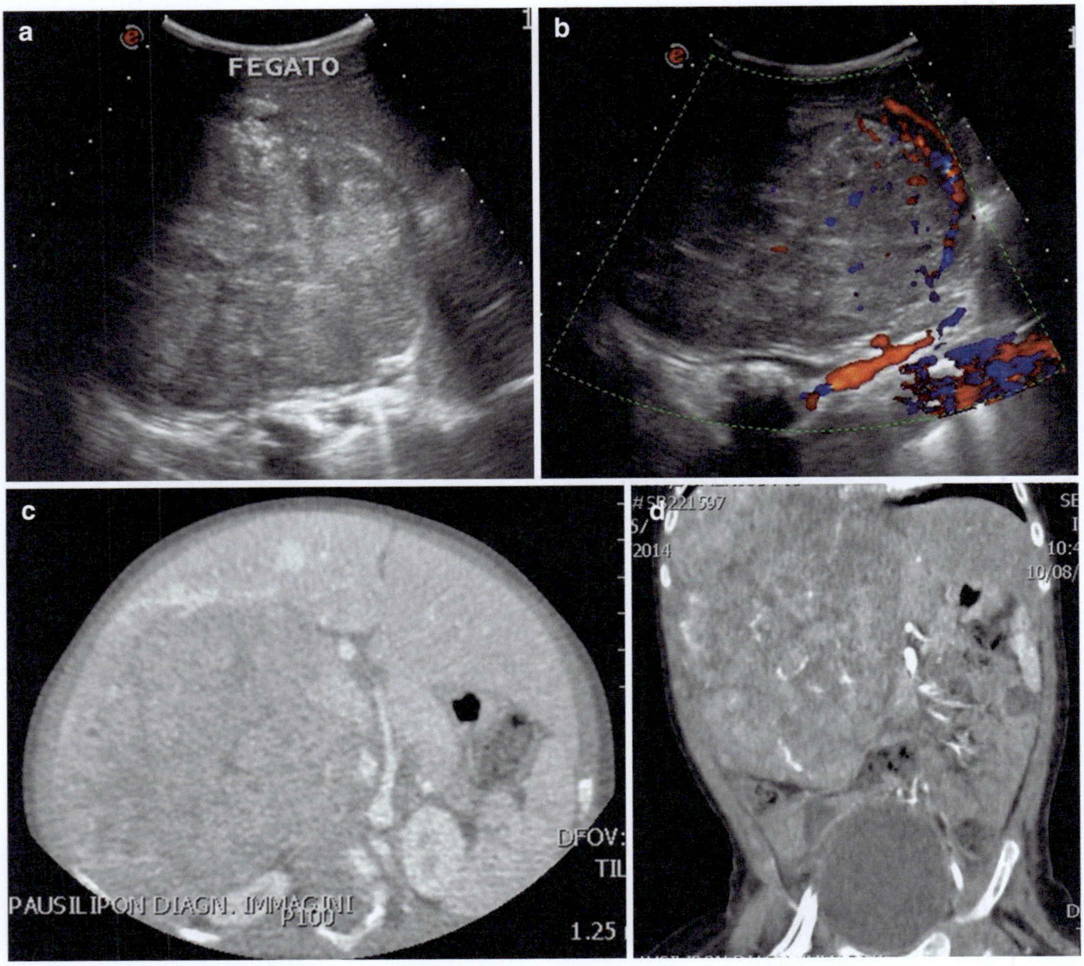

Fig. 21.9 Male, 2 years old. Child with an abdominal palpable mass and distension. US (**a**, **b**) shows a heterogeneous hyperechoic right hepatic mass, with intralesional vessel signals at colour Doppler exam (**b**). MDCT axial scan (**c**) and MPR coronal reconstruction (**d**); a very large and heterogeneous hepatic mass was depicted, with dislocation of the aorta and its branches. Hepatoblastoma was demonstrated at histological examination

The most common presentation of a child with hepatoblastoma in emergency department is an asymptomatic abdominal mass, sometimes associated with distension. Anorexia, pain or weight loss is seen in only 15–20 % of children at diagnosis. The laboratory tests in these cases include a CBC (thrombocytosis is common), urinalysis, chemistry panel including liver transaminases, electrolytes, coagulation studies (to check synthetic liver function) and hepatitis panel. Serum alpha-fetoprotein, elevated in essentially all patients with hepatoblastoma, is helpful for diagnosis and as a marker to follow during and after therapy.

Histologically the tumour presents as a large, usually solitary solid mass. It may contain fibrous bands, leading to a "spoked-wheel appearance". It can either be epithelial or mixed type and has a tendency to invade hepatic and portal veins.

21.6.3.1 Imaging

The first approach is ultrasound exam (US); on US it is detected as a solid mass with similar signal intensity compared with the surrounding liver parenchyma (Fig. 21.9). Calcifications are present in 55 % of cases and may cause acoustic shadowing. Areas of intralesional necrosis or

Table 21.2 Wilms tumour staging

Stage	Characteristics
Stage I	Tumour is limited to the kidney, renal capsule intact with or without rupture, no evidence of tumour beyond resection margin (complete resection)
Stage II	Tumour extends beyond the kidney. If there was spillage before or during surgery, it was confined to the flank, and the peritoneal surface is not involved. There is regional extension of the tumour with penetration through the capsule, invading the renal sinus or blood vessels outside the kidney. After resection, there is no evidence of tumour beyond the resection margins (complete resection)
Stage III	Gross residual tumour confined to the abdomen including any of the following: tumour penetrating the peritoneal surface, implants on the peritoneal surface, subtotal resection of tumour for any reason including infiltration into vital organs (gross or microscopic residual, or tumour spill that is beyond the flank, whether pre- or postoperative)
Stage IV	Metastases from haematogenous or lymphatic dissemination
Stage V	Bilateral renal disease, although each kidney should be staged separately (I, II or III)

tumour thrombi in the portal vein or hepatic veins may be depicted.

On unenhanced CT hepatoblastoma may have different features (Feusner et al. 1997; Miele et al. 1998b); it generally appears as a relatively well-defined, heterogeneous mass, slightly hypodense compared with liver tissue, with or without calcifications (Figs. 21.9 and 21.10). On contrast-enhanced CT, it reveals a heterogeneous enhancement and generally appears hyperdense compared with liver parenchyma in the early arterial post contrast phase and usually iso- or hypodense on delayed images. Invasion of the portal vein and thrombosis of portal or hepatic veins are well depicted by CT. Metastasis may be seen in lymph nodes and lung parenchyma, rarely in the bones and brain.

On MR hepatoblastoma is iso- or slightly hyperintense on T2w images and iso- or hypointense compared with liver parenchyma on T1w. Central necrosis may show a high T2 signal. The contrast enhancement of hepatoblastoma is similar compared with CT and quite non-specific.

Staging of hepatoblastoma depends on the extent of disease and the resectability: stage I tumours are fully resected with negative margins, stage II tumours have microscopic residual disease, stage III tumours have gross residual disease or may be only biopsied and stage IV hepatoblastoma is metastatic disease.

Therapy is surgical resection of liver disease; for large tumours or those associated with metastatic disease, chemotherapy often can finally make a total resection possible; metastatic disease without resection has a worse prognosis. If the resection is extensive, orthotopic liver transplant has been performed to cure the patient.

Chemotherapy for hepatoblastoma usually includes doxorubicin, cisplatin, vincristine, 5-fluorouracil and ifosfamide (Douglass et al. 1993).

21.6.4 Germ Cell Tumour

Paediatric germ cell tumours (GCTs) are rare tumours that include a heterogeneous group of neoplasms arising from variation of normal differentiation of germ cells; they could be benign, malignant or immature neoplasms in children and adolescent.

Eighty percent of GCTs are benign, while only 20 % are malignant representing about 2–3 % of all malignant paediatric tumours. They can develop in the gonads or in extragonadal sites (>50 %) including the retroperitoneum (Figs. 21.10, 21.11, 21.12, 21.13, 21.14, and 21.15), mediastinum or brain (Rescorla 2012).

Teratoma is the most common type with benign (mature) or immature histological features but rarely malignant. It could be classified in mature teratoma when it is composed of differentiated tissue from one or more embryonic germ layers or immature teratoma when it contains also immature epithelial or stromal tissue (Billmire 2006).

The most frequent and aggressive malignant entity in young children is yolk sac tumour (YCT) also known as endodermal sinus tumour. It can arise in all sites and can metastasize to the

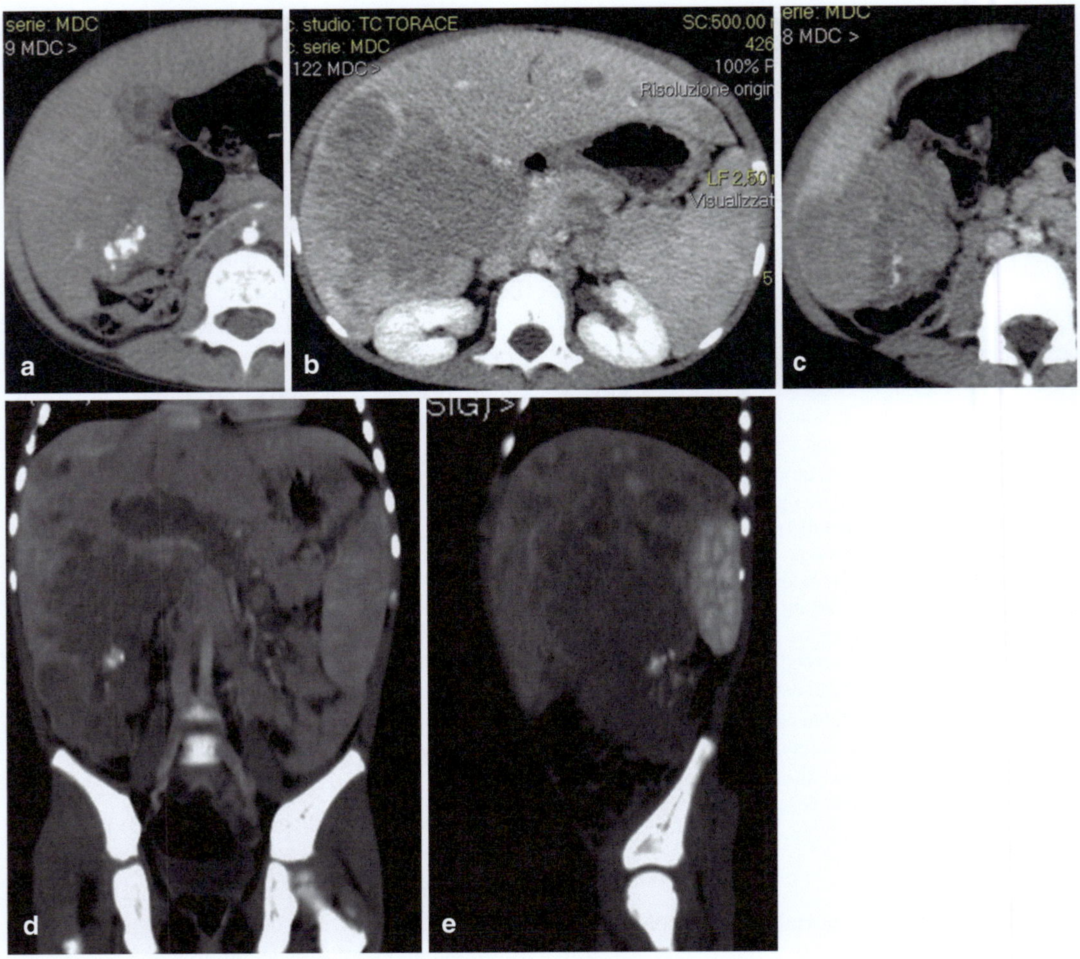

Fig. 21.10 Male, 3 years with abdominal distension and anorexia. Axial CT scan without CE (**a**) shows a hypodense hepatic area with calcifications. In MDCT scans (**b**, **c**) and MPR coronal and sagittal reconstructions (**d**, **e**), a heterogeneous hepatic lesion, relatively hypodense with inhomogeneous CE, was demonstrated. Other hepatic nodules were present. It was a hepatoblastoma

regional lymph nodes, liver, lung and brain. It is characterized by secretion of alpha-fetoprotein, a very important serum marker at diagnosis, during and after the treatment.

Other malignant histotypes are less frequent: germinomas (seminoma in males and dysgerminoma in females) are undifferentiated GCTs typical of adolescents; embryonal carcinoma and choriocarcinoma are rare differentiated forms in paediatric age which include trophoblastic cells secreting a specific serum marker, the beta subunit of human chorionic gonadotropin (beta HCG).

The most frequent localization of extragonadal GCT is the sacrococcygeal (the sacrococcygeal teratoma is treated in the session "Neonatal abdominal masses"); in the gonadal GCT, the ovarian represents about 30 % of GCTs and 70 % of all neoplastic ovarian masses (Rescorla 2008).

21.6.4.1 Ovarian GCTs

They are the most common ovarian neoplasms in children and teenagers, with a peak of incidence in early adolescence (Caruso et al. 1971).

Pathology: all the histological subtypes of GCTs may be reported in the ovary. Benign and

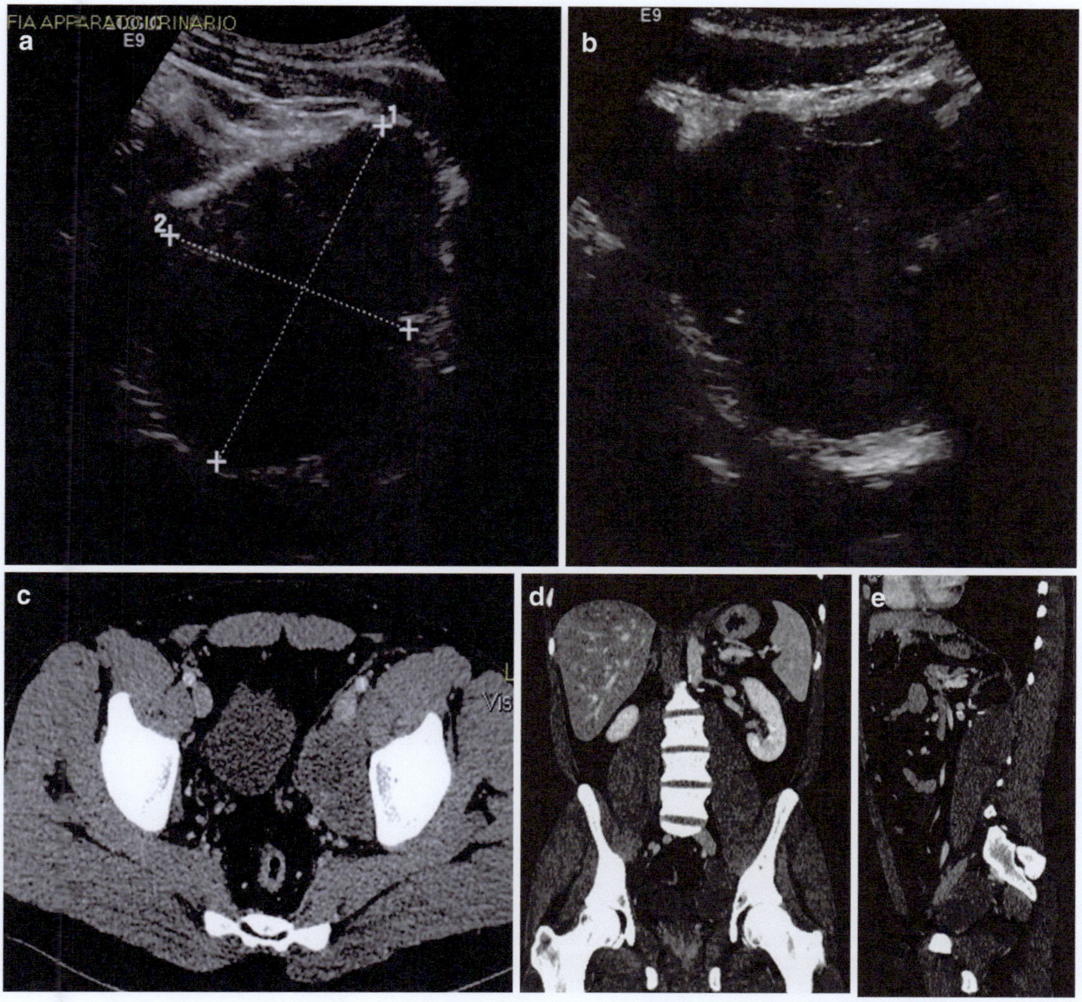

Fig. 21.11 Male, 14 years old. He presents with lower abdominal weight and pain. US (**a**, **b**) shows an inhomogeneous mass in left hemipelvic region. MDCT scan (**c**) and MPR coronal and sagittal reconstruction show the presence of solid tissue in retroperitoneal left iliac region. An extragonadic germ cell tumour was detected

immature teratomas represent about 80 % of all ovarian GCTs, bilateral in 5 % of cases. The incidence of malignant forms is reported in about 20 % and increases during adolescence (Rescorla 2012). The most common malignant entity in young people is the YSCT; dysgerminoma is the most frequent ovarian malignant GCTs in female adolescents and may be bilateral in 10 % of cases. Gonadoblastoma is rare.

The pathologic appearance of mature cystic teratomas is characteristic. In 88 % of cases, they are unilocular, filled with sebaceous material (Caruso et al. 1971). Hair follicles, skin glands, muscle and other tissues lie within the wall. There is often a raised protuberance projecting into the cyst cavity known as Rokitansky nodule. Most of the hair typically arises from this nodule. When the bone or teeth are present, they tend to be located within the protuberance (Matz 1961).

Ectodermal tissue (skin derivatives and neural tissue) is always present, mesodermal tissue (bone, cartilage, bone, fat) is seen in over 90 % of cases (Figs. 21.13, 21.14 and 21.15), and

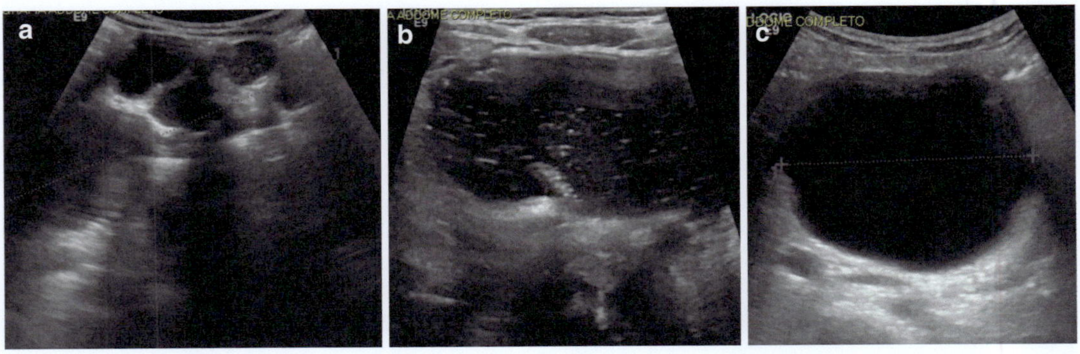

Fig. 21.12 Female, 7 years old. Presenting symptoms: constipation and abdominal distension. An US was performed as the first step, and a retroperitoneal heterogeneous mass, with a predominant sovrafluid composition, was depicted

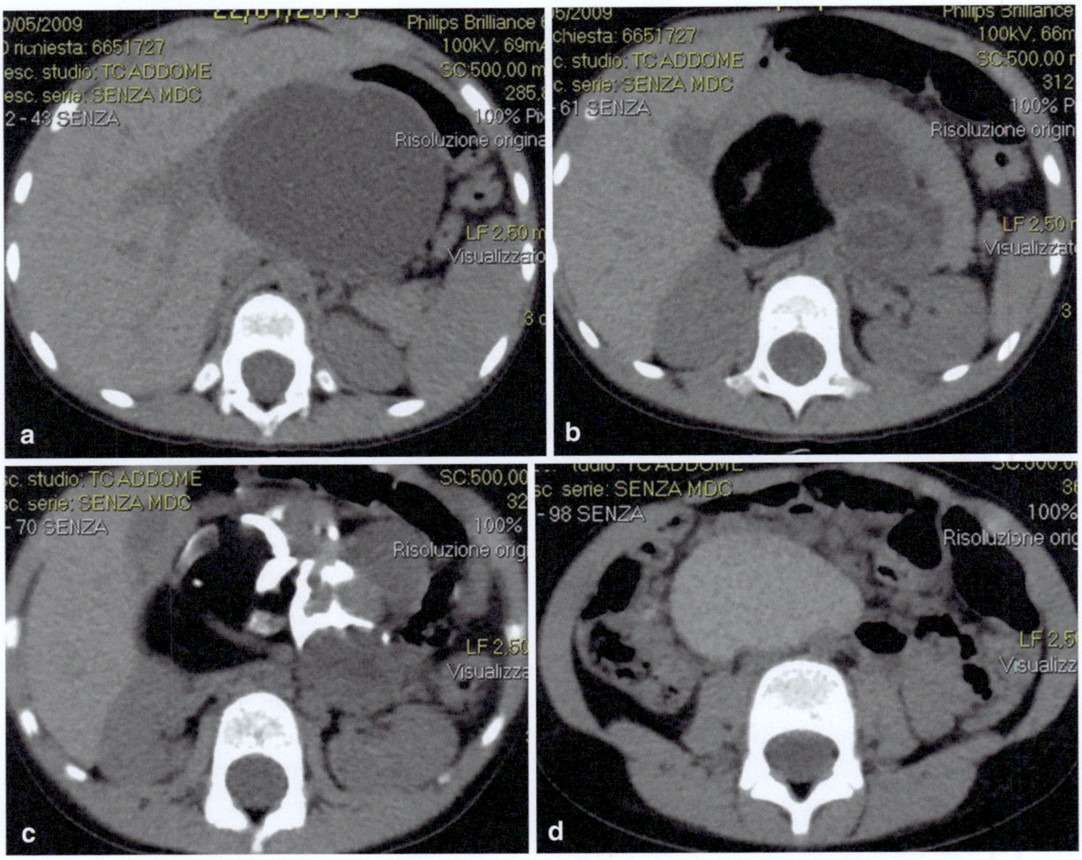

Fig. 21.13 A CT was than performed. In these unenhanced axial scans, a large retroperitoneal mass with cystic, fat, bone and sebaceous components is depicted. A retroperitoneal mature cystic teratoma was diagnosed

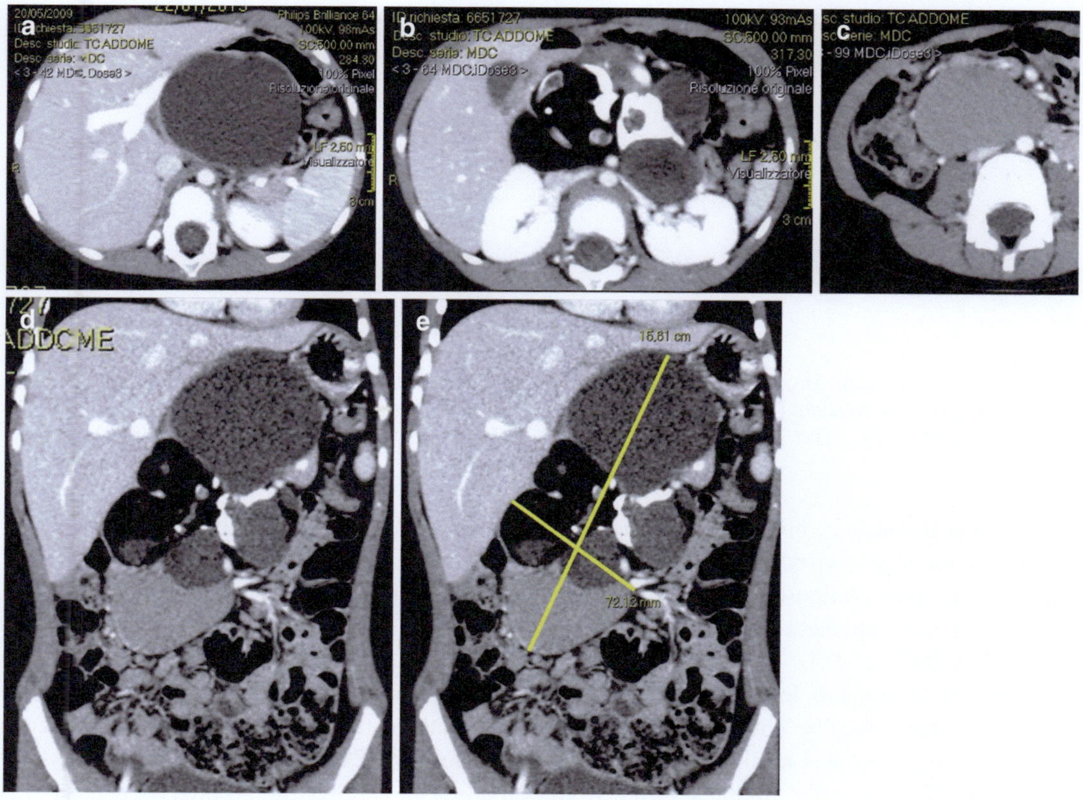

Fig. 21.14 Contrast-enhanced axial CT (**a–c**) and MPR coronal reconstructions (**d**, **e**) well demonstrate the large retroperitoneal mature cystic teratoma with its different components

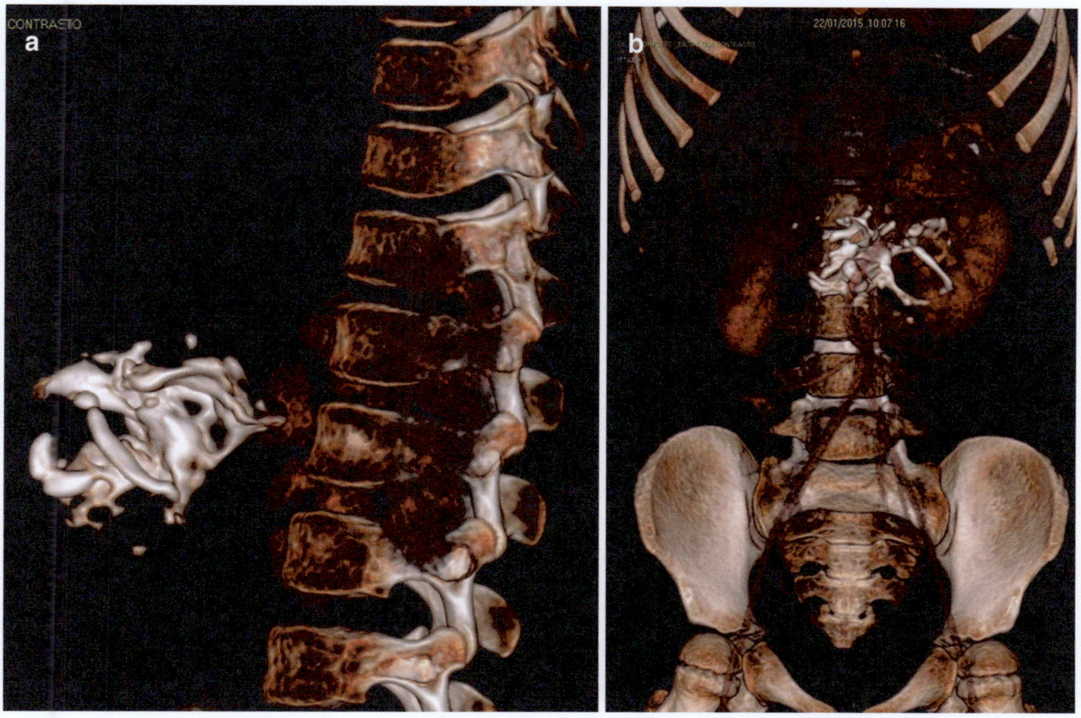

Fig. 21.15 Retroperitoneal mature cystic teratoma. VR reconstructions: the cartilaginous and bone components of the tumour seem to be rib and vertebral sketches

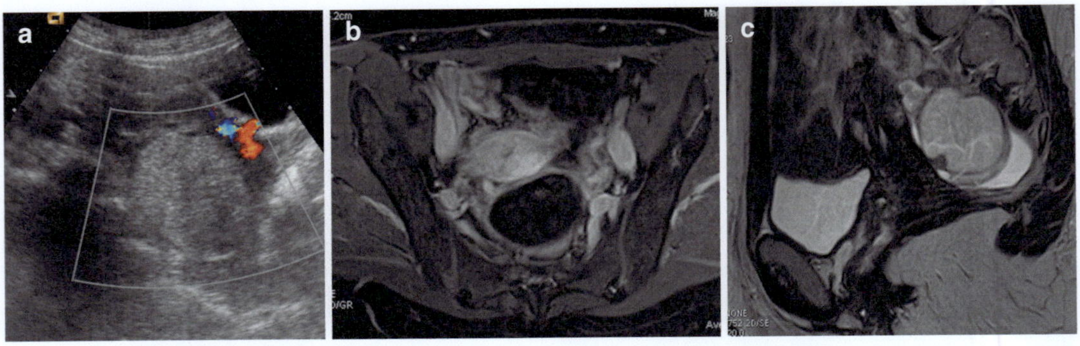

Fig. 21.16 (**a**) US scan. An oval, regular hyperechoic mass in the pelvis is detected. (**b**) Axial T1 fat sat scan after gadolinium eV. The lesion appears highly hypointense due to its fat content, with enhanced wall. In T2w sequence (**c**), a small perilesional free fluid was depicted. A dermoid ovarian cyst was diagnosed

endodermal tissue (e.g. bronchial and gastrointestinal epithelium, thyroid tissue) is seen in the majority of cases. Adipose tissue is present in 67–75 % of cases and teeth in 31 % (Caruso et al. 1971; Matz 1961).

Immature teratoma is less common, affects a younger group (usually during the first two decades of life) and has a clinically malignant behaviour. Histologically findings differ from mature teratoma in the presence of immature or embryonic tissues (Talerman 1994). They are typically larger (14–25 cm), solid or with a predominant solid composition than mature teratoma (Rescorla 2008; Talerman 1994). The cystic areas are usually filled with serous or mucinous fluid or fatty sebaceous material. A frequent perforation of the mass capsule is depicted (Talerman 1994).

Clinical presentation: abdominal pain and lower abdominal mass are the most presenting symptoms, both in malignant and in benign lesions. Constipation, amenorrhoea and vaginal bleeding are less frequent.

Beta HCG produced by choriocarcinoma can cause premature breast enlargement and pubic hair.

For the tumour with malignant components, the pattern of regional spread of malignant cells may include ascites and peritoneal metastases.

Imaging: the diagnostic workup of a young female who arrives in emergency department with a solid pelvic mass and abdominal pain usually starts with an abdominal and pelvic ultrasound (US). The US diagnosis of mature cystic teratoma may be complicated by the variety of appearances of this tumour. The tumour could appear as a cystic lesion with a very echogenic tubercle (Rokitansky nodule) into the cyst lumen or as a diffusely or partially echogenic mass with sound attenuation for the presence of sebaceous material (Fig. 21.12) and hair within the cyst or finally with multiple thin, echogenic bands (hair) in the cyst cavity. Sebum into the cyst could be hypoechoic or anechoic (Malkasian et al. 1965; Quinn et al. 1985; Patel et al. 1998). Fluid-fluid levels may be depicted (Patel et al. 1998).

More simple is the diagnosis of mature cystic teratoma by CT or MR because these modalities are more sensitive for fat. At CT fat attenuation within a cyst, with or without calcification in the wall, is suggestive for mature cystic teratoma (Figs. 21.13, 21.14, and 21.15) (Dodd and Budzik 1990; Occhipinti et al. 1993; Buy et al. 1989). At MR imaging the sebaceous component of dermoid cysts has a very high signal intensity on T1w images. The imaging appearance on T1w and T2w images may be similar to some haemorrhagic lesions (as endometrioma). Chemical shift sequences, gradient echo imaging with an echo time in which the water and fat are in opposite phase and sequences with frequency-selective for saturation help to detect fat in the lesion, distinguishing dermoid cyst and mature cystic teratoma from haemorrhagic lesions (Togashi et al. 1987; Guinet et al. 1993; Imaoka et al. 1993) (Figs. 21.16 and 21.17).

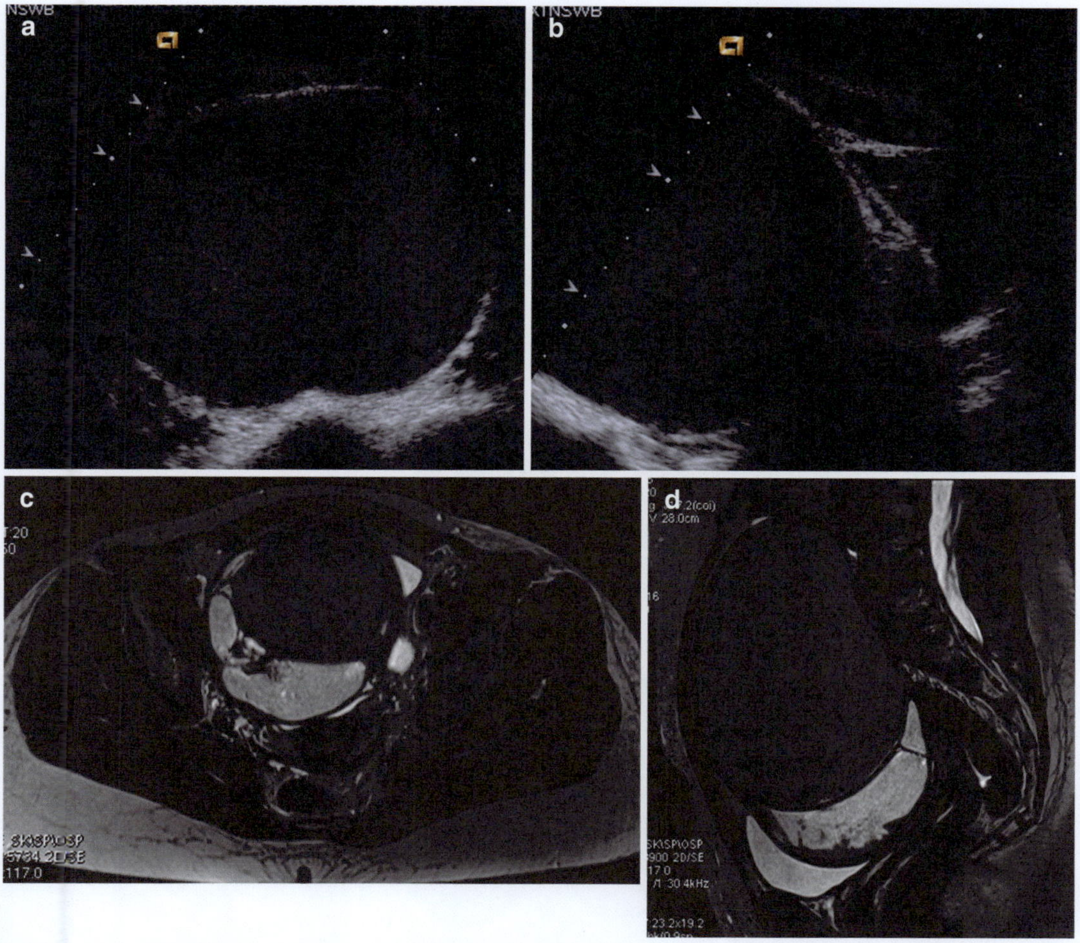

Fig. 21.17 Female, 16 years old. (**a**, **b**) Abdominal sonography: (**a**) axial scan, (**b**) longitudinal scan: huge fluid corpuscular mass completely filling the pelvic space. Bladder displaced inferiorly. (**c**, **d**) MRI, (**c**) axial and (**d**) sagittal T2w sequences confirm the ovarian neoplasm, which includes liquid and fat tissue. Mature ovarian teratoma

Mature cystic teratoma can be associated with complications from rupture (Miele et al. 2002), malignant degeneration or (most commonly) torsion in the larger mass. Findings suggestive for torsion are deviation of the uterus to the twisted side, engorged blood vessels on the twisted side, high signal intensity of the mass on T1w sequences, low signal intensity torsion knot and thick blood vessels around the lesion with complete absence of enhancement (Kimura et al. 1994).

Also immature teratomas are non-specific US appearance (Sutton et al. 1992). They are typically heterogeneous masses, with a predominant solid composition, generally with scattered calcifications. Small fat foci may be difficult to recognize. At CT and MR imaging, these tumours have a characteristic appearance: a large, irregular mainly solid mass with calcifications, small foci of fat and often hemorrhagic areas (Figs. 21.18 and 21.19) (Brammer et al. 1990; Outwater and Dunton 1995).

Laboratory tests: evaluation of serum markers may address the nature of the tumour; alpha-fetoprotein or beta HCG means the presence of malignancy (the first is raised in over 90 % of the malignant tumour, while beta HCG in 30 % of cases). Other markers as LDH and NSE or those typical for epithelial tumours (CEA, CA 125)

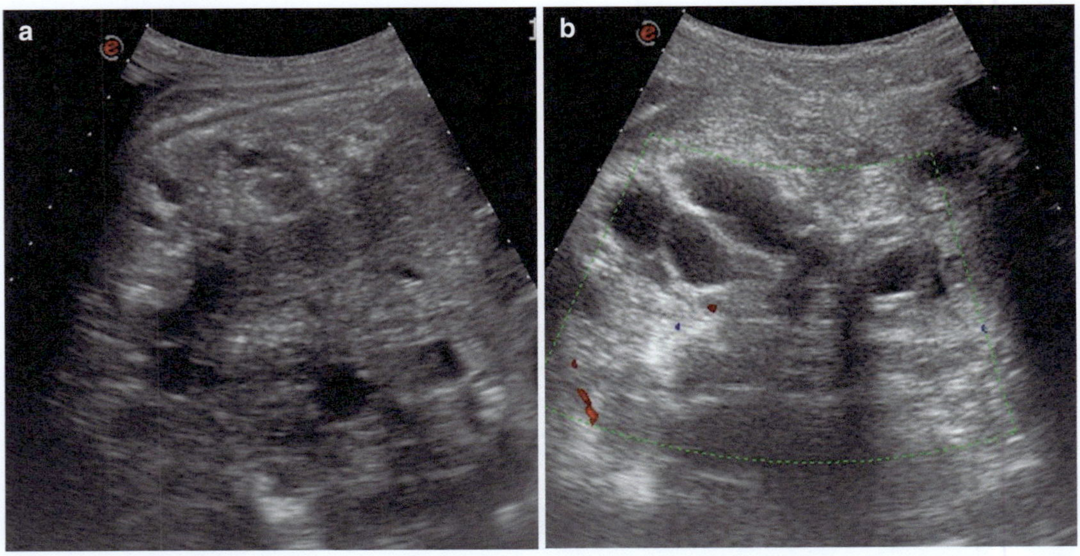

Fig. 21.18 Ovarian immature teratoma. Abdominal ultrasound. (**a**, **b**) The complex mass completely fills the pelvic space

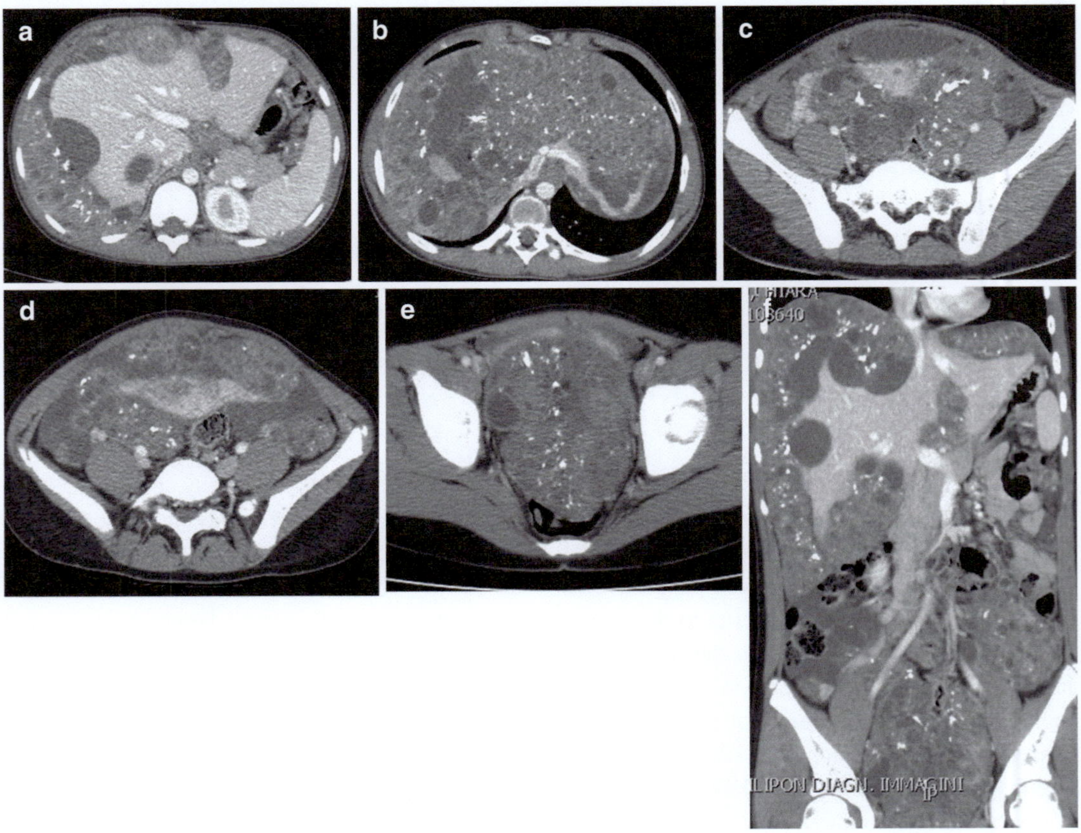

Fig. 21.19 Same patient of Fig. 21.17. CT (**a**–**e**). Bulky pelvic mass, with numerous internal calcifications. Presence of metastases to the liver, root of the mesentery, peritoneum and omentum. Ovarian immature teratoma with multiple metastases

may be elevated in patients with mixed tumours (Von Allmend 2005).

Treatment: ovariectomy and ovarosalpingectomy are the treatment of choice in malignant GCTs However, since malignant GCTs are very chemosensitive, primary excision should be attempted only when it represents a complete but non-mutilating procedure. Generally the mass becomes surgically resectable after chemotherapy. So that this operation is not demolitive (Rescorla 2012; Billmire 2006).

The surgical technique should include well-defined intraoperative staging procedure (Rescorla 2012; Billmire 2006; Von Allmend 2005):

1. Inspection and palpation of the contralateral ovary with a biopsy of suspected areas
2. Collection of peritoneal fluid for cytology
3. Intact removal of the ovary without violation of the tumour capsule. Sparing the fallopian tube only if not adherent
4. Examination of the omentum, the peritoneal surface and the liver with removal of any abnormal areas
5. Examination of iliac and aorto-caval nodes with biopsy of any abnormal nodes

If imaging exams show involvement of neighbouring organs (i.e. the bladder, uterus and vagina) or in case of bilateral malignant GCTs, a tumour biopsy is the best option.

In case of bilateral tumours, most authors recommended to attempt ovarian preservation if possible on chemotherapy which has been proven not effective (Billmire et al. 2004).

Staging: there are two main staging systems for paediatric ovarian malignant tumours, the staging system suggested by the Children's Oncology Group (COG) and the International Federation of Gynaecology and Obstetrics (FIGO) staging system. Both of them are based on the results of the imaging investigations and on the findings of the first surgical approach (Outwater and Dunton 1995; Von Allmend 2005). COG staging system is reported in Table 21.3 (Billmire et al. 2004).

Table 21.3 COG staging system for ovarian MGCTs

Stage	Characteristics
Stage I	Disease limited to the ovary and completely excised; negative peritoneal washing. No clinical, surgical or histological evidence of disease extending beyond the ovary and tumoural markers and/or hormonal levels in range after surgery
Stage II	Microscopic residuals, spillage or nodes affected by disease (<2 cm); negative peritoneal washing. Tumoural markers positive or negative
Stage III	Macroscopic residuals or initial biopsy only; local invasion (omentum, bowel, bladder); positive peritoneal washing; nodes affected (>2 cm). Tumoural markers positive or negative
Stage IV	Distant metastases. Negative or positive markers
Hidden disease	Stage I but tumoural markers persistently out of normal range after a complete surgery

Treatment of benign and immature GC: they are generally well-defined masses with larger cystic components as compared with malignant forms and do not show elevated levels of alpha FP or beta HCG.

In the first months of life, most ovarian lesions are benign and often detected an antenatal ultrasound (Bagolan et al. 1992). Most of them are observed for some months after birth until the spontaneous regression. If the lesions are very huge (more than 5 cm in size) or symptomatic, a more aggressive therapeutic approach is recommended.

The only effective therapy is the complete removal (Templeman and Fallat 2005); the procedure often requires the ovariectomy, or in selected cases with small tumours, the enucleation of the lesion can be possible. Since most GCTs are mixed tumours with mature and immature elements inside, it is sometimes impossible to know whether the lesion is malignant or not before surgery; so that intraoperative staging procedures are recommended.

Chemotherapy may be suggested only if there is the suspect of malignant transformation (Green 2008).

Ovarian torsion of an ovarian mass, often of a benign mass, may present as an acute abdomen which requires an emergent procedure usually with a laparoscopic approach

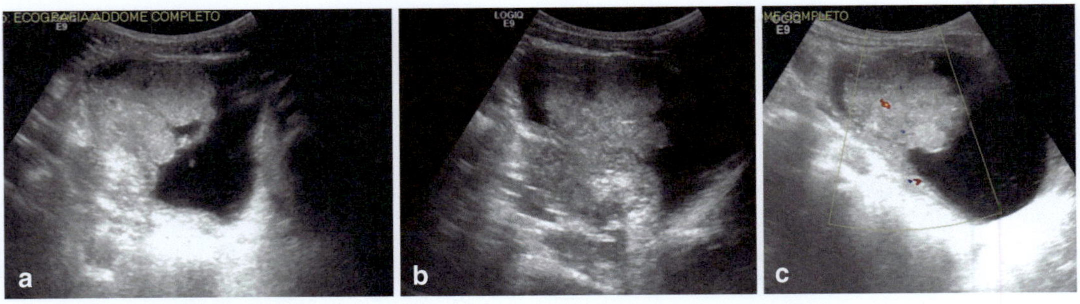

Fig. 21.20 Female, 10 years old. She reports decrease urinary output. US images show a vegetant polylobulate mass in the bladder. Bladder rhabdomyosarcoma

(Di Giacomo et al. 2015). Immediate ovariectomy is necessary only in the setting of an ischemic or necrotic ovary.

21.6.5 Rhabdomyosarcoma

Rhabdomyosarcoma (RMS) is one of the most common malignant solid tumours of childhood, after neoplasms of the central nervous system, neuroblastoma and Wilms tumours (Agrons et al. 1997). The genitourinary tract is the second most common site of RMS, behind the head and neck.

The median age at presentation is 7 years, with variability in presentation secondary to the different sites of origin within the genitourinary tract (the bladder, prostate, testes, paratesticular region, penis, vagina, perineum and uterus). Bladder RMS may cause hydroureteronephrosis, gross haematuria and decreased urinary output with a rapid progression to anuria.

Most of patients with RMS have metastasis at the time of diagnoses at lungs, cortical bone and lymph nodes.

Sonography of the genitourinary system and the other abdominal organs can be helpful to detect the site of origin and the invasion of adjacent or remote structures. The sonographic, CT and MRI appearance of the tumour is variable, generally is solid mass, with haemorrhage or necrotic areas inside (Fig. 21.20, 21.21 and 21.22).

Treatment is surgical excision, often after adjuvant chemotherapy to reduce primary tumour size (Agrons et al. 1997; Maurer et al. 1988).

21.7 Neonatal Abdominal Masses (Younger than 1 Year of Age)

21.7.1 Congenital Mesoblastic Nephroma

Congenital mesoblastic nephroma (CMN) is the most common abdominal neoplasm in the neonate, typically presenting in children at a mean of 3 months as a palpable abdominal mass (Pinto and Guinard 1995; Marsden and Lawler 1983). CMN is generally a benign lesion with some malignant potential; so nephrectomy and complete resection are necessary.

Sonographic findings of this tumour include a large solid renal mass with heterogeneous or low echogenicity (Fig. 21.24), with internal flow at colour Doppler exam. A central hypoechoic area of necrosis can be depicted. The mass may extend beyond the capsule but does not typically involve the renal vein (Riccabona 2003).

The following exam with CT or MR is mandatory when this renal mass was found in ultrasound exam (Fig. 21.23) to exclude metastasis, because they may rarely occur in the case of cellular type pathology.

CMN can have a similar appearance to Wilms tumour, but Wilms tumour is statistically less frequent in neonates.

21.7.2 Haemangioendothelioma

Hepatic haemangioendothelioma is the most commonly diagnosed symptomatic tumour

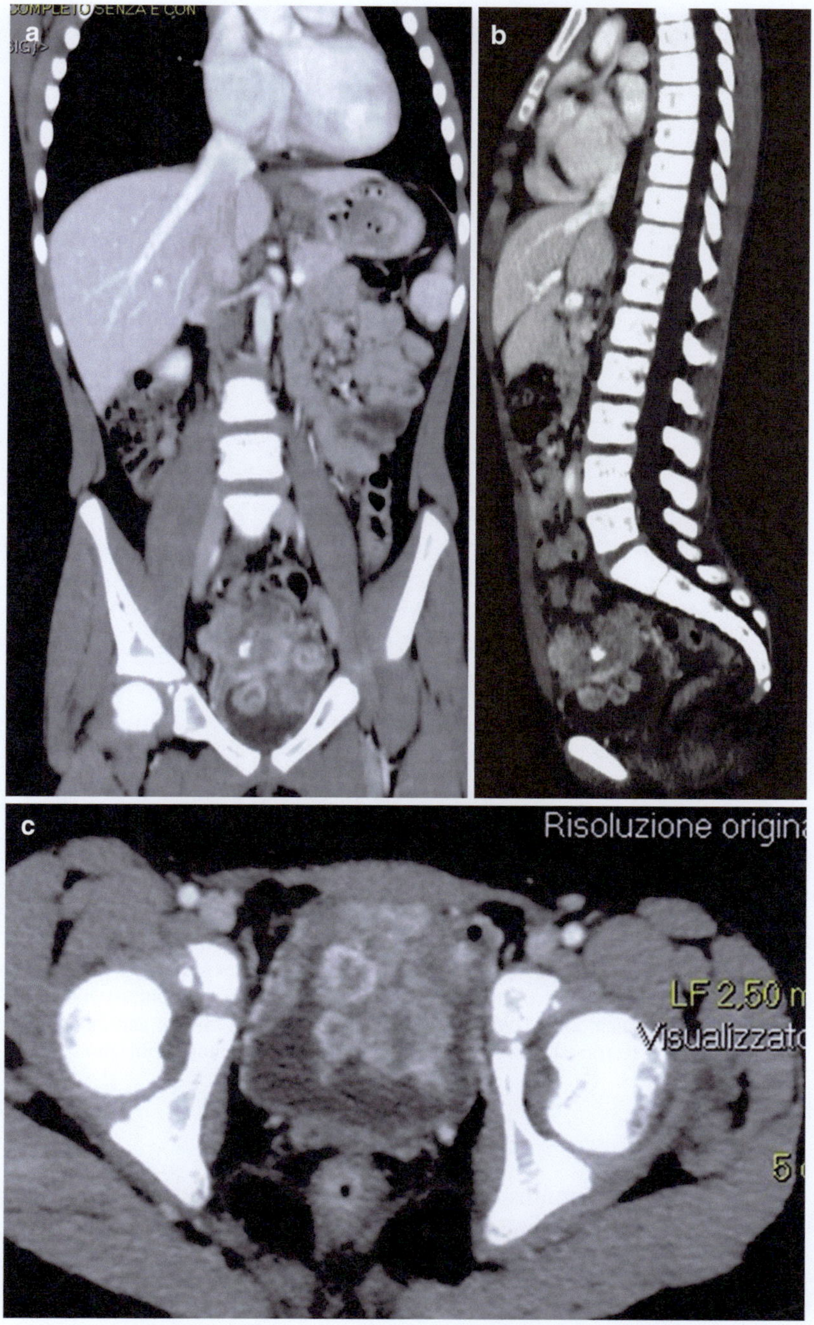

Fig. 21.21 MDCT (**a**, **b**, coronal and sagittal MPR reconstructions; **c**, axial scan) detects the polylobulate heterogeneous mass inside the bladder with necrotic areas inside. A diagnosis of bladder rhabdomyosarcoma was then demonstrated

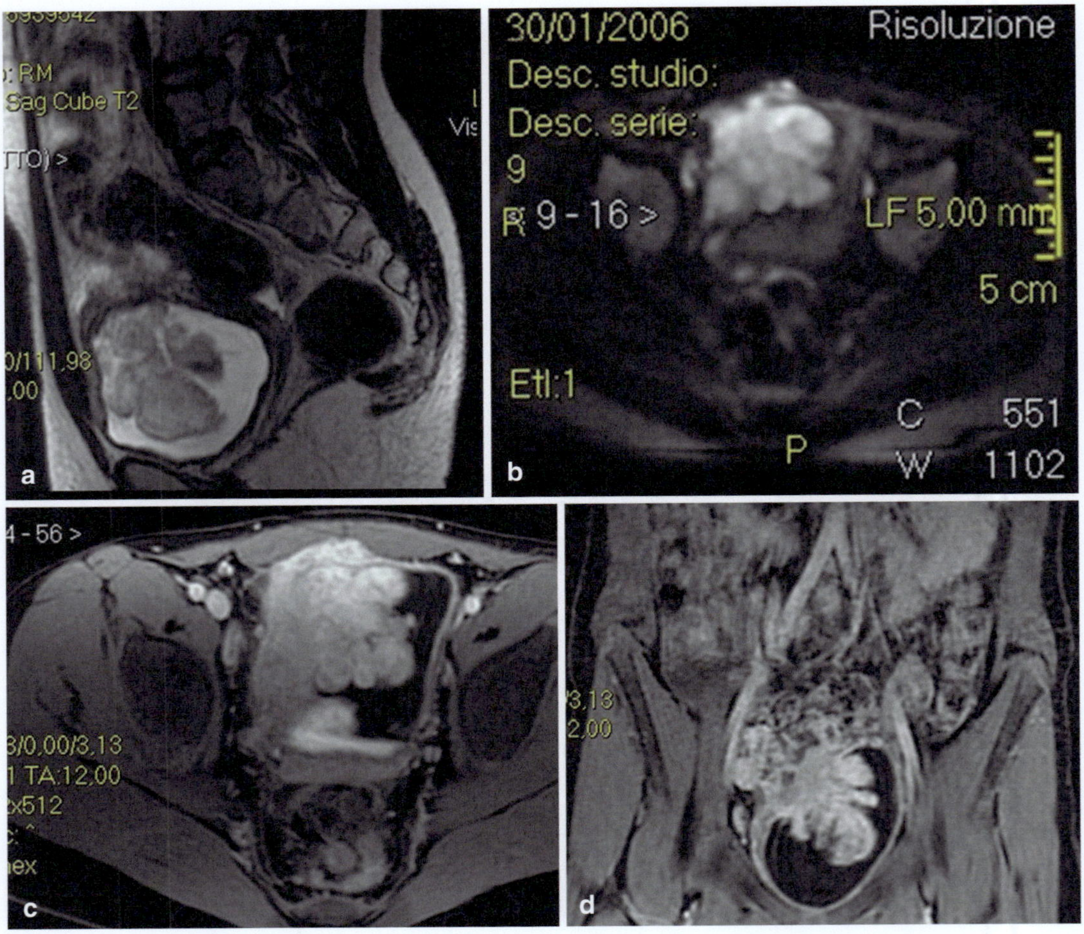

Fig. 21.22 Bladder rhabdomyosarcoma on MR images. Sagittal T2w scan (**a**) shows a isointense mass protruding into the bladder lumen; axial DWI image with b value of 600 (**b**) shows a restricted diffusion of the mass which appears bright on diffusion-weighted images. Axial and coronal contrast-enhanced T1w images (**c**, **d**) demonstrate an intense and inhomogeneous enhancement after gadolinium eV injection

in infants under 6 months of age (Selby et al. 1994; Roos et al. 2003) and represents approximately 12 % of all paediatric hepatic neoplasm. The typical presentation is a palpable right-upper quadrant mass; many infants also have cutaneous haemangiomas, leading to investigation of non-palpable liver lesions. It represents a spectrum of disease from asymptomatic mass to major arteriovenous shunting, which may lead to congestive heart failure. The Kasabach-Merritt phenomenon, which may be associated with this tumour, is the combination of thrombocytopenia, consumptive coagulopathy and haemolytic anaemia.

On US exam haemangioendothelioma typically appears as complex solid hepatic lesions with a heterogeneous echotexture, but predominantly hypoechoic (Roos et al. 2003). Doppler colour flow may be marked, depending on the amount of AV shunting (Fig. 21.24). During involution the mass can increase in echogenicity as it decreases in size. Haemoperitoneum may be present. If multiple haemangioendotheliomas are present in the liver, the disease has an unfavourable prognosis.

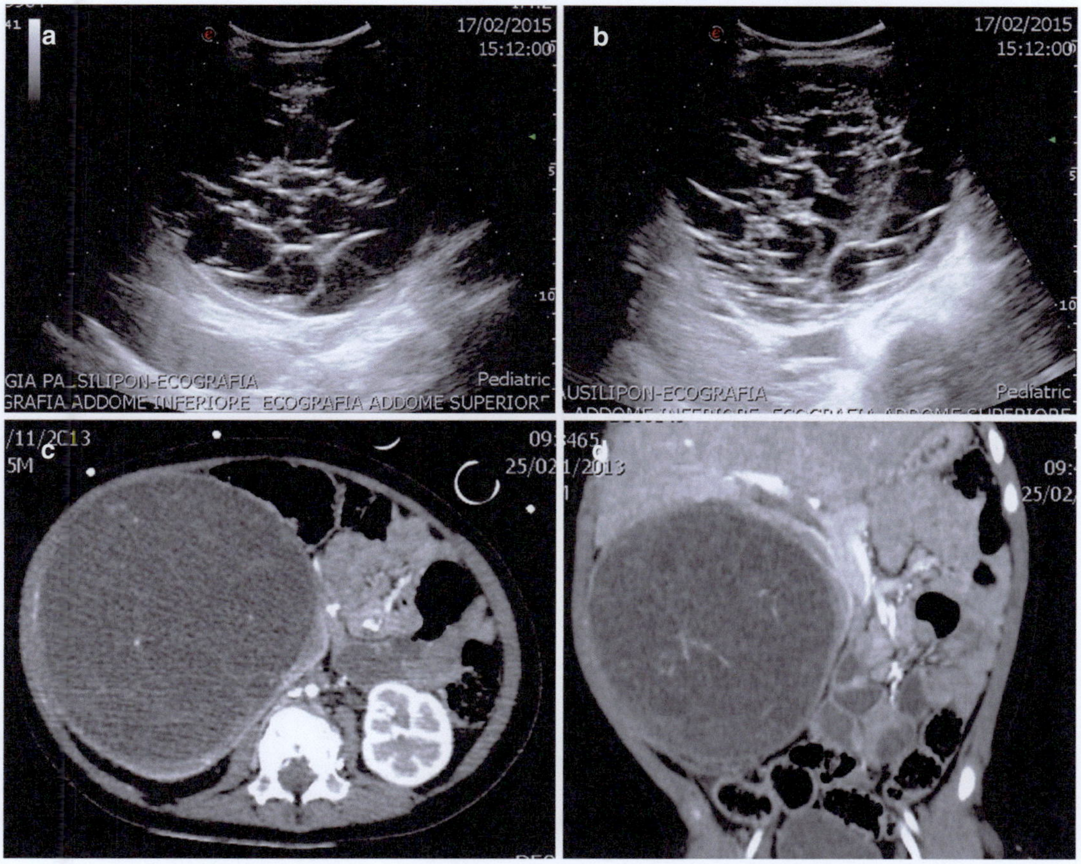

Fig. 21.23 Male, 2 years old, arrives in emergency department with a palpable mass in the right abdomen. US images (**a**, **b**): a pluriconcamerate cystic mass with right renal origin is depicted. CT scans (**c**) and MPR coronal reconstruction (**d**) show a low-attenuation cystic right renal mass with thick septations. A right renal cystic nephroblastoma was discovered

Spontaneous regression is common in patients who have a single hepatic haemangioendothelioma (Selby et al. 1994).

Various therapeutic approaches could be considered: steroids, interferon and chemotherapy; embolization and surgery are reserved for patients who have severe complications.

21.7.3 Sacrococcygeal Teratoma

Sacrococcygeal teratoma (ST) is often diagnosed prenatally because of the typical exophytic component protruding from the foetal buttock; it has a female predilection of at least 3:1 (Pantoja et al. 1976).

STs are classified by the presence or absence of internal (presacral) or external components. Serum alpha-fetoprotein levels are typically elevated with ST.

On US, CT and MR exams, ST shows variable patterns of solid and cystic areas, typically with foci of calcification and fat, and portions of cystic or necrotic areas (Figs. 21.25 and 21.26). The imaging appearance of ST cannot definitively be used to predict histology; however generally benign tumours are more likely to be cystic and malignant tumours are more likely to be solid (Keslar et al. 1994; Miele et al. 1999).

Surgical excision is the recommended treatment, with the addition of chemotherapy when malignancy is established.

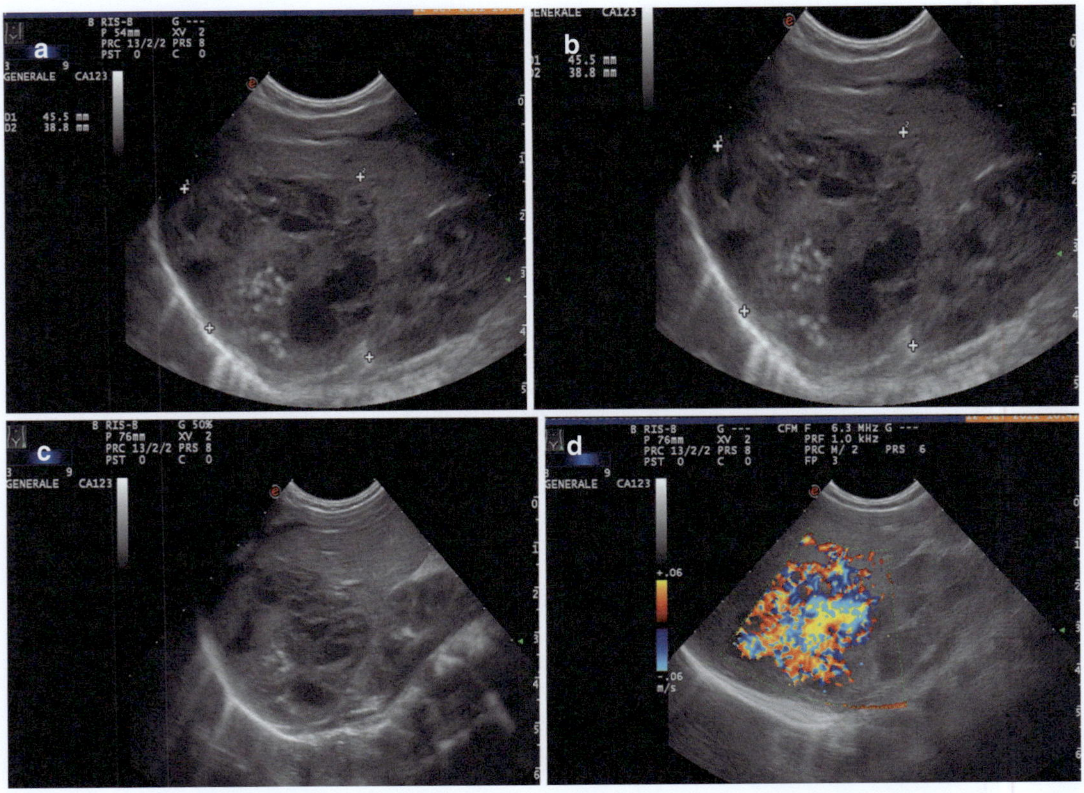

Fig. 21.24 Male, 8-day years old. He arrives with a palpable right-upper quadrant mass and a prenatal diagnoses of adrenal mass. The US images show a solid hepatic lesion with a heterogeneous echotexture, but predominantly hypoechoic. Doppler colour flow (**d**) is marked for the presence of multiple AV shuntings

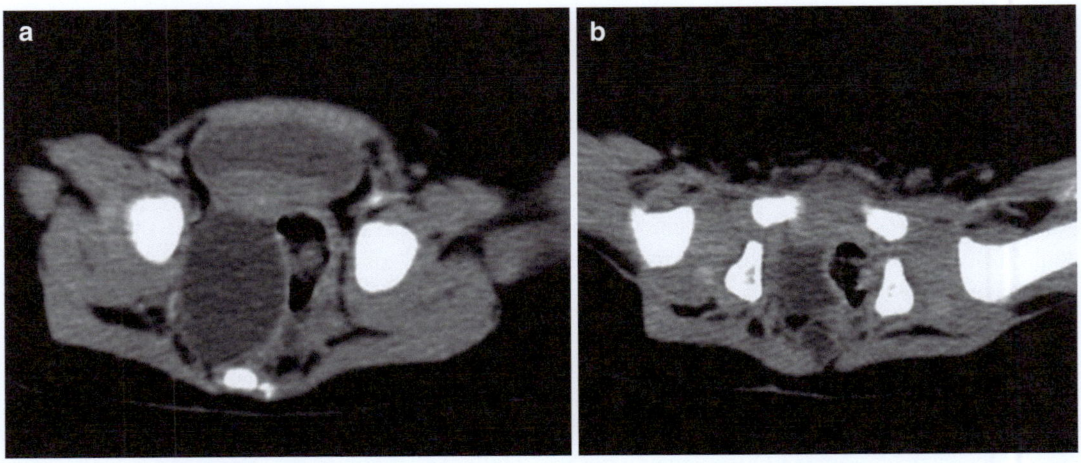

Fig. 21.25 Female, 11-month years old. CT images show a predominantly cystic sacrococcygeal mass. A sacrococcygeal teratoma was then diagnosed

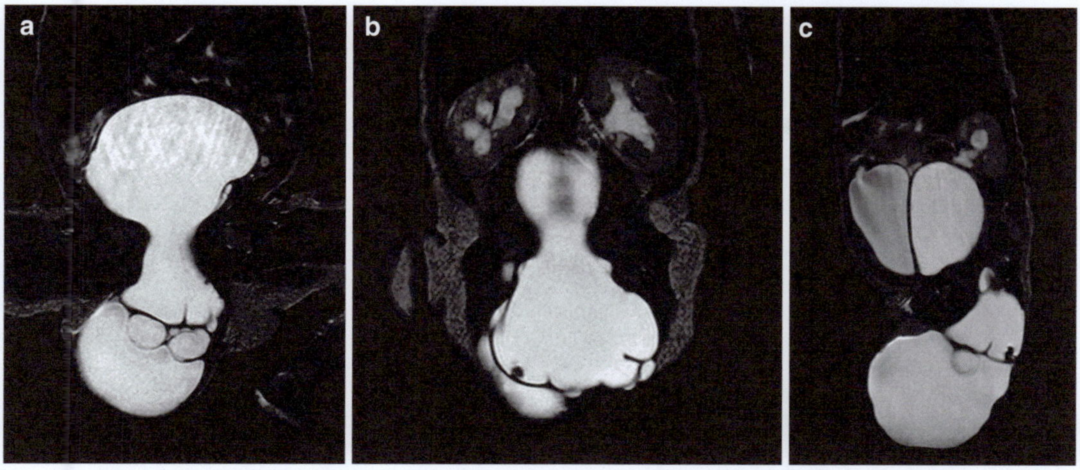

Fig. 21.26 Female. 1 year old. T2w coronal (**a**, **b**) and sagittal (**c**) images show a very large, pluriconcamerate, cystic mass with sacrococcygeal origin, extended to the mesogastrium. A sacrococcygeal teratoma was demonstrated

References

Abramson SJ (1997) Adrenal neoplasms in children. Radiol Clin North Am 35:1415–1453

Agrons GA, Wagner BJ, Lonergan GJ et al (1997) Genitourinary rhabdomyosarcoma in children: radiologic-pathologic correlation. Radiographics 17:919–937

Andrich MP, Shalaby-Rana E, Movassaghi N, Majd M (1996) The role of 131 iodine-metaiodobenzylguanidine scanning in the correlative imaging of patients with neuroblastoma. Pediatrics 97:246–250

Aronson MR, Smoker WR, Oetting GM (1995) Hemorrhagic intracranial parenchymal metastases from primary retroperitoneal neuroblastoma. Pediatr Radiol 25:284–285

Bagolan P, Rivosecchi M et al (1992) Prenatal diagnosis and clinical outcome of ovarian cysts. J Pediatr Surg 27:879–881

Beckwith JB (1998) Children at increased risk for Wilms tumor: monitoring issues. J Pediatr 132:377–379

Berthold F, Brandies WE, Lampert F (1996) Neuroblastoma: diagnostic advances and therapeutic results in 370 patients. Monogr Paediatr 18:206–223

Biasotti S, Garaventa A, Villavecchia GP, Cabria M, Nantron M, De Bernardi B (2000) False-negative metaiodobenzylguanidine scintigraphy at diagnosis of neuroblastoma. Med Pediatr Oncol 35:153–155

Billmire DF (2006) Malignant germ cell tumors in childhood. Semin Pediatr Surg 15:30–36

Billmire D, Vinocur C, Rescorla F et al (2004) Children's Oncology Group (COG) Outcome and staging evaluation in malignant germ cell tumors of the ovary in children and adolescents: An intergroup study. J Pediatr Surg 39:424–429

Black CT (1998) Neuroblastoma. In: Andrassy R (ed) Pediatric surgical oncology. WB Saunders, Philadelphia, pp 175–211

Brammer HM III, Buck JL, Haye WS et al (1990) From the archives of the AFIP. Malignant germ cell tumors of the ovary: radiologic-pathologic correlation. RadioGraphics 10:715–724

Breslow NE, Olson J, Moksness J (1996) Familial Wilms' tumor: a descriptive study. Med Pediatr Oncol 27:398–403

Brodeur GM (1995) Molecular basis for heterogeneity in human neuroblastomas. Eur J Cancer 31A:505–510

Brodeur GM, Seeger RC, Barrett A (1988) International criteria for diagnosis, staging and response to treatment in patients with neuroblastoma. J Clin Oncol 6:1874–1881

Broduer GM, Seeger RC, Schwab M et al (1994) Amplification of N-myc in untreated human neuroblastomas correlates with advanced disease stage. Science 224:1121–1124

Broduer GM, Maris JM, Yamashiro DJ et al (1997) Biology and genetics of human neuroblastomas. J Pediatr Hematol Oncol 19:93–101

Brouder GM, Pritchard J, Berthold F et al (1993) Revisions in the international criteria for neuroblastoma diagnosis, staging and response to treatment. J Clin Oncol 11:1466–1477

Buy JN, Ghossain MA, Moss AA et al (1989) Cystic teratoma of the ovary: CT detection. Radiology 171:697–701

Calisti A, Oriolo L, Molle P, Miele V, Spagnol L (2012) Neonatal adrenal masses: do we have reliable criteria for differential diagnosis and expectant management? Minerva Pediatr 64:313–318

Caruso PA, Marsh MR et al (1971) An intense clinicopathological study of 305 teratomas of the ovary. Cancer 27:343–348

Charles AK, Vujanic GM, Berry PJ (1998) Renal tumours of childhood. Histopathology 32:293–309

Couanet D, Geoffray A, Hartmann O, Leclere JG, Lumbroso JD (1988) Bone marrow metastases in children's neuroblastoma studied by magnetic resonance imaging. Prog Clin Biol Res 271:547–555

Crist WM, Kun LE (1991) Common solid tumors of childhood. N Engl J Med 324:461–471

Di Giacomo V, Trinci M, Van der Byl G, Catania VD, Calisti A, Miele V (2015) Ultrasound in newborns and children suffering from nontraumatic acute abdominal pain: imaging with clinical and surgical correlation. J Ultrasound 18:385–393. doi:10.1007/s40477-014-0087-4. Epub 2014 Apr 9

Dietrich RB, Kangarloo H, Lenarsky C, Feig SA (1987) Neuroblastoma: the role of MR imaging. AJR Am J Roentgenol 148:937–942

Dodd GD, Budzik RF (1990) Lipomatous tumors of the pelvis in women: spectrum of imaging findings. AJR Am J Roentgenol 155:317–322

Douglass EC, Reynolds M, Finegold M et al (1993) Cisplatin, vincristine, and fluorouracil therapy for hepatoblastoma: a Pediatric Oncology Group study. J Clin Oncol 11:96–99

Dresler S, Harvey DG, Levisohn PM (1979) Retroperitoneal neuroblastoma widely metastatic to the central nervous system. Ann Neurol 5:196–198

Evans AE, Siber JH, Shipilsky A et al (1996) Successful management of low stage neuroblastoma without adjuvant therapies: a comparison of two decades, 1972 through 1981 and 1982 through 1992, in a single institution. J Clin Oncol 14:2504–2510

Feusner JH, Ortega J, Haas J, Quinn J, King A, Ablin A et al (1997) Hepatoblastoma in premature infants. Proc Am Soc Clin Oncol 16:525a

Fishman EK, Harman DS, Goldman SM et al (1983) The CT appearance of Wilms' tumor. J Comput Assist Tomogr 7:659–665

Fragkandrea I, Nixon JA, Panagopoulou P (2013) Signs and symptoms of childhood cancer: a guide for early recognition. Am Fam Physician 88:185–192

Frappaz D, Giammarile F, Thiesse P et al (1997) False positive MIBG scan. Med Pediatr Oncol 29:589–592

Ganguly A, Gribble J, Tune B et al (1973) Renin-secreting Wilms' tumor with severe hypertension: report of a case and brief review of renin-secreting tumors. Ann Intern Med 79:835–837

Gilday DL, Ash JM, Reilly BJ (1977) Radionuclide skeletal survey for pediatric neoplasms. Radiology 123:399–406

Golden CB M.D., Feusner JH M.D. (2002) Malignant abdominal masses in children: quick guide to evaluation and diagnosis. Pediatr Clin N Am 49:1369–1392

Graham-Pole J, Salmi T, Anton AH et al (1983) Tumor and urine catecholamines (CATS) in neurogenic tumors. Correlations with other prognostic factors and survival. Cancer 51:834–839

Green DM (2008) Chemotherapy for the treatment of children and adolescents with malignant germ cells tumors (GCT). J Clin Oncol 20:3297–3298

Green DM, D'Angio GL, Beckwith JB et al (1996) Wilms' tumor. CA Cancer J Clin 46:46–63

Grundy P, Koufos A, Morgan K et al (1988) Familial predisposition to Wilms' tumor does not map to the short arm of chromosome 11. Nature 336:374–376

Guinet C, Buy JN, Ghossain MA et al (1993) Fat suppression technique in MR imaging of mature ovarian teratomas: comparison with CT. Eur J Radiol 17:117–121

Hattner RS, Huberty JP, Engelstad BL, Gooding CA, Ablin AR (1984) Localization of m-iodo(131I)-benzylguanidine in neuroblastoma. AJR Am J Roentgenol 143:373–374

Heisel MA, Miller JH, Reid BS, Siegel SE (1983) Radionuclide bone scan in neuroblastoma. Pediatrics 71:206–209

Imaoka I, Sugimura K, Okizuka H et al (1993) Ovarian cystic teratomas: value of chemical fat saturation magnetic resonance imaging. Br J Radiol 66:994–997

Joshi VV, Cantor AB, Altshuler G et al (1992) Age-linked prognostic categorization based on a new histologic grading system of neuroblastomas: a clinopathologic study of 211 cases from the Pediatric Oncology Group. Cancer 69:2197–2211

Kammer BF, Matthay KK, Pacharn P et al (2001) Pulmonary metastases at diagnosis of neuroblastoma in pediatric patients: CT findings and prognosis. AJR Am J Roentgenol 176:755–759

Kenny BJ, Pizer BL, Duncan AW, Foreman NK (1995) Cystic cerebral neuroblastoma. Pediatr Radiol 25(suppl 1): S97–S98

Keslar PJ, Buck JL, Suarez ES (1994) Germ cell tumors of the sacrococcygeal region: radiologic pathologic correlation. Radiographics 14:607–620

Kimura I, Togashi K et al (1994) Ovarian torsion: CT and MRI imaging appearances. Radiology 190: 337–341

King D, Goodman J, Hawk T, Boles ET, Sayers MP (1975) Dumbbell neuroblastomas in children. Arch Surg 110:888–891

Kingston JE, Herbert A, Draper GJ et al (1983) Association between hepatoblastoma and polyposis coli. Arch Dis Child 58:959–962

Kinnier-Wilson LM, Draper GJ (1974) Neuroblastoma, its natural history and prognosis: a study of 487 cases. BMJ 3:301–307

Kramer K, Kushner B, Heller G et al (2001) Neuroblastoma metastatic to the central nervous system. Cancer 91:1510–1519

Kushner BH, Cheung NK, LaQuaglia P et al (1996) Survival from locally invasive or widespread neuroblastoma without cytotoxic therapy. J Clin Oncol 14:373–381

Laug WE, Siegel SE, Shaw KNF et al (1978) Initial urinary catecholamine metabolite concentrations and prognosis in neuroblastoma. Pediatrics 62:77–83

Li FP, Thurber WA, Seddon J et al (1987) Hepatoblastoma in families with polyposis coli. JAMA 257:2475–2477

Lonergan GJ, Martinez-Leon MI, Agrons GA, Montemarano H, Suarez ES (1998) Nephrogenic rests,

nephroblastomatosis, and associated lesions of the kidney. RadioGraphics 18:947–968
Malkasian GD, Symmonds GD, Dockerty MB (1965) Malignant ovarian teratomas. Obstet Gynecol 25: 810–814
Marsden HB, Lawler W (1983) Primary renal tumors in the first year of life. A population-based review. Virchows Arch A Pathol Anat Histopathol 399:1–9
Marten DF, Kirks DR (1985) Diagnostic imaging of pediatric abdominal masses. Pediatr Clin North Am 32: 1397–1425
Matthay KK (1995) Neuroblastoma: a clinical challenge and biologic puzzle. CA Cancer J Clin 45:179–192
Matthay KK, Sather HN, Seeger RC et al (1989) Excellent outcome of stage II neuroblastoma is independent of residual disease and radiation therapy. J Clin Oncol 7:236–244
Matthay KK, Lukens J et al (1994) Outcome and prognostic factors for 1008 children with neuroblastoma treated from 1989–1995 on Children's Cancer Group (CCG) protocols. 6th symposium on Advances in Neuroblastoma Research. Philadelphia, PA, May 13–15, 1993. Prog Clin Biol Res 385:1–448
Matz MH (1961) Benign cystic teratomas of the ovary. Obstet Gynecol Surv 16:591–605
Maurer HM, Beltangady M, Gehan EA et al (1988) The intergroup rhabdomyosarcoma study I: a final report. Cancer 61:209–220
Menichini G, Sessa B, Trinci M, Galluzzo M, Miele V (2015) Accuracy of contrast-enhanced ultrasound in the identification and characterization of traumatic solid organ lesions in children: a retrospective comparison with baseline-US and CE-MDCT. Radiol Med 120:989–1001
Miele V, Di Giampietro I (2014) Diagnostic Imaging in Emergency. Salute e Società, (2EN):127–138. doi: 10.3280/SES2014-002010EN
Miele V, Morucci M, Bibbolino C, Calisti A, De Medici L, Valenti M (1996) Imaging diagnosis in a case of adrenal cystic ganglioneuroblastoma in a child. Radiol Med 91:485–458
Miele V, Galluzzo M, Bellussi A, Valenti M (1998a) Spiral computerized tomography in the study of renal neoplasms in children. Radiol Med 95:486–492
Miele V, Galluzzo M, Cortese A, Patti G, Bellussi A (1998b) Spiral CT study in a case of multifocal hepatoblastoma with atypical features. Radiol Med 95:386–388
Miele V, Stasolla A, Sergi D, Adami L, Calisti A (1999) A neonatal sacrococcygeal teratoma studied by spiral computed tomography. A case report. Radiol Med 98:401–403
Miele V, Andreoli C, Cortese A, De Cicco ML, Luzietti M, Stasolla A, David V (2002) Hemoperitoneum following ovarian cyst rupture: CT usefulness in the diagnosis. Radiol Med 104:122–126
Miele V, Andreoli C, Grassi R (2006) The management of emergency radiology: key facts. Eur J Radiol 59:311–314
Miele V, Di Giampietro I, Ianniello S, Pinto F, Trinci M (2015) Diagnostic imaging in pediatric polytrauma management. Radiol Med 120:33–49
Miele V, Piccolo CL, Sessa B, Trinci M, Galluzzo M (2016a) Comparison between MRI and CEUS in the follow-up of patients with blunt abdominal trauma managed conservatively. Radiol Med 121:27–37
Miele V, Piccolo CL, Galluzzo M, Ianniello S, Sessa B, Trinci M (2016b) Contrast enhanced ultrasound (CEUS) in blunt abdominal trauma. Br J Radiol 89(1061):20150823. doi:10.1259/bjr.20150823Epub2016Jan8
Miele V, Piccolo CL, Trinci M, Galluzzo M, Ianniello S, Brunese L (2016c) Diagnostic imaging of blunt abdominal trauma in pediatric patients. Radiol Med 121:409–430. doi:10.1007/s11547-016-0637-2. Epub 2016 Apr 13
Morris JA, Shcochat SJ, Smith EI et al (1995) Biological variables in thoracic neuroblastoma: a pediatric oncology group study. J Pediatr Surg 30:296–302, discussion: 302-303
Nitschke R, Smith EI, Shochat S et al (1988) Localized neuroblastoma treated by surgery: a Pediatric Oncology Group study. J Clin Oncol 6:1271–1279
Occhipinti KA, Frankel SD, Hricak H (1993) The ovary: computed tomography and magnetic resonance imaging. Radiol Clin North Am 31:1115–1132
Outwater EK, Dunton CJ (1995) Imaging of the ovary and adnexa: clinical issues and applications of MR imaging. Radiology 194:1–18
Pantoja E, Llobet R, Gonzalez-Flores B (1976) Retroperitoneal teratoma: histological review. J Urol 115:520–523
Patel MD, Feldstein VA, Lipson SD et al (1998) Cystic teratomas of the ovary: diagnostic value of sonography. AJR Am J Roentgenol 171:1061–1065
Perez CA, Matthay KK et al (2000) Biologic variables in the outcome of stages I and II neuroblastoma treated with surgery as primary therapy: a Children's Cancer Group study. J Clin Oncol 18:18–26
Pinto E, Guinard JP (1995) Renal masses in the neonate. Biol Neonate 68:175–184
Pinto F, Miele V, Scaglione M, Pinto A (2014) The use of contrast-enhanced ultrasound in blunt abdominal trauma: advantages and limitations. Acta Radiol 55:776–784
Pinto F, Valentino M, Romanini L, Basilico R, Miele V (2015) The role of CEUS in the assessment haemodynamically stable patients with blunt abdominal trauma. Radiol Med 120:3–11
Quinn SF, Erickson S, Black WC (1985) Cystic ovarian teratomas: the sonographic appearance of the dermoid plug. Radiology 155:477–478
Rescorla FJ (2008) Malignant germ cell tumors. In: Carachi R, Grosfeld JL, Azmy AF (eds) The surgery of childhood tumors, 2nd edn. Springer –Verlag, Heidelberg, pp 261–273
Rescorla FJ (2012) Pediatric germ cell tumors. Semin Pediatr Surg 21:51–60

Riccabona M (2003) Imaging of renal tumours in infancy and childhood. Eur Radiol 13(Suppl 4):L116–L129

Roos JE, Pfiffner R, Stallmacj T et al (2003) Infantile hemangioendothelioma. Radiographics 23:1649–1655

Schnater JM, Kohler SE, Lamers WH et al (2003) Where do we stand with hepatoblastoma? A review. Cancer 98:668–678

Seeger RC, Brodeur GM, Sather H et al (1985) Association of multiple copies of the N-myc oncogene with rapid progression of neuroblastomas. N Engl J Med 313:1111–1116

Selby DM, Stocker JT, Waclawiw MA et al (1994) Infantile hemangioendothelioma of the liver. Hepatology 20:39–45

Sessa B, Trinci M, Ianniello S, Menichini G, Galluzzo M, Miele V (2015) Blunt abdominal trauma: role of contrast-enhanced ultrasound in the detection and staging of abdominal traumatic lesions compared with US and CE-MDCT. Radiol Med 120: 180–189

Shalaby-Rana E, Majd M, Andrich MP, Movassaghi N (1997) In-111 pentetreotide scintigraphy in patients with neuroblastoma: comparison with I-131 MIBG, Nmyc oncogene amplification, and patient outcome. Clin Nucl Med 22:315–319

Shimada H, Ambros IM, Dehner LP (1999) The international neuroblastoma pathology classification (the Shimada system). Cancer 86:364–372

Shulkin BL, Shapiro B, Hutchinson RJ (1992) Iodine-131-metaiodobenzylguanidine and bone scintigraphy for the detection of neuroblastoma. J Nucl Med 33:1735–1740

Siegel MJ, Jamroz GA, Glazer HS, Abramson CL (1986) MR imaging of intraspinal extension of neuroblastoma. J Comput Assist Tomogr 10:593–595

Stark DD, Moss AA, Brasch RC et al (1983) Neuroblastoma: diagnostic imaging and staging. Radiology 148:101–105

Sutton CL, McKinney CD et al (1992) Ovarian masses revisited: radiologic and pathologic correlation. Radiographics 12:853–877

Talerman A (1994) Germ cell tumors of the ovary. In: Kurman RJ (ed) Blaustein's pathology of the female genital tract, 4th edn. Springer, New York, pp 849–914

Templeman CL, Fallat ME (2005) Benign ovarian masses. Semin Pediatr Surg 14:93–99

Togashi K, Nisghimura K, Itoh K et al (1987) Ovarian cystic teratomas: MR imaging. Radiology 162:669–673

Von Allmend D (2005) Malignant lesions of the ovary in childhood. Semin Pediatr Surg 14:100–105

White KS, Grossman H (1991) Wilms' and associated renal tumors of childhood. Pediatr Radiol 21:81–88

MDCT and MRI Protocols in Pediatric Non-traumatic Abdominal Emergencies

22

Michele Scialpi, Maria Elena Latini, Sara Riccioni, Valeria Rondoni, Riccardo Torre, Lucia Mariotti, Alfredo D'Andrea, Raffaele Schiavone, and Lucia Manganaro

22.1 Introduction

Non-traumatic acute abdominal processes include spectrum of medical and surgical conditions in pediatric patient presenting with severe abdominal pain that develops over a period of hours (Stoker et al. 2009).

The causes of these abdominal emergencies include inflammation and ischemia of abdominal organs, obstruction and perforation of a hollow organ, and gastrointestinal bleeding. Children with acute abdomen often present with acute abdominal pain, but vomiting, rectal blood loss, and even sepsis may be the first symptom of severe abdominal pathology. Children are often not able to provide the desired information, which makes recognition of the cause of abdominal complaints more difficult; the consequences of a missed diagnosis may be particularly devastating at a young age (Van Heurn et al. 2014; Carty 2002). Accurate and rapid diagnosis of these conditions helps in reducing related complications (Tseng et al. 2008). Medical and surgical diseases causing abdominal pain in pediatric patients, separate into age groups, are reported in Table 22.1 (Van Heurn et al. 2014; Balachandran et al. 2013).

Imaging is an important part in the evaluation of a child with acute abdomen.

Plain abdominal X-rays and contrast studies may be useful in many situations.

Usually ultrasonography (US) represents first-level method of choice (Stoker et al. 2009; Van Heurn et al. 2014).

Multidetector-row computed tomography (MDCT) is an imaging technique that provides otherwise unobtainable information in US due to the highest sensitivity and specificity in pediatric patients with acute abdominal pain (Tseng et al. 2008). Specific CT imaging protocols, as split-bolus MDCT technique, are designed for children to reduce radiation exposure significantly in comparison to the conventional bi- or multiphasic CT protocols (Scialpi et al. 2015).

Magnetic resonance imaging (MRI) is an attractive modality in patients for whom the risks of

M. Scialpi, MD (✉) • M.E. Latini, MD
S. Riccioni, MD • V. Rondoni, MD • R. Torre, MD
L. Mariotti, MD
Division of Radiology 2 and Nuclear Medicine, Department of Surgical and Biomedical Sciences, Perugia University, S. Maria della Misericordia Hospital, S. Andrea delle Fratte, Perugia, Italy
e-mail: michelescialpi1@gmail.com; michelescialpi@libero.it

A. D'Andrea, MD
Department of Radiology, San Giuseppe Moscati Hospital, Aversa, Caserta, Italy

R. Schiavone, MD
Department of Radiology, Meyer Children Hospital, Firenze, Italy

L. Manganaro, MD
Department of Radiological Oncological and Anatomopathological Sciences Policlinico Umberto I, La Sapienza University of Rome, Viale Regina Elena 324, Rome, Italy

V. Miele, M. Trinci (eds.), *Imaging Non-traumatic Abdominal Emergencies in Pediatric Patients*,
DOI 10.1007/978-3-319-41866-7_22

Table 22.1 Common causes of acute abdomen pain

	Birth to 1 year	Two to 5 years	Six to 11 years	12–18 years
Medical	Infantile colic Gastroenteritis Constipation Urinary tract infection	Gastroenteritis Lower lobe pneumonia Constipation Pharyngitis Urinary tract infection Sickle cell crisis Mesenteric lymphadenitis Henoch-Schönlein purpura	Gastroenteritis Constipation Abdominal tuberculosis Bowel disease Functional pain Lower lobe pneumonia Pharyngitis Urinary tract infection Pneumonia Henoch-Schönlein purpura Mesenteric lymphadenitis Sickle cell crisis	Gastroenteritis constipation Lower lobe pneumonia Pharyngitis Dysmenorrhea Mittelschmerz Pelvic inflammatory disease Inflammatory bowel disease
Surgical	Intussusception Volvulus/malrotation Incarcerated hernia Hirschsprung's disease Necrotizing enterocolitis	Appendicitis Intussusception Volvulus	Appendicitis Cholecystitis Testicular torsion	Appendicitis Ectopic pregnancy Ovarian/testicular torsion

radiation or the potential nephrotoxicity of iodinated contrast agents is major such as pediatric patients. In addition, MRI is an excellent problem-solving modality in certain conditions such as assessment for choledocholithiasis, adnexal and ovarian torsion, appendicitis, and inflammatory bowel disease (Singh et al. 2007; Moore et al. 2016).

We report MDCT and MRI protocols in children with non-traumatic abdominal emergencies.

22.2 Conventional MDCT Protocols

MDCT represents the imaging of the choice in non-traumatic abdominopelvic emergency having significant effects on patient management, and its cost-effectiveness has been proven (Stoker et al. 2009).

Conventional MDCT body protocols in pediatric patients are scarcely reported in the literature (Table 22.2) due to many variables such as different body weight and age, techniques for intravenous contrast material (CM) administration, and variable delays in onset of scanning (Bae 2010; Ruess et al. 1998; Frush et al. 1999, 2001; Roche et al. 1996; Siegel 2008; Bae et al. 2008).

According to these ones, contrast material concentration varies from 240 to 350 mgI/mL, with a concentration for kilogram (kg) of weight variable from 1.5 to 3 mgI/kg (mean 2 mgI/kg), a maximum volume of 120 mL, and flow rates variable from 0.3 to 3 mL/s (mean 2 mL/s).

As regards saline solution, few data are available: Bae et al. suggest 15–20 mL of saline flush after contrast material administration. The rate of contrast material injection is 3–4 mL/s for a 20-G catheter, 1.5–2.5 mL/s for a 22-G catheter, and 1–1.5 mL/s for 24-G catheter (Siegel 2008). In patients with central venous access (double- or triple-lumen catheters or subcutaneous reservoirs with tip in the superior vena cava or right atrium), the contrast material is administered by this way (Frush et al. 1999).

About the use of tracking technique, there is a large variability among the various authors. Despite even more intrinsic variability in contrast enhancement in children and infants, this technique has not been systematically studied in this group. Some authors (Frush et al. 1999; Silverman et al. 1995) conclude that, although

Table 22.2 Conventional CT protocols for pediatric patients

Authors	CM concentration (mgI/mL)	CM (mgI/kg)	Maximum volume CM (mL)	Injection rate (mL/s)	Saline flush (mL)	Bolus tracking	Fixed delay scan for hepatic enhancement
Roche et al. (1996)	320	2	–	1.7–2	–	–	60–70 s from the start of the injection
Ruess et al. (1998)	240	2–3	100–120	1–2	–	Important role optimizing liver imaging	10 s at flow rate of 2 mL/s or 0 s at flow rate of 3 mL/s after the end of the injection
Frush et al. (1999)	300	2	–	0.3–3.5 (mean 1.23) for 20–24 G	–	Helpful but not necessary	10–20 s from the end of the injection
Frush et al. (2001)	300	2	–	2	–	–	20 s after the end of the injection
Siegel et al. (2008)	–	2	125	3–4 (for 20G) 1.5–2.5 (mean 2 for 22 G) 1–1.5 (for 24 G)	–	Suggest for angiographic studies	Chest: 30–40 s from the start of injection or >10 s after the end of the injection Abdomen: 50–60 s from the start of the injection or 10–15 s after the end of the injection
Bae et al. (2008)	350	1.5–1.8	80	2	15–20 (at same injection rate of C.M.	–	60 s from the start of the injection or 20 s after the end of the injection

CM contrast material

bolus tracking is not necessary for obtaining good scans in pediatric patients, it is helpful in infants and young children, particularly those with multisystem disease, by allowing a greater and more consistent hepatic enhancement. Due to the increased radiation exposure, this technique is not routinely used. Some authors restrict the use of bolus tracking to angiographic studies using an enhancement threshold of 100–120 Hounsfield unit (HU) (Siegel 2008).

The timing of hepatic arterial and venous enhancement peak depends on the injection duration. A shorter injection duration (either rapid rate or low-volume injection) results in earlier hepatic enhancement peak, whereas a longer injection duration (slow rate or high-volume injection) produces later hepatic enhancement peak (Siegel 2008).

Hepatic arterial enhancement peak usually occurs within 10 s after the completion of the contrast material injection and hepatic parenchymal enhancement peak within 30 s (Ruess et al. 1998).

Several investigators (Roche et al. 1996; Frush et al. 2001; Bae et al. 2008) recommended an empiric scan delay of 60 s after the start or 15–20 s after the end of the contrast material injection to obtain an excellent hepatic enhancement (an increase of at least 50 HU over baseline unenhanced liver parenchyma) in children between 18 months and 12 years old.

CT scans without contrast material administration are not routinely needed, but they may be helpful in selected instances. Indications for non-contrast studies include identification of calcifications or acute hemorrhage and determination of the attenuation value of a parenchymal lesion, which may be useful in its characterization.

22.3 Split-Bolus MDCT Protocols

In last years, split-bolus MDCT has become an alternative to standard multiphasic or monophasic portal venous phase (PVP), MDCT protocols, and its application in pediatric patients (Miglioretti et al. 2013).

Split-bolus MDCT by splitting intravenous injection of contrast material in double or triple boluses, provides synchronous phase set of images on a single image acquisition maintaining the diagnostic performance of CT and reducing dose radiation to patient.

Recently Thomas et al. (2015) presented a dual bolus intravenous (DBI) contrast technique for single-acquisition imaging of the chest, abdomen, and pelvis, with evaluation of multicompartmental vascular enhancement. A larger initial bolus (two-thirds volume) is followed by a smaller bolus (one-third volume) before imaging the chest, abdomen, and pelvis in a single acquisition, 45–65 s after the start of initial injection. Flow rates and second bolus timing were tailored to the patient weight and contrast volume, using five weight categories. This study demonstrates that a weight-stratified DBI contrast technique improves image quality in pediatric multicompartmental vascular and parenchymal enhancement, avoiding "dual-phase" imaging (Thomas et al. 2015).

We optimized and applied split-bolus single-pass CT protocol in pediatric patients determining both the volume of contrast material and the injection duration for the first and second bolus based on patient weight, similar to Thomas et al., and on the broad clinical experience (Bae 2010; Ichikawa et al. 2006). The total volume of contrast material (2 mL/kg) (the maximum volume used is 110 mL for 55 kg weighing patient) is injected in two boluses providing synchronous hepatic arterial phase (HAP) and hepatic parenchymal enhancement during PVP set of images on a single image acquisition (Scialpi et al. 2014).

The volume of contrast material and first and second bolus of contrast material related to patient weight for single-pass SB-MDCT technique of the abdomen-pelvis are reported in Table 22.3.

The volume of contrast material for the first bolus determines a consistent enhancement of the hepatic parenchyma (always above 50 HU compared to unenhanced CT). This is related to the effects of contrast material recirculation. We obtained an adequate enhancement of liver parenchyma using, as first bolus, 1.2 mL/kg of contrast material containing 320 mgI/mL, with a total dose of 384 mgI/kg (a dose significantly lower than that reported in literature for standard MDCT protocols) (Scialpi et al. 2015; Prokop and van der Molen 2003).

The amount of the second bolus was calculated in pediatric patients with body weight from 15 to 55 kg and ranged from 10 to 44 mL (0.8 mL/kg).

The injection rate differs between the two boluses. The injection rate of the first bolus ranged from 1.0 to 1.5 mL/s, while the second bolus is administered at a rate ranging from 1.5 to 3 mL/s. Each bolus of contrast material is followed by the administration of saline (NaCl 0.9 %) at the same rate of the each bolus. Saline flush improves the contrast enhancement and the efficiency of contrast material use (Scialpi et al. 2015; Prokop and van der Molen 2003).

In the urologic emergencies, MDCT split in dual bolus or MDCT split in triple bolus can be performed. MDCT in triple bolus consist in the injection of three boluses of contrast material (I bolus – half of the amount of the second bolus – followed after 7–8 min by the injection of two boluses) in a single-pass synchronous corticomedullary phase (CMP), nephrographic phase (NP), and excretory phase (EP) is obtained.

22.4 Acquisition Parameters

For split-bolus 64-detector-row CT protocol, the following acquisition parameters were used: slice thickness 2.0–2.5 mm, gantry rotation time 0.75 s, reconstruction interval 1.0–1.25, collimation 64×0.625 mm, pitch 0,935:1 without ECG gating, and 80–100 kVp tube current that was set to the automatic milliampere setting on the bases of the patient's weight. MDCT examinations

Table 22.3 Schematic representation of single-pass SB-MDCT technique of the abdomen-pelvis

<table>
<tr><td>55 kg</td><td>110 mL total volume of CM
66 mL of CM (first bolus) at 1.5 mL/s
15 mL of saline at 1.5 mL/s
44 mL of CM (second bolus) at 3.0 mL/s
15 mL of saline at 3.0 mL/s</td><td>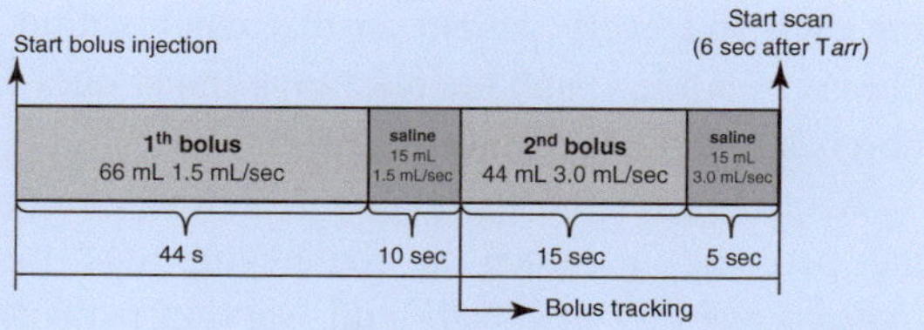
</td></tr>
<tr><td>45 kg</td><td>90 mL total volume of CM
54 mL of CM (first bolus) at 1.3 mL/s
15 mL of saline at 1.3 mL/s
36 mL of CM (second bolus) at 3.0 mL/s
15 mL of saline at 3.0 mL/s</td><td>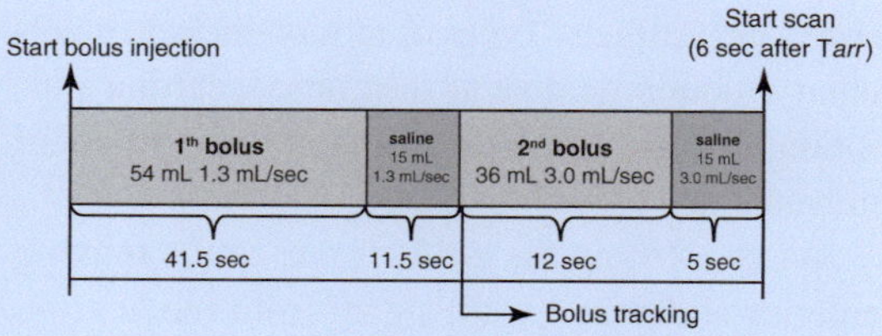
</td></tr>
<tr><td>35 kg</td><td>70 mL total volume of CM
42 mL of CM (first bolus) at 1.2 mL/s
10 mL of saline at 1.2 mL/s
28 mL of CM (second bolus) at 2.0 mL/s
10 mL of saline at 2.0 mL/s</td><td>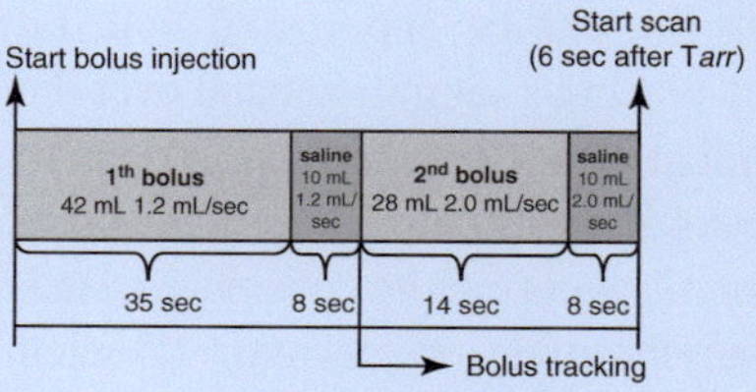
</td></tr>
<tr><td>25 kg</td><td>50 mL total volume of CM
30 mL of CM (first bolus) a 1.0 mL/s
10 mL of saline at 1.0 mL/s
20 mL of CM (second bolus) at 1.5 mL/s
10 mL of saline at 1.5 mL/s</td><td>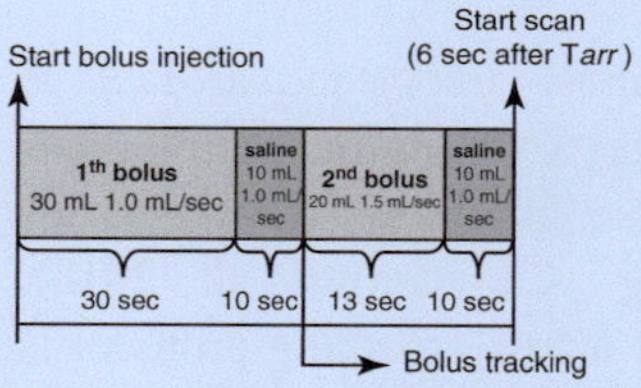
</td></tr>
<tr><td>15 kg</td><td>30 mL total volume of CM
20 mL of CM (first bolus) a 1.0 mL/s
5 mL of saline at 1.0 mL/s
10 mL of CM (second bolus) at 2.0 mL/s
5 mL of saline at 2.0 mL/s</td><td>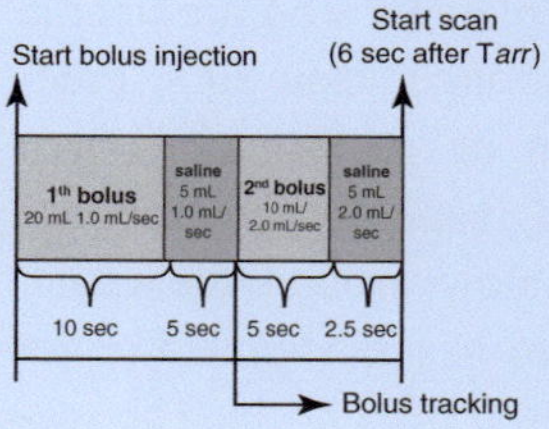
</td></tr>
</table>

CM contrast material, *Tarr* time of the arrival of the CM into the aorta

were completed with sagittal, coronal, and curved multiplanar reconstructions (MPR).

22.5 Dosimetry and Data Storage

Split-bolus MDCT technique, by reduction of the acquisitions, allows an imaging of diagnostic quality with a significant reduction of radiation dose (potentially up to 70 %) and significant reduction from 35 % to 70 % of the number of images produced, compared to the multiphasic techniques, with a twofold important practical impact: (1) reduction of the time of reporting for a minor amount of images to evaluate without affecting the diagnosis and (2) sending to the RIS/PACS of a lower number of images for each patient with obvious advantages in terms of storage and costs.

22.6 MRI Protocols

MRI is a radiation-free imaging tool that allows for acquiring images with a high spatial resolution and excellent soft tissue contrast throughout the body (Nievelstein and Littooij 2016). It is essential to tailor the MRI examination protocol for each and every patient so that examination time is minimized and the relevant clinical question is answered (Singh et al. 2007).

Acquiring diagnostic-quality MR images on the pediatric abdomen is challenging due to motion, inability to breath-hold, varying patient sizes, and artifacts. Types of motion include involuntary motion relative to respiration, cardiac pulsation, or bowel peristalsis and voluntary patient movements.

As concerning the artifacts due to the moving anterior abdominal wall, signal from moving tissues, including fat, can be suppressed with fat saturation or by placing a saturation band over the anterior abdominal wall (Chavhan et al. 2013). To reduce the bowel motility, intravenous injection of an antiperistaltic agent can be considered, such as hyoscine butylbromide or glucagon (Gutzeit et al. 2012).

However, the most important artifact is related to breath, and a variety of motion-compensation technique are now available for abdominal imaging (Chavhan et al. 2013). Actually, the use of a free-breathing protocol is preferable for pediatric patients who are unable to hold their breath for longer than 20 s. Free-breathing protocols can be performed in two ways. In the first method, respiratory tracings are obtained by tying it below around the chest. Images are then acquired in a designated phase of respiration in each respiratory cycle. The second method for respiratory triggering is the navigator technique. In this technique, the position of the diaphragm is detected with a navigator prepulse, and signal acquisition is prospectively or retrospectively gated to a stable portion of the respiratory cycle, typically end expiration. The navigator technique is theoretically more accurate (Chavhan et al. 2013).

With the use of free breathing, the most reproducible position is at the end of expiration. Magnetization-prepared T1-weighted sequences and single-excitation half-Fourier T2-weighted sequences (HASTE) are the mainstay of free-breathing protocols (Singh et al. 2007).

Breath-hold protocols remain the best option for eliminating movement artifacts but need cooperative pediatric patients. Faster sequences like single-shot fast spin-echo (FSE), balanced steady-state free precession (SSFP), and T1-weighted three-dimensional (3D) gradient-echo (GRE) sequences can be performed within short breath-hold times. Faster sequences also have their own limitations. In general, they have reduced signal-to-noise ratio (SNR) and low resolution in comparison with longer sequences (Chavhan et al. 2013).

In the past, MR imaging required long examination times. Currently, with recently introduced high-speed techniques, MR imaging protocols for patients with acute abdominal pain involve examination times shorter than 15 min. A protocol should contain a combination of some longer-acquisition-time higher-resolution sequences and some faster sequences, to keep overall time within reasonable limits (Chavhan et al. 2013).

A typical MR imaging protocol for emergency evaluation of the abdomen includes:

- T1-weighted 2D or 3D GRE
- T2-weighted FSE
- T2-weighted single-shot FSE (half-Fourier rapid acquisition)
- T2-weighted short inversion time inversion recovery (STIR)

T1-weighted sequences are used to define hemorrhagic collections, which have high signal intensity on T1-weighted images. Artifacts due to air, metallic objects, hemosiderin, and calcium deposits are more visible on T1-weighted images obtained with longer echo times (Singh et al. 2007).

T1-weighted 2D GRE (fast low-angle shot [FLASH], spoiled gradient-recalled [SPGR] imaging, T1-weighted turbo field echo [TFE]) can be performed with multiple breath-holds or respiratory triggering (Chavhan et al. 2013).

T1-weighted 3D GRE (volumetric interpolated breath-hold examination [VIBE], liver acquisition with volume acquisition [LAVA], THRIVE) is the fastest T1-weighted sequence and can be performed within a breath-hold. T1-weighted 2D and 3D GRE are usually the best choices for coronal T1-weighted imaging (Chavhan et al. 2013).

Table 22.4 Acquisition parameter at 1.5 T for emergency evaluation of the abdomen in childhood

Sequence	Axial T2-weighted Propeller	Axial T2-weighted FS Propeller	Axial T1-weighted SE Pre-GDTPA with respiratory compensation	Sagittal T2-weighted SS FSE	Coronal T2-weighted SS FSE	Axial T1-weighted SE FS Post-GDTPA with respiratory compensation
Slice thickness (mm)	5.0	5.0	5.0	4.0	4.0	5.0
Gap	0.5	0.5	0.5	0.4	0.4	0.5
Repetition time	11,250	11,250	500	800 (minimum)	800 (minimum)	500
Echo time (ms)	87	87	Min full	102	102	Min full
Field of view (mm)[a]	30	30	30	32	32	30
Matrix	288	288	Freq. 256 Phase 192	Freq. 288 Phase 224	Freq. 288 Phase 224	Freq. 256 Phase 192
NEX	2	2	2	2	2	2
Echo train length	28	28	–	–	–	–

NEX number of excitations, *FS* fat sat, *SE* spin-echo, *SS FSE* single-shot fast spin-echo, *GD-DTPA* gadopentetate dimeglumine

[a]Depends on the patient's body

T2-weighted images of the abdomen are useful for lesion detection and characterization, allowing demonstration of edema and assessment of fluid collections or iron depositions. In fact, T2-weighted images provide excellent depiction of the pancreaticobiliary tree, ascites, pleural effusion, hydronephrosis, and fluid-filled bowel (Singh et al. 2007; Chavhan et al. 2013). T2-weighted sequences, which can be used for abdominal imaging, include T2-weighted FSE, T2-weighted single-shot FSE, and STIR.

STIR and T2-weighted FSE are usually performed with respiratory gating and take a long acquisition time. STIR sequence has lower SNR than T2-weighted FSE but provides more homogeneous fat suppression. Single-shot FSE can be performed during a breath-hold or with respiratory gating, and it is relatively motion insensitive. However, it has lower SNR and less contrast between tissues due to decreased T2 differences (Schneider et al. 2006; Vu et al. 2010; Vasanawala and Lustig 2011). For solid organ imaging of the abdomen, T2-weighted FSE with fat saturation should be preferred over single-shot FSE, whenever feasible (Chavhan et al. 2013). For coronal T2-weighted imaging, STIR with respiratory gating works well in small children and provides better SNR than does single-shot FSE. However, in older children, it does not work as well, due to heavier breathing, and single-shot FSE is a better choice (Chavhan et al. 2013).

In Table 22.4 are the reported acquisition parameters at 1.5 T for emergency evaluation of the abdomen.

Gadolinium-based contrast agents are routinely used intravenously in child, and T1-weighted images with fat saturation are obtained before and after its administration. Gadopentetate dimeglumine-DTPA (GD-DTPA) is not necessary in all patients, and specific sequences may be necessary. In these cases, the evaluation using morphological unenhanced sequences (T1 weighted and T2 weighted) can represent the only modality such as for appendicitis (Singh et al. 2007).

22.7 MR Urography

MR urography (MRU) has been widely accepted as a substitute to intravenous urography (IVU) for urologic emergency (e.g., hydronephrosis) in children after preliminary assessment by US and voiding cystourethrography (VCUG) (Emad-Eldin et al. 2015). MRU allows comprehensive evaluation of the kidneys and urinary tract in children, by providing both morphological and functional information in a one-stop-shop manner without the use of ionizing radiation (Servaes and Epelman 2013; Dickerson et al. 2015).

Pediatric MRU can be used to thoroughly evaluate renal and urinary tract abnormalities that are difficult to identify or fully characterize with other imaging techniques. Common indications for pediatric MRU include evaluation of complex renal and urinary tract anatomy, suspected urinary tract obstruction, complicated infection, tumors, cystic disease, and operative planning.

In the assessment of urinary tract emergencies using MRU, the potential advantages are as follows: multiplanar capabilities, offering excellent anatomic resolution and soft tissue contrast, and not using ionizing radiation (Cerwinka and Kirsch 2010).

Static MRU depicts dilated or obstructed urinary systems, whereas excretory MRU post-contrast imaging (GD-DTPA-enhanced T1-weighted gradient-echo imaging of the kidneys and urinary system) depicts not dilated or not obstructed urinary systems; in addition post-contrast MRU also allows a functional evaluation of the kidneys and urinary tract that includes estimation of differential renal function (Dickerson et al. 2015; Riccabona et al. 2010).

22.8 MR Urography Techniques

Static MRU technique provides axial T2-FSE sequence (TR/TE -/80–110, NEX=3) with fat suppression and respiratory triggering for motion artifact suppression and coronal T2-weighted SS FSE sequence (TR/TE min/90 ms, NEX=1) performed in a slightly angulated coronal orientation over the kidneys, ureters, and bladder.

Excretory MRU technique provides a 1 mg/kg of furosemide given 1 min before contrast material. (CM). A bolus of 0.1 mmol/kg of GD-DTPA is administered followed by 10 mL saline injection. Sequences: axial before CM and coronal T1-weighted fat-suppressed gradient-echo (GRE) sequence or liver acquisition with volume acceleration (LAVA) (TR/TE = min/2.2 ms, flip angle = 15°, NEX=1) before and after the administration of CM to enhance the conspicuity of the ureters. Multiphasic images (corticomedullary phase (CMP), nephrographic phase (NP), and excretory phase (EP) at 8–10 min) are acquired. Images can be obtained during continuous breathing (infant and young children) or during breath-hold (in older cooperative children). The total examination duration was approximately of 30 min. Recently, split-bolus MRU has been proposed providing synchronous visualization of vascular and excretory phase enhancement (Battal et al. 2015). MRU, using contrast material as two separate bolus injections can be used to determine several vascular and urinary collecting system abnormalities (e.g. nutcracker syndrome, crossing renal vessels and retroiliac ureters) (Battal et al. 2015).

In Table 22.5 are the reported acquisition parameters at 1.5 T for MR urography in childhood.

22.9 MR Cholangiopancreatography in Childhood

Small caliber of the pediatric bile ducts and motion artifacts makes difficult to obtain high-quality MR cholangiopancreatographic images. Improved coil technology, increased acquisition speed, refinement in respiratory compensation techniques, and new sequences allow an imaging of diagnostic quality. T2-weighted fast spin-echo (FSE) and single-shot FSE MR imaging sequences with long echo times are used to image biliary and pancreatic ducts. Fat saturation (FS) FIESTA (fast imaging employing steady-state acquisition) sequences tend to highlight biliary fluid.

The use of MR cholangiopancreatography in children is limited by the need for sedation or

Table 22.5 Acquisition parameter at 1.5 T for MR urography in childhood

Sequence	Axial T2-weighted RT Propeller	Coronal T2-weighted SS FSE	Coronal 3D RT SS FSE	Axial 3D LAVA PRE	Coronal 3D LAVA PRE	Coronal 3D LAVA POST
Slice thickness (mm)	5.0	4.0	1.6	4.0	4.0	4.0
Gap	1.0	0–1.0	0	0	0	0
Repetition time (ms)	11,250	Min	[a]	6.8	6.9	6.9
Echo time (ms)	80–110	102	1000	2.1	2.1	2.1
Matrix	288	Freq. 288 Phase 224	Freq. 320 Phase 256	Freq. 320 Phase 224	Freq. 320 Phase 224	Freq. 320 Phase 224
NEX	2	2	1	1	1	1
Field of view (mm)[b]	30	30	30	30	30	30
SAT	Fat	–	Fat	Fat ideal	Fat ideal	Fat ideal
Scan time	2.15 min	00.43 s	–	23 s	23 s	23 s
Flip angle	–	–	–	12–15	12–15	12–15

NEX number of excitations, *SAT* saturation, *RT* respiration triggered, *SS FSE* single-shot fast spin-echo, *LAVA* liver acquisition with volume acceleration
[a]Depends on the patient's breath
[b]Depends on the patient's body

Table 22.6 Acquisition parameter at 1.5 T for MR cholangiopancreatography in childhood

Sequence	Axial T2-weighted RT Propeller	Coronal 3D RT	MRCP T2-weighted SS FSE radial
Slice thickness (mm)	4	1.6	10.0
Gap	0.4	0.0	0.0
Repetition time (ms)	11,250	[a]	6000.0
Echo time (ms)	89	600	900
Field of view (mm)[b]	30	At least 30	At least 30
Scan time	2.15 min	–	1.00 min
Flip angle	–	80	–
Matrix	*288*	Freq. 320 Phase 256	Freq. 192 Phase 192
NEX	2	1	1
Echo train length	28	–	–

NEX number of excitations, *RT* respiration triggered, *SS FSE* single-shot fast spin-echo, *MRCP* magnetic resonance cholangiopancreatography
[a]Depends on the patient's breath
[b]Depends on the patient's body

anesthesia, high cost, limited availability, and long scanning times. Nonetheless, this modality can be a viable alternative to endoscopic retrograde cholangiopancreatography (ERCP).

MR cholangiopancreatography (MRCP) can be useful in the evaluation of various pathologic entities such as choledocholithiasis, choledochal cyst, pancreatitis, Caroli disease, sclerosing cholangitis, adrenal hemorrhage, varices, biliary atresia, and abnormal union of pancreaticobiliary junction (Chavhan et al. 2008).

In Table 22.6 are the reported acquisition parameters at 1.5 T for MR cholangiopancreatography in childhood.

Conclusion

Imaging techniques are becoming increasingly important in the diagnosis of non-traumatic abdominal emergencies of children. In patients with acute abdominal pain, when conventional radiology and US are nondiagnostic or equivocal, MDCT is required, owing to the highest sensitivity and specificity. Only in critical patients an MDCT should be performed without a prior US.

The choice of imaging modality is driven mainly by reducing the radiation dose as much as possible. In this prospective, the interest for split-bolus MDCT, a novel emerging injection protocol, is growing up considering simultaneous and adequate vascular and parenchymal enhancement in single-pass that can be used in non-traumatic abdominal emergencies with lower-dose radiation than conventional multiphasic MDCT (Scialpi et al. 2015).

MR imaging is an attractive modality for diagnostic imaging but is not currently utilized extensively for imaging patients with acute abdominal pain.

Recent studies have demonstrated that MRI is sufficiently accurate to diagnose appendicitis, ureterolithiasis, choledocholithiasis, and inflammatory bowel disease (Singh et al. 2007; Moore et al. 2016). The advantage of MRI over MDCT is that no administration of contrast media is necessary and that there is no ionizing radiation exposure. Disadvantages of MR imaging include its high cost, the limited availability of MR imaging systems and trained radiologists, and the incompatibility of MR imaging systems and the equipment used for intensive care and monitoring of patient status (Singh et al. 2007). The downside is poor literature supporting the use of MRI for abdominopelvic emergencies.

There is a strong need for large prospective cohort studies to better validate the role and cost-effectiveness of split-bolus MDCT and MRI in children with non-traumatic abdominal emergencies both for diagnosis and therapy.

Acknowledgements The authors thank Domenico Mezzasoma, technician in radiology, for his valuable assistance in technical parameters.

References

Bae KT (2010) Intravenous contrast medium administration and scan timing in CT: considerations and approaches. Radiology 256:32–61

Bae KT, Shah AJ, Shang SS, Wang JH, Chang S, Kanematsu M, Hildebolt CF (2008) Aortic and hepatic contrast enhancement with abdominal 64-MDCT in pediatric patients: effect of body weight and iodine dose. AJR Am J Roentgenol 191(5):1589–1594

Balachandran B, Singhi S, Lal S (2013) Emergency management of acute abdomen in children. Indian J Pediatr 80(3):226–234

Battal B, Kocaoğlu M, Akgün V, İnce S, Gök F, Taşar M. Split-bolus MR urography: synchronous visualization of obstructing vessels and collecting system in children. Diagn Interv Radiol 2015;21(6):498–502

Carty HM (2002) Paediatric emergencies: non-traumatic abdominal emergencies. Eur Radiol 12(12): 2835–2848

Cerwinka WH, Kirsch AJ (2010) Magnetic resonance urography in pediatric urology. Curr Opin Urol 20(4):323–329

Chavhan GB, Babyn PS, Manson D, Vidarsson L (2008) Pediatric MR cholangiopancreatography: principles, technique, and clinical applications. Radiographics 28(7):1951–1962

Chavhan GB, Babyn PS, Vasanawala SS (2013) Abdominal MR imaging in children: motion compensation, sequence optimization, and protocol organization. Radiographics 33(3):703–719

Dickerson EC, Dillman JR, Smith EA, DiPietro MA, Lebowitz RL, Darge K (2015) Pediatric MR urography: indications, techniques, and approach to review. Radiographics 35(4):1208–1230

Emad-Eldin S, Abdelaziz O, El-Diasty TA (2015) Diagnostic value of combined static-excretory MR urography in children with hydronephrosis. J Adv Res 6(2):145–153

Frush DP, Spencer EB, Donnelly LF, Zheng JY, DeLong DM, Bisset GS 3rd (1999) Optimizing contrast-enhanced abdominal CT in infants and children using bolus tracking. AJR Am J Roentgenol 172(4): 1007–1013

Frush DP, Donnelly LF, Bisset GS 3rd (2001) Effect of scan delay on hepatic enhancement for pediatric abdominal multislice helical CT. AJR Am J Roentgenol 176(6):1559–1561

Gutzeit A, Binkert CA, Koh DM, Hergan K, von Weymarn C, Graf N, Patak MA, Roos JE, Horstmann M, Kos S, Hungerbühler S, Froehlich JM (2012) Evaluation of the anti-peristaltic effect of glucagon and hyoscine on the small bowel: comparison of intravenous and intramuscular drug administration. Eur Radiol 22(6):1186–1194

Ichikawa T, Erturk SM, Araki T (2006) Multiphasic contrast-enhanced multidetector-row CT of liver: contrast-enhancement theory and practical scan protocol with a combination of fixed injection duration and patients' body-weight-tailored dose of contrast material. Eur J Radiol 58(2):165–176

Miglioretti DL, Johnson E, Williams A, Greenlee RT, Weinmann S, Solberg LI, Feigelson HS, Roblin D, Flynn MJ, Vanneman N, Smith-Bindman R (2013) The use of computed tomography in pediatrics and the associated radiation exposure and estimated cancer risk. JAMA Pediatr 167(8):700–707

Moore MM, Kulaylat AN, Hollenbeak CS, Engbrecht BW, Dillman JR, Methratta ST (2016) Magnetic resonance imaging in pediatric appendicitis: a systematic review. Pediatr Radiol 46(6):928–939

Nievelstein RA, Littooij AS (2016) Whole-body MRI in paediatric oncology. Radiol Med 121(5):442–453

Prokop M, van der Molen AJ (2003) Preparazione del paziente ed impiego dei mezzi di contrasto. In: Prokop M, Galanski M (eds) Tomografia computerizzata spirale e multistrato. Elsevier, Masson, pp 99–109

Riccabona M, Avni FE, Dacher JN, Damasio MB, Darge K, Lobo ML, Ording-Müller LS, Papadopoulou F, Willi U, ESPR uroradiology task force and ESUR paediatric working group (2010) ESPR uroradiology task force and ESUR paediatric working group: imaging and procedural recommendations in paediatric uroradiology, part III. Minutes of the ESPR uroradiology task force minisymposium on intravenous urography, uro-CT and MR-urography in childhood. Pediatr Radiol 40(7):1315–1320

Roche KJ, Genieser NB, Ambrosino MM (1996) Pediatric hepatic CT: an injection protocol. Pediatr Radiol 26(8):502–507

Ruess L, Bulas DI, Kushner DC, Silverman PM, Fearon TC (1998) Peak enhancement of the liver in children using power injection and helical CT. AJR Am J Roentgenol 170:677–681

Schneider G, Grazioli L, Saini S (2006) Techniques for liver imaging. In: Schneider G, Grazioli L, Saini S (eds) MRI of liver: imaging technique, contrast enhancement and differential diagnosis, 2nd edn. Springer, New York, pp 1–15

Scialpi M, Palumbo B, Pierotti L, Gravante S, Piunno A, Rebonato A, D'Andrea A, Reginelli A, Piscioli I, Brunese L, Rotondo A (2014) Detection and characterization of focal liver lesions by split-bolus multidetector-row CT: diagnostic accuracy and radiation dose in oncologic patients. Anticancer Res 34(8):4335–4344

Scialpi M, Schiavone R, D'Andrea A, Palumbo I, Magli M, Gravante S, Falcone G, De Filippi C, Manganaro L, Palumbo B (2015) Single-phase whole-body 64-MDCT split-bolus protocol for pediatric oncology: diagnostic efficacy and dose radiation. Anticancer Res 35(5):3041–3048

Servaes S, Epelman M (2013) The current state of imaging pediatric genitourinary anomalies and abnormalities. Curr Prob Diagn Radiol 42(1):1–12

Siegel MJ (2008) Practical CT techniques. In: Siegel MJ (ed) Pediatric body CT. 2. Lippincott Williams & Wilkins, Philadelphia, pp 1–32

Silverman PM, Brown B, Wray H et al (1995) Optimal contrast enhancement of the liver using helical (spiral) CT: value of SmartPrep. AJR 164:1169–1171

Singh A, Danrad R, Hahn PF, Blake MA, Mueller PR, Novelline RA (2007) MR imaging of the acute abdomen and pelvis: acute appendicitis and beyond. Radiographics 27(5):1419–1431

Stoker J, van Randen A, Laméris W, Boermeester MA (2009) Imaging patients with acute abdominal pain. Radiology 253(1):31–46

Thomas KE, Mann EH, Padfield N, Greco L, Bendavid G, Alzahrani A (2015) Dual bolus intravenous contrast injection technique for multiregion paediatric body CT. Eur Radiol 25(4):1014–1022

Tseng YC, Lee MS, Chang YJ, Wu HP (2008) Acute abdomen in pediatric patients admitted to the pediatric emergency department. Pediatr Neonatol 49(4):126–134

Van Heurn LW, Pakarinen MP, Wester T (2014) Contemporary management of abdominal surgical emergencies in infants and children. Br J Surg 101(1):e24–e33

Vasanawala SS, Lustig M (2011) Advances in pediatric body MRI. Pediatr Radiol 41(suppl 2):549–554

Vu TL, Qureshi W, Turan N, Yonkers S, Stallings C, Semelka RC (2010) Pediatric body MR imaging: our approach. Appl Radiol 39(4):3–19

23 The Radioprotection of the Child in Emergency Radiology

Andrea Magistrellli

23.1 Why Radiation Protection Is Important in Children?

Diagnostic radiation is an effective tool that can save lives, especially in emergency settings. Anyway, ionizing radiation could be detrimental for humans. Furthermore, it is universally recognized that children are not small adults (Strauss 2006). Over the past two decades, special issues have arisen regarding the protection of children undergoing radiological examinations.

In fact children results to be more sensitive than adult, due to fast-growing cells (e.g., high number of cells in mitotic phase), more sensitive tissues (e.g., red narrow in long bones and skull), and long life expectancy during which effect of ionizing radiation can emerge.

Brenner et al. (2001) estimated one death for radiation-induced cancer every 1,200 abdominal or head CT scans, reporting a significant radiosensitivity of children (females more than males) if compared to adult population, particularly at very low doses, with the risk increasing with decreasing age.

Berrington de Gonzales et al. (2009) estimated that 29,000 future cancers and 14,500 future deaths could develop due to radiation from the 72 million CT scans performed in the United States in 2007 (cancer incidence = 0.04 %).

Other more recent retrospective cohort studies on large series (Pearce et al. 2012; Mathews et al. 2013; Miglioretti et al. 2013) correlate CT scans to an increased incidence of leukemia and brain tumors in children. All these studies' conclusions rely on some currently unverified scientific assumptions (e.g., a linear relationship between radiation dose and risk even at very low exposures), and their results could be affected by reverse causation or confounding by indication.

The undoubtful fact is that they highlight the need to maintain radiation doses "as low as reasonably achievable" (ALARA principle) when obtaining justified diagnostic information.

23.1.1 Principles of Medical Radiation Protection

In practice radiation protection of patients relies on meeting requirements that apply two principles adopted in most regulatory systems throughout the world:

- Justification of the practices involved
- Optimization of protection and safety in practices involved in terms of risks, costs, benefits, etc.

A. Magistrellli
Department of Imaging, Ospedale Pediatrico Bambino Gesù, Children's Hospital Bambino Gesù, Rome, Italy
e-mail: andrea.magistrelli@opbg.net

V. Miele, M. Trinci (eds.), *Imaging Non-traumatic Abdominal Emergencies in Pediatric Patients*,
DOI 10.1007/978-3-319-41866-7_23

As reported by the International Commission on Radiological Protection (ICRP), medical exposure might cause an individual detriment so that the principal aim of medical exposures is to do more good than harm to the individual patient (ICRP 103 2007).

Due to that, the cornerstones of medical radiation protection principles (justification and optimization) are an ethical duty of the practitioner, and dosimetry represents a quality index of the individual medical exposure.

All individual medical exposures must be performed under the clinical responsibility of a practitioner that takes into account the efficacy, benefits, and risks of available alternative techniques having the same objective but involving no or less exposure to ionizing radiation.

Individual justification is particularly important in special practices (such as children exposure, CT, or diagnostic/interventional fluoroscopy).

The most effective means to decrease radiation dose associated with pediatric imaging is not to perform unnecessary or inappropriate procedures. In fact, we should consider that justification leads to a 100 % dose savings in not appropriate medical exposure while optimization can only determine a partial ("as low as reasonably achievable") dose reduction.

Evidence-based imaging referral guidelines help radiologists for justification of imaging (Perez 2015), and comparable guidance in different regions of the world could be found (e.g., RCR iRefer 2012, ACR Appropriateness Criteria 2015).

Once examinations are justified, they need to be optimized. The basic aim of the optimization of a radiological procedure is to "taylor" imaging parameters to the individual patient and to the clinical question in such a way that images are obtained with the lowest possible radiation dose and net benefit is maximized. Optimization of the examination involves at least three main aspects: radiological equipment, technical parameters, and their knowledge by operators.

The ICRP has recommended that dose limits not be applied to medical exposures, pediatric radiology included.

Once justified, the exposed individual will derive benefit from the procedure, and medical procedures must lead to a diagnostic result. Using insufficient radiation may increase the risk of misdiagnosis or repeat testing with the attendant exposure to even more radiation (Fig. 23.1).

23.1.2 Effects of Ionizing Radiation

Energy absorbed in tissues and organs exposed to radiation may induce damage to DNA. Despite robust DNA repair mechanisms within the body, radiation exposure can induce cell death or nonlethal transformation of cells.

Most adverse health effects of radiation exposure may be grouped in two general categories:

(a) Deterministic effects, due in large part to the killing/malfunction of cells following high doses and characterized by a threshold dose.
(b) Stochastic effects, such as cancer and heritable effects that are indistinguishable from those caused by other factors.

23.1.2.1 Deterministic Effects

The deterministic effects are clinically observable when the absorbed dose is above a threshold and their magnitude depends on several factors such as the linear energy transfer of the radiation, the dose rate, and the volume of the irradiated part of the organ or tissue. Typical examples are the eye lens cataract, skin erythema, and infertility.

Such effect requires high-absorbed doses, and the probability of its occurrence will rise to 100 % above the threshold dose. Due to these, the deterministic effects can occur in radiation therapy, complex interventional procedures, or "nonoptimized" fluoroscopic procedures.

23.1.2.2 Stochastic Effects

The risks associated with the use of ionizing radiation in diagnostic imaging include almost exclusively *stochastic* effects (e.g., cancer or genetic modifications). These effects are also called "probabilistic" because under certain exposure conditions, these effects may or may not occur,

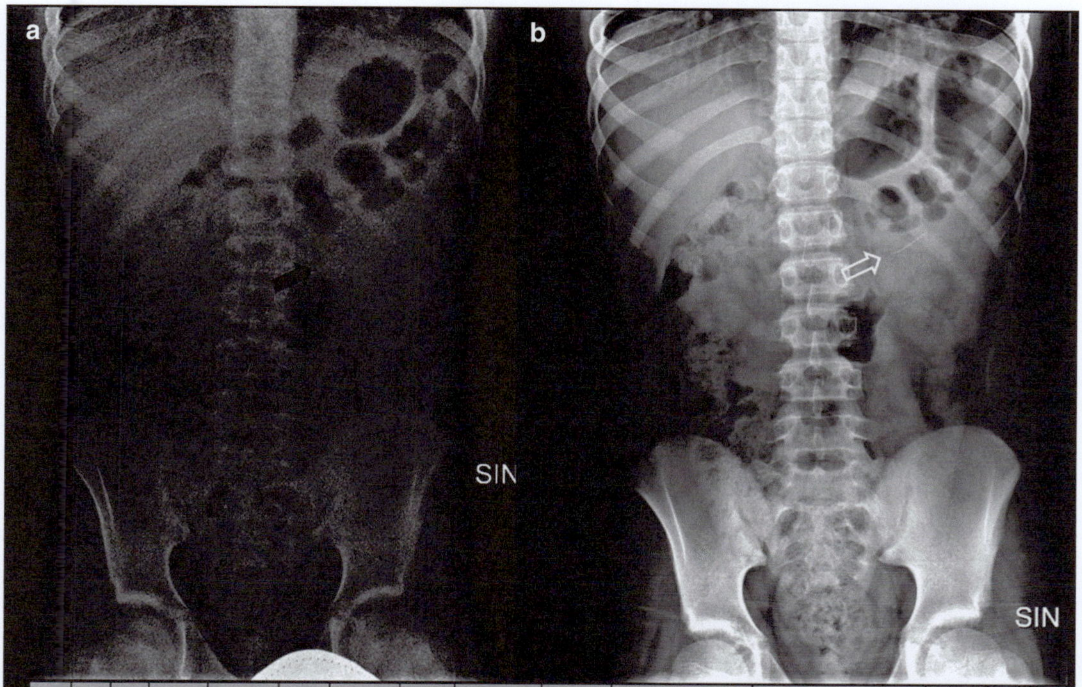

	kV	mAs	ms	Livello...	Lunghezza...	CampoM	Filtro Cu	Formato	Correzione an...	Curva caratt..	Data e ora	Nome programma d'organo	DAP	EXI	Dose p...
a	120.[illegible]	0.5	9	1123	1	m	Cu 0.3 mm	RAD	-2		25-10-2013 22.58.16	RAD_Addome AP_CORPO EST...	1.91	51	102
b	72.[illegible]	25.1	30.9		1		Cu 0.0 mm	RAD	0		25-10-2013 23.09.29	RAD_Addome AP (ADDOME)	133.70	485	7200

Fig. 23.1 Foreign body ingestion. In (**a**) an example of false negative due to an excessive reduction of dose (high kV and low mAs technique, DAP 1.9 cGy*cm^2). In (**b**) repeating exam with standard technique (72.9 kV, 25,1 mAs; DAP 133.7 cGy*cm^2; kV *kilovoltage*, mAs *milliAmperage second*, DAP *Dose-Area Product*) shows the presence of metallic foreign body in the small bowel (*white arrow*), not evident in the previous examination (*black arrow* in **a**)

and there is no threshold. It is assumed that the probability of having these effects is proportional to the absorbed dose, not to its severity.

Indeed, despite the fact that x-rays are officially classified as a carcinogen by the World Health Organization's International Agency for Research on Cancer (Amis et al. 2007), epidemiological and experimental studies provide evidence of cancer radiation risk at doses about 100 mSv (NAS/NRC 2006; Preston et al. 2003, 2012; UNSCEAR 2000).

Below this threshold, there are many uncertainties, and up today it's not feasible to determine, on epidemiological grounds alone, if there is or not an increased risk of cancer following doses less than 100 mSv.

The practical system of radiological protection recommended by the ICRP, based upon dose-response model generally known as "linear non-threshold" (LNT) model, remains a prudent basis for the practical purposes of radiological protection at low doses and low dose rates.

23.1.3 How to Manage the Dose: The DRL Role

The management of the dose is important to have a reference point. To help in the optimization process of medical exposure to patients, the concept of DRLs has been introduced by the ICRP. The IAEA International Basic Safety Standards (BSS) mandate their use (International Atomic Energy Agency 2014).

DRL values are not a dose limit or a dose constrain but advisory values, taken as the third quartile value of national DRL, to establish whether practice is reasonable or not.

In the absence of dose limits, DRLs applicable to pediatric patients need to be considered by radiologists and other practitioners. In practice, they tend to be set so that if the local DRL values involved are exceeded, the radiological procedure involved needs to be investigated.

Currently in Europe, there is a complete lack of national pediatric DRLs in many countries for many examinations, in particular for all pediatric interventional procedures.

Anyway in the near future, all the European countries must review their national DRLs following the new directive 2013/59/Euratom (European Council Directive 2013/59/Euratom 2014) and the draft "European diagnostic reference levels for paediatric imaging PiDRL" sponsored by the European Community (EuroSafe Imaging 2015).

The PiDRL drafts several practical methods to establish pediatric DRLs. The most important are for:

- The dose quantities that should be an easily measurable quantity such as dose index provided by equipment (e.g., Entrance surface dose (ESD) in conventional radiography, Kerma in Aria Product (KAP) in fluoroscopy, Computed-tomography dose-index volume (CTDIvol) and Dose-length product (DLP) in computed tomography)
- The grouping of patients that needs to consider the weight of patients and not their age (e.g., <5 kg, 5–15 kg, etc.)
- Technical equipment parameters

23.2 Technical Aspect of Radiation Protection in Conventional Radiology and Fluoroscopy

23.2.1 General Consideration

Ideally, equipment specifically designed for pediatric patients should be installed; anyway most of the imaging equipments are structured to handle adult patients.

When purchasing new radiographic/fluoroscopic equipment, especially for pediatric use, the following dose reduction measures should be considered: removable grids, last-image hold (LIH), copper filters, pulsed fluoroscopy, and virtual collimation.

Organ protocols with appropriate technique factors (tailored upon child size) for common types of x-ray/fluoroscopic examinations should be pre-installed in each equipment (Fig. 23.2a).

Pediatric patients' size varies in practice, from as small as 500 g to in excess of 100 kg. In order to obtain a diagnostic examination (minimizing the dose), a correct radiographic positioning and use of correct collimation of the primary beam are essential.

23.2.2 Immobilization and Collimation

In uncooperative children, immobilization is required when performing radiographic studies.

A proper immobilization allows a correct beam centering and collimation with a proper shielding of the non-examined parts of the body (Fig. 23.3).

In addition, blurring and motion artifacts are reduced.

Several devices, such as sandbags or sponges, may be used with newborns or toddlers. If the assistance of a person is needed for immobilization, this has to be done by a parent and not, routinely, by a hospital staff.

For individuals directly involved in comforting and caring (not young children or pregnant), the ICRP Publication 103 (2007) indicates that a dose constraint of 1 mSv per episode is reasonable (5 mSv for the duration of a given release after radionuclide therapy).

It is important to use collimation to expose only the area intended for examination (Fig. 23.3).

A too large field will result in unnecessary radiation dose outside the area of interest and increase the scattered radiation, impairing the image contrast and resolution. On the other hand, a too small field may require a second exposure, so that a certain degree of tolerance may be necessary to ensure that the entire field of interest is included.

After child positioning and his immobilization, operators need to collimate the field of view through the "light" for the beam centering (Fig. 23.2d, e).

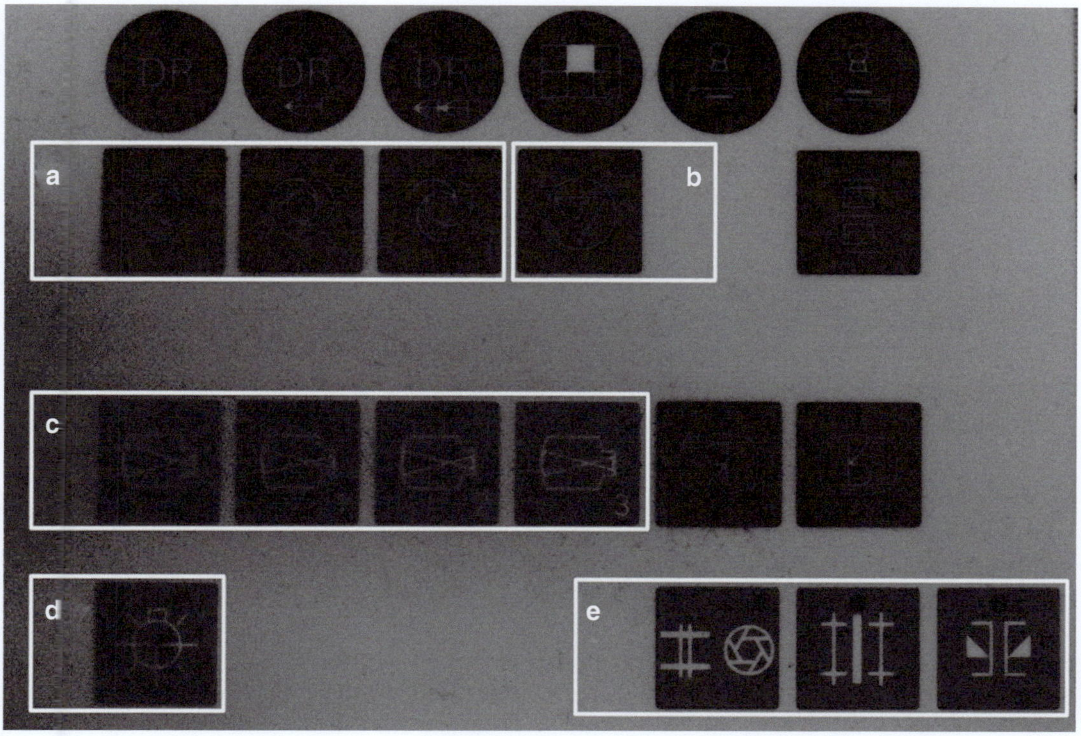

Fig. 23.2 Example of fluoroscopic equipment console. The main functions for the optimization of the procedure are indicated: (**a**) three different kid-size presets, (**b**) block of the technical parameters based upon LIH, (**c**) four different magnification settings (*tip: use larger FOV*), (**d**) "light" beam, a useful tool to optimize collimation without radiation exposure (**e**) different types of shielding

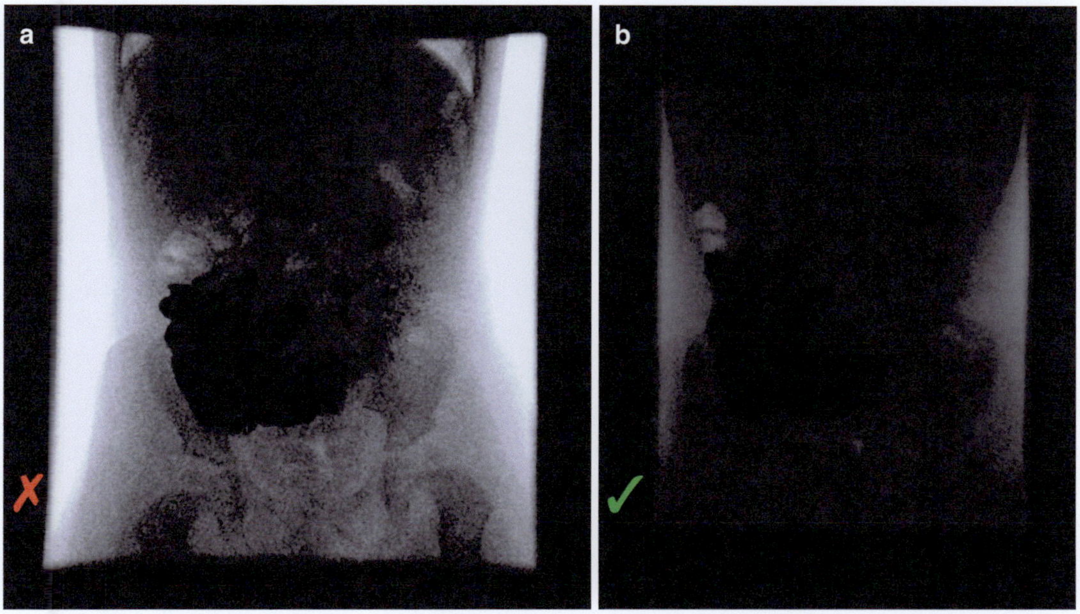

Fig. 23.3 An example of improper (**a**) and correct (**b**) collimation. Note in (**b**) the best image quality due to automatic brightness control (ABC) system, other settings were not modified. A proper collimation avoids the exposure of radiosensitive organs such as the breast and gonads, without the needing of lead shielding

The use of post-processing collimation (e.g., uncollimated examination), fluoroscopy before x-ray examination, or collimation "on the way" during radiation exposure are malpractices that should be avoided, leading to unnecessary radiation exposure.

In particular, the use of post-processing technique, such as manual collimation, can create an image sent to the viewer for interpretation that does not indicate how much of the original picture was actually exposed (cropped out). This has no effect on image quality and patient-absorbed dose but can "crop out" important diagnostic information (Fig. 23.4).

23.2.3 Additional Spectral Filters

The x-ray spectrum includes low-energy photons that are completely absorbed in the patient's skin and do not contribute to image generation. Additional filters could "remove" the low-energy photons reducing the nonproductive radiation and thus patient dose.

Most of x-ray/fluoroscopic equipments used for pediatric have a minimum filtration of 2.5 mm of aluminum. These equipments should have the capacity to add additional filtration (usually copper filters) and to change it easily when appropriate.

Generally an additional copper filtration of 0.1(–0.2) mm in x-ray examinations and 0.2(–0.3) mm in fluoroscopic procedures is adequate. Consider that for standard tube voltages each 0.1 mm of copper is equivalent to approximately 3 mm of aluminum (ICRP 121 2013).

Nicholson et al. (2000) have shown that the addition of 0.1–0.3 mm of copper reduced the skin dose by 30–50 %.

23.2.4 Anti-scatter Grids

Anti-scatter grids increase contrast but also increase radiation dose to the adult patient.

In children anti-scatter grids are normally not necessary due to the smaller size of children (e.g., relatively low scatter radiation produced in the

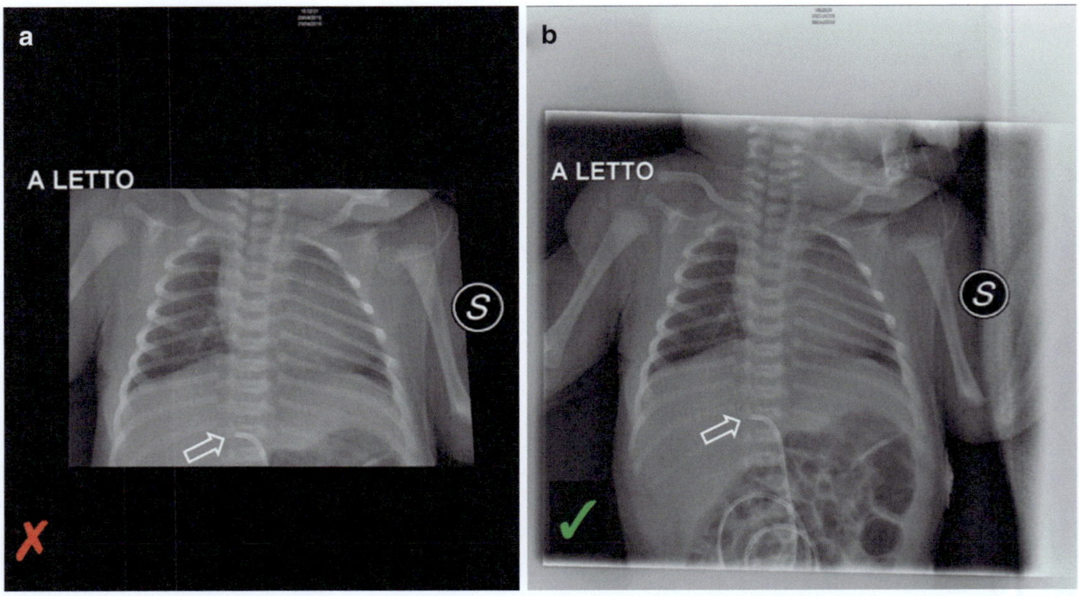

Fig. 23.4 An example of improper use of post-processing manual collimation in chest x-ray. In (**a**) important diagnostic information are cropped out by manual collimation (*white arrow*); in the original image (**b**) a misplacement of umbilical vein catheter in the left intrahepatic portal branch was evident. *Tip: the anatomical parts of the body, once exposed, must not to be cropped out*

irradiated volume) so that removable anti-scatter grid needs to be available (Cook 2001).

They are usually not advisable for abdominal examinations in patients under 3 years of age or, with optimization, younger than 8 years of age (Schneider et al. 2000).

Not using them avoids unnecessary exposure and results in an approximately 50 % reduction in dose (Cook 2001).

23.3 Practical Aspect and Pitfalls in Conventional Radiology

Computed-radiography (CR) and Digital-radiography (DR) offer substantial benefits compared to screen-film radiography (SFR), such as readily available electronic archive and image post-processing that can compensate for under-exposure or overexposure to produce acceptable images. That means a reduced repeat rate of CR/DR images but also a risk of unwitting increase of the patient dose.

Overexposed SFR appears too dark and the examination must be repeated while digital technology can compensate this overexposure by altering brightness and contrast after acquisition, without any recognizable artifact on images (Fig. 23.5).

In DR systems, a feedback regarding the radiographic techniques for a specific exam is given by the exposure index (EI) displayed on images, so that operators need to be confident with them to evaluate whether the image is technically correct or not (Seibert and Morin 2011).

Unfortunately each vendor uses different exposure index values and methods so that radiologists should be confident with them.

The use of automatic exposure control (AEC) system with pediatric patients should be carefully evaluated.

If used pediatric AEC devices need to be selected with respect to the most important region

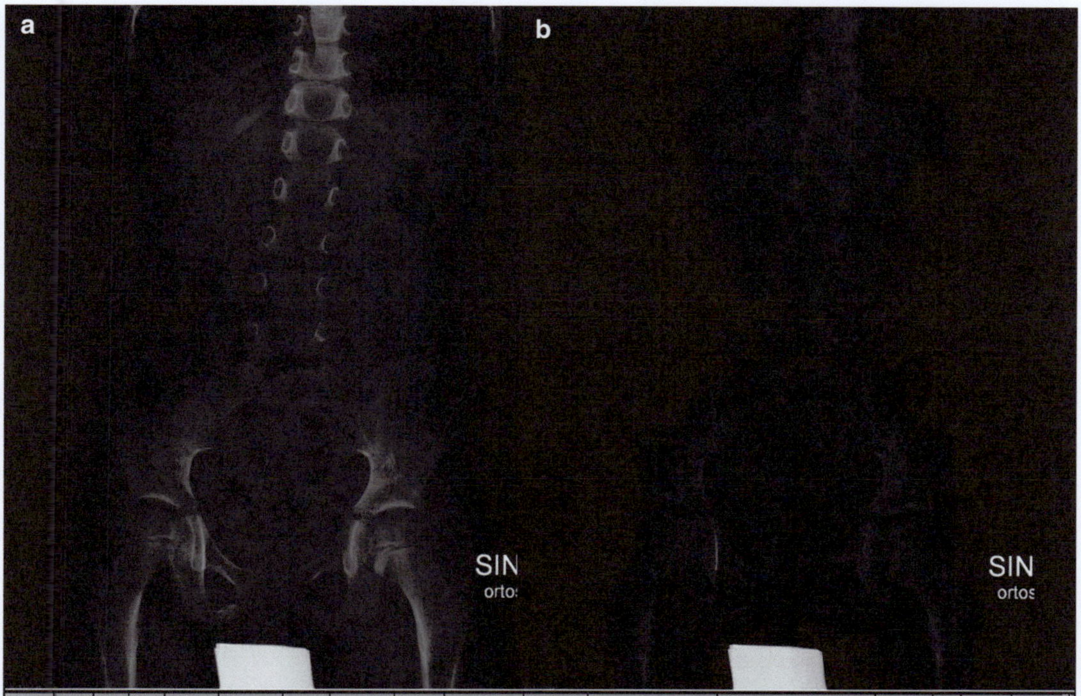

No. i...	kV	mAs	ms	Livello ...	Lunghezza...	CampoM	Filtro Cu	Formato	Correzione an...	Curva caratt.	Data e ora	Nome programma d'organo	DAP	EXI	Dose p...	Fuoco
1	72.9	25.1	31.7		1		Cu 0.0 mm	RAD	0	C70	16-03-2015 4.42.09	RAD_Addome AP (ADDOME)	159.09	1508	8570	Grande

Fig. 23.5 An example of DR overexposure in abdominal x-ray of a 5-year-old male child. Note in (**a**) how the post-processing can compensate the original overexposed image (**b**). *Tip: routinely check the exposure index reported on the images to identify over- or underexposure technique*

of interest, they are very sensitive to patient movement and could length the minimal exposure time affecting image quality and patient dose.

In small children exposure charts corresponding to radiographic techniques (weight based for the trunk or patient size based for the extremities) are easy to use and safer.

Other pitfalls in CR/DR can be caused by unfamiliarity with post-processing algorithms that could decrease displayed image quality.

See Tables 23.1, 23.2, 23.3, and 23.4 for suggested abdominal and chest x-ray technique in children.

23.4 Practical Aspect and Pitfalls in Fluoroscopy

23.4.1 Tube/Image Intensifier Positioning

Radiation dose can be reduced by keeping

1. The tube as far as possible from patient to reduce skin entrance dose
2. The image intensifier as close as possible to the patient (Hiorns et al. 2006)

Table 23.1 Suggested abdominal x-ray AP/PA technique

Age (years)	Kg	Focal spot	Total filtration	kV	mAs	DAP	Grid	AEC
Newborn	<4	Fine	2.5 mm Al + 0.1 mm Cu	65	2	0.4	No	No
Newborn–1	4–10	Fine	2.5 mm Al + 0.1 mm Cu	70	3	0.9	No	No
1–3	10–14	Fine	2.5 mm Al + 0.1 mm Cu	75	3	1.7	No	No
3–5	14–30	Broad	2.5 mm Al + 0.1 mm Cu	85	4	3	Yes	No
5–10	30–50	Broad	2.5 mm Al + 0.1 mm Cu	75	6	7.4	Yes	No
10–15	>50	Broad	2.5 mm Al + 0.1 mm Cu	95	8	36	Yes	No

Table 23.2 Suggested chest x-ray AP/PA technique

Age (years)	Kg	Focal spot	Total filtration	kV	mAs	DAP	Grid	AEC
Newborn	<4	Fine	2.5 mm Al + 0.1 mm Cu	70	2	0.2	No	No
Newborn–1	4–10	Broad	2.5 mm Al + 0.1 mm Cu	73	2.5	0.3	No	No
1–3	10–14	Broad	2.5 mm Al + 0.1 mm Cu	75	2.5	0.5	No	No
3–5	14–29	Broad	2.5 mm Al + 0.1 mm Cu	75	2.5	0.5	No	No
5–10	30–50	Broad	2.5 mm Al + 0.1 mm Cu	75	3.5	1.6	No	No
10–15	>50	Broad	2.5 mm Al + 0.1 mm Cu	80	3	2.9	No	No

Table 23.3 Suggested mobile chest x-ray AP technique in neonatal intensive care units (NICU)

Age (years)	Kg	Focal spot	Total filtration	kV	mAs	DAP	Grid	AEC
Newborn	<1	Fine	2.5 mm Al	60	0.6	–	No	No
Newborn	1–1.5	Fine	2.5 mm Al	62	0.8	–	No	No
Newborn	1.5–2	Fine	2.5 mm Al	64	0.8	–	No	No
Newborn	2–2.5	Fine	2.5 mm Al	65	0.8	–	No	No
Newborn	2.5–3	Fine	2.5 mm Al	68	0.8	–	No	No

Table 23.4 Suggested mobile abdominal x-ray AP technique in neonatal intensive care units (NICU)

Age (years)	Kg	Focal spot	Total filtration	kV	mAs	DAP	Grid	AEC
Newborn	<1	Fine	2.5 mm Al	60	0.5	–	No	No
Newborn	1–1.5	Fine	2.5 mm Al	64	0.5	–	No	No
Newborn	1.5–2	Fine	2.5 mm Al	66	0.5	–	No	No
Newborn	2–2.5	Fine	2.5 mm Al	66	0.8	–	No	No
Newborn	2.5–3	Fine	2.5 mm Al	68	0.5	–	No	No

Usually an undercouch tube positioning is suggested; that positioning minimizes the patient radiation dose and the scattered radiation to the staff. Anyway in children an overcouch tube positioning may have some advantage, it's less frightening for a child and it makes access to the child easier for both the operator and comforters.

If shielding is used for patient protection, it needs to be strategically placed over the patient if an overcouch tube is used or under the patient if an undercouch tube is used.

23.4.2 Ionizing Chamber

Generally a certain amount of radiation (exposure) needs to reach each point on the x-ray detector to maintain an adequate signal/noise ratio on images.

Modern fluoroscopic equipment uses three focal spots, spatial and spectral beam profiling, and system of entrance exposure regulation (Fig. 23.6)

Anyway the use of automatic exposure control (AEC) system or automatic brightness control (ABC) system in fluoroscopy with pediatric patients should be carefully evaluated.

An excessive collimation could exclude lateral focal points with an involuntary overexposure of the patient. A real-time monitoring of the position, shape, and size of the ionization chambers can be done on the LIH image displayed on the monitor (Fig. 23.7).

For the same reason if shielding is used, it should not be placed in the direct beam, as this

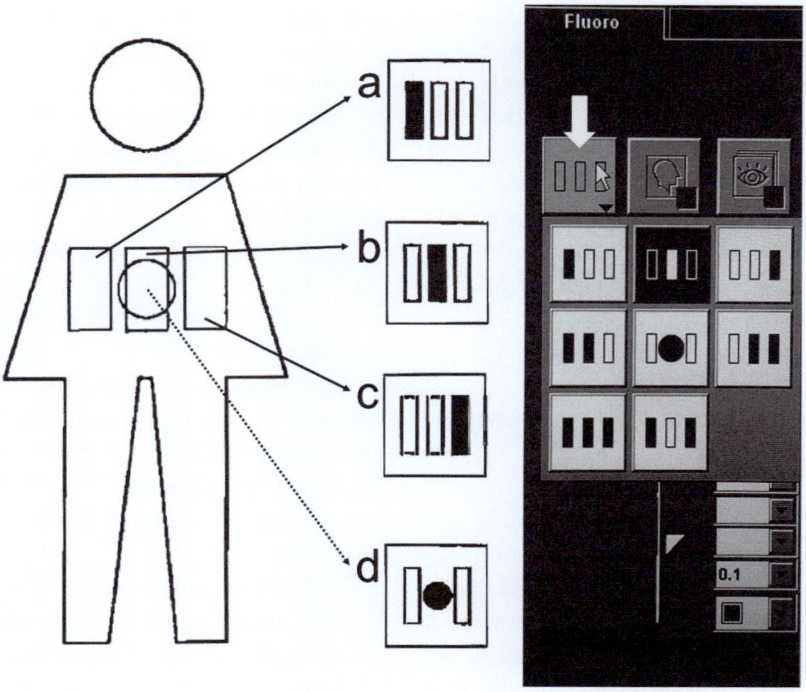

Fig. 23.6 Schematic representation of focal spots used by systems of entrance exposure regulation. These can be manually selected by the operator, as shown on the right (*white arrow*). Anyway in x-ray examination if lateral focal spots (**a** or **c**) are excluded from excessive collimation, the central circular focal spot (**d**) is usually automatically selected; the same situation in fluoroscopic examination could unawares increase the radiation dose due to AEC/ABC system

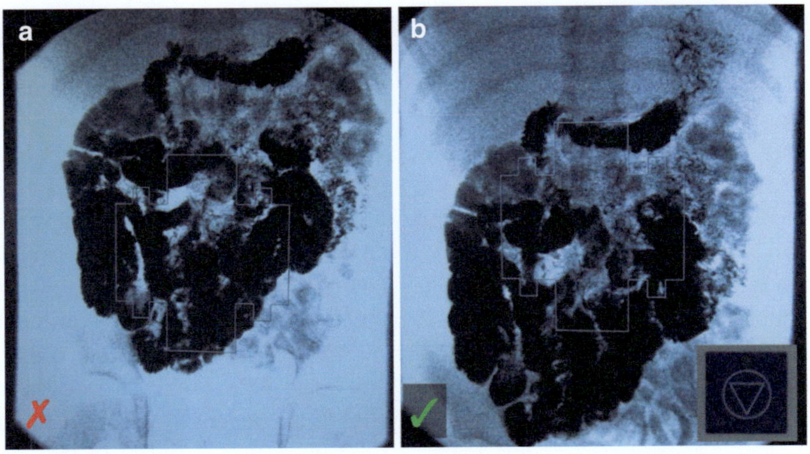

Fig. 23.7 An example of ionizing chamber (IC) displayed on the monitor of the fluoroscopic examination. Note how the positioning of IC changes the image quality (and radiation dose). In (**a**) the IC is positioned on contrast-filled bowel and ABC system significantly increase the dose; poor details are displayed on image. In (**b**) the IC is placed on less dense areas where more details are evident on the image. Remember that operators could block IC settings with the proper command showed on the *bottom right*, in (**b**)

will tend to increase the entrance skin doses for those units using AEC features.

To avoid excessive dose rates, ABC system should be switched off during fluoroscopic examinations where there are relatively large areas with positive contrast material (e.g., contrast-filled bladder or small bowel). Alternatively, it's possible to "block" the technical parameter (kV, mAs) of the fluoroscopy at the beginning of the procedure, using the dedicated command in the equipment console (Figs. 23.2b and 23.6).

23.4.3 Pulsed Fluoroscopy and Last-Image Hold

Pulsed fluoroscopy is a standard feature of modern equipment, and it can be the most effective and easiest way in reducing dose. Pulsed fluoroscopy reduces fluoroscopic radiation dose by limiting the time during which the patient was exposed to the x-ray beam, using reduction in the number of exposures per second. Most fluoroscopy units have a range of 3–30 pulses/s. The lowest setting of three pulses/s is satisfactory for many diagnostic procedures and can be increased to higher settings (7.5–10 pulses/s) in uncooperative children.

The use of pulsed fluoroscopy can lead to tenfold reduction without significant reduction of contrast or spatial resolution in pediatric radiology (Lederman et al. 2002).

With equivalent perceptibility levels, Aufrichtig et al. (1994) showed average dose savings of 22 %, 38 %, and 49 % at 15, 10, and 7.5 pulses/s, respectively.

Last-image hold is another useful feature, whereby the last image is digitally "frozen" on the monitor after x-ray exposure is terminated. That allows physicians to contemplate (and store) images without additional radiation exposure.

LIH capture avoids additional exposure.

Still images acquired using last-image hold should be captured avoiding additional exposure.

Image acquisition runs should only be performed if necessary for diagnosis (Fig. 23.8).

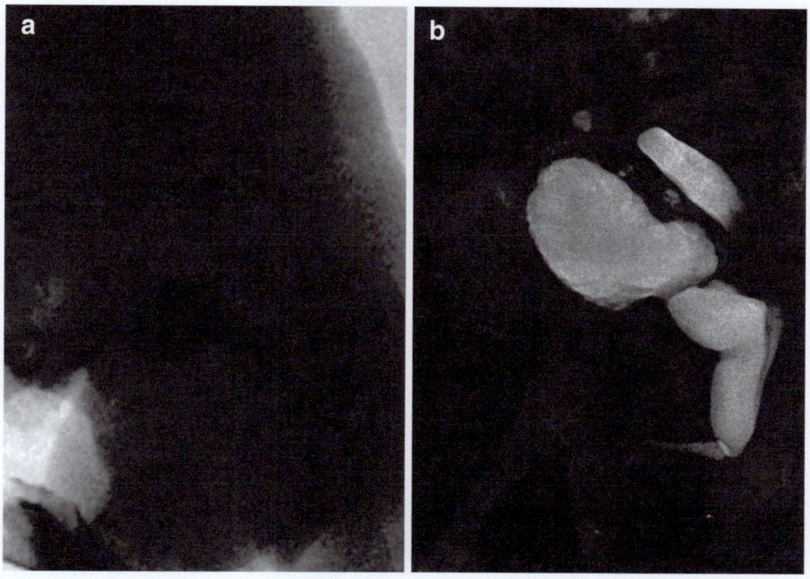

Fig. 23.8 The use of LIH capture reduces significantly the dose without affecting the clinical information on images, as depicted in (**a**). Due to particular clinical settings, in which detailed images are needed, fluorography runs could be used, as shown in (**b**)

23.4.4 Electronic Magnification

The ability to create magnified images can be clinically very useful, and there could be an increased need to use magnification, especially in small-sized children. Anyway this can further increase dose when electronic magnification is unnecessarily used (Connolly et al. 2006).

In fact dose increases with greater electronic magnification. Modern fluoroscopes have at least three (till five) electronic magnification modes, each with a unique field of view and unique dose level (Fig. 23.2c).

For example, the radiation dose increases by the square of the ratio of the image intensifier diameters, so that if the entrance skin exposure is 100 units for a 32-cm field of view, the radiation entrance dose increases to 400 units when the field of view is reduced to 16 cm $(32/16)^2$ (Mahesh 2001).

Most of the procedures do not require magnification that could be kept to a minimum.

Images obtained using the lowest magnification could be "magnified" in post-processing.

23.4.5 Patient Dose Monitoring Methods: "Alert" Systems and Staff Training

Fluoroscopic procedures will result in exposures that vary over several orders of magnitude, depending on patient's factors (age, sex, body mass, body thickness, and cooperation of the child), clinical question, equipment settings, and operator technique.

Modern fluoroscopy equipments are generally featured with cumulative timing device alerts and air kerma-area product (KAP) meter, to help the acknowledging of the operators in monitoring and in minimizing doses in the procedure. In particular KAP should be recorded, but also it needs to be checked during the procedure and compared with local and national DRL.

Each fluoroscopic procedure (diagnostic or interventional) needs to be preplanned, and all the staff should be aware how the procedure will be held (e.g., number and timing of acquisitions, contrast parameters, patient positioning) and which are the main goal of it.

Tips and Tricks in Gastrointestinal System

Food bolus impaction

- Acquire single frame of the chest and then "lock" technical parameter.
- Use adequate frame/rate (at least 7.5 pulses/s) to easily identify non-radiopaque foreign body into the esophagus.

Barium enema for intussusception

- Acquire single frame of the abdomen and then "lock" technical parameter.
- Set the lowest frame/rate as possible (three pulses/s) and adjust it during the procedure, depending on situation.
- Alternate fluoroscopy and ultrasound to monitor the procedure and to minimize the dose.

Foreign body (FB) ingestion

- Perform frontal projection of the chest, including the neck, and abdomen.
- Consider fluorospot images if more projections are needed for the location of FB (Figs. 23.9 and 23.10).

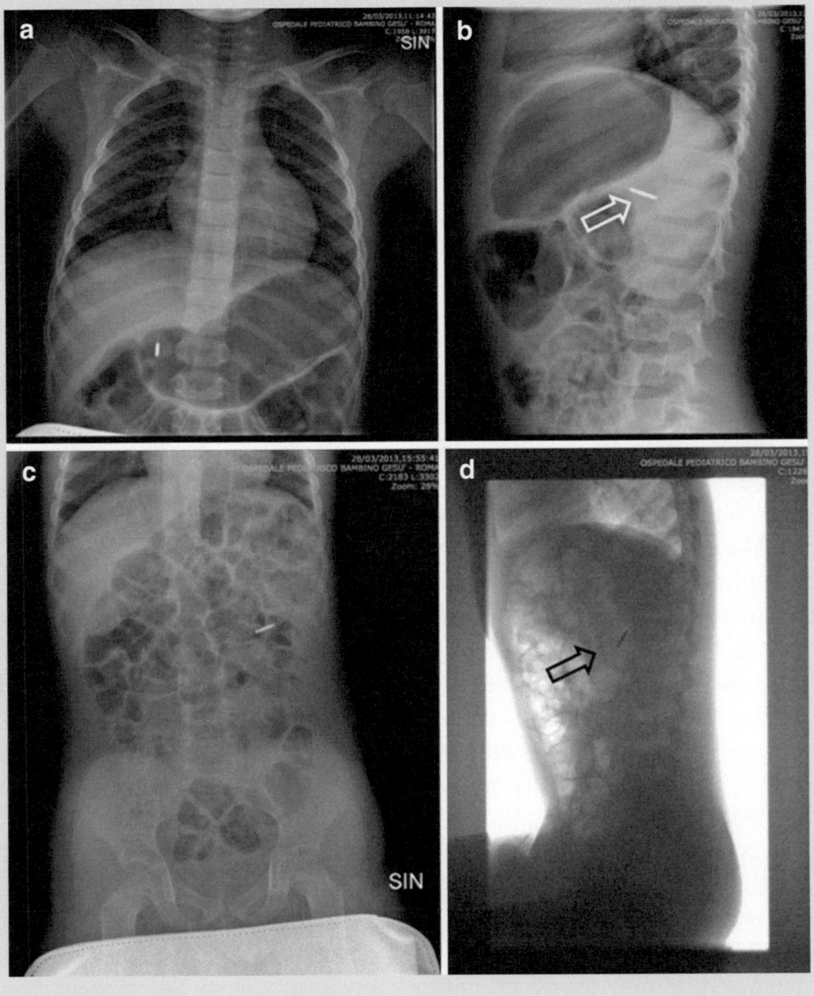

Fig. 23.9 Needle FB ingestion. In case of harmful radiopaque FB ingestions, two projection (AP and LL) are needed to evaluate its localization and complications, as depicted in (**a**) and (**b**). If other controls are needed, consider the use of high kV (**c**) or fluoroscopic (**d**) technique to minimize the radiation dose (respectively, 16.62 cGy*cm² and 1 cGy*cm²) without affecting the diagnostic information

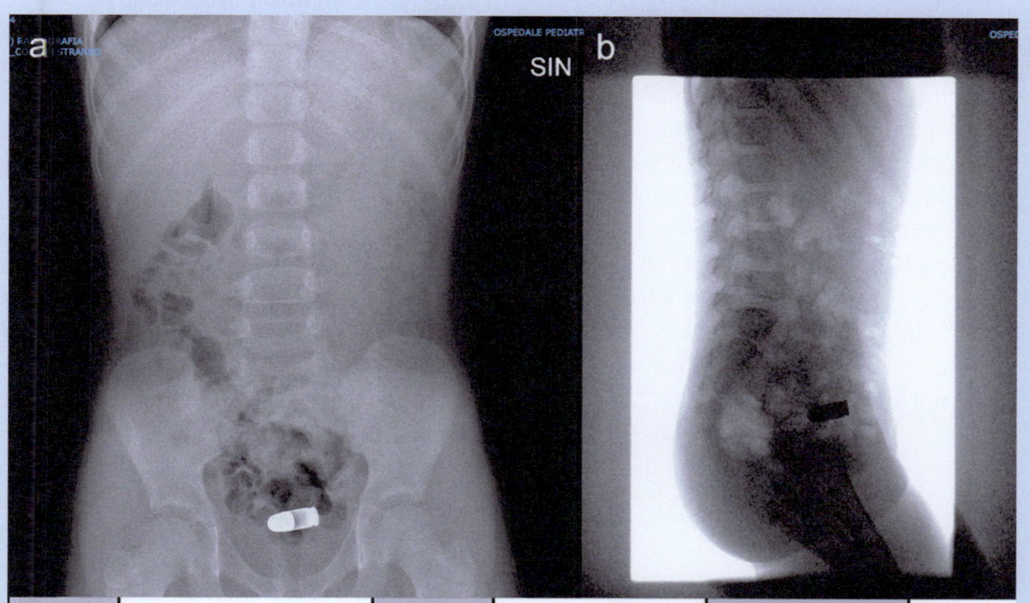

• Reparto		• Nome istituto	OSPEDALE PEDIATRICO BAMBINO GESU - ROMA	•+ Prod. area-dose (µGy*m²)	0.57
				•+ Dose ingresso (mGy)	

kV	mAs	ms	Livello ...	Lunghezza...	CampoM	Filtro Cu	Formato	Correzione an...	Curva caratt.	Data e ora	Nomo programma d'organo	DAP	EXI	Dose p...	Fuoco	No. i...
[illegible]	0.2	3.5	1123	1	m	Cu 0.3 mm	RAD	-2		10-02-2013 10.56.20	RAD_Addome AP_CORPO EST...	0.42	68	22	Grande	2
[illegible]				1		Cu 0.2 mm	42.6 cm			10-02-2013 10.57.21	CP_RAD_POSMONING (ADDOME)					LIH 3

Fig. 23.10 In case of certainly radiopaque FB ingestions, a high kV technique can be used in AP projection (**a**). Fluoroscopic technique can be used if additional projections (e.g., latero-lateral projection) are needed, as showed in (**b**)

Tips and Tricks in Genitourinary System

Voiding cystourethrography (VCUG)

- Acquire single frame of the abdomen and then "lock" technical parameter.
- Set the lowest frame/rate as possible (three pulses/s).
- "Step lightly" on the fluoroscopy pedal (one frame is enough to check for the presence/absence of vesicoureteral reflux).
- Look at the child or to the infusion line for the voiding phase, minimizing the use of fluoroscopy.

Tips and Tricks in Abdominal X-ray

In suspected pneumoperitoneum or intestinal occlusion of newborns and toddlers, the lateral decubitus position can be performed as alternative to conventional frontal and dorsal decubitus position. The examination is able to depict free peritoneal air or air-fluid levels (Fig. 23.11), and it can be performed at the patient's location, such as the NICU, with a mobile x-ray unit.

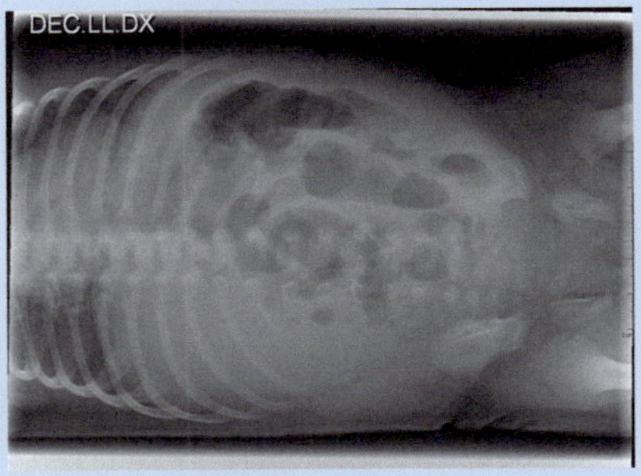

Fig. 23.11 Suspected intestinal occlusion in a female newborn. The right lateral decubitus abdominal x-ray shows some small bowel air-fluid levels in central abdominal quadrant

23.5 Main Issues in Emergency Radiation Protection

23.5.1 To Shield or Not to Shield?

A good radiographic technique includes standard use of lead or equivalent shielding when radiosensitive organs such as the thyroid, breasts, and/or gonads lie within 5 cm of the primary beam (ICRP 34 1982; Njeh et al. 1997).

Anyway the use of lead shielding should not compromise the clinical goals of the examinations.

Furthermore the absorbed dose by tissues outside the primary beam arises from the internal scattered radiation that cannot be shielded or attenuated by a properly placed shield (European Commission 16261 1996; Njeh et al. 1997).

23.5.1.1 CXR and Fluoroscopy

The routine use of gonadal shields in abdominal x-ray is controversial, especially in females. On one hand, it represents a dose-saving strategy in pediatric radiography or fluoroscopy; on the other hand, important diagnostic information can be obscured (see Fig. 23.12) (Winfeld et al. 2013).

In addition if poorly placed, such lead shielding may worsen image quality and/or may not be appropriate (Dauer et al. 2007; Bardo et al. 2009) (Fig. 23.13).

In males there is no reason to include gonads within the primary radiation field for abdominal/lumbar spine x-ray, contrast/barium enema, upper GI studies, and micturating cystourethrograms. A proper collimation of the field and the use of properly adjusted capsules reduce the absorbed dose in the testes by up to 95 % (ICRP 121 2013).

In females' abdominal or pelvic x-rays, the gonad protection may not be possible because shielding may mask important pathology. Anyway with proper technique selection, collimation, and added filtration, the gonadal absorbed dose could be significantly reduced (in newborn 25–50 μGy for boys and 13–25 μGy for girls) also without lead shielding, especially in females where a thicker layer of tissues naturally shields the female gonads (Slovis and Strauss 2013).

In any case gonadal shielding should never be used as a substitute for careful patient positioning, the use of correct technique factors or proper collimation, because this could result in unnecessary doses to other sensitive tissues (e.g., breast) and could adversely affect the quality of the radiograph (Fig. 23.14).

23.5.1.2 CT

Recently, the use of lead shielding in MDCT has been virtually abandoned due to several reasons, including an important reduction in image quality and accuracy (streak and beam-hardening artifacts in suboptimally placed shielding; see Fig. 23.15) and the development of alternative methods for reducing dose to peripheral organs in CT scanning, such as "virtual shielding" techniques by some manufacturers. If bismuth shields

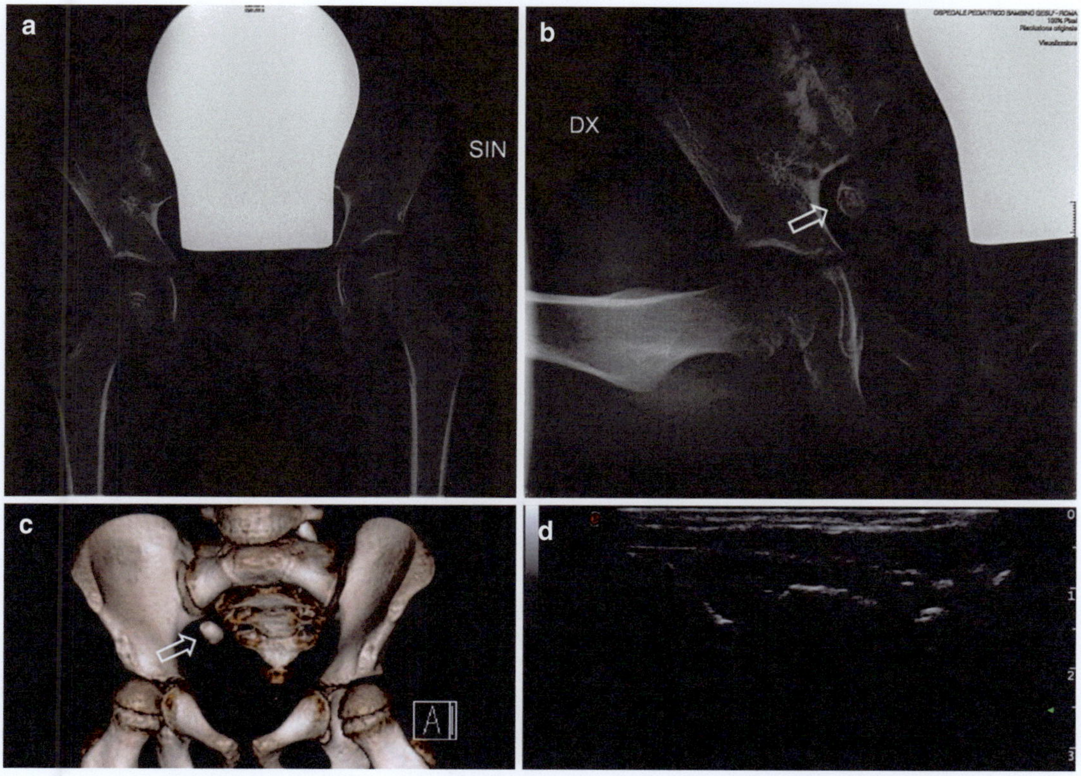

Fig. 23.12 Limping child. The AP pelvis x-ray (**a**) does not show significant findings, while in the axial projection (**b**), a gross calcification into the pelvis (previously masked by lead shield) is well evident. It is identified as appendicolith on CT (**c**) and US (**d**). The patient underwent surgical appendectomy with resolution of the pain to the right hip

are not properly used can even increase radiation dose (Coursey et al. 2008; Leswick et al. 2008).

In 2012, the American Association of Physicists in Medicine (AAPM) edited an interesting position statement on the use of bismuth shielding in CT scanning. AAPM points out that bismuth protection should only be placed after the scout view (or AEC prescanning) is performed and that anyway their usage should be tested specifically for each scanner because one approach is not appropriate for all scanners and/or manufacturers (AAPM 2012).

23.5.2 Pregnancy

Several renowned documents require to observe a special protection during pregnancy or in potentially pregnant patients (Radiation Protection 100 1998; ICRP 84 2000).

The general provisions of the new BSS, the Directive 2013/59/Euratom, confirm that need of protection (European Council Directive 2013/59/Euratom 2014).

Although usually not considered, pregnancy can occur in girls of childbearing age after the menarche. Precautions for this group have to be taken for exposures that may involve a fetus, in particular if abdominal and pelvic regions are involved.

Before an exposure, it is important to determine whether a female patient of childbearing age may be pregnant or not. The last menstrual period should be documented, and the “ten-day rule” needs to be considered in female who are menstruating, especially when high-exposure procedures are involved.

In doubtful cases, a pregnancy test could be ordered also if they are of little value in excluding early pregnancy.

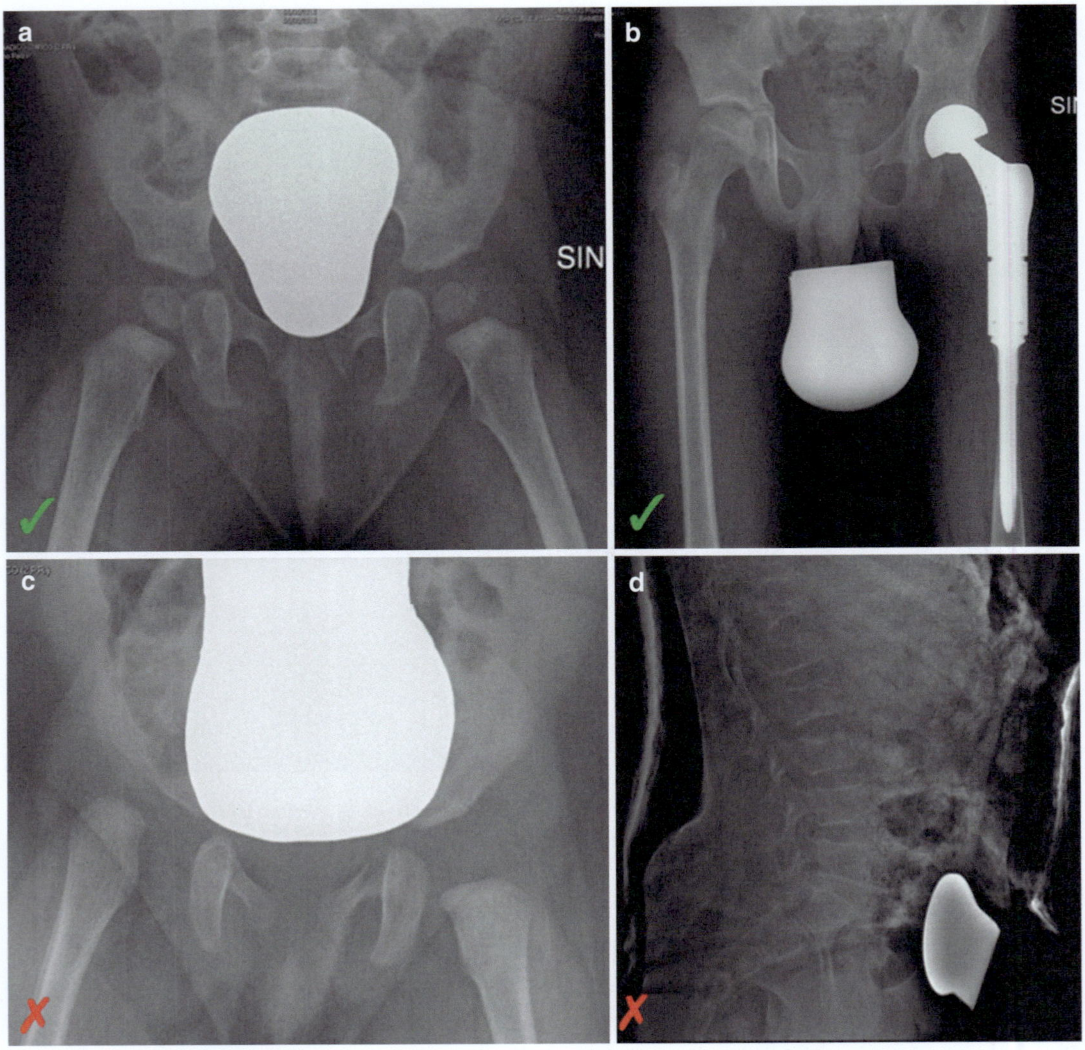

Fig. 23.13 The correct positioning of the shields in female (**a**) and male (**b**) child is shown. In (**c**) the shield is oversized and misplaced, limiting the diagnostic information of pelvis x-ray. In (**d**) the shield used for the frontal projection was not removed and its presence influences the image post-processing

A careful approach is that pregnancy is assumed in females of childbearing age in whom pregnancy cannot be explicitly excluded (Health Protection Agency 2009).

Obviously in emergency, the referring clinician may override these concerns, but special attention should be given to justification and optimization, taking into account both the patient and the fetus.

If a pregnant patient is exposed (due to clinical reasons or unintentionally), the absorbed dose to the embryo/fetus, including the scattering component, must be estimated by a medical physics expert. The ICRP Publication 103 (2007) indicates that absorbed doses below 100 mGy to the embryo/fetus should not be considered a reason for terminating a pregnancy.

23.5.3 Communication in Emergency

Communicating the benefits and risks of justified medical procedures is an essential component of medical care, and this includes communicating

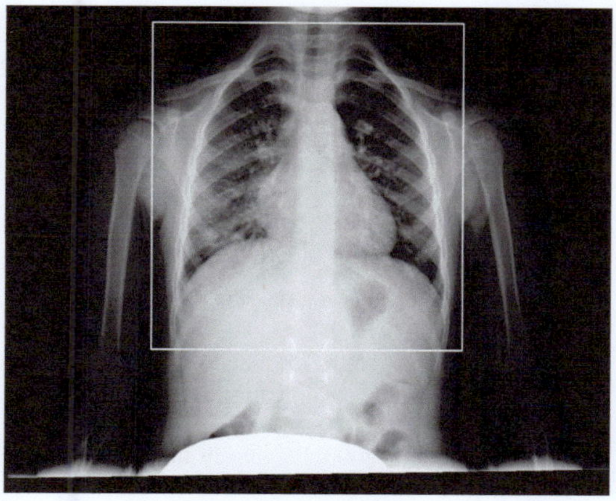

Fig. 23.14 An example of wrong collimation in chest x-ray; the *white square* shows the right field of view. The lead shielding is correctly positioned to shield the females' gonads, but it would be useless if the examination was properly collimated

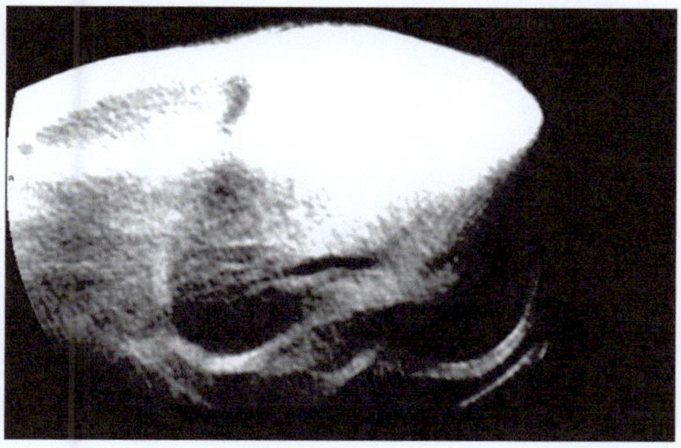

Fig. 23.15 An example of streak artifacts due to a misplaced breast bismuth shielding in a thorax CT scan

benefits of radiological procedures and radiation risks (Levetown 2008).

Parents of some children may desire to have information about radiation risk, in particular for high-dose examinations, and it is important to ensure that they receive the information they need in a way that they can understand (Dauer et al. 2011; McCollough et al. 2015).

It's important to focus key messages on relevant information that will reassure the parents (e.g., benefits of the procedure, availability of quality control, and dose management mechanisms) rather than by information on radiation doses provided throughout the customary language of radiation protection (dose units, risks, nominal probabilities, and coefficients for stochastic effects) (Picano 2004).

If the information is not properly provided, some parents may misinterpret radiation risk and may refuse a potentially lifesaving procedure for fear of radiation.

The iconic example used by Wagner (2011) is exhaustive: "After a pelvic CT scan of a pregnant woman, which statement delivers the most appropriate message about risk? 'This study could perhaps double the risk that your child will develop cancer before age 19 (0.6 % vs 0.3 %),' or 'The risk of adverse outcome is very small and the likelihood of normal development is nearly the same as it is for any child (96.7 % vs 96.4 %).'"

Both statements are technically accurate and transmit the same data. But the first one focuses on the risk magnification that could result from the procedure, while the latter reassure the patient about the likelihood of a normal outcome. There is evidence that explaining the risk in a proper way will not dissuade patients from undergoing the examination (Boutis et al. 2013).

Recently the World Health Organization (WHO) (2016) published an exhaustive free downloadable document on this topic.

References

AAPM (2012) PP 26-A use of bismuth shielding for the purpose of dose reduction in CT scanning. Available via http://www.aapm.org/publicgeneral/BismuthShielding.pdf

ACR (2015) American College of radiology's appropriateness criteria®. http://www.acr.org/quality-safety/appropriateness-criteria. Accessed 26 Dec 2015

Amis ES Jr, Butler PF, Applegate KE, Birnbaum SB, Brateman LF, Hevezi JM, Mettler FA, Morin RL, Pentecost MJ, Smith GG, Strauss KJ, Zeman RK (2007) American college of radiology white paper on radiation dose in medicine. J Am Coll Radiol 4:272–284

Aufrichtig R, Xue P, Thomas CW, Gilmore GC, Wilson DL (1994) Perceptual comparison of pulsed and continuous fluoroscopy. Med Phys 21:245–256

Bardo DME, Black M, Schenk K, Zaritzky MF (2009) Location of the ovaries in girls from newborn to 18 years of age: reconsidering ovarian shielding. Pediatr Radiol 39:253–259

Berrington de Gonzales A, Mahesh M, Kim KP, Bhargavan M, Lewis R, Mettler F, Land C (2009) Projected cancer risks from computed tomographic scans performed in the United States in 2007. Arch Intern Med 169:2071–2077

Boutis K, Cogollo W, Fischer J, Freedman SB, Ben David G, Thomas KE (2013) Parental knowledge of potential cancer risks from exposure to computed tomography. Pediatrics 132:305–311

Brenner D, Elliston C, Hall E, Berdon W (2001) Estimated risks of radiation-induced fatal cancer from pediatric CT. AJR Am J Roentgenol 176(2):289–296

Connolly B, Racadio J, Towbin R (2006) Practice of ALARA in the pediatric interventional suite. Pediatr Radiol 68(S2):163–167

Cook V (2001) Radiation protection and quality assurance in paediatric radiology. Imaging 13:229–238

Coursey C, Frush DP, Yoshizumi T, Toncheva G, Nguyen G, Greenberg SB (2008) Pediatric chest MDCT using tube current modulation: effect on radiation dose with breast shielding. AJR Am J Roentgenol 190(1):W54–W61

Dauer LT, Casciotta KA, Rothenberg LN (2007) Radiation dose reduction at a price: the effectiveness of a male gonadal shield during helical CT scans. BMC Med Imaging 7:5

Dauer LT, Thornton RH, Hay JL, Balter R, Williamson MJ, St Germain J (2011) Fears, feelings, and facts: interactively communicating benefits and risks of medical radiation with patients. AJR Am J Roentgenol 196:756–761

Don S (2004) Radiosensitivity of children: potential for overexposure in CR and DR and magnitude of doses in ordinary radiographic examinations. Pediatr Radiol 34(S3):S167–S172

European Commission 16261 (1996) European guidelines on quality criteria for diagnostic radiographic images in paediatrics. Office for Official Publications of the European Communities, Luxembourg

European Council Directive 2013/59/Euratom (2014) European Council Directive 2013/59/Euratom on basic safety standards for protection against the dangers arising from exposure to ionising radiation and repealing directives 89/618/Euratom, 90/641/Euratom, 96/29/Euratom, 97/43/Euratom and 2003/122/Euratom. OJ of the EU. L13; 57:1–73 Accesible via https://ec.europa.eu/energy/sites/ener/files/documents/CELEX-32013L0059-EN-TXT.pdf

EuroSafe imaging (2015) PiDRL project – European diagnostic reference levels for paediatric imaging. Available via http://www.eurosafeimaging.org/wp/wp-content/uploads/2015/09/European-Guidelines-on-DRLs-for-Paediatric-Imaging_FINAL-for-workshop_30-Sept-2015.pdf

Health Protection Agency (2009) Protection of pregnant patients during diagnostic medical exposures to ionising radiation. Advice from the Health Protection Agency, The Royal College of radiologists and the college of radiographers. HPA Radiation, Chemical and Environmental Hazards RCE-9. Oxfordshire

Hiorns MP, Saini A, Marsden PJ (2006) A review of current local dose-area product levels for paediatric fluoroscopy in a tertiary referral centre compared with national standards. Why are they so different? Br J Radiol 79:326–330

ICRP Publication 103 (2007) The 2007 recommendations of the international commission on radiological protection. Elsevier: Ann ICRP 37(2–4)

ICRP Publication 121 (2013) Radiological protection in paediatric diagnostic and interventional radiology. Elsevier: Ann ICRP 42(2)

ICRP Publication 34 (1982) Protection of the patient in diagnostic radiology. Pergamon Press, Oxford, Ann ICRP 9 (2/3)

ICRP Publication 84 (2000) Pregnancy and medical radiation. Pergamon Press, Oxford, Ann ICRP 30(1)

International Atomic Energy Agency (2014) Radiation protection and safety of radiation sources: international basic safety standards. Edition IAEA safety standards no: general safety requirements part 3, Vienna

Lederman HM, Khademian ZP, Felice M, Hurh PJ (2002) Dose reduction fluoroscopy in pediatrics. Pediatr Radiol 32:844–848

Leswick DA, Hunt MM, Webster ST, Fladeland DA (2008) Thyroid shields versus z-axis automatic tube current modulation for dose reduction at neck CT. Radiology 249(2):572–580

Levetown M (2008) Communicating with children and families: from everyday interaction to skill in conveying distressing information. Pediatrics 121(5): e1441–e1460

WHO Library (2016) Communicating radiation risks in paediatric imaging: information to support health care discussions about benefit and risk. ISBN 978 92 4 151034 9. Accessible via http://www.who.int/ionizing_radiation/pub_meet/radiation-risks-paediatric-imaging/en/

Mahesh M (2001) Fluoroscopy: patient radiation exposure issues. Radio Graph 21:1033–1045

Mathews JD, Forsythe AV, Brady Z, Butler MW, Goergen SK, Byrnes GB, Giles GG, Wallace AB, Anderson PR, Guiver TA, McGale P, Cain TM, Dowty JG, Bickerstaffe AC, Darby SC (2013) Cancer risk in 680,000 people exposed to computed tomography scans in childhood or adolescence: data linkage study of 11 million Australians. BMJ 346:f2360–f2378

McCollough CH, Bushberg JT, Fletcher JG, Eckel LJ (2015) Answers to common questions about the use and safety of CT scans. Mayo Clin Proc 90(10):1380–1392

Miglioretti DL, Johnson E, Williams A, Greenlee RT, Weinmann S, Solberg LI, Feigelson HS, Roblin D, Flynn MJ, Vanneman N, Smith-Bindman R (2013) Pediatric computed tomography and associated radiation exposure and estimated cancer risk. JAMA Pediatr 167:700–707

NAS/NRC (2006) Health risks from exposure to low levels of ionizing radiation: BEIR VII phase 2. Board on radiation effects research. National Research Council of the National Academies. The National Academies Press, Washington, DC

Nicholson R, Tuffee F, Uthappa MC (2000) Skin sparing in interventional radiology: the effect of copper filtration. Br J Radiol 73:36–42

Njeh CF, Wade JP, Goldstone KE (1997) The use of lead aprons in chest radiography. Radiography 3:143–147

Pearce MS, Salotti JA, Little MP, McHugh K, Lee C, Kim KP, Howe NL, Ronckers CM, Rajaraman P, Craft AW, Parker L, Berrington de González A (2012) Radiation exposure from CT scans in childhood and subsequent risk of leukaemia and brain tumours: a retrospective cohort study. Lancet 380:499–505

Perez MR (2015) Referral criteria and clinical decision support: radiological protection aspects for justification. Ann ICRP 44(1):276–287

Picano E (2004) Informed consent and communication of risk from radiological and nuclear medicine examinations: how to escape from a communication inferno. BMJ 329(7470):849–851

Preston DL, Shimizu Y, Pierce DA, Suyama A, Mabuchi K (2003) Studies of mortality of atomic bomb survivors. Report 13: solid cancer and non-cancer disease mortality 1950–1997. Radiat Res 160:381–407

Preston DL, Shimizu Y, Pierce DA, Suyama A, Mabuchi K (2012) Studies of mortality of atomic bomb survivors. Report 13: solid cancer and noncancer disease mortality: 1950–1997. 2003. Radiat Res 178(2): AV146–1472

Radiation Protection 100 (1998) European commission guidance for protection of unborn children and infants irradiated due to parental medical exposures. Office for Official Publications of the European Communities, Luxembourg

RCR (2012) iRefer: making the best use of clinical radiology, 7th edn. The Royal College of Radiologists, London, (http://www.rcr.ac.uk/content.aspx?PageID=995. Accessed 23 Dec 2015

Schneider K, Perlmutter N, Arthur R, Cook V, Horwitz AE, Thomas P, Kramer P, Montagne JP, Ernst G, Kohn MM, Panzer W, Wall B (2000) Micturition cystourethrography in paediatric patients in selected children's hospitals in Europe: evaluation of fluoroscopy technique, image quality criteria and dose. Radiat Prot Dosimetry 90:197–201

Seibert JA, Morin RL (2011) The standardized exposure index for digital radiography: an opportunity for optimization of radiation dose to the pediatric population. Pediatr Radiol 41:573–581

Slovis TL, Strauss KJ (2013) Gonadal shielding for neonates. Pediatr Radiol 43:1265–1266

Strauss K (2006) Pediatric interventional radiography equipment: safety considerations. Pediatr Radiol 36(S2): 126–135

UNSCEAR (2000) Sources and effects of ionizing radiation. United Nations scientific committee on the effects of atomic radiation report to the general assembly with scientific annexes, vol II, Effects. United Nations, New York

Wagner LK (2011) Toward a holistic approach in the presentation of benefits and risks of medical radiation. Health Phys 101(5):566–571

Winfeld M, Strubel N, Pinkney L, Lala S, Milla S, Babb J, Fefferman N (2013) Relative distribution of pertinent findings on portable neonatal abdominal radiographs: can we shield the gonads? Pediatr Radiol 43:1295–1302

24 Informed Consent and Medicolegal Issues Related to the Imaging of Pediatric Non-traumatic Emergencies

Antonio Pinto, Giuseppe Lo Re, Fabio Pinto, and Luigia Romano

24.1 Introduction

Pediatric non-traumatic emergencies may be due to a large spectrum of lesions.

Multitude of several indications exists for non-traumatic head imaging in the emergency department (ED) among children, most common of which is headache. Other common indications comprise seizures, syncope, ataxia, or a focal neurologic deficit. For many of these reasons, a non-contrast head computed tomography (CT) is often performed.

Non-traumatic thoracic emergencies in children are very frequent, and they usually present with breathing difficulties. Associated symptoms may be feeding or swallowing problems or less specific general symptoms such as fever, sepsis, or chest pain. The emergencies always need a quick diagnosis in order to establish the correct medical or surgical treatment, and radiological imaging often plays a key role. Prompt interpretation of the radiological findings is of crucial importance in diagnosing and monitoring the illness and in avoiding serious complications (de Lange 2011).

Acute abdominal pain is a common complaint in pediatric emergency departments. A complete evaluation is the key factor approaching the disease and should include the patient's age, the onset and chronicity of the pain, the associated symptoms, and a meticulous physical examination. The possible etiologies include acute surgical disease, intra-abdominal medical disorders, extra-abdominal conditions, systemic illness, and, commonly, functional abdominal pain. A timely diagnosis is necessary for preventing further complications and, of course, the possible legal problems (Yang et al. 2013).

Polls among emergency physicians show that delivering prehospital emergency care to children causes anxiety and emotional stress (Meyburg et al. 2009). Many diagnostic and therapeutic techniques are considered to be especially difficult in children, particularly in the case of small children. Furthermore, as pediatric emergencies account for only 2–10 % of all medical emergencies (Bernhard et al. 2006), it seems difficult to acquire adequate experience in a realistic period of time merely by performing one's job as a prehospital emergency care physician.

A. Pinto (✉) • L. Romano
Department of Diagnostic Radiological Imaging, A. Cardarelli Hospital, Naples, Italy
e-mail: antopin68@libero.it

G.L. Re
Radiology Section, DIBIMED, University of Palermo, Palermo, Italy

F. Pinto
Department of Diagnostic Imaging, Marcianise Hospital, ASL, Caserta, Italy

V. Miele, M. Trinci (eds.), *Imaging Non-traumatic Abdominal Emergencies in Pediatric Patients*, DOI 10.1007/978-3-319-41866-7_24

24.2 Informed Consent in the Pediatric Patient

Informed consent represents a communication method that is ethically required before the beginning of any procedure or treatment (Berkowitz et al. 2004). It provides important information concerning the diagnosis and the treatment of a patient. Consent is considered "valid" or "real" when it is given voluntary without any act of coercion by a person with capacity and competence to provide the consent; moreover, consent should include a minimum level of adequate information in relation to the nature of procedure to which he/she is consenting (Kaushik et al. 2010).

Effective physician-patient communication is a permanent process. Consent to medical intervention infers a deep relationship between the patient and physician which cannot be compressed into a short encounter. It is a process which implies the doctor's duty to inform patients of the benefits and potential risks of the treatment options, to answer their questions openly and honestly, to help patients in their choice, and, finally, to accept that choice (Pomara et al. 2015).

The essential components of consent include voluntariness (willingness of the patient to undergo treatment), capacity (the patient is able to understand the nature of the treatment), and knowledge (adequate information about the nature of treatment are disclosed to the patient) (Kaushik et al. 2010). Basic elements related to the content of the informed consent form that may be addressed before the beginning of any treatment or procedure are the following: nature and need of procedure, risks, benefits, alternatives, and consequences of refusal of treatment.

The legal implications and ethics of consent related to practice involving children are complex, especially in the ED. Minors (persons under the age of legal consent as defined by state law) frequently require care in the prehospital environment and present to the ED with acute conditions. Children occasionally present to the ED unaccompanied by a parent or legal guardian. Healthcare professionals should desist from providing nonurgent testing and treatment to children who present to medical facilities unaccompanied by a custodial parent or legal guardian. If an emergency medical condition exists, the performance of the medical screening examinations and the stabilization of the pediatric patient must not be delayed (Pinto and Romano 2015). If a parent or legal guardian is present or available, the healthcare professional treating the child should make every reasonable effort to obtain and document informed consent (Committee on Pediatric Emergency Medicine and Committee on Bioethics 2011).

If an emergency medical condition exists, including life- or limb-threatening conditions, severe pain, and surgical or nonsurgical conditions with the potential for severe harm or dysfunction if left untreated, the performance of the medical screening examinations and the stabilization of the pediatric patient, with an identified emergency medical condition, must not be delayed. Medical screening examination might require the use of extensive ED resources, including laboratory testing, diagnostic imaging, and subspecialty consultations, as needed for a correct diagnosis.

The use of medical imaging techniques, including those using ionizing radiation, has increased exponentially over the past decades. Due to the evolving knowledge of the potential carcinogenic effects associated with radiation, imaging procedures that do not deliver ionizing radiation, such as MRI and ultrasound, should be optimized and used whenever possible and also in emergency situations, in the pediatric population (Pinto and Romano 2015). The ethical basis for this approach is based in the professional's duty to search for the best interest of the child. The legal basis for taking action in an emergency when consent is not available is known as the "emergency exception rule" (Committee on Pediatric Emergency Medicine and Committee on Bioethics 2011).

Under the emergency exception rule, a medical professional may presume consent and proceed with correct treatment and transport if the following four conditions are met:

1. The child is suffering from an emergent medical or surgical condition that places his or her life or health in danger.
2. The child's legal guardian is absent, unavailable, or unable to provide consent for treatment or transport.
3. Treatment or transport cannot be safely delayed until consent can be obtained.
4. The professional administers only treatment for emergent conditions (Committee on Pediatric Emergency Medicine and Committee on Bioethics 2011).

The emergency exception exists to protect the healthcare professional from liability with the postulation that if the parents were present, they would consent to the treatment (American Academy of Pediatrics, Committee on Bioethics 1995).

If radiologic procedures are nonemergent, the final responsibility for ensuring informed consent rests with the radiologist. The radiologist is the one performing and interpreting the examination and being compensated for doing so (Karsli et al. 2009). The radiologist usually has the best understanding of the proposed procedure and other imaging alternatives.

A particularly challenging condition occurs when the healthcare professional is faced with a legal guardian who refuses to give consent for treatment of a child in situations in which such treatment is considered indispensable to the child's well-being. When a legal guardian refuses to consent to medical care or transport that is necessary and likely to prevent death, disability, or serious harm to the child, it might be necessary to notify the police and enlist their assistance in placing the child in temporary protective custody (Pinto and Romano 2015).

In a life-threatening emergency, it might be necessary to involve hospital security so that emergent evaluation and treatment can begin while child-protective services and the police are notified (Committee on Pediatric Emergency Medicine and Committee on Bioethics 2011).

If a language obstacle exists, informed consent for medical treatment should, when clinical circumstances permit, be obtained through a trained medical interpreter. Using an interpreter not only increases the likelihood of truly informed consent but also enhances the possibility of optimal medical treatment by allowing the professional to obtain accurate information about the child's underlying medical conditions, allergies, current medications, or other relevant and essential information (Pinto and Romano 2015).

Healthcare of older children and adolescents is complex as they are in the phase of developing competence to take part in decision-making on their health. A child's agreement to medical procedures in situations where he or she is not legally authorized or lacks sufficient understanding for giving consent competently is called "assent" (Pinto and Romano 2015). Children are considered to be "assent" when they have sufficient competence to understand the nature, risks, and benefits of a procedure but not enough competence to give fully informed consent (Foreman 1999).

24.3 Medicolegal Issues

The last three decades have produced an enormous era of technical advance, data acquisition, and data transfer. Radiology has been intimately involved with these changes, especially those pertaining to imaging. This has resulted in significant changes in protocols for imaging of various symptom complexes. Computed tomography (CT) is one of the most important technological developments of the late twentieth century as far as medical technology is concerned, starting with a single 10 mm slice machine in the early 1970s and evolving to multidetector CT (MDCT) systems that obtain simultaneously 2,561 or 3,202 slices of the human body.

Justification should be the first principle to be applied when a request for CT examination is received by the radiologist. This is not only needed for CT but for all radiological procedures. However, inadequate effort has been applied to justification, and there is paucity of information on evaluation of results of these efforts. Some of the main reasons for this situation, according to the International Atomic Energy Agency (IAEA) report, include a culture of the use of radiology for the purpose of defensive medicine, economic and political drivers favoring continuation of weak justification including target-driven processes, clinical pathways, self-referrals, reimbursement patterns, financial models for the development of radiological services, as well as significant and systematic communication failures between healthcare professionals and both patients and public (Tsapaki et al. 2010).

In the evaluation of the pediatric patient with non-traumatic emergences, it is important that the radiologists use only the necessary amount of radiation in performing imaging studies of children. Significant progress has been made in radiation protection for children during the last 10 years. However, many challenges remain. These include the need for continued education and change of practice at adult-focused hospitals where many pediatric CT exams are performed and the need for increased emphasis on appropriateness of pediatric imaging and outcome research to validate the performance of CT studies (Goske et al. 2011).

Conclusions

In the assessment of the pediatric patient with non-traumatic emergences, radiologists have the responsibility to adequately inform clinical colleagues and patients about the risks and benefits of radiologic examinations. Efforts should be directed toward improved information and communication.

References

American Academy of Pediatrics, Committee on Bioethics (1995) Informed consent, parental permission, and assent in pediatric practice. Pediatrics 95:314–317

Berkowitz KA, Foglia MB, Chanko BL (2004) Informed consent. Chest 125:2367–2368

Bernhard M, Hilger T, Sikinger M et al (2006) Patientenspektrum im Notarztdienst. Was hat sich in den letzten 20 Jahren geändert? Anaesthesist 55:1157–1165

Committee on Pediatric Emergency Medicine and Committee on Bioethics (2011) Consent for emergency medical services for children and adolescents. Pediatrics 128:427–433

de Lange C (2011) Radiology in paediatric non-traumatic thoracic emergencies. Insights Imaging 2:585–598

Foreman DM (1999) The family rule: a framework for obtaining ethical consent for medical interventions from children. J Med Ethics 25:491–496

Goske MJ, Applegate KE, Bulas D et al (2011) Image gently: progress and challenges in CT education and advocacy. Pediatr Radiol 41(Suppl 2):461–466

Karsli T, Kalra MK, Self JL et al (2009) What physicians think about the need for informed consent for communicating the risk of cancer from low-dose radiation. Pediatr Radiol 39:917–925

Kaushik JS, Narang M, Agarwal N (2010) Informed consent in pediatric practice. Indian Pediatr 47:1039–1046

Meyburg J, Bernhard M, Hoffmann GF et al (2009) Principles of pediatric emergency care. Dtsch Arztebl Int 106:739–747

Pinto A, Romano L (2015) Informed consent and medicolegal issues related to the imaging of pediatric traumatic emergencies. In: Miele V, Trinci M (eds) Imaging trauma and polytrauma in pediatric patients. Springer International Publishing, Cham, pp 185–188, chapter 8

Pomara C, Pascale N, Maglietta F et al (2015) Use of contrast media in diagnostic imaging: medico-legal considerations. Radiol Med 120:802–809

Tsapaki V, Rehani M, Saini S (2010) Radiation safety in abdominal computed tomography. Semin Ultrasound CT MRI 31:29–38

Yang WC, Chen CY, Wu HP (2013) Etiology of non-traumatic acute abdomen in pediatric emergency departments. World J Clin Cases 1:276–284

MIX
Papier aus verantwortungsvollen Quellen
Paper from responsible sources
FSC® C105338
FSC
www.fsc.org

If you have any concerns about our products,
you can contact us on
ProductSafety@springernature.com

In case Publisher is established outside the EU,
the EU authorized representative is:
Springer Nature Customer Service Center GmbH
Europaplatz 3, 69115 Heidelberg, Germany

Printed by Libri Plureos GmbH
in Hamburg, Germany